Crohn's Disease: A Diagnostic and Therapeutic Approach

Crohn's Disease: A Diagnostic and Therapeutic Approach

Editor: Sophia Cook

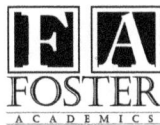

FOSTER ACADEMICS

www.fosteracademics.com

www.fosteracademics.com

FA
FOSTER
ACADEMICS

Cataloging-in-Publication Data

Crohn's disease : a diagnostic and therapeutic approach / edited by Sophia Cook.
   p. cm.
Includes bibliographical references and index.
ISBN 978-1-63242-958-2
1. Crohn's disease. 2. Crohn's disease--Diagnosis. 3. Crohn's disease--Treatment.
4. Inflammatory bowel diseases. I. Cook, Sophia.
RC862.E52 C76 2020
616.344--dc23

© Foster Academics, 2020

Foster Academics,
118-35 Queens Blvd., Suite 400,
Forest Hills, NY 11375, USA

ISBN 978-1-63242-958-2 (Hardback)

Contents

Preface

The inflammatory bowel disease affecting any part of the gastrointestinal tract is referred to as Crohn's disease. It is believed to arise due to a combination of several genetic, immune, environmental and bacterial factors. In this condition, the immune system of the body attacks the gastrointestinal tract. Crohn's disease can occur in men and women of any age group but typically sets in between 15 and 30 years of age. Affected people may experience Crohn's related symptoms for years before the diagnosis. They may have recurring periods of remission and flare-ups. Abdominal pain, diarrhea, bloating, flatulence, nausea, vomiting, etc. can occur in affected people. Many systemic symptoms such as growth failure in children and weight loss in adults may also be seen. The diagnosis of Crohn's disease is considered challenging and requires a number of tests for a diagnosis to be established. Several medications, lifestyle changes and dietary regimes, activity and exercise seek to control its relapse. This book presents a diagnostic and therapeutic approach to the study of Crohn's disease. It includes some of the vital pieces of work being conducted across the world, on various topics related to this condition. Coherent flow of topics, student-friendly language and extensive use of examples make this book an invaluable source of knowledge.

Significant researches are present in this book. Intensive efforts have been employed by authors to make this book an outstanding discourse. This book contains the enlightening chapters which have been written on the basis of significant researches done by the experts.

Finally, I would also like to thank all the members involved in this book for being a team and meeting all the deadlines for the submission of their respective works. I would also like to thank my friends and family for being supportive in my efforts.

Editor

Defective Apoptosis in Intestinal and Mesenteric Adipose Tissue of Crohn's Disease Patients

Cilene Bicca Dias[1,2,3], **Marciane Milanski**[2], **Mariana Portovedo**[2], **Vivian Horita**[4], **Maria de Lourdes Setsuko Ayrizono**[1], **Núria Planell**[5], **Cláudio Saddy Rodrigues Coy**[1], **Lício Augusto Velloso**[2], **Luciana Rodrigues Meirelles**[4], **Raquel Franco Leal**[1,2]*

1 Coloproctology Unit, Surgery Department, University of Campinas (UNICAMP), Medical School, Sao Paulo, Brazil, 2 Laboratory of Cell Signaling, Internal Medicine Department, University of Campinas (UNICAMP), Medical School, Sao Paulo, Brazil, 3 Doctoral CAPES fellowship, Post graduate Program in Surgery Sciences, Faculty of Medical School, University of Campinas, Sao Paulo, Brazil, 4 Department of Pathology, University of Campinas (UNICAMP), Medical School, Sao Paulo, Brazil, 5 Department of Gastroenterology and Bioinformatics Platform, CIBERehd, Barcelona, Spain

Abstract

Background: Crohn's disease (CD) is associated with complex pathogenic pathways involving defects in apoptosis mechanisms. Recently, mesenteric adipose tissue (MAT) has been associated with CD ethiopathology, since adipose thickening is detected close to the affected intestinal area. However, the potential role of altered apoptosis in MAT of CD has not been addressed.

Aims: To evaluate apoptosis in the intestinal mucosa and MAT of patients with CD.

Methods: Samples of intestinal mucosa and MAT from patients with ileocecal CD and from non-inflammatory bowel diseases patients (controls) were studied. Apoptosis was assessed by TUNEL assay and correlated with the adipocytes histological morphometric analysis. The transcriptional and protein analysis of selected genes and proteins related to apoptosis were determined.

Results: TUNEL assay showed fewer apoptotic cells in CD, when compared to the control groups, both in the intestinal mucosa and in MAT. In addition, the number of apoptotic cells (TUNEL) correlated significantly with the area and perimeter of the adipose cells in MAT. Transcriptomic and proteomic analysis reveal a significantly lower transcript and protein levels of Bax in the intestinal mucosa of CD, compared to the controls; low protein levels of Bax were found localized in the *lamina propria* and not in the epithelium of this tissue. Furthermore, higher level of Bcl-2 and low level of Caspase 3 were seen in the MAT of CD patients.

Conclusion: The defective apoptosis in MAT may explain the singular morphological characteristics of this tissue in CD, which may be implicated in the pathophysiology of the disease.

Editor: Fabio Cominelli, CWRU/UH Digestive Health Institute, United States of America

Funding: FAPESP (Foundation for Research Support of the Sao Paulo State) for financial support and CAPES-Brazil for research fellowship (C.B. Dias). The funders had no role in study design, data collection and analysis, decision to publish, or preparation of the manuscript.

Competing Interests: The authors have declared that no competing interests exist.

* E-mail: rafranco.unicamp@gmail.com

Introduction

The pathophysiology of CD is not yet completely elucidated, but environmental factors and inappropriate responses of the immune system in genetically-susceptible individuals have been proposed as possible causes of the disease. [1–3] A common feature in chronic CD with transmural inflammation is hypertrophy of the mesenteric adipose tissue (MAT), close to the affected intestinal area; furthermore, the potential involvement of this phenomenon in the disease's pathophysiology has been recently suggested. This alteration extends from the mesentery, partially covers the circumference, presents an outer layer of intestinal fat and may involve the small and large bowel. [4] Differential expression of adipocytokines and pro-inflammatory cytokines, as well as, histological alterations have been previously described in the MAT of CD individuals. [5–8] However, no studies regarding apoptosis pathways in this tissue have been yet reported.

Apoptosis is a known physiological process of programmed cell death and is essential for the development and homeostasis of tissues and organs as well as the elimination of hazards and abnormal cells. [9,10] In the past 30 years, due to the importance of this cellular mechanism in many diseases, methods have been developed for the detection of apoptosis and of the proteins involved in the process. Apoptosis can be induced by two main pathways: the intrinsic (mitochondrial), in which Bax is one of the most important pro-apoptotic protein, and the extrinsic pathways. [11] In addition, there is a close relationship between these apoptosis-related pathways and inflammatory pathways. TNF-α, an important pro-inflammatory cytokine, is involved in the

TUNEL

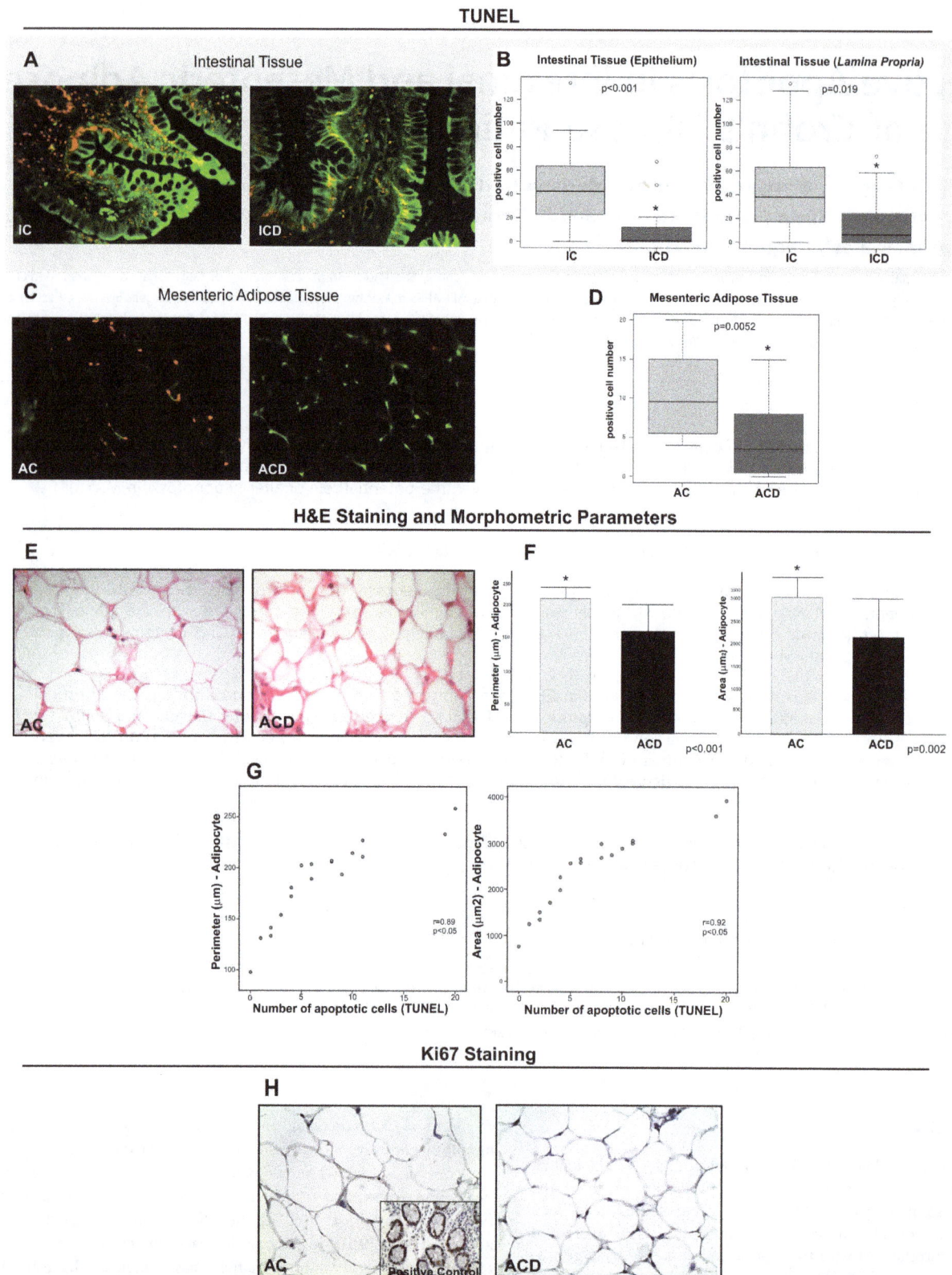

A Intestinal Tissue

B Intestinal Tissue (Epithelium) | Intestinal Tissue (*Lamina Propria*)

C Mesenteric Adipose Tissue

D Mesenteric Adipose Tissue

H&E Staining and Morphometric Parameters

E

F

G

Ki67 Staining

H

Figure 1. TUNEL assay shows different patterns in the intestinal mucosa (ICD) and in the mesenteric adipose tissue (MAT) of Crohn's disease (ACD), compared to the respective control biopsy samples (IC and AC). (A) Enterocyte and *lamina propria* cell apoptosis are shown by immunofluorescence staining (overlay image); TUNEL+ cells are showed in orange (co-labeled by PI and FITC). Low numbers of TUNEL+ enterocytes and *lamina propria* cells were detected in the ICD group compared to IC. (C) Adipocyte apoptosis, shown by immunofluorescence staining (overlay image); TUNEL+ cells are showed in orange (co-labeled by PI and FITC). Low numbers of TUNEL+ adipocytes were detected in the ACD group compared to AC. Note the high density of TUNEL+ adipocytes, in orange, in the control (AC). Images were obtained using a 40x objective. (B) and (D) Quantitative analysis of TUNEL staining in the ICD and ACD groups, compared to the respective controls (IC and AC). The graphs of intestinal tissue show the quantitative analysis for the epithelium and *lamina propria* TUNEL staining, separately. For ICD, n = 10; for ACD, n = 10; for IC, n = 8; and, for AC, n = 8, *p<0.05 vs control. (E) Representative hematoxylin-eosin (H&E) staining of fixed paraffin-embedded MAT from AC and ACD groups shows lower area and perimeter of the adipocytes in the ACD group, compared to the control (AC). Images were obtained using a 40x objective. (F) Quantitative morphometric histological analysis in the mesenteric adipose tissue (MAT) of Crohn's disease (ACD), compared to the respective control group (AC). The graphs show the decreased perimeter (μm) and area (μm²) of the adipocytes from the MAT of Crohn's disease, compared to the control biopsy samples. For ACD, n = 10; for AC, n = 8, *p<0.05 vs control. (G) The graphs dispersion show a significant correlation between the perimeter (μm) and the number of apoptotic cells (TUNEL+), (r = 0.89, p<0.05) and also between the area (μm²) and the number of apoptotic cells (TUNEL+), (r = 0.92, p<0.05). (H) Immunohistochemical staining of Ki67 in the mesenteric adipose tissue (MAT) of the Crohn's disease group (ACD), compared to the control biopsy samples (AC); no evidence of proliferation were found in all samples (ACD, n = 10; AC, n = 8). Images were obtained using a 40x objective. The positive control was from tissue section of intestinal mucosa.

activation of apoptosis, while NF-κB has an anti-apoptotic function, activating the expression of other members of the Bcl-2 family, such as Bcl-2, which prevents cell death [12,13].

While apoptosis in MAT has not yet been investigated in CD, studies regarding apoptosis in the intestinal tissue of CD patients, and in other inflammatory bowel diseases, such as, ulcerative colitis (UC) and in the ileal pouch of UC patients, have been previously published. [14–16] Reports show that the T cells of CD

mucosa exhibit resistance to a variety of signals that induce apoptosis, including the differential expression of proteins from the Bcl-2 family and differences in the ratio between pro and anti-apoptotic proteins [10,17], suggesting that apoptosis may be one of the mechanisms involved in CD pathophysiology. Furthermore, defective apoptosis in immune cells, such as macrophages and neutrophils, has been reported [18,19].

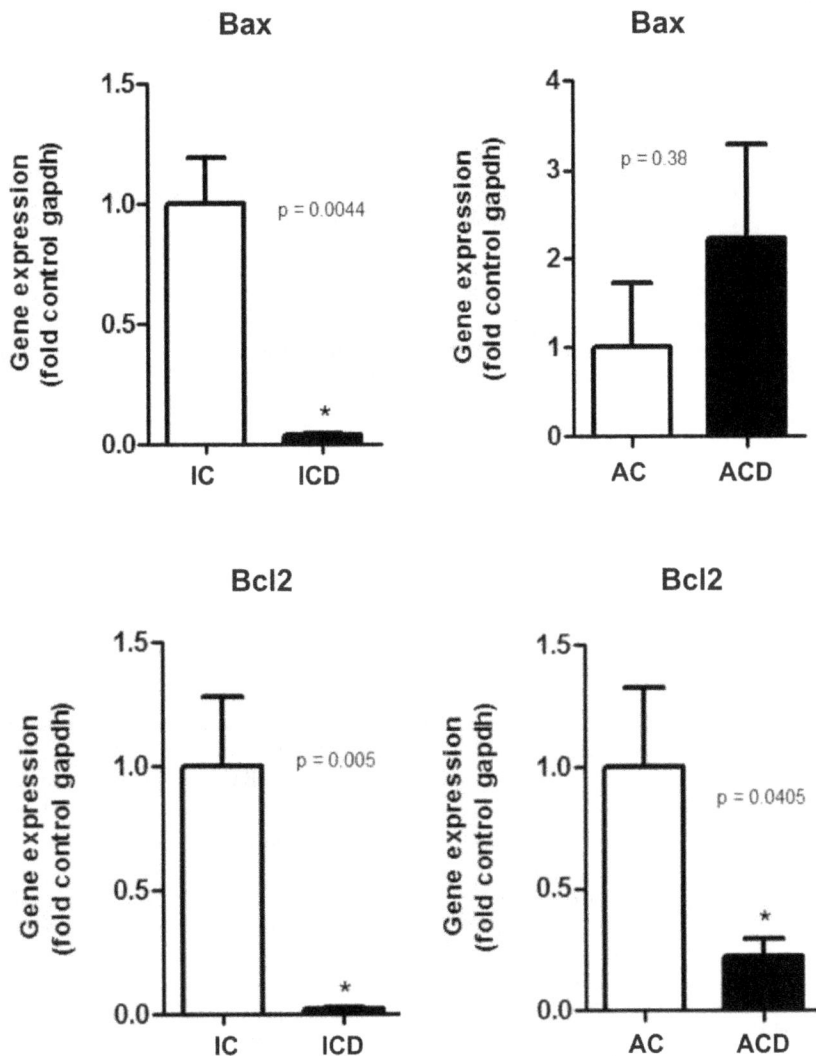

Figure 2. Bax and Bcl2 gene expressions, as determined by RT-PCR; low transcript levels of Bax and Bcl2 are observed in the intestinal mucosa of the Crohn's disease group (ICD), compared to the respective control (IC). Low transcript levels of Bcl2 are also seen in the mesenteric adipose tissue (MAT) of the Crohn's disease group (ACD), compared to the respective control (AC), while no differences in Bax transcripts were found in the MAT groups. For ICD, n = 10; for ACD, n = 10; for IC, n = 8; and, for AC, n = 8, *p<0.05 vs control.

Bax

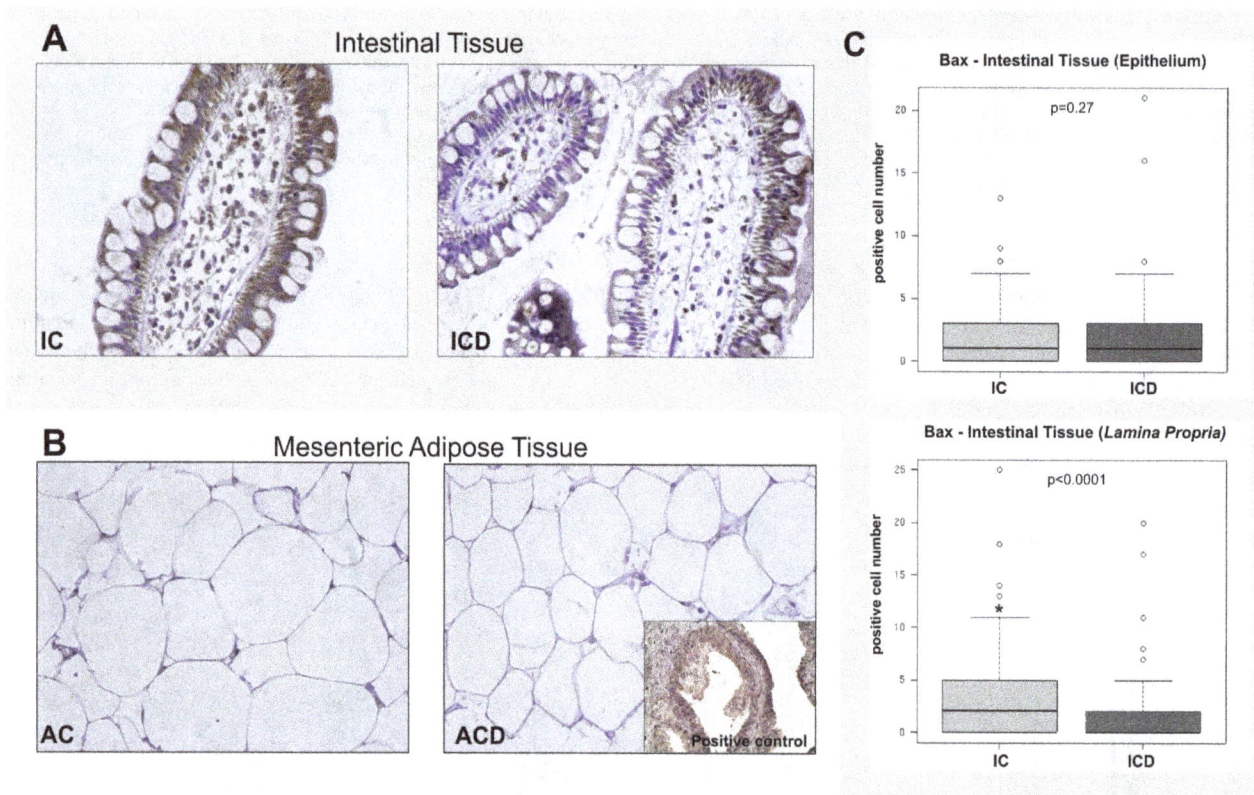

Figure 3. Immunohistochemical staining of Bax in the intestinal tissue (epithelium and *lamina propria*) of the Crohn's disease group (ICD) and in the mesenteric adipose tissue (MAT) of the Crohn's disease group (ACD), compared to the respective control biopsy samples (IC and AC). (A) Representative staining of fixed paraffin-embedded tissue of terminal ileum from IC and ICD groups showing fewer positive cells (brown) in the *lamina propria* of ICD, compared to the IC group. (B) Representative staining of fixed paraffin-embedded mesenteric adipose tissue in the AC and ACD groups; no differences were found among the groups. Images were obtained using a 40x objective. The positive control was from tissue section of prostatic cancer. For ACD, n = 10; and for AC, n = 8. (C) Quantitative analysis of immunohistochemical staining for Bax in the intestinal mucosa of the Crohn's disease group (ICD), compared to the respective control (IC). The graphs show the quantitative analysis for the epithelium and *lamina propria* immunostainings separately. For ICD, n = 10; for IC, n = 8, *p<0.05 vs control.

Materials and Methods

Sample Collection

Intestinal mucosal and MAT samples, located near the affected intestinal area, were taken from 10 patients with ileocecal CD who underwent surgical resection [median age, 34.9 (range, 14–60) years; 50% male]. We labeled as ICD group for intestinal mucosa of CD patients and ACD for MAT of these patients. The presence of disease activity was assessed by colonoscopy before surgery and all patients had a Crohn's disease activity index (CDAI) [22] of more than 250 points. The control groups were composed of 8 patients who underwent intestinal resection for non-inflammatory disease, with normal distal ileum (MAT control group – AC group) [median age, 55.6 (range, 39–70) years; 62.5% male; 37.5% female], and 8 patients with normal ileocolonoscopy (control intestinal tissue group – IC group) [median age, 50.4 (range, 33–60) years; 37.5% male; 62.5% female]. All CD patients and healthy controls had body mass index, (weight in kilograms (kg) divided by height in meters squared) (BMI) less than 25 points.

Whether the thickening of MAT acts as a barrier to the inflammatory process, or is a secondary factor that maintains the inflammatory process, resulting in the transmural aspect of CD, is unknown. [4,20,21] Therefore, this study aimed to evaluate the potential contribution of apoptosis in accumulation of MAT, as well as the relationship between altered apoptosis in MAT and in intestinal tissue involved by CD. To do this, we detected apoptotic DNA strand breaks using the TUNEL assay, in addition to analyzing the transcriptional and protein expressions of selected molecules, to determine the pathways potentially involved in altered apoptosis.

TUNEL Apoptosis Detection Analysis

For detection and quantification of apoptosis in the intestinal mucosa and MAT samples, the TUNEL Apoptosis Detection assay was performed (Terminal deoxynucleotidyl transferase mediated dUTP nick end labelling) [23], using a kit from Millipore (Billerica, MA). This assay is based on the marking of DNA strand breaks by the technique of labelling of DNA with terminal dUTP (FITC-conjugated). We used the protocol recommended by the manufacturer. The nuclear staining was performed with propidium iodide (PI). Photomicrographs were taken using a Leica DM 4500B microscope and Leica DFC 290 digital camera system with Leica Application Suite version 3.8 Software (Leica Microsystems, Wetzlar). Three fields for each sample were captured. Any cell type showing nuclear co-labeling (FITC+PI)

Bcl-2

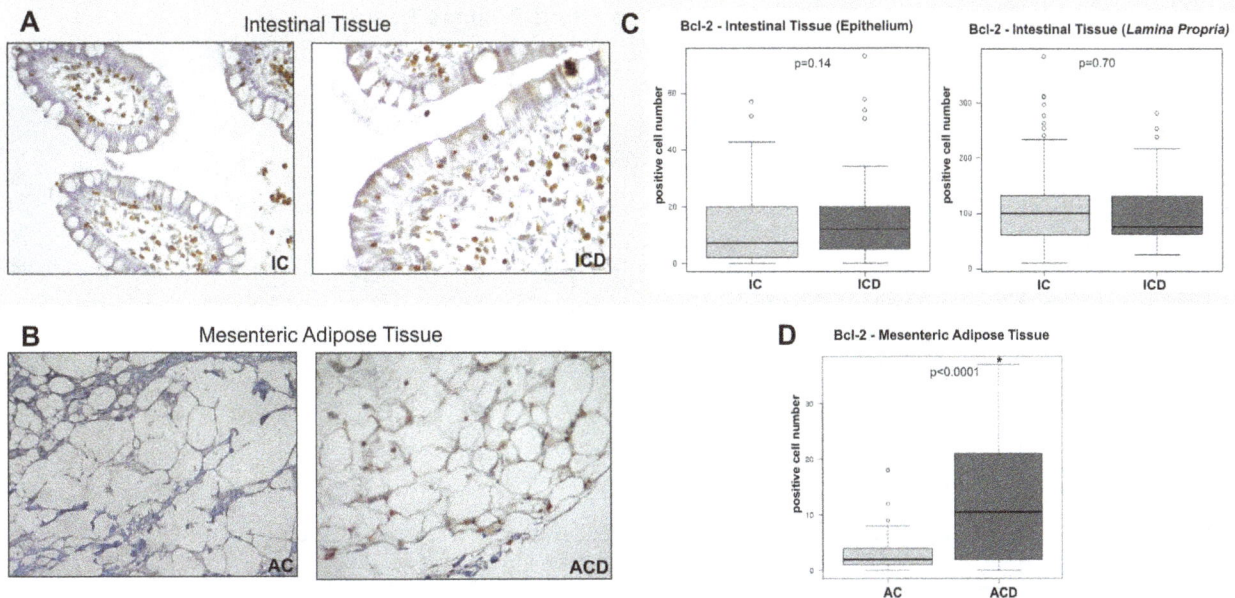

Figure 4. Immunohistochemical staining of Bcl-2 in the intestinal tissue (epithelium and *lamina propria*) of the Crohn's disease group (ICD) and in the mesenteric adipose tissue (MAT) of the Crohn's disease group (ACD), compared to the respective control biopsy samples (IC and AC). (A) Representative staining of fixed paraffin-embedded tissue of terminal ileum from IC and ICD groups showing similar numbers of positive cells (brown) in the ICD and IC groups. (B) Representative staining of fixed paraffin-embedded mesenteric adipose tissue from the AC and ACD groups, showing a higher intensity in the ACD group, compared to the control (AC). Images were obtained using a 40x objective. (C) and (D) Quantitative analysis of immunohistochemical staining for Bcl-2 of ICD and ACD groups, compared to the respective control groups (IC and AC). The graphs of intestinal tissue show the quantitative analysis for the epithelium and *lamina propria* immunostainings separately. For ICD, n = 10; for ACD, n = 10; for IC, n = 8; and for AC, n = 8, *p<0.05 vs control.

was considered positive for quantitative analysis, which was analyzed by a blinded observer (C.B.D.), in a panchromatic objective field of higher magnification 40X.

Histological Analysis (Hematoxylin - Eosin)

Biopsies from the mucosa of the terminal ileum and from the MAT, near the affected intestinal area, were embedded in paraffin blocks for histological analysis. Sections of 5 µm were cut and stained with hematoxylin and eosin dye.

Photomicrographs were taken using a Zeiss Axiophot microscope and Cannon Power Shot G5 digital camera system (Cannon Inc., Tokyo). Fifty fields of higher magnification (40X) were scanned for each sample and 10 random fields were analyzed. The number of adipocytes was counted and their area and perimeters were obtained. The morphometric results were quantified by a blinded observer (C.B.D.) using the software Image J (Image Processing and Analysis in Java, public domains, *rsbweb.nih.gov/ij/21*).

Bax, Bcl-2 and Ki67 Immunohistochemical Staining

Histological sections of 5 µm were also performed for immunostaining procedures of samples included in paraffin blocks. Endogenous peroxidase was blocked with 3% hydrogen peroxide/10 mM PBS pH 6.0 for 15 min. Afterwards, the sections were microwaved in 3% milk buffer for 30 min and incubated overnight with primary antibodies; anti-Bax (DAKO A/S Denmark; N-20 5c493, rabbit polyclonal), anti-Bcl-2 (DAKO A/S Denmark; N-19 5c492, mouse polyclonal), anti-Ki67 (DAKO A/S Denmark; F0788, mouse monoclonal) with dilutions of 1:600, 1:150 and 1:500 respectively at 20°C. The sections were incubated

with post primary block and secondary antibodies (Novocastra Laboratories Ltd; Novolink RE 7260-K) for 1 h, and processed using the DAB reaction (0.5 mg/ml, Sigma, USA, St Louis). Any cell type showing cytoplasmic staining was considered positive for quantitative analysis [11,24], which was performed by a blinded observer (C.B.D.). The microscope and the software used to capture images for quantitative analysis were the same as those used for the hematoxylin and eosin study.

Caspase 3 Immunofluorescence Staining

Histological sections of 5 µm were also performed for immunofluorescence procedures of samples included in paraffin blocks. The preparation of slides was performed (deparaffinization and hydration), followed by antigen retrieval. The tissue was incubated in primary antibody anti-Caspase 3 (Santa Cruz CA; H-277: sc-7148, rabbit polyclonal), with a dilution of 1:200 at 4°C overnight and after with secondary antibody conjugated with FITC (goat anti-rabbit IgG-FITC: sc-2012) in the same concentration for 1 hour. DAPI was used for nuclear staining. Any cell type showing co-labeling in the cytosol for FITC were considered positive for quantitative analysis [11], which was performed by a blinded observer (C.B.D.). The microscope and the software used to capture images for quantitative analysis were the same as those used for the TUNEL study.

RT-PCR Analysis

Biopsies from the mucosa of the terminal ileum and from the MAT, located near the affected intestinal area, were snap-frozen in liquid nitrogen and stored at −80°C until use. Total RNA was extracted using Trizol (Invitrogen), according to the manufactur-

Bax

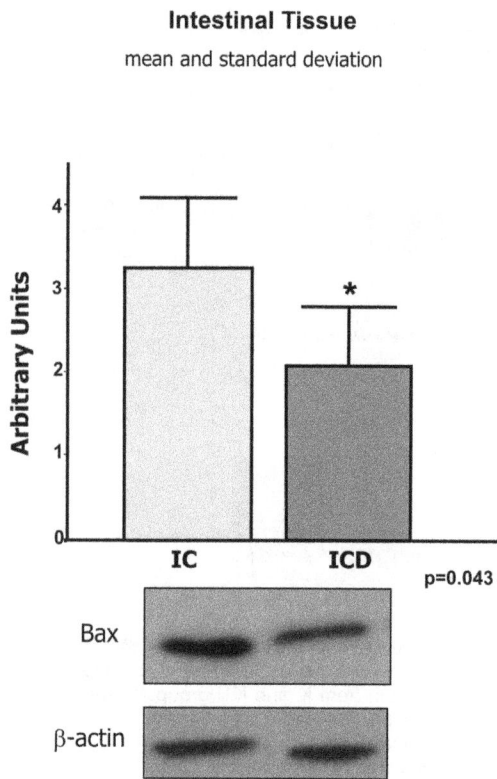

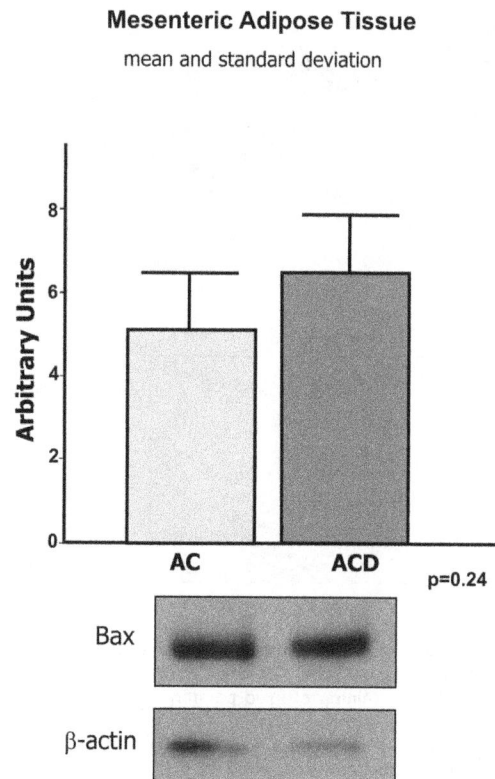

Bcl-2

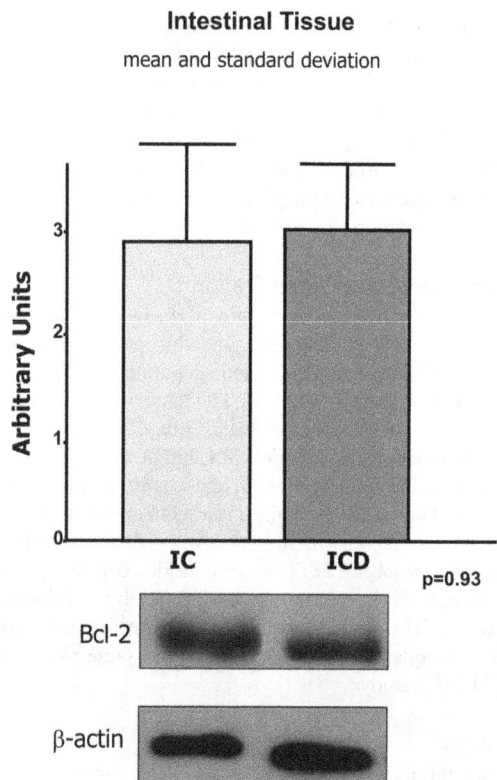

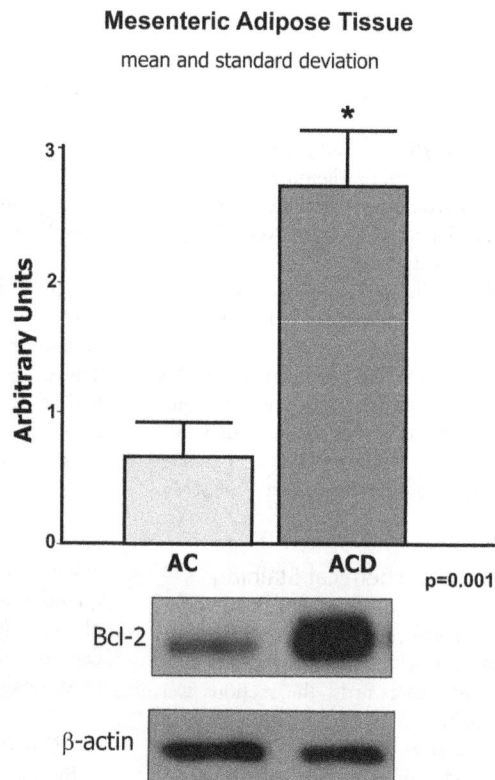

Figure 5. Representative Western blot analyses and determination of Bax and Bcl-2 protein expression in the intestinal tissue (mucosa) of the Crohn's disease group (ICD) and in the mesenteric adipose tissue (MAT) of the Crohn's disease group (ACD),

compared to the respective controls (IC and AC). Decreased expression of Bax was observed in ICD group, compared to the control group (IC), and higher expression of Bcl-2, an anti-apoptotic protein, was observed in the MAT of Crohn's disease (ACD) compared to the control group (AC). For illustration purposes, each band represents one patient. For ICD, n = 10; for ACD, n = 10; for IC, n = 8; and, for AC, n = 8, *p<0.05 vs control.

er's instructions. RNA purity and concentration were determined by UV spectrophotometry at 260 nm. RNA was treated with RNase-free Dnase (RQ1 RNase-free Dnase, Promega) and then reverse transcribed using oligo (dT) primers and reverse transcriptase (RevertAid Kit, Fermentas). The reaction mixture (20 μl) was incubated at 42°C for 60 min, then for 10 min at 70°C, and cooled on ice. RT-PCR was performed on resulting cDNA, using the manufacturer's protocol, in a 25 μl reaction volume per capillary. Gene-specific primers (Applied Biosystems) were: Hs00180269_m1 (Bax); Hs00608023_m1 (Bcl2); NM_002046.3 (GAPDH). RT-PCR amplification consisted of an initial denaturation step (50°C for 2 min and 95°C for 10 min), 40 cycles of denaturation (95°C for 15 s), annealing (53°C for 20 s) and extension (72°C for 20 s), followed by a final incubation at 60°C for 1 min. All measurements were normalized by the expression of GAPDH gene, considered as a stable housekeeping

gene. Gene expression was determined using the delta-delta Ct method: $2^{-\Delta\Delta CT}$ ($\Delta\Delta CT = [Ct(\text{target gene})-Ct(\text{GAPDH})]_{\text{patient}}-[Ct(\text{target gene})-Ct(\text{GAPDH})]_{\text{control}}$).

Real-time PCR analysis of gene expression was performed in a 7500 SDS sequence detection system (Applied Biosystems). The optimal concentration of cDNA and primers, as well as the maximum efficiency of amplification, were obtained by five-point, two-fold dilution curve analysis for each gene. Real-time data were analyzed using the Sequence Detector System 1.7 (Applied Biosystems).

Immunoblotting – Gel Electrophoresis

For total protein extract preparation, the fragments of MAT, which were previously snap-frozen and stored at −80°C, were homogenized in solubilization buffer at 4°C [1% Triton X-100, 100 mM Tris-HCl (pH 7.4), 100 mM sodium pyrophosphate,

Caspase 3

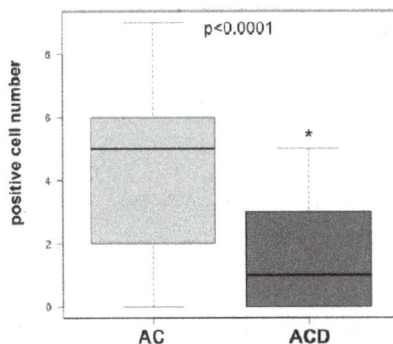

Figure 6. Immunofluorescence staining of Caspase 3 in the mesenteric adipose tissue (MAT) of the Crohn's disease group (ACD) compared to the respective control biopsy samples (AC). (A) Representative staining of fixed paraffin-embedded mesenteric adipose tissue from the AC and ACD groups, showing a higher number of positive cells for FITC (green-fluorescent) in the cytosol, co-labeled with DAPI (nuclear staining: blue-fluorescent) in the ACD group, compared to the control (AC). The arrows show the positive cells. Images were obtained using a 40x objective. (B) Quantitative analysis of immunofluorescence staining for Caspase 3 of ACD group compared to the respective control group (AC). For ACD, n = 10; for AC, n = 8, *p<0.05 vs control.

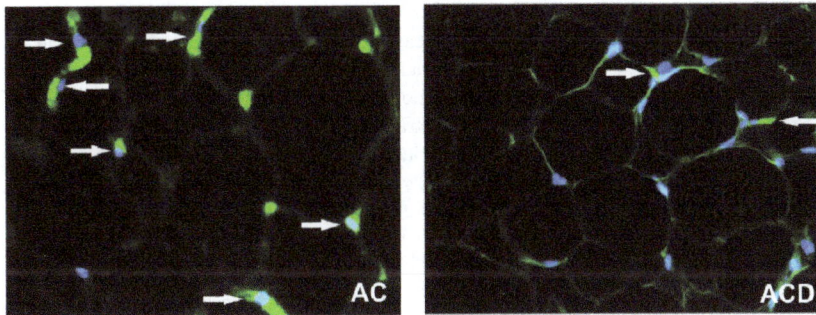

100 mM sodium fluoride, 10 mM EDTA, 10 mM sodium orthovanadate, 2.0 mM phenylmethylsulfonyl fluoride (PMSF), and 0.1 mg aprotinin/ml] with a Polytron PTA 20S generator (model PT 10/35; Brinkmann Instruments, Westbury, NY) operated at maximum speed for 30 sec. Insoluble material was removed by centrifugation (20 min at 11000 rpm at 4°C). The protein concentrations of the supernatants were determined by the Bradford dye binding method. [25] Aliquots of the resulting supernatants containing 50 μg total proteins were separated by SDS-PAGE, transferred to nitrocellulose membranes and blotted with anti-Bax and anti-Bcl-2 antibodies [26].

Reagents for SDS-PAGE and immunoblotting were from Bio-Rad Laboratories (Richmond, CA). Phenylmethylsulfonyl fluoride, aprotinin, Triton X-100, Tween 20, and glycerol were from Sigma (St. Louis, MO). Nitrocellulose paper (BA85, 0.2 μm) was from Amersham (Aylesbury, UK). The anti-Bax (sc-493, rabbit polyclonal) and anti-Bcl-2 (sc-492, rabbit polyclonal) antibodies were from Santa Cruz Biotechnology, Inc. (Santa Cruz, CA). Molecular weights of proteins were assessed using the PageRulerTM from Fermentas (Glenburnie, MD). The signal was detected by a chemiluminescent reaction (SuperSignal West Pico Chemiluminescent Substrate from Pierce Biothecnology, Inc. Rockford, IL).

The results of blots are presented as direct comparisons of bands in autoradiographs and were quantified by densitometry using the Gel-Pro Analyzer 6.0 software (Exon-Intron Inc., Farrell, MD). All results were normalized by β-actin.

Statistical Analysis

The Pearson's regression coefficient (r) was used for correlations between TUNEL results and morphometric data. A non-parametric test (Mann-Whitney U, unpaired) was performed using R Statistics Software (version 2.15.0) for statistical analyses to compare the MAT of the CD group and its respective adipose control group. The intestinal tissue of the CD group and its respective intestinal control group were also compared separately. The level of significance was set at $p < 0.05$.

Ethical Considerations

The study was performed in accordance with the Declaration of Helsinki and was approved by the Institutional Ethics Committee of the Clinical Hospital of the Faculty of Medical Sciences (University of Campinas, Sao Paulo, Brazil). All biopsies were obtained after patients gave their written informed consent. In the case of minors/teenagers enrolled in our study, parents or guardians signed the informed consent on their behalf. All consents forms are kept as hard copy. The study was carried out in the Coloproctology Unit of the Surgery Department, and at the Cell Signaling Laboratory of the Department of Internal Medicine, University of Campinas.

Results

TUNEL Assay Reveals Altered Apoptosis in the Intestinal Mucosa and in MAT of CD Individuals

The macroscopic increase of MAT close to the affected intestinal area is a common feature in CD, in contrast to observations in other inflammatory bowel diseases. Therefore, our first objective was to determine, using TUNEL assay, the overall rate of apoptotic cells in intestinal mucosa and MAT samples of CD, and compare with their respective controls. This analysis showed a significantly lower number of apoptotic cells in the ICD and ACD groups, when compared to the respective control groups (IC and AC) ($p < 0.05$). A representative image of TUNEL assay is shown in Figure 1 (A and C), where the apoptotic cells are well

identified in orange in the different groups. Figure 1 (B and D) shows the quantitative analysis for all assessed samples.

Since we found an impaired apoptosis in the MAT of CD group compared to controls, one of our aims was also to analyze the morphometric characteristics of MAT, near the intestinal affected area, and correlate these findings with the apoptotic index (TUNEL). Figure 1 (E and F) demonstrates the histological aspect (hematoxilin and eosin) and the mean perimeter and area of the adipose cells of the AC and ACD groups. The adipocytes of the ACD group presented a lower mean area and perimeter, when compared to the controls (AC group) ($p < 0.05$). There was a strong positive correlation between the adipocyte area and perimeter with the apoptotic index, as shown in Figure 1G. In addition, immunohystochemistry for Ki67 was performed in all samples from ACD and AC groups to access the proliferation rate of the adipocytes and verify if this could be related to the morphometric characteristics of MAT. However, no evidence of proliferation was verified in MAT from both groups (Figure 1H).

Transcriptional Expression of Apoptosis-related Genes in the Intestinal Mucosa and in MAT Reveals differences between CD and Controls

Since alterations were detected in overall rate of apoptosis by TUNEL in intestinal mucosa and in MAT of CD patients compared to the controls, we decide to explore the molecular mechanisms involved. Two relevant genes related to apoptosis pathway were studied; Bax and Bcl2, which encode for a pro-apoptotic and an anti-apoptotic protein, respectively. We found a significant decrease of Bax transcriptional expression in the intestinal mucosa of patients with CD, compared to the control ($p < 0.05$), while no differences were detected in MAT ($p > 0.05$). In addition, Bcl2 transcriptional expression was significantly decreased in the intestinal mucosa and in MAT in CD, when compared to the respective controls ($p < 0.05$). These findings are shown in Figure 2.

Protein Analysis by Immunohistochemistry Confirms Transcriptional Expression of Bax in the Intestinal Mucosa of CD Patients

In order to validate our transcriptional finding we used immunohistochemistry in the same samples used in PCR analysis. Figure 3 (A and B) shows a representative picture of Bax staining for intestinal tissue and MAT. A clear positive immunoreactivity was observed for intestinal tissue, while MAT samples were all negative. The quantitative analysis reveals a significant decrease in Bax expression restricted in the *lamina propria* of CD patients, clearly shown in Figure 3 (A and C), according with transcriptional results. However, no differences were found in epithelium from intestinal mucosa.

Immunohistochemical Protein Analysis Revealed a Higher Expression of Bcl-2 in MAT of CD Patients

CD patients presented significantly higher protein expression of Bcl-2 in MAT, compared to the controls, as seen in Figure 4 (B and D). Positive immunoreactivity for Bcl-2 was also observed in the intestinal mucosa (Figure 4A); however, quantitative analysis showed no statistical difference between the groups ($p > 0.05$) (Figure 4C).

Confirmation of the Expression of Bax and Bcl-2 Proteins in the Intestinal Mucosa and in MAT of CD Patients by Immunoblotting

Due to the conflicting data for Bcl2 transcriptional expression and the immunohistochemistry study of Bcl-2, we assessed protein expression by immunoblotting. The Bcl-2 anti-apoptotic protein was found to be significantly more expressed in the MAT of CD patients (ACD group), when compared to controls (AC group) (p< 0.05). No differences were detected in the intestinal mucosa between the ICD and IC groups (p>0.05). See Figure 5.

Immunoblotting for Bax, shown in Figure 5, was also performed in intestinal mucosa and MAT from CD and controls. The levels of Bax were in accordance to the transcriptional results.

Caspase 3 Expression Confirms Defective Apoptosis in MAT of CD Patients

To confirm the TUNEL and protein-related apoptosis expression results, immunofluorescence for Caspase 3 was performed. The Caspase 3 was significantly less expressed in the MAT of CD patients (ACD group), when compared to controls (AC group) (p< 0.05). Figure 6 illustrates this finding.

Discussion

Although phenotypic variation occurs in CD patients, some common macroscopic aspects can be observed, especially with regard to the thickening of the MAT close to the affected intestinal area. This feature is not seen in patients with UC who develop a superficial inflammatory process in the intestinal wall that is usually restricted to the intestinal mucosa and submucosa layers. [7,27] The adipose tissue is considered an important endocrine organ, responsible for the production and release of hormones and cytokines. [28] It is known that mesenteric adipocytes of normal individuals are able to synthesize several pro-inflammatory and anti-inflammatory cytokines, and express Toll-Like Receptor 4 for the recognition of bacterial antigens. [29] These studies revealed abnormalities in the MAT of CD patients, including the infiltration of macrophages and T cells, perivascular inflammation, fibrosis and differences in adipocytes number and size.

There are currently no studies regarding apoptosis in the MAT of CD individuals, nor in the animal model of hypertrophied MAT with associated colitis. [30] With this purpose in mind, we used TUNEL assay to evaluate apoptosis in the intestinal mucosa and in MAT, which revealed significantly fewer apoptotic cells in CD, when compared to the control groups, not only in the intestinal mucosa, but also in MAT. Intestinal barrier is maintained due to balance rates of epithelial cell proliferation and cell death. The literature has shown that healthy intestinal mucosa has high rates of cell proliferation at the base of the epithelium (crypt), with inhibition of signals to apoptosis, whereas epithelial cells that compound the intestinal villi shows cell death activation. This mechanism is not totally understood, but it seems to be a shedding cell associated to cell death. [31–33] This explains the high turn-over of the intestinal epithelial cells in homeostasis conditions. In the present study, we found a low amount of TUNEL-positive epithelial cells in CD compared to controls. This may be explained by the presence of damaged mucosa consequent to inflammation, where most part of the villi are lost. In this situation, the remaining cells may be the ones that show low rate of apoptosis and high rate of proliferation in order to recover the affected area and restore function. Concerning the decreased apoptosis in *lamina propria* cells of CD compared to the controls, and the fact that part of these cells are immune cells, this confirms previous published results in the literature [10,17].

In addition, the main novelty of our study was the correlation of the number of apoptotic cells in MAT, as evidenced by TUNEL, with reduced adipocyte size. Peyrin-Biroulet et al. [8] previously described the morphometric features of the adipocytes from hypertrophied CD MAT relating that these cells were small in size and four times higher in number when compared to control adipose tissue. However, these authors did not correlate these findings with apoptosis. Figure 1G shows the significant correlation between the morphometric parameters (perimeter and area) of the adipose cells and the number of the apoptotic cells in the MAT of CD and controls. These findings may explain, at least in part, the intriguing features of MAT in CD: the thickening of this tissue may be due to a resistance of adipose cells to undergo apoptosis, leading to an increased number of adipocytes that exhibit a lower perimeter and area than the control group. NF-KB activation is one of the mechanisms described that can inhibit apoptosis by inducing Bcl-2 expression (anti-apoptotic protein). [34,35] High levels of NF-KB activation are verified in CD [36,37]. This factor is responsible for activate transcription of a large number of genes related to inflammation, among them, TNF-α transcription. This may explain the resistance to apoptosis in MAT of CD patients. We did not verify positivity for Ki67 in MAT from CD patients and controls. This result is in accordance with what is described in the literature concerning fat cell turn over in humans. In non-obese conditions, adipose cells are not prone to proliferation. Adipocytes proliferation (hyperplasia) occurs only in severe cases of obesity, while hypertrophy occurs across all obese states. [38] All CD patients included in the present study, as well as the healthy controls were not obese, presenting BMI (body mass index) less than 25.

To describe the molecular mechanisms involved with the defective apoptosis detected by TUNEL, we studied Bax and Bcl2 transcripts and also the respective encoded proteins in the intestinal mucosa and MAT of CD patients. Itoh et al. found low levels of Bax in CD *lamina propria* T cells, using flow cytometric analysis, when compared to UC and controls, indicating a resistance to apoptosis in CD. [10] In the present study, we report findings of low transcript and protein levels of Bax in the intestinal mucosa of CD, compared to the control intestinal mucosa. Moreover, we observed that the low protein levels of Bax (as seen by immunohistochemistry) were localized in the *lamina propria*, and not in the epithelium. Although there was low transcriptional expression of Bcl2 in the ICD group, no differences were observed with regard to Bcl-2 protein expression, as analyzed by immunohistochemistry in this group. These findings reinforce the data of Itoh et al. [10] and Santaolalla et al. [17], who associated the defective apoptosis in the *lamina propria* to the Bax-related pathways.

A defective apoptosis was also seen in the MAT of CD. This apoptosis correlated significantly with high levels of Bcl-2 and Caspase 3, and not with Bax protein expression. The low Bcl2 transcriptional expression observed in association with higher protein MAT levels of Bcl-2 (as detected by immunohistochemistry and immunoblotting) in the ACD group could be explained by cytosine methylation, which greatly increases the stability of the Bcl2 promoter (as described by Lin et al. [39]). Another possibility is that high Bcl-2 protein levels could induce a negative feedback control of Bcl2 gene transcription. The decreased expression of Caspase 3 in MAT of ACD group compared to the control (AC group) confirmed an altered apoptosis in this tissue.

The point of our study is to present new data that may help to explain the singular characteristics of MAT in CD patients. Given the current emphasis that has been given to the role of adipose tissue in gut homeostasis and inflammation [40], the defective apoptosis of MAT in CD may explain the high survival rate of these cells, which in large amount may express higher levels of pro-inflammatory mediators. For instance, significantly higher expression of C-reactive protein (CRP), an inflammatory marker, was detected in the MAT of CD compared to UC and controls. [41] Moreover, a comparison of adipocyte gene expression from MAT of CD and in healthy individuals showed up-regulation of pro-inflammatory genes and decrease of genes involving lipid metabolism [21].

MAT may have an important role in the maintenance of inflammation in CD, since the altered balance between pro-inflammatory and anti-inflammatory factors in this tissue, as well as defective autophagy, have been previously reported in the literature. [5,42–48] Among these studies, one of them verified lower levels of adiponectin (anti-inflammatory properties) in peripheral serum and in MAT of active CD patients, revealing deficient anti-inflammatory conditions. [43] Moreover, this tissue may be involved in the maintenance of inflammation in the late stages of the disease, and in the mechanism that leads to relapses during the course of the disease. Therefore, the decreased apoptosis revealed in the present study, associated with already

published previous data that have shown the capacity of the adipose cells to produce cytokines and its plasticity [42,44,49], could lead to insights for further research that may explain the complete role of MAT in CD.

Acknowledgments

We thank FAPESP (Foundation for Research Support of the Sao Paulo State) for financial support and CAPES-Brazil for research fellowship (C.B.D.). We thank Dr. A. Salas and Dr. J. Panés for their review of our manuscript, Ms. A.C.S. Piaza for assistance in the immunohistochemical staining, Dr. J. Contin for assistance in TUNEL assay and N. Conran for English review.

Author Contributions

Conceived and designed the experiments: RFL MM LRM LAV. Performed the experiments: CBD MP VH. Analyzed the data: CBD RFL MM NP CSRC. Contributed reagents/materials/analysis tools: MM LAV LRM RFL. Wrote the paper: CBD RFL. Performed the colonoscopy examinations/surgeries and participated in sample collection: MLSA CSRC RFL.

References

1. Hisamatsu T, Kanai T, Mikami Y, Yoneno K, Matsuoka K, et al. (2013) Immune aspects of the pathogenesis of inflammatory bowel disease. Pharmacol Ther 137(3): 283–97.
2. Brazil JC, Louis NA, Parkos CA (2013) The role of polymorphonuclear leukocyte trafficking in the perpetuation of inflammation during inflammatory bowel disease. Inflamm Bowel Dis 19(7): 1556–65.
3. Chuo JH (2008) The genetics and immunopathogenesis of inflammatory bowel disease. Nature 8: 458–466.
4. Yamamoto K, Kiyohara T, Murayama Y, Kihara S, Okamoto Y, et al. (2005) Production of adiponectin, an anti-inflammatory protein, in mesenteric adipose tissue in Crohn's disease. Gut 54: 789–796.
5. Jung SH, Saxena A, Kaur K, Fletcher E, Ponemone V, et al. (2013) The role of adipose tissue-associated macrophages and T lymphocytes in the pathogenesis of inflammatory bowel disease. Cytokine 61: 459–468.
6. Schäffler A, Schölmerich J (2009) The role of adiponectin in inflammatory gastrointestinal diseases. Gut 58: 317–22.
7. Sheehan AL, Warren BF, Gear MW, Shepherd NA (1992) Fat-wrapping in Crohn's disease: pathological basis and relevance to surgical practice. Br J Surg 79: 955–8.
8. Peyrin-Biroulet L, Chamaillard M, Gonzalez F, Beclin E, Decourcelle C, et al. (2007) Mesenteric fat in Crohn's disease: a pathogenetic hallmark or an innocent bystander? Gut 56: 577–583.
9. Ziegler U, Groscurth P (2004) Morphological features of cell death. News Physiol Sci 19: 124–128.
10. Itoh J, de La Motte C, Strong SA, Levine AD, Fiocchi C, et al. (2001) Decreased Bax expression by mucosal T cells favours resistance to apoptosis in Crohn's disease. Gut 49(1): 35–41.
11. Huerta S, Goulet EJ, Huerta-Yepez S, Livingston EH (2007) Screening and detection of apoptosis. J Surg Res 139: 143–156.
12. Deveraux QL, Schendel SL, Reed JC (2001) Antiapoptotic proteins: The Bcl-2 and inhibitor of apoptosis protein families. Card Clin 19(1): 57–74.
13. Vermeulen K, Van Bockstaele DR, Bernemann ZN (2005) Apoptosis: mechanisms and relevance in cancer. Ann Hematol 84: 627–639.
14. Ueyama H, Kiyohara T, Sawada N, Isozaki K, Kitamura S, et al. (1998) High Fas ligand expression on lymphocytes in lesions of ulcerative colitis. Gut 43: 48–55.
15. Di Sabatino A, Ciccocioppo R, Luinetti O, Ricevuti L, Morera R, et al. (2003) Increased enterocyte apoptosis in inflamed areas of Crohn's disease. Dis Colon Rectum 46(11): 1498–1507.
16. Coffey JC, Bennett MW, Wang JH, O'Connell J, Neary P, et al. (2001) Upregulation of Fas-Fas-L (CD95/CD95L)- mediated ephitelial apoptosis – a putative role in pouchitis? J Surg Res 98: 27–32.
17. Santaolalla R, Mañé J, Pedrosa E, Lorén V, Fernández-Bañares F, et al. (2011) Apoptosis resistance of mucosal lymphocytes and IL-10 deficiency in patients with steroid-refractory Crohn's disease. Inflamm Bowel Dis 17(7): 1490–500.
18. Palmer CD, Rahman FZ, Sewell GW, Ahmed A, Ashcroft M, et al. (2009) Diminished macrophage apoptosis and reactive oxygen species generation after phorbol ester stimulation in Crohn's disease. PLoS One 12(11): e7787.
19. Catarzi S, Marcucci T, Papucci L, Favilli F, Donnini M, et al. (2008) Apoptosis and Bax, Bcl-2, Mcl-1 expression in neutrophils of Crohn's disease patients. Inflamm Bowel Dis 14(6): 819–25.
20. Karmiris K, Koutroubakis IE, Kouroumalis EA (2008) Leptin, adiponectin, resistin, and ghrelin - Implications for inflammatory bowel disease. Mol Nutr Food Res 52: 855–866.
21. Zulian A, Cancello R, Micheletto G, Gentilini D, Gilardini L, et al. (2012) Visceral adipocytes: old actors in obesity and new protagonists in Crohn's disease? Gut 61: 86–94.
22. Best WR, Becktel JM, Singleton JW, Kern F Jr. (1976) Development of a Crohn's disease activity index. National Cooperative Crohn's disease Study. Gastroenterology 70(3): 439–444.
23. Sanders EJ, Wride MA (1996) Ultrastructural identification of apoptotic nuclei using the TUNEL technique. Histochem J 28: 275–281.
24. Hsu SM, Raine L, Fanger H (1981) Use of Avidin-Biotin-Peroxidase Complex (ABC) in immunoperoxidase techniques: a comparison between ABC and unlabeled antibody (PAP) procedures. J Histochem Cytochem 29: 577–580.
25. Bradford MM (1976) A rapid and sensitive method for the quantitation of microgram quantities of protein utilizing the principle of protein-dye binding. Anal Biochem 72: 248–254.
26. Velloso LA, Folli F, Sun XJ, White MF, Saad MJ, et al. (1996) Cross-talk between the insulin and angiotensin signaling systems. Proc Natl Acad Sci USA 93: 12490–12495.
27. Schäffler A, Herfarth H (2005) Creeping fat in Crohn's disease: travelling in a creeper lane of research. Gut 54: 742–744.
28. Karmiris K, Koutrobakis IE, Kouroumalis EA (2005) The emerging role of adipocytokines as inflammatory mediators in inflammatory bowel disease. Inflamm Bowel Dis 11(9): 847–855.
29. Pietsch J, Batra A, Stroh T, Fedke I, Glauben R, et al. (2006) Toll-like receptor expression and response to specific stimulation in adipocytes and preadipocytes: on the role of fat in inflammation. Ann N Y Acad Sci 1072: 407–9.
30. Olivier I, Théodorou V, Valet P, Castan-Laurell I, Guillou H, et al. (2011) Is Crohn's creeping fat an adipose tissue? Inflamm Bowel Dis 17(3): 747–757.
31. Barker N (2014) Adult intestinal stem cells: critical drivers of epithelial homeostasis and regeneration. Nat Rev Mol Cell Biol 15(1): 19–33.
32. Bullen TF, Forrest S, Campbell F, Dodson AR, Hershman MJ, et al. (2006) Characterization of epithelial cell shedding from human small intestine. Lab Invest 86: 1052–63.
33. Marchiando AM, Shen L, Graham WV, Edelblum KL, Duckworth CA, et al. (2011) The epithelial barrier is maintained by in vivo tight junction expansion during pathologic intestinal epithelial shedding. Gastroenterology 140: 1208–18.
34. Wang CY, Guttridge DC, Mayo MW, Baldwin AS Jr. (1999) NF-κB induces expression of the Bcl-2 homologue A1/Bfl-1 to preferentially suppress chemotherapy-induced apoptosis. Mol Cell Biol 19(9): 5923.
35. Sun XFl, Zhang H (2007) NFKB and NFKBI polymorphisms in relation to susceptibility of tumour and other diseases. Histol Histopathol 22(12): 1387–98.
36. Rogler G, Brand K, Vogl D, Page S, Hofmeister R, et al. (1998) Nuclear factor kappaB is activated in macrophages and epithelial cells of inflamed intestinal mucosa. Gastroenterology 115: 357–69.
37. Schreiber S, Nikolaus S, Hampe J (1998) Activation of nuclear factor kappa B inflammatory bowel disease. Gut 42: 477–84.
38. Arner P, Spalding KL (2010) Fat cell turnover in humans. Biochem Biophys Res Commun 396(1): 101–4.
39. Lin J, Hou JQ, Xiang HD, Yan YY, Gu YC, et al. (2013) Stabilization of G-quadruplex DNA by C-5-methyl-cytosine in bcl-2 promoter: implications for epigenetic regulation. Biochem Biophys Res Commun 433(4): 368–73.

40. Drouet M, Dubuquoy L, Desreumaux P, Bertin B (2012) Visceral fat and gut inflammation. Nutrition 28(2): 113–7.
41. Peyrin-Biroulet L, Gonzalez F, Dubuquoy L, Rousseaux C, Dubuquoy C, et al. (2012) Mesenteric fat as a source of C reactive protein and as a target for bacterial translocation in Crohn's disease. Gut 61: 78–85.
42. Curat CA, Miranville A, Sengenès C, Diehl M, Tonus C, et al. (2004) From blood monocytes to adipose tissue-resident macrophages: induction of diapedesis by human mature adipocytes. Diabetes 53: 1285–92.
43. Rodrigues VS, Milanski M, Fagundes JJ, Torsoni AS, Ayrizono ML, et al. (2012) Serum levels and mesenteric fat tissue expression of adiponectin and leptin in patients with Crohn's disease. Clin Exp Immunol 170(3): 358–64.
44. Batra A, Zeitz M, Siegmund B (2009) Adipokine signaling in inflammatory bowel disease. Inflamm Bowel Dis 15(12): 1897–1905.
45. Barbier M, Vidal H, Desreumax P, Dubuquoy L, Bourreille A, et al. (2005)

46. Overexpression of leptin mRNA in mesenteric adipose tissue in inflammatory bowel diseases. Gastroenterol Clin Biol 27: 1–5.
46. Sitaraman S, Liu X, Charrier L, Gu LH, Ziegler TR, et al. (2004) Colonic leptin: source of a novel pro-inflammatory cytokine involved in inflammatory bowel disease. J FASEB 18(6): 696–698.
47. Paul G, Schäffler A, Neumeier M, Fürst A, Bataillle F, et al. (2006) Profiling adipocytokine secretion from creeping fat in Crohn's Disease. Inflamm Bowel Dis 12: 47–477.
48. Leal RF, Coy CS, Velloso LA, Dalal S, Portovedo M, et al. (2012) Autophagy is decreased in mesenteric fat tissue but not in intestinal mucosae of patients with Crohn's disease. Cell Tissue Res 350(3): 549–52.
49. Charrière G1, Cousin B, Arnaud E, André M, Bacou F, et al. (2003) Preadipocyte conversion to macrophage. Evidence of plasticity. J Biol Chem 278(11): 9850–5.

2

The Role of Osteopontin (*OPN/SPP1*) Haplotypes in the Susceptibility to Crohn's Disease

Jürgen Glas[1,2,3,◑], Julia Seiderer[1,◑], Corinna Bayrle[2], Martin Wetzke[4], Christoph Fries[1,2], Cornelia Tillack[1], Torsten Olszak[1,5], Florian Beigel[1], Christian Steib[1], Matthias Friedrich[1,2], Julia Diegelmann[1,2], Darina Czamara[6], Stephan Brand[1]*

1 Department of Medicine II - Grosshadern, Ludwig-Maximilians-University, Munich, Germany, 2 Department of Preventive Dentistry and Periodontology, Ludwig-Maximilians-University, Munich, Germany, 3 Department of Human Genetics, Rheinisch-Westfälische Technische Hochschule (RWTH), Aachen, Germany, 4 Department of Pediatrics, Hannover Medical School, Hannover, Germany, 5 Division of Gastroenterology, Brigham and Women's Hospital, Harvard Medical School, Boston, Massachusetts, United States of America, 6 Max-Planck-Institute of Psychiatry, Munich, Germany

Abstract

Background: Osteopontin represents a multifunctional molecule playing a pivotal role in chronic inflammatory and autoimmune diseases. Its expression is increased in inflammatory bowel disease (IBD). The aim of our study was to analyze the association of osteopontin (*OPN/SPP1*) gene variants in a large cohort of IBD patients.

Methodology/Principal Findings: Genomic DNA from 2819 Caucasian individuals (n = 841 patients with Crohn's disease (CD), n = 473 patients with ulcerative colitis (UC), and n = 1505 healthy unrelated controls) was analyzed for nine *OPN* SNPs (rs2728127, rs2853744, rs11730582, rs11739060, rs28357094, rs4754 = p.Asp80Asp, rs1126616 = p.Ala236Ala, rs1126772 and rs9138). Considering the important role of osteopontin in Th17-mediated diseases, we performed analysis for epistasis with IBD-associated *IL23R* variants and analyzed serum levels of the Th17 cytokine IL-22. For four *OPN* SNPs (rs4754, rs1126616, rs1126772 and rs9138), we observed significantly different distributions between male and female CD patients. rs4754 was protective in male CD patients (p = 0.0004, OR = 0.69). None of the other investigated *OPN* SNPs was associated with CD or UC susceptibility. However, several *OPN* haplotypes showed significant associations with CD susceptibility. The strongest association was found for a haplotype consisting of the 8 *OPN* SNPs rs2728127-rs2853744-rs11730582-rs11439060-rs28357094-rs112661-rs1126772-rs9138 (omnibus p-value = 2.07×10^{-8}). Overall, the mean IL-22 secretion in the combined group of *OPN* minor allele carriers with CD was significantly lower than that of CD patients with *OPN* wildtype alleles (p = 3.66×10^{-5}). There was evidence for weak epistasis between the *OPN* SNP rs28357094 with the *IL23R* SNP rs10489629 (p = 4.18×10^{-2}) and between *OPN* SNP rs1126616 and *IL23R* SNP rs2201841 (p = 4.18×10^{-2}) but none of these associations remained significant after Bonferroni correction.

Conclusions/Significance: Our study identified *OPN* haplotypes as modifiers of CD susceptibility, while the combined effects of certain *OPN* variants may modulate IL-22 secretion.

Editor: Jan-Hendrik Niess, Ulm University, Germany

Funding: J. Glas was supported by a grant from the Broad Medical Foundation (IBD-0126R2). J. Seiderer and J. Diegelmann were supported by grants from the Ludwig-Maximilians-University Munich (FöFoLe Nr. 422; Habilitationsstipendium, LMU Excellent to J.S. and Promotionsstipendium to J.D.); J. Seiderer was also supported by the Robert-Bosch-Foundation and the Else Kröner-Fresenius-Stiftung (81/08//EKMS08/01). S. Brand was supported by grants from the DFG (BR 1912/6-1), the Else Kröner-Fresenius-Stiftung (Else Kröner Exzellenzstipendium 2010; 2010_EKES.32), and by grants of Ludwig-Maximilians-University Munich (Excellence Initiative, Investment Funds 2008 and FöFoLe program). The funders had no role in study design, data collection and analysis, decision to publish, or preparation of the manuscript.

Competing Interests: The authors have declared that no competing interests exist.

* E-mail: Stephan.Brand@med.uni-muenchen.de

◑ These authors contributed equally to this work.

Introduction

The pathogenesis of inflammatory bowel diseases (IBD) such as Crohn's disease (CD) and ulcerative colitis (UC) is only partially understood. Currently, these diseases are assumed to be triggered by an exaggerated immune response to intestinal bacteria in a genetically susceptible host. In addition to the nucleotide-binding oligomerization domain 2/caspase recruitment domain-containing protein 15 (*NOD2/CARD15*) [1,2], various novel susceptibility loci such as the interleukin-23 receptor (*IL23R*) [3,4], the *ATG16L1*

(autophagy-related 16-like 1) gene [5,6] and variants in the 5p13.1 region [7] have been identified as susceptibility variants in CD patients. Based on new insights in the genetic background of CD, there is raising evidence for a key role of innate immunity and CD-related inflammatory pathways such as IL-23/IL-17 mediated T cell responses [8]. Recently, osteopontin (OPN, also known as Eta-1), an extracellular matrix glycosylated phosphoprotein produced by immune cells, epithelial cells and osteoblasts has been identified as an important molecule involved in tissue repair, inflammation and autoimmunity as well as tumour growth [9,10,11,12]. So far, two forms of osteopontin have been identified - secreted osteopontin (sOPN) seems to be involved in the production of pathogenetic Th1 and Th17 cells, while an intracellular form of osteopontin (iOPN) is a key regulator for Toll like receptor-9 (TLR9) and/or TLR7-dependent interferon-α (IFN-α) expression by plasmacytoid dendritic cells (DCs) and Th17 development [13]. There is evidence for a key role of osteopontin in Th1- and Th17-mediated diseases [10,14,15] such as rheumatoid arthritis [16,17,18], psoriasis [19] and multiple sclerosis [20,21,22,23]. In addition, osteopontin has also shown to be involved in granuloma formation [10], cell migration [24,25,26], and IL-12 production [27,28,29].

Osteopontin is expressed in the terminal ileum of CD patients [30] and seems to be closely involved in the Th1 immune response associated with CD [31,32,33,34]. Moreover, it has also been reported to play an important role in the pathogenesis of UC [35,36,37,38]. Analyzing the exact role of osteopontin in a murine model of acute colitis, a recent study demonstrated that $Opn^{-/-}$ mice showed increased serum levels of TNF-α but also reduced mRNA expression of IL-1β and matrix metalloproteinases as well as decreased blood levels of IL-22 [39]. In contrast, in a chronic DSS model, $Opn^{-/-}$ mice were protected from mucosal inflammation showing lower serum IL-12 levels compared to wildtype mice and neutralization of OPN in wildtype mice abrogated colitis [39]. These findings implicate a dual function of osteopontin in intestinal inflammation characterized by activation of innate immunity and Th17 cytokines such as IL-22 initiating mucosal repair in acute inflammation; while under conditions of chronic intestinal inflammation it may promote the Th1 response and thereby enhancing inflammation [39]. Further investigations by daSilva et al. in a DSS model demonstrated that osteopontin administration reduced the disease activity index, improved red blood cell counts, and reduced gut neutrophil activity compared with the DSS-treated wildtype mice [37]. Interestingly, the study by Heilmann et al. demonstrated a significant correlation of osteopontin serum levels with disease activity in human CD [39].

In this study, we aimed to analyze the role of OPN gene variants on IBD disease susceptibility and phenotype. We also investigated for potential epistasis with IBD-associated $IL23R$ gene variants. In total, we genotyped nine common single nucleotide polymorphisms (SNPs) in the OPN gene, which were previously shown to be associated with other immune-mediated diseases [40,41,42,43]. Last, based on the important role demonstrated for IL-22 in colitis experiments in $Opn-/-$ mice [39], we analyzed the effect of OPN gene variants on IL-22 serum levels.

Methods

Ethics statement

Written, informed consent was obtained from all patients prior to inclusion into the study. In the case of minors, the consent was provided by the parents. This study was approved by the Ethics committee of the Medical Faculty of Ludwig-Maximilians-University Munich. The study protocol adhered to the ethical principles for medical research involving human subjects of the Helsinki Declaration (as described in detail under: http://www.wma.net/en/30publications/10policies/b3/index.html).

Study population

Our study population comprised 2819 individuals of Caucasian origin including n = 841 patients with CD, n = 473 patients with UC and n = 1505 healthy unrelated controls. All phenotypic data were collected blind to the results of genotyping and included detailed demographic and clinical parameters (disease behaviour, anatomic manifestation of IBD, complications, surgical or immunosuppressive therapy). The diagnosis of CD and UC was based on established guidelines according to endoscopic, radiological, and histopathological parameters. For classification of CD patients, the Montreal classification [44] based on age at diagnosis (A), location (L), and behaviour (B) of disease was used. In patients with UC, anatomic location was also based on the Montreal classification, based on the criteria ulcerative proctitis (E1), left-sided UC (distal UC; E2), and extensive UC (pancolitis; E3). Patients with indeterminate colitis were excluded from the study. The clinical characteristics of the IBD study population are shown in Table 1.

DNA extraction

From all study participants, blood samples were taken and genomic DNA was isolated from peripheral blood leukocytes using the DNA blood mini kit from Qiagen (Hilden, Germany) according to the manufacturer's guidelines.

Genotyping of OPN gene variants

Nine OPN SNPs (rs2728127, rs2853744, rs11730582, rs11739060, rs28357094, rs4754 = p.Asp80Asp, rs1126616 = p.Ala236Ala, rs1126772 and rs9138) were genotyped by PCR and melting curve analysis using a pair of fluorescence resonance energy transfer (FRET) probes in a LightCycler® 480 Instrument (Roche Diagnostics, Mannheim, Germany) as previously described in detail [45,46,47,48]. The selection of these SNPs was based on previous studies in which associations for several of these OPN variants with autoimmune and Th1- and Th17-mediated diseases

Table 1. Demographic characteristics of the IBD study population.

	Crohn's disease	Ulcerative colitis	Controls
	n = 841	n = 473	n = 1505
Gender			
Male (%)	49.2	47.3	62.6
Female (%)	50.8	52.7	37.4
Age (yrs)			
Mean ± SD	39.4±13.1	41.7±14.4	45.9±10.7
Range	10–80	7–85	18–71
Body mass index			
Mean ± SD	23.1±4.2	23.9±4.1	
Range	13–40	15–41	
Age at diagnosis (yrs)			
Mean ± SD	27.9±11.7	31.9±13.4	
Range	7–71	9–81	
Disease duration (yrs)			
Mean ± SD	12.2±8.4	11.0±7.7	
Range	0–44	1–40	
Positive family history of IBD (%)	16.1	16.0	

have been shown [40,41,42,43,49,50,51,52,53]. The donor fluorescent molecule (fluorescein) at the 3′-end of the sensor probe (or the anchor probe in the case of rs2853744 and rs11730582) is excited at its specific fluorescence excitation wavelength (533 nm) and the energy is transferred to the acceptor fluorescent molecule at the 5′-end (LightCycler Red 610, 640 or 670) of the anchor probe (or the sensor probe in the case of rs2853744 and rs11730582). The specific fluorescence signal emitted by the acceptor molecule is detected by the optical unit of the LightCycler. The sensor probe is exactly matching to one allele of each SNP, preferentially to the rarer allele, whereas in the case of the other allele, there is a mismatch resulting in a lower melting temperature. The total volume of the PCR was 5 µl containing 25 ng of genomic DNA, 1× Light Cycler 480 Genotyping Master (Roche Diagnostics), 2.5 pmol of each primer and 0.75 pmol of each FRET probe (TIB MOLBIOL, Berlin, Germany). In the case of rs11739060, the concentration of the forward primer, and in the case of rs1126772, the concentration of the reverse primer was reduced to 0.5 pmol. The PCR comprised an initial denaturation step (95°C for 10 min) and 45 cycles (95°C for 10 sec, primer annealing temperature as given in the Supplementary data (Table S1) for 10 sec, 72°C for 15 sec). The melting curve analysis comprised an initial denaturation step (95°C for 1 min), a step rapidly lowering the temperature to 40°C and holding for 2 min, and a heating step slowly (1 acquisition/°C) increasing the temperature up to 95°C and continuously measuring the fluorescence intensity. The results of the melting curve analysis have been confirmed by analyzing two patient samples for each possible genotype using sequence analysis. For sequencing, the total volume of the PCR was 100 µl containing 250 ng of genomic DNA, 1× PCR buffer (Qiagen, Hilden, Germany), a final MgCl$_2$ concentration of 2 mM, 0.5 mM of a dNTP mix (Sigma, Steinheim, Germany), 2.5 units of HotStar Plus Taq^{TM} DNA polymerase (Qiagen) and 10 pmol of each primer (TIB MOL-BIOL). The PCR comprised an initial denaturation step (95°C for 5 min), 35 cycles (denaturation at 94°C for 30 sec, primer annealing at 60°C for 30 sec, extension at 72°C for 30 sec) and a final extension step (72°C for 10 min). The PCR products were purified using the QIAquick PCR Purification Kit (Qiagen) and sequenced by a commercial sequencing company (Sequiserve, Vaterstetten, Germany). All sequences of primers and FRET probes and primer annealing temperatures used for genotyping and for sequence analysis are given in Tables S1 and S2.

Genotyping of IL23R gene variants

Genotypes of 10 IBD-associated IL23R gene variants (rs1004819, rs7517847, rs10489629, rs2201841, rs11465804, rs11209026 = p.Arg381Gln, rs1343151, rs10889677, rs11209032, rs1495965) were available for all study patients and controls from previous studies [4,54].

Analysis of IL-22 serum levels in CD patients

In order to investigate a potential correlation between IL-22 serum expression and OPN/SPP1 genotype, IL-22 serum levels were determined in a subcohort of CD patients, in which serum samples and genomic DNA was available. IL-22 serum levels for the majority of these patients were available from a previous study [55]. For the ELISA analysis, the human IL-22 Quantikine Elisa Kit (R&D Systems, Minneapolis, MN) was used following the manufacturer's guidelines. The following steps were performed: First, all reagents, working standards, and samples were prepared as outlined in the manufacturer's guidelines. Next, 100 µL of assay diluent RD1-88 were added to each well. After this step, 100 µL of standard, control, or sample were added per well and incubated

for two hours at room temperature. Then, each well was aspirated and washed four times. 200 µL of a mouse monoclonal antibody against IL-22 conjugated to horseradish peroxidase were added and the plates were incubated for two hours at room temperature. After this, wells were aspirated and washed four times. Next, 200 µL of substrate solution were added to each well. The plates were incubated for 30 minutes at room temperature to allow colour development while being protected from light. Next, 50 µL of stop solution were added to each well and the optical density of each well was determined within 30 minutes, using a microplate reader set to 450 nm. IL-22 serum levels (pg/ml) were calculated from a standard curve of known IL-22 concentrations.

Statistical analyses

Each genetic marker was tested for Hardy-Weinberg equilibrium in the control population. Single-marker allelic tests were performed with Fisher's exact test. All tests were two-tailed, considering p-values<0.05 as significant. Odds ratios were calculated for the minor allele at each SNP. For multiple comparisons, Bonferroni correction was applied where indicated. rs4754 deviated from the Hardy-Weinberg equilibrium in the control population (p = 0.0005) and was therefore excluded from the haplotype analysis. Haplotype analysis was conducted with PLINK (http://pngu.mgh.harvard.edu/~purcell/plink/) and the –hap-logistic option using a sliding-window approach with 2 up to 8 included SNPs. Interaction between different polymorphisms were also tested with PLINK and the –epistasis command. For analyzing potential differences of IL-22 serum levels between the carriers of the different OPN gene variants, the mean IL-22 serum level of carriers of the wildtype allele of each SNP was compared with the mean IL-22 serum level of carriers of the minor allele (= combined group of heterozygous and homozygous carriers) using Student's t-test.

Results

Frequency distribution of OPN gene variants and their role in IBD susceptibility

For all three subgroups (CD, UC, and controls), the minor allele frequencies of the nine OPN SNPs (rs2728127, rs2853744, rs11730582, rs11739060, rs28357094, rs4754 = p.Asp80Asp, rs1126616 = p.Ala236Ala, rs1126772 and rs9138) are summarized in Table 2. With the exception of rs4754, no significant differences in the allele frequencies were observed comparing CD and UC patients to healthy controls (Table 2). Our analysis revealed a weak association of SNP rs4754 (p.Asp80Asp) with CD susceptibility (p = 1.28×10^{-2}; OR (95% CI) 0.85 [0.74–0.96]). Similar to CD, rs4754 (p.Asp80Asp) decreased susceptibility to UC, although this association did not reach significance in univariate analysis (p = 5.25×10^{-2}; OR (95% CI) 0.85 [0.70–1.00]) (Table 2). Moreover, both associations of rs4754 (regarding CD and UC susceptibility) were not statistically significant after Bonferroni correction, suggesting that these OPN variants are not major contributors to IBD susceptibility on their own. In addition, rs4754 deviated from the Hardy-Weinberg equilibrium in the control population (p = 0.0005) and was therefore excluded from the haplotype analysis. However, several OPN haplotypes were associated with CD susceptibility. As shown in table 3, the strongest association was found for a haplotype consisting of the 8 OPN SNPs rs2728127-rs2853744-rs11730582-rs11439060-rs28357094-rs112661-rs1126772-rs9138 with an omnibus p-value of 2.07×10^{-8} (Table 3); if rs4754 would be included into this haplotype block, the omnibus p-value would increase further to

Table 2. Associations of *OPN/SPP1* gene markers in CD and UC case-control association studies.

Cohort		Crohn's disease			Ulcerative colitis			Controls
Number of individuals		n = 841			n = 473			n = 1505
Gene marker	Minor allele	MAF	p value	OR [95% CI]	MAF	p value	OR [95% CI]	MAF
rs2728127	G	0.295	0.841	0.98 [0.86–1.12]	0.274	0.162	0.89 [0.75–1.05]	0.298
rs2853744	T	0.071	0.520	0.92 [0.73–1.16]	0.080	0.725	1.05 [0.80–1.38]	0.076
rs11730582	C	0.503	0.125	1.09 [0.97–1.24]	0.495	0.430	1.06 [0.92–1.23]	0.479
rs11739060	insG	0.290	0.815	0.98 [0.86–1.12]	0.274	0.266	0.91 [0.77–1.07]	0.294
rs28357094	G	0.223	0.437	1.06 [0.92–1.23]	0.198	0.358	0.91 [0.76–1.10]	0.213
rs4754 = p.Asp80Asp	C	0.281	**0.013**	**0.85 [0.74–0.96]**	0.282	0.053	0.85 [0.70–1.00]	0.316
rs1126616 = p.Ala236Ala	T	0.279	0.892	0.99 [087–1.13]	0.285	0.804	0.97 [0.82–1.14]	0.281
rs1126772	G	0.220	0.852	1.01 [0.87–1.17]	0.213	0.783	0.97 [0.81–1.17]	0.218
rs9138	C	0.278	0.919	1.01 [0.88–1.15]	0.280	0.868	1.02 [0.86–1.20]	0.276

Minor allele frequencies (MAF), allelic test *P*-values, and odds ratios (OR, shown for the minor allele) with 95% confidence intervals (CI) are depicted for both the CD and UC case-control cohorts. rs4754 deviated from the Hardy-Weinberg equilibrium (HWE) in the control population (p = 0.0005) and was therefore excluded from further analysis.

$p = 3.67 \times 10^{-12}$. In contrast, there were no associations of certain *OPN* haplotypes with UC susceptibility (Table 4).

Analysis for gender-specific differences in *OPN* variants

Previous studies demonstrated significant gender-specific effects of *OPN* variants in systemic lupus erythematosus (SLE) and type 1-diabetes, particularly in male patients [43,50]. Considering the deviation of rs4754 from the Hardy-Weinberg equilibrium, we therefore investigated potential gender-specific effects in IBD susceptibility. For four *OPN* SNPs (rs4754, rs1126616, rs1126772 and rs9138), we observed significantly different distributions between male and female CD patients. Interestingly, for these SNPs, there was an opposite direction of the association results for males and females (rs4754: p = 0.0004, OR = 0.69 [95% CI: 0.56–0.85] (males), p = 0.7693, OR = 1.03 (females); rs1126616: p = 0.1187, OR = 0.85 (males), p = 0.2676, OR = 1.12 (females); rs1126772: p = 0.1679, OR = 0.85 (males), p = 0.0893, OR = 1.21 (females); rs9138: p = 0.1256, OR = 0.85 (males), p = 0.0864, OR = 1.19 (females)). Given that the most pronounced difference between male and female CD patients was found for rs4754, which deviated from the Hardy-Weinberg equilibrium in the control population, we next investigated if the deviation from Hardy-Weinberg equilibrium is based on a gender-specific effect. This analysis revealed that there was significant deviation from Hardy-Weinberg equilibrium in male controls (n = 917; p = 0.0018), but not in female controls (n = 547; p = 0.1347), confirming the gender-specific effect of this *OPN* SNP found in CD patients.

Analysis for epistasis between *OPN* variants and *IL23R* variants

To investigate if *OPN* variants modify IBD susceptibility by epistatic interaction with other Th17-related IBD susceptibility genes, we next analyzed for potential epistasis of *OPN* variants with main IBD-associated *IL23R* variants. We found evidence of weak epistasis between the *OPN* SNP rs28357094 with the *IL23R* SNP rs10489629 ($p = 4.18 \times 10^{-2}$) and between *OPN* SNP rs1126616 and *IL23R* SNP rs2201841 ($p = 4.18 \times 10^{-2}$) but none of these associations remained significant after Bonferroni correction (Table 5).

Correlation between *OPN* variants and IL-22 serum levels in CD patients

Based on the recent data of Heilmann et al. [39] demonstrating decreased blood levels of IL-22 in acute colitis in *Opn−/−* mice, we next investigated a potential association of *OPN* variants and IL-22 serum levels in a subcohort of CD patients. No correlation was found between *OPN* SNPs and IL-22 serum levels (Table 6). However, overall the IL-22 serum levels tended to be lower in the carriers of *OPN* minor alleles, which was statistically significant when the mean IL-22 expression level of carriers of the 9 investigated *OPN* SNPs minor alleles (homo- and heterozygous carriers) were compared to the homozygous carriers of the wildtype allele ($p = 3.6 \times 10^{-5}$). Interestingly, for 7 out of 8 *OPN* SNPs forming the haplotype rs2728127-rs2853744-rs11730582-rs11439060-rs28357094-rs112661-rs1126772-rs9138, which was strongly associated with CD susceptibility (omnibus p-value 2.07×10^{-8}), the IL-22 serum levels were nominally lower in CD carriers of the minor allele than in wildtype carriers, although these differences were for each SNP only small and statistically not significant (Table 6).

Discussion

The presented study represents the first detailed analysis of *OPN* gene variants in IBD patients. In this study, there were no significant associations of single *OPN* SNPs with CD or UC susceptibility after Bonferroni correction for multiple testing; however, several *OPN* haplotypes were associated with CD susceptibility. The strongest association was found for a haplotype consisting of the 8 *OPN* SNPs (rs2728127-rs2853744-rs11730582-rs11439060-rs28357094-rs112661-rs1126772-rs9138; omnibus p-value 2.07×10^{-8}). However, considering the strength of the association signals found for a number of other recently identified IBD susceptibility genes [56,57], this argues against a major role for *OPN* in the genetic susceptibility for IBD. Given the strong association of osteopontin with Th1- and Th17-mediated diseases, the finding of an association of *OPN* haplotypes with CD, a Th1- and Th17-mediated disease, but not UC susceptibility is not surprising. In contrast, UC has been associated with a predominantly modified Th2 response but partially also with a Th17 immune response. The results of our haplotype analysis suggest

Table 3. Haplotypes of *OPN* SNPs in Crohn's disease (CD) case-control sample (846 cases and 1510 controls) and omnibus p-values for association with CD susceptibility.

Haplotype combination	Omnibus p-value
rs2728127-rs2853744	9.09×10^{-1}
rs2853744-rs11730582	2.74×10^{-1}
rs11730582-rs11439060	6.87×10^{-2}
rs11439060-rs28357094	2.25×10^{-1}
rs28357094-rs1126616	6.11×10^{-1}
rs1126616-rs1126772	1.81×10^{-1}
rs1126772-rs9138	4.71×10^{-1}
rs2728127-rs2853744-rs11730582	1.95×10^{-1}
rs2853744-rs11730582-rs11439060	1.34×10^{-1}
rs11730582-rs11439060-rs28357094	5.37×10^{-2}
rs11439060-rs28357094-rs1126616	2.72×10^{-1}
rs28357094-rs1126616-rs1126772	3.72×10^{-1}
rs1126616-rs1126772-rs9138	6.45×10^{-1}
rs2728127-rs2853744-rs11730582-rs11439060	**2.15×10^{-2}**
rs2853744-rs11730582-rs11439060-rs28357094	1.62×10^{-1}
rs11730582-rs11439060-rs28357094-rs1126616	1.35×10^{-1}
rs11439060-rs28357094-rs1126616-rs1126772	2.74×10^{-1}
rs28357094-rs1126616-rs1126772-rs9138	6.77×10^{-1}
rs2728127-rs2853744-rs11730582-rs11439060-rs28357094	**3.77×10^{-2}**
rs2853744-rs11730582-rs11439060-rs28357094-rs1126616	1.98×10^{-1}
rs11730582-rs11439060-rs28357094-rs1126616-rs1126772	6.95×10^{-2}
rs11439060-rs28357094-rs1126616-rs1126772-rs9138	3.84×10^{-1}
rs2728127-rs2853744-rs11730582-rs11439060-rs28357094-rs112661	5.03×10^{-2}
rs2853744-rs11730582-rs11439060-rs28357094-rs1126616-rs1126772	6.86×10^{-2}
rs11730582-rs11439060-rs28357094-rs1126616-rs1126772-rs9138	5.75×10^{-2}
rs2728127-rs2853744-rs11730582-rs11439060-rs28357094-rs112661-rs1126772	**1.44×10^{-7}**
rs2853744-rs11730582-rs11439060-rs28357094-rs1126616-rs1126772-rs9138	**2.76×10^{-5}**
rs2728127-rs2853744-rs11730582-rs11439060-rs28357094-rs112661-rs1126772-rs9138	**2.07×10^{-8}**

Significant p-values<0.05 are depicted in bold. All significant p-values remained significant after 10.000 permutations.

that certain rare haplotypes significantly contribute to the genetic risk of CD. This is in agreement with recent results of the International IBD Genetics Consortium which identified a total of 71 CD susceptibility loci [56]. These 71 susceptibility loci explain only slightly more than 20% of CD heritability. Therefore, it is assumed that a number of rare SNPs and haplotypes contribute to the overall CD risk such as recently shown by us for *PXR* gene variants [58]. In addition, most likely a high number of common CD risk genes with small effect size are still unidentified but for their identification very large cohorts would be required.

So far, genetic variants in the *OPN* gene have shown to be involved in susceptibility to other immune-mediated diseases such as SLE [59,60], oligoarticular juvenile idiopathic arthritis [61] and sarcoidosis [51]. Despite promising functional data, previous genotype analyses could not confirm *OPN* as significant disease-modifying gene in classical Th17-mediated diseases such as multiple sclerosis [62,63] and rheumatoid arthritis [64]. Investigating the role of *OPN* as a susceptibility gene in SLE, a recent study demonstrated a significant association in male patients [50] – a phenomenon also seen in a study investigating *OPN* variants in type-1 diabetes, implicating a potential gender-specific mechanism acting in the autoimmune process [43]. Similarly, our analysis

demonstrated gender-specific effects for four *OPN* SNPs, particularly for rs4754 which deviated from the Hardy-Weinberg equilibrium in male controls. Moreover, there was a significant association of this SNP with CD in male but not in female patients.

While osteopontin is closely involved in the Th1- and Th17-mediated immune response associated with CD [31,32,33,34], its role in murine colitis models is controversially discussed. In one study, osteopontin deficiency protected mice from DSS-induced colitis [38], while in another study, osteopontin administration in *Opn−/−* mice reduced the disease activity index, improved red blood cell counts, and reduced gut neutrophil activity compared with the DSS-treated wildtype mice [37]. Interestingly, a recent study demonstrated that *Opn−/−* mice showed decreased blood levels of IL-22 [39]. Since we recently demonstrated that IL-22 serum levels are increased in CD and correlate with disease activity and the *IL23R* genotype [55], we next analyzed a potential association between *OPN* genotypes and IL-22 serum levels in CD patients. Overall, we observed lower IL-22 serum levels in the carriers of *OPN* minor alleles (homo- and heterozygous carriers), which was statistically significant when the mean IL-22 expression level of carriers of the 9 investigated *OPN* SNPs minor alleles was compared to the mean IL-22 serum level of the carriers of the

Table 4. Haplotypes of *OPN* SNPs in ulcerative colitis (UC) case-control sample (501 cases and 1510 controls) and omnibus p-values for association with UC susceptibility.

Haplotype combination	Omnibus p-value
rs2728127-rs2853744	5.62×10^{-1}
rs2853744-rs11730582	3.72×10^{-1}
rs11730582-rs11439060	7.01×10^{-1}
rs11439060-rs28357094	9.54×10^{-1}
rs28357094-rs1126616	8.08×10^{-1}
rs1126616-rs1126772	2.80×10^{-1}
rs1126772-rs9138	2.65×10^{-1}
rs2728127-rs2853744-rs11730582	5.24×10^{-1}
rs2853744-rs11730582-rs11439060	6.86×10^{-1}
rs11730582-rs11439060-rs28357094	8.62×10^{-1}
rs11439060-rs28357094-rs1126616	7.28×10^{-1}
rs28357094-rs1126616-rs1126772	3.86×10^{-1}
rs1126616-rs1126772-rs9138	3.02×10^{-1}
rs2728127-rs2853744-rs11730582-rs11439060	8.26×10^{-1}
rs2853744-rs11730582-rs11439060-rs28357094	4.98×10^{-1}
rs11730582-rs11439060-rs28357094-rs1126616	8.39×10^{-1}
rs11439060-rs28357094-rs1126616-rs1126772	1.97×10^{-1}
rs28357094-rs1126616-rs1126772-rs9138	5.24×10^{-1}
rs2728127-rs2853744-rs11730582-rs11439060-rs28357094	5.02×10^{-1}
rs2853744-rs11730582-rs11439060-rs28357094-rs1126616	8.25×10^{-1}
rs11730582-rs11439060-rs28357094-rs1126616-rs1126772	5.07×10^{-1}
rs11439060-rs28357094-rs1126616-rs1126772-rs9138	3.01×10^{-1}
rs2728127-rs2853744-rs11730582-rs11439060-rs28357094-rs112661	7.27×10^{-1}
rs2853744-rs11730582-rs11439060-rs28357094-rs1126616-rs1126772	5.85×10^{-1}
rs11730582-rs11439060-rs28357094-rs1126616-rs1126772-rs9138	5.36×10^{-1}
rs2728127-rs2853744-rs11730582-rs11439060-rs28357094-rs112661-rs1126772	5.86×10^{-1}
rs2853744-rs11730582-rs11439060-rs28357094-rs1126616-rs1126772-rs9138	5.95×10^{-1}
rs2728127-rs2853744-rs11730582-rs11439060-rs28357094-rs112661-rs1126772-rs9138	5.00×10^{-1}

None of the haplotypes was significantly associated with UC susceptibility (p>0.05).

Table 5. Analysis for epistatic interactions between *OPN* SNPs and *IL23R* SNPs regarding CD susceptibility (based on 1510 controls and 704 cases).

OPN SNPs	rs2728127	rs2853744	rs11730582	rs11439060	rs28357094	rs1126616	rs1126772	rs9138
IL23R SNPs								
rs1004819	5.45×10^{-1}	1.34×10^{-1}	3.00×10^{-1}	8.83×10^{-1}	5.93×10^{-1}	3.69×10^{-1}	2.86×10^{-1}	4.52×10^{-1}
rs7517847	4.52×10^{-1}	7.94×10^{-1}	2.53×10^{-1}	5.96×10^{-1}	3.98×10^{-1}	8.57×10^{-1}	4.97×10^{-1}	5.79×10^{-1}
rs10489629	1.90×10^{-1}	3.31×10^{-1}	5.54×10^{-1}	2.32×10^{-1}	$\mathbf{4.18 \times 10^{-2}}$	8.05×10^{-1}	4.31×10^{-1}	6.28×10^{-1}
rs2201841	2.49×10^{-1}	2.18×10^{-1}	2.43×10^{-1}	1.74×10^{-1}	5.91×10^{-2}	$\mathbf{4.71 \times 10^{-2}}$	6.46×10^{-2}	8.10×10^{-2}
rs11465804	8.02×10^{-1}	5.97×10^{-1}	5.98×10^{-1}	7.45×10^{-1}	9.86×10^{-2}	6.19×10^{-1}	4.54×10^{-1}	6.18×10^{-1}
rs11209026 = p.Arg381Gln	6.71×10^{-1}	8.056×10^{-1}	2.466×10^{-1}	6.64×10^{-1}	5.17×10^{-1}	8.87×10^{-1}	6.29×10^{-1}	9.76×10^{-1}
rs1343151	6.65×10^{-1}	2.25×10^{-1}	9.68×10^{-1}	7.34×10^{-1}	1.23×10^{-1}	9.98×10^{-1}	3.32×10^{-1}	8.79×10^{-1}
rs10889677	2.49×10^{-1}	3.09×10^{-1}	3.29×10^{-1}	1.53×10^{-1}	6.05×10^{-2}	5.88×10^{-2}	8.51×10^{-2}	9.73×10^{-2}
rs11209032	4.46×10^{-1}	2.92×10^{-1}	2.71×10^{-1}	3.58×10^{-1}	2.71×10^{-1}	1.91×10^{-1}	3.46×10^{-1}	3.75×10^{-1}
rs1495965	1.79×10^{-1}	2.77×10^{-1}	9.52×10^{-2}	1.34×10^{-1}	1.11×10^{-1}	1.94×10^{-1}	2.82×10^{-1}	2.39×10^{-1}

Significant p-values<0.05 are depicted in bold. However, these associations did not remain significant after Bonferroni correction.

Table 6. *OPN* gene variants modulate IL-22 serum levels in CD patients.

OPN SNP	IL-22 serum levels in *OPN* wildtype carriers [pg/ml]	IL-22 serum levels in *OPN* minor allele carriers* [pg/ml]	p-value
rs2728127	39.72	37.28	0.537
rs2853744	38.24	39.54	0.854
rs11730582	42.07	37.18	0.341
rs11439060	39.72	37.28	0.537
rs28357094	39.23	37.36	0.614
rs4754 = p.Asp80Asp	40.19	36.78	0.380
rs1126616 = p.Ala236Ala	40.19	36.59	0.357
rs1126772	41.04	34.96	0.106
rs9138	40.35	36.59	0.333
Mean	**40.08**	**37.06**	**3.66×10^{-5}**

The mean IL-22 serum level was analyzed for each *OPN* variant in a subgroup of 151 CD patients for which DNA for genotyping and serum for ELISA analysis was available. P values are given for the comparison of the mean IL-22 serum levels of carriers of the minor allele (*homozygous and heterozygous) compared to cytokine levels in homozygous wild-type carriers.

homozygous wildtype alleles ($p = 3.6 \times 10^{-5}$). In 7 out of 8 *OPN/SPP1* SNPs forming the haplotype rs2728127-rs2853744-rs11730582-rs11439060-rs28357094-rs112661-rs1126772-rs9138, which was strongly associated with CD susceptibility, the IL-22 serum levels were nominally lower in CD carriers of the minor allele than in homozygous wildtype carriers, although these differences were for each SNP only small and statistically not significant. Similarly, there were no significant associations with CD or UC susceptibility with single *OPN* SNPs after Bonferroni correction, suggesting that only the combined effect of certain *OPN* SNPs and haplotypes leads to decreased basal IL-22 levels and increased CD susceptibility. We therefore hypothesize that certain *OPN* variants may increase the CD risk via decreased basal expression of IL-22, for which we and others demonstrated strong epithelial-protective properties [65,66,67,68]. However, given the multitude of functions mediated by osteopontin, other disease-modulating properties of *OPN* haplotypes are likely and need further functional investigation.

In addition to increased wound healing, IL-22 mediates also early host defense against attaching and effacing bacterial pathogens [69,70]. In line with the data of Heilmann et al. [39] demonstrating a dual role of osteopontin in intestinal inflammation, one might therefore hypothesize that carriers of *OPN* minor alleles with lower IL-22 serum levels are at high risk of developing intestinal inflammation due to the lack of IL-22-induced mucosal protection. Interestingly, *Opn−/−* mice demonstrated altered wound healing [71], which may be also related to decreased expression of IL-22, which is a strong enhancer of intestinal wound healing [65].

Recent studies in mice showed that osteopontin is involved in Th17 cell differentiation [72] and *Opn*-expressing DCs induce IL-17 production in T cells [21]. On the other hand, osteopontin expression in DCs is repressed by IFN-α and IFN-γ [73,74]. This decreased osteopontin expression is associated with high produc-tion of IL-27, a Th17 cell-inhibiting cytokine that favors regulatory T cell development [75]. We recently demonstrated that IL-27 is also a protective factor for the intestinal epithelial barrier [76]. IL-27 induces anti-inflammatory and antibacterial responses in intestinal epithelial cells and increases cell restitution after wounding [76]. In mice with *Opn*-deficient DCs, substantially elevated levels of IL-27 are produced and *Opn−/−* mice develop delayed experimental autoimmune encephalitis with a Th1 rather than Th17-dominated response [73]. *Opn−/−* mice display a stronger Th1-mediated proinflammatory response during chronic inflammation while a reduced Th17 response during acute colitis protects them from mucosal inflammation [39], further strengthening the dual role of osteopontin in intestinal inflammation.

In summary, our study identified certain *OPN* haplotypes to be associated with CD susceptibility. *OPN* variants may modulate IL-22 secretion which is consistent with data in *Opn−/−* mice, in which low levels of the epithelial-protective cytokine IL-22 predispose to intestinal inflammation. However, the rather weak association signals found in this study argue against a significant role for *OPN* as major IBD susceptibility gene which is consistent with the recent IBD meta-analyses [56,57]. Further functional analysis of large cohorts and detailed fine mapping is required to clarify the role of *OPN* variants in the genetic susceptibility to IBD.

Author Contributions

Conceived and designed the experiments: JG SB. Performed the experiments: JG CB MW CF JG. Analyzed the data: DC JG SB. Contributed reagents/materials/analysis tools: CS JD TO DC MF CS JG SB. Wrote the paper: JS JG SB. Collected phenotype data and DNA samples: JS JG CT TO JD FB CS SB.

References

1. Hugot JP, Chamaillard M, Zouali H, Lesage S, Cezard JP, et al. (2001) Association of NOD2 leucine-rich repeat variants with susceptibility to Crohn's disease. Nature 411: 599–603.

2. Ogura Y, Bonen DK, Inohara N, Nicolae DL, Chen FF, et al. (2001) A frameshift mutation in NOD2 associated with susceptibility to Crohn's disease. Nature 411: 603–606.

3. Duerr RH, Taylor KD, Brant SR, Rioux JD, Silverberg MS, et al. (2006) A genome-wide association study identifies IL23R as an inflammatory bowel disease gene. Science 314: 1461–1463.

4. Glas J, Seiderer J, Wetzke M, Konrad A, Torok HP, et al. (2007) rs1004819 is the main disease-associated IL23R variant in German Crohn's disease patients: combined analysis of IL23R, CARD15, and OCTN1/2 variants. PLoS ONE 2: e819.

5. Hampe J, Franke A, Rosenstiel P, Till A, Teuber M, et al. (2007) A genome-wide association scan of nonsynonymous SNPs identifies a susceptibility variant for Crohn disease in ATG16L1. Nat Genet 39: 207–211.

6. Glas J, Konrad A, Schmechel S, Dambacher J, Seiderer J, et al. (2008) The ATG16L1 gene variants rs2241879 and rs2241880 (T300A) are strongly associated with susceptibility to Crohn's disease in the German population. Am J Gastroenterol 103: 682–691.

7. Libioulle C, Louis E, Hansoul S, Sandor C, Farnir F, et al. (2007) Novel Crohn disease locus identified by genome-wide association maps to a gene desert on 5p13.1 and modulates expression of PTGER4. PLoS Genet 3: e58.

8. Brand S (2009) Crohn's disease: Th1, Th17 or both? The change of a paradigm: new immunological and genetic insights implicate Th17 cells in the pathogenesis of Crohn's disease. Gut 58: 1152–1167.

9. Kawamura K, Iyonaga K, Ichiyasu H, Nagano J, Suga M, et al. (2005) Differentiation, maturation, and survival of dendritic cells by osteopontin regulation. Clin Diagn Lab Immunol 12: 206–212.

10. O'Regan A, Berman JS (2000) Osteopontin: a key cytokine in cell-mediated and granulomatous inflammation. Int J Exp Pathol 81: 373–390.

11. Giachelli CM, Steitz S (2000) Osteopontin: a versatile regulator of inflammation and biomineralization. Matrix Biol 19: 615–622.

12. Mori R, Shaw TJ, Martin P (2008) Molecular mechanisms linking wound inflammation and fibrosis: knockdown of osteopontin leads to rapid repair and reduced scarring. J Exp Med 205: 43–51.

13. Uede T (2011) Osteopontin, intrinsic tissue regulator of intractable inflammatory diseases. Pathol Int 61: 265–280.

14. Lund SA, Giachelli CM, Scatena M (2009) The role of osteopontin in inflammatory processes. J Cell Commun Signal 3: 311–322.

15. Renkl AC, Wussler J, Ahrens T, Thoma K, Kon S, et al. (2005) Osteopontin functionally activates dendritic cells and induces their differentiation toward a Th1-polarizing phenotype. Blood 108: 946–955.

16. Ohshima S, Yamaguchi N, Nishioka K, Mima T, Ishii T, et al. (2002) Enhanced local production of osteopontin in rheumatoid joints. J Rheumatol 29: 2061–2067.

17. Bazzichi L, Ghiadoni L, Rossi A, Bernardini M, Lanza M, et al. (2009) Osteopontin is associated with increased arterial stiffness in rheumatoid arthritis. Mol Med 15: 402–406.

18. Sennels H, Sorensen S, Ostergaard M, Knudsen L, Hansen M, et al. (2008) Circulating levels of osteopontin, osteoprotegerin, total soluble receptor activator of nuclear factor-kappa B ligand, and high-sensitivity C-reactive protein in patients with active rheumatoid arthritis randomized to etanercept alone or in combination with methotrexate. Scand J Rheumatol 37: 241–247.

19. Buommino E, Tufano MA, Balato N, Canozo N, Donnarumma M, et al. (2009) Osteopontin: a new emerging role in psoriasis. Arch Dermatol Res 301: 397–404.

20. Vogt MH, Ten Kate J, Drent RJ, Polman CH, Hupperts R (2010) Increased osteopontin plasma levels in multiple sclerosis patients correlate with bone-specific markers. Mult Scler 16: 443–449.

21. Murugaiyan G, Mittal A, Weiner HL (2008) Increased osteopontin expression in dendritic cells amplifies IL-17 production by CD4+ T cells in experimental autoimmune encephalomyelitis and in multiple sclerosis. J Immunol 181: 7480–7488.

22. Braitch M, Nunan R, Niepel G, Edwards LJ, Constantinescu CS (2008) Increased osteopontin levels in the cerebrospinal fluid of patients with multiple sclerosis. Arch Neurol 65: 633–635.

23. Niino M, Kikuchi S, Fukazawa T, Yabe I, Tashiro K (2003) Genetic polymorphisms of osteopontin in association with multiple sclerosis in Japanese patients. J Neuroimmunol 136: 125–129.

24. Standal T, Borset M, Sundan A (2004) Role of osteopontin in adhesion, migration, cell survival and bone remodeling. Exp Oncol 26: 179–184.

25. Zohar R, Cheifetz S, McCulloch CA, Sodek J (1998) Analysis of intracellular osteopontin as a marker of osteoblastic cell differentiation and mesenchymal cell migration. Eur J Oral Sci 106 Suppl 1: 401–407.

26. Begum MD, Umemura M, Kon S, Yahagi A, Hamada S, et al. (2007) Suppression of the bacterial antigen-specific T cell response and the dendritic cell migration to the lymph nodes by osteopontin. Microbiol Immunol 51: 135–147.

27. O'Regan AW, Hayden JM, Berman JS (2000) Osteopontin augments CD3-mediated interferon-gamma and CD40 ligand expression by T cells, which

results in IL-12 production from peripheral blood mononuclear cells. J Leukoc Biol 68: 495–502.

28. Koguchi Y, Kawakami K, Kon S, Segawa T, Maeda M, et al. (2002) Penicillium marneffei causes osteopontin-mediated production of interleukin-12 by peripheral blood mononuclear cells. Infect Immun 70: 1042–1048.

29. Koguchi Y, Kawakami K, Uezu K, Fukushima K, Kon S, et al. (2003) High plasma osteopontin level and its relationship with interleukin-12-mediated type 1 T helper cell response in tuberculosis. Am J Respir Crit Care Med 167: 1355–1359.

30. Gassler N, Autschbach F, Gauer S, Bohn J, Sido B, et al. (2002) Expression of osteopontin (Eta-1) in Crohn disease of the terminal ileum. Scand J Gastroenterol 37: 1286–1295.

31. Agnholt J, Kelsen J, Schack L, Hvas CL, Dahlerup JF, et al. (2007) Osteopontin, a protein with cytokine-like properties, is associated with inflammation in Crohn's disease. Scand J Immunol 65: 453–460.

32. Gordon JN, MacDonald TT (2005) Osteopontin: a new addition to the constellation of cytokines which drive T helper cell type 1 responses in Crohn's disease. Gut 54: 1213–1215.

33. Sato T, Nakai T, Tamura N, Okamoto S, Matsuoka K, et al. (2005) Osteopontin/Eta-1 upregulated in Crohn's disease regulates the Th1 immune response. Gut 54: 1254–1262.

34. Mishima R, Takeshima F, Sawai T, Ohba K, Ohnita K, et al. (2007) High plasma osteopontin levels in patients with inflammatory bowel disease. J Clin Gastroenterol 41: 167–172.

35. Masuda H, Takahashi Y, Asai S, Hemmi A, Takayama T (2005) Osteopontin expression in ulcerative colitis is distinctly different from that in Crohn's disease and diverticulitis. J Gastroenterol 40: 409–413.

36. Masuda H, Takahashi Y, Asai S, Takayama T (2003) Distinct gene expression of osteopontin in patients with ulcerative colitis. J Surg Res 111: 85–90.

37. da Silva AP, Ellen RP, Sorensen ES, Goldberg HA, Zohar R, et al. (2009) Osteopontin attenuation of dextran sulfate sodium-induced colitis in mice. Lab Invest 89: 1169–1181.

38. Zhong J, Eckhardt ER, Oz HS, Bruemmer D, de Villiers WJ (2006) Osteopontin deficiency protects mice from Dextran sodium sulfate-induced colitis. Inflamm Bowel Dis 12: 790–796.

39. Heilmann K, Hoffmann U, Witte E, Loddenkemper C, Sina C, et al. (2008) Osteopontin as two-sided mediator of intestinal inflammation. J Cell Mol Med 13: 1162–1174.

40. Barizzone N, Marchini M, Cappiello F, Chiocchetti A, Orilieri E, et al. (2011) Association of osteopontin regulatory polymorphisms with systemic sclerosis. Hum Immunol 81: 930–934.

41. Chiocchetti A, Orilieri E, Cappellano G, Barizzone N, S DA, et al. (2010) The osteopontin gene +1239A/C single nucleotide polymorphism is associated with type 1 diabetes mellitus in the Italian population. Int J Immunopathol Pharmacol 23: 263–269.

42. Schmidt-Petersen K, Brand E, Telgmann R, Nicaud V, Hagedorn C, et al. (2009) Osteopontin gene variation and cardio/cerebrovascular disease phenotypes. Atherosclerosis 206: 209–215.

43. Marciano R, D'Annunzio G, Minuto N, Pasquali L, Santamaria A, et al. (2009) Association of alleles at polymorphic sites in the Osteopontin encoding gene in young type 1 diabetic patients. Clin Immunol 131: 84–91.

44. Silverberg MS, Satsangi J, Ahmad T, Arnott ID, Bernstein CN, et al. (2005) Toward an integrated clinical, molecular and serological classification of inflammatory bowel disease: Report of a Working Party of the 2005 Montreal World Congress of Gastroenterology. Can J Gastroenterol 19 Suppl A: 5–36.

45. Glas J, Seiderer J, Nagy M, Fries C, Beigel F, et al. (2010) Evidence for STAT4 as a common autoimmune gene: rs7574865 is associated with colonic Crohn's disease and early disease onset. PLoS ONE 5: e10373.

46. Glas J, Seiderer J, Fries C, Tillack C, Pfennig S, et al. (2011) CEACAM6 gene variants in inflammatory bowel disease. PLoS ONE 6: e19319.

47. Glas J, Seiderer J, Tillack C, Pfennig S, Beigel F, et al. (2010) The NOD2 single nucleotide polymorphisms rs2066843 and rs2076756 are novel and common Crohn's disease susceptibility gene variants. PLoS ONE 5: e14466.

48. Glas J, Stallhofer J, Ripke S, Wetzke M, Pfennig S, et al. (2009) Novel genetic risk markers for ulcerative colitis in the IL2/IL21 region are in epistasis with IL23R and suggest a common genetic background for ulcerative colitis and celiac disease. Am J Gastroenterol 104: 1737–1744.

49. Chiocchetti A, Comi C, Indelicato M, Castelli L, Mesturini R, et al. (2005) Osteopontin gene haplotypes correlate with multiple sclerosis development and progression. J Neuroimmunol 163: 172–178.

50. Han S, Guthridge JM, Harley IT, Sestak AL, Kim-Howard X, et al. (2008) Osteopontin and systemic lupus erythematosus association: a probable gene-gender interaction. PLoS One 3: e0001757.

51. Maver A, Medica I, Salobir B, Tercelj M, Peterlin B (2009) Genetic variation in osteopontin gene is associated with susceptibility to sarcoidosis in Slovenian population. Dis Markers 27: 295–302.

52. Kariuki SN, Moore JG, Kirou KA, Crow MK, Utset TO, et al. (2009) Age- and gender-specific modulation of serum osteopontin and interferon-alpha by osteopontin genotype in systemic lupus erythematosus. Genes Immun 10: 487–494.

53. Forton AC, Petri MA, Goldman D, Sullivan KE (2002) An osteopontin (SPP1) polymorphism is associated with systemic lupus erythematosus. Hum Mutat 19: 459.

54. Seiderer J, Elben I, Diegelmann J, Glas J, Stallhofer J, et al. (2007) Role of the novel Th17 cytokine IL-17F in inflammatory bowel disease (IBD): Upregulated colonic IL-17F expression in active crohn's disease and analysis of the IL17F p.His161Arg polymorphism in IBD. Inflamm Bowel Dis 14: 437–445.

55. Schmechel S, Konrad A, Diegelmann J, Glas J, Wetzke M, et al. (2008) Linking genetic susceptibility to Crohn's disease with Th17 cell function: IL-22 serum levels are increased in Crohn's disease and correlate with disease activity and IL23R genotype status. Inflamm Bowel Dis 14: 204–212.

56. Franke A, McGovern DP, Barrett JC, Wang K, Radford-Smith GL, et al. (2010) Genome-wide meta-analysis increases to 71 the number of confirmed Crohn's disease susceptibility loci. Nat Genet 42: 1118–1125.

57. Anderson CA, Boucher G, Lees CW, Franke A, D'Amato M, et al. (2011) Meta-analysis identifies 29 additional ulcerative colitis risk loci, increasing the number of confirmed associations to 47. Nat Genet 43: 246–252.

58. Glas J, Seiderer J, Fischer D, Tengler B, Pfennig S, et al. (2011) Pregnane X receptor (PXR/NR1I2) gene haplotypes modulate susceptibility to inflammatory bowel disease. Inflamm Bowel Dis 17: 1917–1924.

59. D'Alfonso S, Barizzone N, Giordano M, Chiocchetti A, Magnani C, et al. (2005) Two single-nucleotide polymorphisms in the 5′ and 3′ ends of the osteopontin gene contribute to susceptibility to systemic lupus erythematosus. Arthritis Rheum 52: 539–547.

60. Xu AP, Bai J, Lu J, Liang YY, Li JG, et al. (2007) Osteopontin gene polymorphism in association with systemic lupus erythematosus in Chinese patients. Chin Med J (Engl) 120: 2124–2128.

61. Marciano R, Giacopelli F, Divizia MT, Gattorno M, Felici E, et al. (2006) A polymorphic variant inside the osteopontin gene shows association with disease course in oligoarticular juvenile idiopathic arthritis. Ann Rheum Dis 65: 662–665.

62. Hensiek AE, Roxburgh R, Meranian M, Seaman S, Yeo T, et al. (2003) Osteopontin gene and clinical severity of multiple sclerosis. J Neurol 250: 943–947.

63. Mas A, Martinez A, de las Heras V, Bartolome M, de la Concha EG, et al. (2007) The 795CT polymorphism in osteopontin gene is not associated with multiple sclerosis in a Spanish population. Mult Scler 13: 250–252.

64. Urcelay E, Martinez A, Mas-Fontao A, Peris-Pertusa A, Pascual-Salcedo D, et al. (2005) Osteopontin gene polymorphisms in Spanish patients with rheumatoid arthritis. J Rheumatol 32: 405–409.

65. Brand S, Beigel F, Olszak T, Zitzmann K, Eichhorst ST, et al. (2006) IL-22 is increased in active Crohn's disease and promotes proinflammatory gene expression and intestinal epithelial cell migration. Am J Physiol Gastrointest Liver Physiol 290: G827–838.

66. Sugimoto K, Ogawa A, Mizoguchi E, Shimomura Y, Andoh A, et al. (2008) IL-22 ameliorates intestinal inflammation in a mouse model of ulcerative colitis. J Clin Invest 118: 534–544.

67. Zenewicz LA, Yancopoulos GD, Valenzuela DM, Murphy AJ, Stevens S, et al. (2008) Innate and adaptive interleukin-22 protects mice from inflammatory bowel disease. Immunity 29: 947–957.

68. Brand S, Dambacher J, Beigel F, Zitzmann K, Heeg MH, et al. (2007) IL-22-mediated liver cell regeneration is abrogated by SOCS-1/3 overexpression in vitro. Am J Physiol Gastrointest Liver Physiol 292: G1019–1028.

69. Aujla SJ, Chan YR, Zheng M, Fei M, Askew DJ, et al. (2008) IL-22 mediates mucosal host defense against Gram-negative bacterial pneumonia. Nat Med 14: 275–281.

70. Zheng Y, Valdez PA, Danilenko DM, Hu Y, Sa SM, et al. (2008) Interleukin-22 mediates early host defense against attaching and effacing bacterial pathogens. Nat Med 14: 282–289.

71. Liaw L, Birk DE, Ballas CB, Whitsitt JS, Davidson JM, et al. (1998) Altered wound healing in mice lacking a functional osteopontin gene (spp1). J Clin Invest 101: 1468–1478.

72. Chen G, Zhang X, Li R, Fang L, Niu X, et al. (2010) Role of osteopontin in synovial Th17 differentiation in rheumatoid arthritis. Arthritis Rheum 62: 2900–2908.

73. Shinohara ML, Kim JH, Garcia VA, Cantor H (2008) Engagement of the type I interferon receptor on dendritic cells inhibits T helper 17 cell development: role of intracellular osteopontin. Immunity 29: 68–78.

74. Murugaiyan G, Mittal A, Weiner HL (2010) Identification of an IL-27/osteopontin axis in dendritic cells and its modulation by IFN-gamma limits IL-17-mediated autoimmune inflammation. Proc Natl Acad Sci U S A 107: 11495–11500.

75. Murugaiyan G, Mittal A, Lopez-Diego R, Maier LM, Anderson DE, et al. (2009) IL-27 is a key regulator of IL-10 and IL-17 production by human CD4+ T cells. J Immunol 183: 2435–2443.

76. Diegelmann J, Olszak T, Göke B, Blumberg RS, Brand S (2011) A novel role for IL-27 as mediator of intestinal epithelial barrier protection mediated via differential STAT signaling and induction of antibacterial and anti-inflammatory proteins. J Biol Chem. Nov 8. [Epub ahead of print].

3

Evidence for Significant Overlap between Common Risk Variants for Crohn's Disease and Ankylosing Spondylitis

Debby Laukens[1], Michel Georges[2], Cécile Libioulle[2], Cynthia Sandor[2], Myriam Mni[2], Bert Vander Cruyssen[3], Harald Peeters[1], Dirk Elewaut[3☯], Martine De Vos[1*☯]

1 Department of Gastroenterology, Ghent University, Ghent, Belgium, 2 Unit of Animal Genomics, GIGA-R and Faculty of Veterinary Medicine, University of Liège, Liège, Belgium, 3 Department of Rheumatology, Ghent University, Ghent, Belgium

Abstract

Background: A multicenter genome-wide association scan for Crohn's Disease (CD) has recently reported 40 CD susceptibility loci, including 29 novel ones (19 significant and 10 putative). To gain insight into the genetic overlap between CD and ankylosing spondylitis (AS), these markers were tested for association in AS patients.

Principal Findings: Two previously established associations, namely with the *MHC* and *IL23R* loci, were confirmed. In addition, rs2872507, which maps to a locus associated with asthma and influences the expression of the *ORMDL3* gene in lymphoblastoid cells, showed a significant association with AS (p = 0.03). In gut biopsies of AS and CD patients, *ORMDL3* expression was not significantly different from controls and no correlation was found with the rs2872507 genotype (Spearman's rho: −0.067). The distribution of p-values for the remaining 36 SNPs was significantly skewed towards low p-values unless the top 5 ranked SNPs (*ORMDL3*, *NKX2–3*, *PTPN2*, *ICOSLG* and *MST1*) were excluded from the analysis.

Conclusions: Association analysis using risk variants for CD led to the identification of a new risk variant associated with AS (*ORMDL3*), underscoring a role for ER stress in AS. In addition, two known and five potentially relevant associations were detected, contributing to common susceptibility of CD and AS.

Editor: Antje Timmer, HelmholtzZentrum München, Germany

Funding: This work was supported by grants from (i) La Direction Générale des Technologies de la Recherche et de l'Energie from the Walloon Region (DGTRE, nr 315422), (ii) The 2nd Excellence Programme from the Walloon Region called CIBLES, (iii) from the Communauté Française de Belgique (Biomod ARC), (iv) the Belgian Science Policy organization (SSTC Genefunc and Biomagnet PAI) and (v) by a concerted action grant BOF07/GOA/002 of Ghent University, Belgium. Cynthia Sandor is a fellow of the Formation à la Recherche dans l'Industrie et dans l'Agriculture (FRIA). The funders had no role in study design, data collection and analysis, decision to publish, or preparation of the manuscript.

Competing Interests: The authors have declared that no competing interests exist.

* E-mail: martine.devos@ugent.be

☯ These authors contributed equally to this work.

Introduction

Genome wide association studies (GWAS) are revealing increasing numbers of common risk variants for a growing list of pathologies. Common themes emerging from GWAS include (i) the polygenic architecture of most common diseases, including many risk variants with individually small effects, (ii) the absence of convincing epistatic interactions between common risk variants, and (iii) the fact that the common variants detected to date typically account for less than 20% of the genetic risk. Association mapping greatly benefits from meta-analyses, as pooling of medium sized cohorts considerably increases the power to detect the mainly small genetic effects [1].

An additional noteworthy outcome of recent GWAS are the connections that are being established between diseases initially considered unrelated, through the identification of shared risk variants. Examples include the association of *IL23R* variants with Crohn's disease (CD), psoriasis and ankylosing spondylitis, of *PTPN2* variants with CD and type 1 diabetes, and of *ORMDL3* variants with asthma and CD [2–7].

Crohn's disease and ankylosing spondylitis (AS) are idiopathic, chronic inflammatory disorders of, respectively, the intestinal tract and the spine and sacroiliac joints [8,9]. Although very distinct and well defined entities, there is clinical and genetic evidence supporting some degree of overlap between the pathogenesis of the two entities. Crohn's disease is associated in up to 30% of the patients with articular pathology including sacroilliitis, spondylitis and/or peripheral arthritis [10]. Prior studies also demonstrated evidence for the presence of asymptomatic chronic intestinal inflammation in a subgroup of patients with spondylarthritis (SpA) associated with an increased risk for the development of CD [11]. *HLA-B27* has been known for a long time to be a major risk factor for AS [12], while the previously suspected influence of the MHC on CD susceptibility has recently been clearly confirmed [7]. As mentioned before, *IL23R* variants have been shown to be associated with both CD and AS [2,4]. Risk variants for CD in *NOD2* have also been shown to increase the risk for chronic gut inflammation in SpA patients [13]. Finally, animal models including HLA-B27/human β2-microglobulin transgenic rats and TNFΔ^ARE mice, support links between articular and gut inflammation [14,15].

Through a meta-analysis involving a total of 6,894 CD cases and 9,316 controls of Caucasian descent, we recently identified 19 novel CD risk loci in addition to 11 previously identified ones.

Moreover, we presented strongly suggestive evidence for at least 10 more loci, for a total of 40 CD risk loci [7]. To further examine the potential overlap between the inherited susceptibility to CD and AS, we genotyped a cohort of 182 AS patients for SNP markers corresponding to 39 of these 40 CD risk loci described in Barrett et al. and evaluated their effect on AS outcome [7]. *NOD2* was not included in the analysis because we and others have shown that none of the three CD-associated SNPs are associated with AS [13,16].

Results

As expected, a highly significant association (p = 0.00004) was found with rs3763313, corresponding to the well established major effect of the *MHC* [12]. In addition, we observed a nominally significant association (p = 0.04) with rs11209026, which is in agreement with the previously described effect on AS of the *IL23R* locus (Supporting Table S1) [4].

Of the remaining 37 SNPs, rs2872507 showed a significant association with AS after Bonferroni correction for 37 new tests (p = 0.03), this being a strong candidate for a novel AS susceptibility locus. Because this SNP has been shown to influence the expression of the *ORMDL3* gene [7], we measured the transcript abundance of this gene in endoscopically healthy intestinal biopsies of patients with AS, CD and ulcerative colitis (UC) (patient characteristics Table 1). No difference was found in *ORMDL3* mRNA expression in the colon or ileum of CD, UC and AS patients as compared to healthy controls. In addition, no correlation was found between the expression of this gene and the rs2872507 genotype AA/AG/GG (Spearman's Rho: −147 for the total group, N = 82; 0.147 for ileal biopsies only, N = 32; 0.138 for colonic biopsies only, N = 50).

None of the other 36 SNPs yielded significant p-values after Bonferroni correction, which was not really a surprise given the small size of the studied AS cohort. However, it is well established that one can gain additional statistical power by examining the distribution of p-values across a series of tests rather than considering each of them individually [17]. Thus, we verified whether the remaining 36 SNPs were showing an excess of low p-values when compared to a typical distribution of p-values expected for 36 true null hypotheses. The sum of $\log(1/p_i)$ values obtained with the 36 SNPs was only reached for 7 out of 10,000 simulations,

thus equating to a p-value of 0.0007, strongly suggesting the occurrence of true alternative hypotheses amongst the 36 remaining SNPs. The same approach was successively applied to the 35, 34, 33, 32, … SNPs with highest p-values, i.e. progressively dropping the SNP with lowest p-values and verifying whether the remaining distributions were still significantly skewed towards low values. The outcome of this analysis is shown in Fig. 1. It indicates that the top four SNPs, at least, are very likely to affect the risk of developing AS.

Discussion

We herein first confirm two previously established associations with the risk to develop AS, respectively with the *MHC* and *IL23R* loci.

In addition, we report a novel association between AS and a SNP mapping at position 35,294,289 of human chromosome 17. Remarkably, rs2872507 maps to a locus shown first to be associated with asthma [6] and subsequently with CD [7]. Rs2872507 was shown to be associated with expression levels of the closely linked *ORMDL3* and *GSDML* genes in lymphoblastoid cell lines, which therefore stood out as prime candidate genes [6,7]. However we could not detect differential expression of *ORMDL3* in whole gut biopsies of patients with CD or AS. Although this polymorphism has been shown to influence the expression of *ORMDL3* in lymphoblastoid cells, it is likely that such influences might play only a marginal role in complex tissue such as gut biopsies. Alternatively, SNPs in LD with rs2872507 might have more profound control on the expression of ORMDL3.

Using a survey of SNPs surrounding the *ORMDL3* gene genotyped in the Welcome Trust case consortium dataset, no association was found with AS (personal communication). The population used in this study might contain a bias towards patients with subclinical gut alterations, since the patients were sampled as the result of a collaboration between the departments of rheumatology and gastroenterology. *HLA-B27*, a well-known risk factor associated with AS, has the tendency to misfold during class I complex formation in the endoplasmic reticulum (ER). As such, *ORMDL3* represents an interesting candidate gene for AS, as this protein resides in the ER and overexpression of this gene facilitates the activation of the unfolded protein response [18].

By applying a method that seeks to extract information from the distribution of p-values rather than individual ones, we provide

Table 1. Clinical features of the patient population recruited for intestinal ORMDL3 gene expression analysis.

	Colonic biopsies				Ileal biopsies			
	control	CD	UC	AS	control	CD	UC	AS
N	21	39	10	14	17	24	11	10
Gender (M/F)	9/12	18/21	7/3	8/6	8/9	12/12	4/7	4/6
Age, yrs (mean, range)	50 (22–69)	38 (11–73)	45 (25–61)	36 (16–51)	51 (27–69)	37 (11–66)	32 (7–51)	35 (16–44)
Age at diagnosis (A1/A2/A3)		3/28/8	0/4/6			3/15/6	1/8/2	
Disease location (L1/L2/L3/L4)		15/5/18/1				4/8/11/1		
Rs2872507 (AA/AG/GG/unknown)	3/6/6/6	9/11/1/18	0/3/0/7	0/7/4/3	2/3/5/7	3/9/1/11	0/1/0/10	0/5/3/2
Medication intake:								
no	21	30	7	2	17	19	10	1
5-aminosalicylates	0	9	3		0	5	1	
NSAID				12				9

A1:0–16 yrs; A2:16–40 yrs; A3: ≥40 yrs; disease location is defined as maximal extension of inflammation before first resection. L1: ileal involvement only, L2: colonic involvement only, L3: ileal and colonic involvement. NSAID: non-steroidal anti-inflammatory drugs.

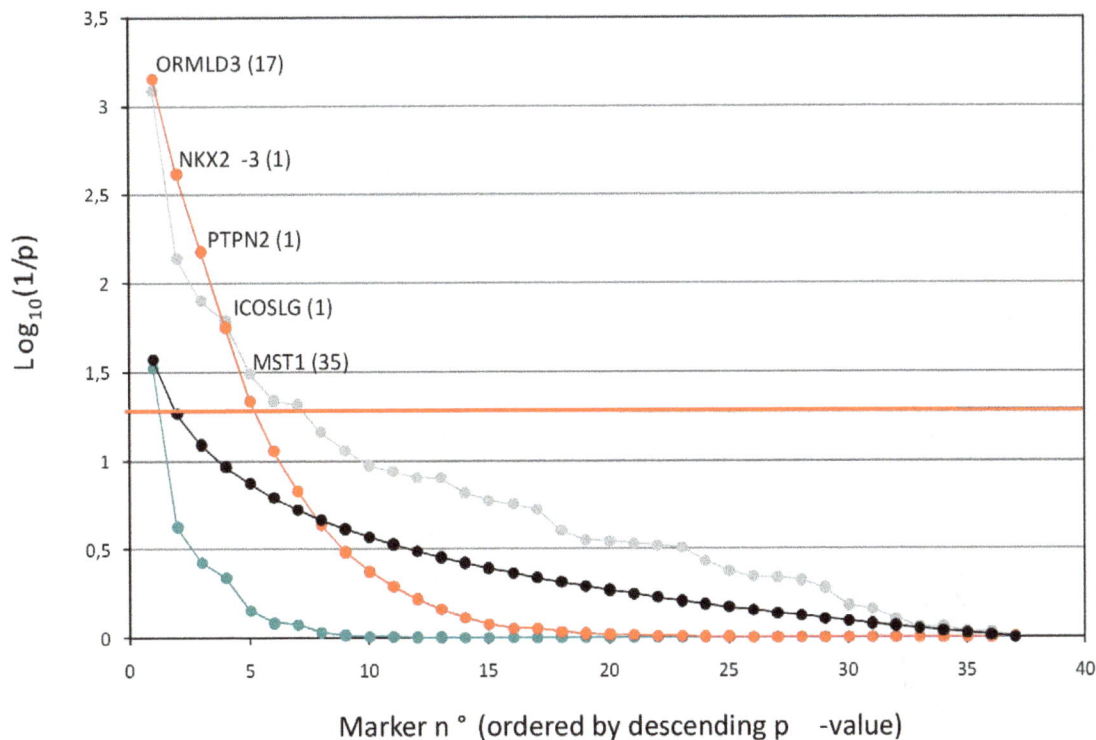

Figure 1. Association of 36 SNPs known to influence CD risk with AS. SNPs are ordered on the X-axis by increasing p-value. Y-axis: $\log_{10}(1/p)$, corresponding to (i) nominal p-values (gray), (ii) Bonferroni corrected p-values (blue), (iii) expected distribution of p-values assuming that all SNPs are true null hypotheses (black), and (iv) the p-value of the distribution of individual p-values for the corresponding marker plus all the less significant ones (red). The horizontal line corresponds to a p-value of 0.05. The names of gene of interest in the vicinity of the associated SNPs as well as the number of genes in the confidence interval (defined according to [7]) are given for the five most interesting SNPs, exceeding the 0.05 significance threshold using the approach that extracts information from the p-value distribution.

evidence for an addition of four novel AS risk loci. The three first of these define an LD-based confidence interval encompassing one gene each: *NKX2-3*, *PTPN2* and *ICOSLG* [7]. As mentioned before, *PTPN2* is particularly interesting as it has been implicated before in the pathogenesis of CD [7] and type I diabetes [19]. The sign of the association is apparently the same for the three diseases, i.e. the same allele increases risk for the three pathologies. *ICOSLG* is also very interesting because of its known involvement in the regulation of immune response [20,21]. The fourth SNP defines a confidence interval encompassing 35 genes, including *MST1* which has recently been implicated in the pathogenesis of CD [22].

One could argue that the observed skewed distribution of p-values reflects population stratification rather than genuine associations. While we cannot formally refute this possibility on the basis of the available data, we consider this to be an unlikely hypothesis. Indeed, the controls originated from the same geographical region as the cases, namely Belgium, and were subjected to the same ethnicity criteria. Moreover, the exact same control cohort has been successfully used as confirmation cohort in an association study for CD based on Belgian cases [7].

In conclusion, we herein provide evidence for an important overlap between the determinants of inherited predisposition to CD and AS. Prior to this study the *MHC* and *IL23R* loci were known to be implicated in the susceptibility to both diseases. We have studied an additional 37 recently defined CD risk loci. Given the limited size of the studied AS cohort, the significance threshold associated with a Type-I error of 5% (accounting for the realization of 37 independent tests), was only exceeded for one

(*ORMLD3*) of the 37 SNPs not previously known to affect AS. However, the distribution of p-values for the remaining 36 SNPs was significantly skewed towards low p-values unless the top 5 SNPs were removed from the analysis, hence supporting at least five novel associations with AS.

Materials and Methods

Ethics Statement

This study was approved by the ethics committee of the University Hospital Ghent (nos. 2000/242 and 2004/242) and each participant obtained a written informed consent form. This form was signed by the participants and approved by the ethics committee.

Patients

All included patients fulfilled the modified New York criteria for definite AS [23], were of self-reported white ancestry, born between 1930 and 1986. Patients were followed at the Rheumatology Department of the University Hospital in Ghent. The male to female ratio was 2.4. Patients with abdominal inflammatory symptoms were not included in this analysis.

Genotyping

Genotyping was performed using the Illumina Golden Gate assay previously used on the Belgian-French cohort in the CD meta-analysis [7]. The genotyping success rate for the AS patients that were retained for analysis was ≥97% and all markers were in Hardy-Weinberg equilibrium in the control population [7].

Quantitative real-time PCR

For *ORMDL3* gene expression analysis, endoscopically healthy biopsies were retrieved during colonoscopy. Total RNA was extracted from the biopsies using the RNeasy Mini Kit (Qiagen Benelux, Venlo, The Netherlands). The quality of each sample was determined using automated gelelectrophoresis (Experion Systems, Maynard, MA, USA, RQI range 7.6–10). Twenty ng of total RNA was converted to cDNA and amplified using the WT-Ovation RNA amplification system (Nugen Technologies, Bemmel, The Netherlands). Ten ng of amplified cDNA was used in SYBRGreen real-time quantitative PCR using automated pipetting (Caliper ALH3000, Caliper Life Sciences, Teralfene, Belgium). Cycling conditions were 95°C for 10 minutes and 44 cycles of 95°C for 10 seconds and 60°C for 30 seconds (Bio-Rad CFX384, Bio-Rad Laboratories, Nazareth, Belgium). Melting curve analysis confirmed primers specificities. The amplification efficiencies of the primer pairs were calculated using a standard curve of reference genomic DNA. Amplification efficiency was determined using the formula $10^{-1/slope}$. *ORMDL3* expression was normalized with the geometric mean value of three reference genes. Primer sequences for *ORMDL3* detection were GTAAAAGGCATGTG-CTGCAA; CCCAACCCCACTACAAGCTA (E = 105% R² = 0.999), for GAPDH TGCACCACCAACTGCTTAGC; GGC-ATGGACTGTGGTCATGAG (E = 110%; R² = 0.990), for HPRT TGACACTGGCAAAACAATGCA; GGTCCTTTTCA-CCAGCAAGCT (E = 111%; R² = 0.998) and for SDHA TGG-GAACAAGAGGGCATCTG; CCACCACTGCATCAAATTC-ATG (E = 105; R² = 0.994).

Statistics

Marker allele frequencies were compared between AS cases and previously described Belgian replication controls, using a one-sided Fisher's exact test imposing an allelic effect with the same sign as observed for CD [7]. For the 36 SNPs that did not exceed Bonferroni-adjusted significance thresholds, we compared the distribution of p-values with that expected for 36 true null hypotheses. This was achieved by comparing $\sum_{i=1}^{35} \log(1/p_i)$ obtained with the real data, with the distribution of 10,000 $\sum_{i=1}^{35} \log(1/r_i)$, where r_i are random numbers drawn between 0 and 1. Gene expression differences between groups were evaluated by the Kruskal-Wallis statistic with Dunn's multiple comparison test.

Author Contributions

Conceived and designed the experiments: DL MG DE MdV. Performed the experiments: CL CS MM. Analyzed the data: CL. Wrote the paper: DL MG. Patient recruitment: BVC HP DE.

References

1. McCarthy MI, Abecasis GR, Cardon LR, Goldstein DB, Little J, et al. (2008) Genome-wide association studies for complex traits: consensus, uncertainty and challenges. Nat Rev Genet 9: 356–69.
2. Duerr RH, Taylor KD, Brant SR, Rioux JD, Silverberg MS, et al. (2006) A genome-wide association study identifies IL23R as an inflammatory bowel disease gene. Science 314: 1461–3.
3. Cargill M, Schrodi SJ, Chang M, Garcia VE, Brandon R, et al. (2007) A large-scale genetic association study confirms IL12B and leads to the identification of IL23R as psoriasis-risk genes. Am J Hum Genet 80: 273–90.
4. Burton PR, Clayton DG, Cardon LR, Craddock N, Deloukas P, et al. (2007) Association scan of 14,500 nonsynonymous SNPs in four diseases identifies autoimmunity variants. Nat Genet 39: 1329–37.
5. Parkes M, Barrett JC, Prescott NJ, Tremelling M, Anderson CA, et al. (2007) Sequence variants in the autophagy gene IRGM and multiple other replicating loci contribute to Crohn's disease susceptibility. Nat Genet 39: 830–2.
6. Moffatt MF, Kabesch M, Liang L, Dixon AL, Strachan D, et al. (2007) Genetic variants regulating ORMDL3 expression contribute to the risk of childhood asthma. Nature 448: 470–3.
7. Barrett JC, Hansoul S, Nicolae DL, Cho JH, Duerr RH, et al. (2008) Genome-wide association defines more than 30 distinct susceptibility loci for Crohn's disease. Nat Genet 40: 955–62.
8. Cho JH (2008) The genetics and immunopathogenesis of inflammatory bowel disease. Nat Rev Immunol 8: 458–66.
9. Brown MA, Wordsworth BP, Reveille JD (2002) Genetics of ankylosing spondylitis. Clin Exp Rheumatol 20: S43–9.
10. de Vlam K, Mielants H, Cuvelier C, De Keyser F, Veys EM, et al. (2000) Spondyloarthropathy is underestimated in inflammatory bowel disease: prevalence and HLA association. J Rheumatol 27: 2860–5.
11. De Vos M (2004) Review article: joint involvement in inflammatory bowel disease. Aliment Pharmacol Ther 20 Suppl 4: 36–42.
12. Brewerton DA, Hart FD, Nicholls A, Caffrey M, James DC, et al. (1973) Ankylosing spondylitis and HL-A 27. Lancet 1: 904–7.
13. Laukens D, Peeters H, Marichal D, Vander Cruyssen B, Mielants H, et al. (2005) CARD15 gene polymorphisms in patients with spondyloarthropathies

identify a specific phenotype previously related to Crohn's disease. Ann Rheum Dis 64: 930–5.
14. Kontoyiannis D, Pasparakis M, Pizarro TT, Cominelli F, Kollias G (1999) Impaired on/off regulation of TNF biosynthesis in mice lacking TNF AU-rich elements: implications for joint and gut-associated immunopathologies. Immunity 10: 387–98.
15. Taurog JD, Maika SD, Simmons WA, Breban M, Hammer RE (1993) Susceptibility to inflammatory disease in HLA-B27 transgenic rat lines correlates with the level of B27 expression. J Immunol 150: 4168–78.
16. Miceli-Richard C, Zouali H, Lesage S, Thomas G, Hugot JP, et al. (2002) CARD15/NOD2 analyses in spondylarthropathy. Arthritis Rheum 46: 1405–6.
17. Storey JD, Tibshirani R (2003) Statistical significance for genomewide studies. Proc Natl Acad Sci U S A 100: 9440–5.
18. Cantero-Recasens G, Fandos C, Rubio-Moscardo F, Valverde MA, Vicente R (2010) The asthma-associated ORMDL3 gene product regulates endoplasmic reticulum-mediated calcium signaling and cellular stress. Hum Mol Genet 19: 111–21.
19. Todd JA, Walker NM, Cooper JD, Smyth DJ, Downes K, et al. (2007) Robust associations of four new chromosome regions from genome-wide analyses of type 1 diabetes. Nat Genet 39: 857–64.
20. Ito T, Yang M, Wang YH, Lande R, Gregorio J, et al. (2007) Plasmacytoid dendritic cells prime IL-10-producing T regulatory cells by inducible costimulator ligand. J Exp Med 204: 105–15.
21. Nakazawa A, Dotan I, Brimnes J, Allez M, Shao L, et al. (2004) The expression and function of costimulatory molecules B7H and B7-H1 on colonic epithelial cells. Gastroenterology 126: 1347–57.
22. Goyette P, Lefebvre C, Ng A, Brant SR, Cho JH, et al. (2008) Gene-centric association mapping of chromosome 3p implicates MST1 in IBD pathogenesis. Mucosal Immunology 1: 131–8.
23. van der Linden S, Valkenburg HA, Cats A (1984) Evaluation of diagnostic criteria for ankylosing spondylitis. A proposal for modification of the New York criteria. Arthritis Rheum 27: 361–8.

4

Genes Involved in the Metabolism of Poly-Unsaturated Fatty-Acids (PUFA) and Risk for Crohn's Disease in Children & Young Adults

Irina Costea[1,2], David R. Mack[3], David Israel[4], Kenneth Morgan[5], Alfreda Krupoves[2,6], Ernest Seidman[7], Colette Deslandres[2,8], Philippe Lambrette[2], Guy Grimard[2,9], Emile Levy[2,10], Devendra K. Amre[2,8]*

1 Public Health Agency of Canada, Montreal, Canada, 2 Research Centre, Sainte-Justine Hospital, Montreal, Canada, 3 Division of Gastroenterology, Hepatology and Nutrition, Children's Hospital of Eastern Ontario, Ottawa, Canada, 4 Department of Gastroenterology, Hepatology and Nutrition, British Columbia's Children's Hospital, Vancouver, Canada, 5 Department of Human Genetics, McGill University and the Research Institute of the McGill University Health Center, Montreal, Canada, 6 Department of Preventive and Social Medicine, University of Montreal, Montreal, Canada, 7 Department of Medicine, McGill University and the Research Institute of the McGill University Health Center, Montreal, Canada, 8 Department of Pediatrics, University of Montreal, Montreal, Canada, 9 Division of Orthopedics, Department of Pediatrics, University of Montreal, Montreal, Canada, 10 Department of Nutrition, University of Montreal, Montreal, Canada

Abstract

Background and Objectives: Epidemiological evidence for the role of polyunsaturated fatty-acids (PUFA) in Crohn's disease (CD) is unclear, although the key metabolite leucotriene B4 (LTB_4) is closely linked to the inflammatory process. We hypothesized that inherited variation in key PUFA metabolic enzymes may modify susceptibility for CD.

Methods and Principal Results: A case-control design was implemented at three pediatric gastroenterology clinics in Canada. Children $\leq$20 yrs diagnosed with CD and controls were recruited. 19 single nucleotide polymorphisms (SNPs) across the ALOX5 (4) CYP4F3 (5) and CYP4F2 (10) genes, were genotyped. Associations between SNPs/haplotypes and CD were examined. A total of 431 cases and 507 controls were studied. The mean ($\pm$SD) age of the cases was 12.4 ($\pm$3.3) years. Most cases were male (56.4%), had ileo-colonic disease (L3$\pm$L4, 52.7%) and inflammatory behavior (B1$\pm$p, 87%) at diagnosis. One genotyped CYP4F3 SNP (rs2683037) not in Hardy-Weinberg Equilibrium was excluded. No associations with the remaining 4 CYP4F3 SNPs with CD were evident. However haplotype analysis revealed associations with a two-marker haplotype (TG) (rs3794987 & rs1290617) (p = 0.02; permuted p = 0.08). CYP4F2 SNPs, rs3093158 (OR (recessive) = 0.56, 95% CI = 0.35–0.89; p = 0.01), rs2074902 (OR (trend) = 1.26, 95% CI = 1.00–1.60; p = 0.05), and rs2108622 (OR (recessive) = 1.6, 95% CI = 1.00–2.57; p = 0.05) were significantly associated whereas rs1272 (OR (recessive) = 0.58, 95% CI = 0.30–1.13; p = 0.10) showed suggestions for associations with CD. A haplotype comprising these 4 SNPs was significantly associated (p = 0.007, permuted p = 0.02) with CD. Associations with SNP rs3780901 in the ALOX5 gene were borderline non-significant (OR (dominant) = 1.29, 95% CI = 0.99–1.67; p = 0.056). A haplotype comprising the 4 ALOX5 SNPs (TCAA, p = 0.036) was associated with CD, but did not withstand corrections for multiple comparisons (permuted p = 0.14).

Conclusions: Inherited variation in enzymes involved in the synthesis/metabolism of LTB_4 may be associated with CD. These findings implicate PUFA metabolism as a important pathway in the CD pathogenesis.

Editor: Antje Timmer, Ludwig Maximilian University of Munich, Germany

Funding: The study was funded by the Canadian Institutes of Health Research (MOP200603). Dr. Amre is supported by a research salary award from the Fonds de la Recherché en Santé du Québec (FRSQ), Québec. Dr. Costea was supported by a doctoral award from the FRSQ. Dr. Krupoves is supported by a scholarship from the Sainte-Justine Hospital Foundation, Montreal and by a scholarship from the PhD Program of the University of Montreal, Montreal. The funders had no role in study design, data collection and analysis, decision to publish, or preparation of the manuscript.

Competing Interests: The authors have declared that no competing interests exist.

* E-mail: devendraamre@hotmail.com

Introduction

Crohn's disease (CD) a chronic inflammatory bowel disease (IBD) is common in children and appears to be on the rise in most developing countries including Canada [1,2]. Children with CD phenotypically differ from adults with CD and present unique clinical challenges relative to their more aggressive disease [3–5].

Recent genome-wide association (GWA) studies both in adults and children [6–9] have provided valuable insights on the potential mechanisms that underlie the chronic inflammation that

is characteristic of CD. Much however remains to be known as GWA studies have accounted for <20% of the inherited variation in CD [7]. CD may represent a group of heterogeneous diseases with unique and overlapping pathophysiologies and in this context, it remains to be explored how environmental factors modify the expression of CD among genetically susceptible individuals.

We have recently shown that in Canadian children an imbalance in consumption of dietary polyunsaturated fatty acids (PUFA) may be associated with risk for CD [10]. In particular the consumption ratio of ω6/ω3 PUFA was observed to be of relevance, as has been proposed by others [11,12]. However, many epidemiological studies [13] and clinical trials [14] using sources of ω fatty acids have not provided consistent results. We hypothesized that inherited variation in the ability to metabolize dietary PUFA may mediate development of CD and may have contributed to the previously observed inconsistent results.

The PUFA metabolic pathway is a complex pathway involving interplay of various enzymes [15]. Key steps relate to the release of arachidonic acid, a ω-6 fatty acid from the cell walls and synthesis of inflammatory mediators known as eicosanoids. A key eicosanoid is leucotriene-B4 (LTB_4), a well recognized mediator of inflammation. Indeed, various studies have shown that LTB_4 levels are associated with CD inflammation [16,17]. Interestingly, a recent study has shown that the levels and activities of various enzymes involved in the PUFA metabolic pathway that leads to production of LTB_4 were related to inflammation in IBD [18]. Three key enzymes are the 5-LO (5-lipoxygenase) that metabolizes arachidonic acid and initiates the pathway and the cytochrome P450 enzymes, CYP4F3 and CYP4F2 that are known de-activators of LTB_4 [19]. In this study we investigated whether DNA variations in these key genes were associated with CD in children.

Methods

Ethics statement

Ethical approval was acquired from the Ethics Review Board of the Ste-Justine Hospital Foundation (HSJ), Montreal; the Children's Hospital of Eastern Ontario (CHEO), Ottawa; and the British Columbia's Children's Hospital, Vancouver. Informed written consent was obtained from all participants (directly from the subject if he/she was an adult or from the parent/guardian if otherwise).

A case-control study was carried out. Cases were children (≤20 yrs of age) diagnosed with CD and recruited from 3 pediatric gastroenterology clinics across Canada (Montreal, Ottawa, Vancouver). Diagnosis of CD was based on established criteria that included clinical, radiological, endoscopic and histological confirmation [20,21]. Disease location and behavior were classified according to the Montreal Classification [22]. Controls were recruited from various sources to parallel population representativeness. These included children visiting the orthopedic clinics for minor trauma (fractures mostly), population-based controls (children) identified using random digit dialing, a birth cohort and a cohort of healthy adults recruited for ongoing genetic epidemiology studies at the Montreal study center. Cases and controls were restricted to those with self-reported European ancestry. Most of these controls have been previously utilized to replicate/validate recent associations reported either in candidate gene or GWA studies [23–28]. Blood and/or saliva were collected as a source for DNA.

Selection of markers, genotyping & statistical analysis

Three genes, ALOX5, CYP4F3 and CYP4F2 were selected for study as they regulate critical *upstream* and *downstream* events that lead to production/metabolism of LTB_4. Relevant markers to genotype were identified using the tag-SNP approach [29]. The following parameters were employed: linkage disequilibrium (LD)>0.80, minor allele frequencies >10%. Genotyping data for populations of European origin housed at the Seattle SNPs data resources (http://gvs.gs.washington.edu/GVS) was utilized to select the tag-SNPs. SNPs were genotyped using the Sequenom platform at the McGill University & Genome Quebec Innovation Center in Montreal. Primers utilized for genotyping the SNP are

listed in table S1. Prior to analysis, Hardy-Weinberg equilibrium (HWE) was examined in the controls. Allelic, genotype and haplotype analysis was carried out using PLINK http://pngu. mgh.harvard.edu/~purcell/plink) and HAPLOVIEW (http:// broad.mit.edu/mpg/HAPLOVIEW). Various models of inheritance (additive, dominant, and recessive) were investigated. Odds ratios (OR) and corresponding 95% confidence intervals (95% CI) were estimated. P-values for the haplotype analysis were corrected using permutation (n = 10000).

Results

A total of 431 cases and 507 controls were investigated (table 1). There were more males and the most common location of disease was the ileo-colonic site (L3±L4). Most children had inflammatory behavior at diagnosis (B1±p).

Four SNPs in the ALOX5 gene, 5 in the CYP4F3 gene and 10 in the CYP4F2 gene were examined (table S1). SNP rs2683037 in the CYP4F3 gene was not in HWE in the controls and was excluded from further analysis. The average genotype rate was >95%. Single SNP analysis did not reveal associations with the CYP4F3 gene (table 2). An haplotype analysis however revealed that the 4 markers were distributed in two blocks (table 3) of LD. A two-marker haplotype (block 1) comprising SNPs rs394987 & rs1290617 was significantly associated with CD (p = 0.02). This association however was borderline non-significant on permutation testing (permuted p = 0.08).

For the ALOX5 gene, there were suggestions for associations with one SNP rs3780901 (OR = 1.29, 95% CI = 0.99–1.67; p = 0.056) under a dominant model (table 4). Haplotype analysis (table 5) comprising the 4 SNPs revealed 5 high frequency (>5%) haplotypes of which haplotype TCAA was significantly associated with CD (p = 0.036). The latter associations however did not withstand corrections for multiple comparisons (permuted p = 0.14).

Of the ten SNPs in the CYP4F2 gene investigated, three were significantly associated with CD (table S2) under various models of inheritance. SNP rs3093158 showed protective associations with CD under the recessive model (OR = 0.56, 95% CI = 0.35–0.89; p = 0.01), SNP rs2074902 was risk conferring under the additive model (OR = 1.26, 95% CI = 1.00–1.60; p = 0.05), and SNP

Table 1. Clinical and demographic characteristics of the CD patients.

Characteristic		Cases (N = 431)
Age at diagnosis (Mean (±SD))		12.4 (±3.3)
Gender (%)	Females	188 (43.6)
	Males	243 (56.4)
Disease location (%)†	L1±L4	77 (17.9)
	L3±L4	227 (52.7)
	L2±L4	123 (28.5)
	Only L4	4 (0.93)
Disease behaviour (%)†	B1±p	375 (87.0)
	B2±p	28 (6.5)
	B3±p	28 (6.5)

†Disease location (L1 = isolated ileal; L2 = isolated colonic; L3 = ileo-colonic; L4 = upper tract) and behaviour (B1 = inflammatory; B2 = stricturing; B3 = penetrating; p = perianal disease) was classified at diagnosis, according to WGO's Montreal classification.

Table 2. Associations between the *CYP4F3* gene and CD in Canadian children.

SNP	Model	Cases	Controls	P-value
rs3794987 (C/T)	TREND	431/453	456/514	0.46
	DOM	322/120	347/138	0.66
	REC	109/333	109/376	0.43
rs1290617 (G/A)	TREND	314/560	373/593	0.23
	DOM	255/182	301/182	0.22
	REC	59/378	72/411	0.54
rs2283612 (T/G)	TREND	393/487	404/562	0.22
	DOM	305/135	320/163	0.32
	REC	88/352	84/399	0.31
rs4646904 (C/T)	TREND	160/726	173/801	0.86
	DOM	145/298	162/325	0.86
	REC	15/428	11/476	0.29

DOM: dominant, REC: recessive, TREND: Cochran-Armitage trend test. For this test, the numbers in the table represent the number of chromosomes that had the minor or the major allele.

Table 4. Associations between the *ALOX5* gene and CD in Canadian children.

SNP	Model	Cases	Controls	P-value
rs2115819 (C/T)	TREND	394/444	437/535	0.39
	DOM	296/123	334/152	0.53
	REC	98/321	103/383	0.43
rs3780901 (C/T)	TREND	256/592	324/652	0.17
	DOM	213/211	276/212	0.056
	REC	43/381	48/440	0.88
rs2291427 (A/G)	TREND	249/599	314/662	0.20
	DOM	209/215	264/224	0.15
	REC	40/384	50/438	0.68
rs10751383 (A/C)	TREND	349/495	435/541	0.17
	DOM	273/149	337/151	0.16
	REC	76/346	98/390	0.43

DOM: dominant, REC: recessive, TREND: Cochran-Armitage trend test. For this test, the numbers in the table represent the number of chromosomes that had the minor or the major allele.

rs2108622 was risk conferring under the recessive model (OR = 1.6, 95% CI = 1.00–2.57; p = 0.05). There were suggestions for associations with a fourth SNP rs1272 under the recessive models (p = 0.10) but these did not achieve nominal statistical significance. Haplotype associations (table 6) using the 4 *CYP4F2* SNPs (rs1272, rs3093158, rs2072902, and rs2108622) indicated significant associations with haplotype GGTC (p = 0.007) and marginally non-significant associations with haplotype GACT (p = 0.06). Associations with haplotype GGTC remained significant (permuted p = 0.02) after corrections for multiple comparisons.

Discussion

In this study we examined whether key enzymes within the fatty-acid metabolic pathway were associated with risk for CD. Although there were suggestions for associations with the *ALOX5* gene at the single marker and haplotype level they did not withstand corrections for multiple comparisons. Similarly for the *CYP4F3* gene associations were evident at the haplotype level that were borderline non-significant on correction for multiple comparisons. Associations were evident, both at the single marker

and haplotype level, with the *CYP4F2* gene, suggesting that variation in this gene may influence risk for CD in children.

PUFA have long been implicated in the pathogenesis of CD. Various epidemiological investigations have been undertaken to examine whether dietary consumption of PUFA was associated with CD [13]. While some studies suggest that ω-3 PUFA may be beneficial and that a higher ratio of ω-3/ω-6 may be associated with lower risks, evidence across studies has been inconsistent. Similarly, potential benefits from dietary supplementation of PUFA, have been equivocal. As individuals will differ in their capacities to metabolize dietary PUFA, we hypothesized that DNA variation in key genes that metabolize PUFA may be important and may modify any associations between dietary PUFA and CD. An important metabolite of PUFA metabolism is the generation of LTB_4 a potent mediator of inflammation. It is generated via the metabolism of arachidonic acid, an ω-6 PUFA which is the first metabolite released from the cell membranes. It is a substrate of the 5-LO enzyme coded by the *ALOX5* gene. LTB_4 derived from the 5-LO metabolic pathway is deactivated mainly by the CYP4F3 (expressed mainly in neutrophils) and CYP4F2 (expressed largely in the liver and kidney) enzymes. We thus selected these three genes for study given their key roles in the metabolic pathway.

Table 3. Association between *CYP4F3* haplotypes and CD.

Blocks	Haplotype	Case	Control	P-value
Block 1	CG	0.51	0.52	0.55
	TA	0.36	0.37	0.44
	TG	0.13	0.10	0.02*†
Block 2	TC	0.55	0.58	0.24
	GC	0.27	0.24	0.23
	GT	0.18	0.17	0.82

Block 1 (rs3794987, rs1290617); Block 2 (rs2283612, rs4646904);
*p-value<0.05;
†permuted p-value=0.08.

Table 5. Associations between *ALOX5* haplotypes and CD.

Haplotype	Cases (%)	Controls (%)	P-value
CTGC	0.30	0.29	0.64
TCAA	0.16	0.20	0.036*†
TTGA	0.15	0.15	0.75
TTGC	0.14	0.13	0.52
CTAC	0.06	0.05	0.39

Haplotypes comprising SNPs: rs2115819, rs3780901, rs2291427, and rs10751383;
*p-value<0.05;
†permuted p-value=0.14.

Table 6. Associations between *CYP4F2* haplotypes and CD.

Haplotype	Cases (%)	Controls (%)	P-value
GATC	0.36	0.36	0.93
CGTC	0.21	0.21	0.84
GACT	0.21	0.18	0.06
GATT	0.12	0.13	0.81
GGTC	0.09	0.13	0.007*†

Haplotypes comprising SNPs rs1272, rs3093158, rs2074902, and rs2108622;
*P-value<0.05,
†permuted p-value=0.02.

The *CYP4F2* & *CYP4F3* genes are located in a cluster on chromosome region 19p13.2. Three genome scans have reported significant linkages to this region in different populations. Rioux et al (2000) [30] using affected sib-pairs reported peak LOD scores of 4.6 for IBD and 3.0 for CD in a Canadian population. In their recent meta-analyses of 10 IBD genome scans among affected relatives, van Heel et al (2004) [31] reported significant linkage of CD to chromosome 19. Low et al (2004) [32] carried out a linkage scan among UK Caucasians (affected sib-pairs) and confirmed linkage of CD to the 19p13.2 region (peak multi-point linkage score of 1.59). The location of the *CYP4F2* & *CYP4F3* genes in the region of significant linkage adds further support to our observations that they may be important candidate genes for CD.

A number of previous studies have implicated LTB$_4$ in the pathogenesis of IBD. The greatly enhanced mucosal synthesis of LTB$_4$ in IBD [16,17] or in rectal diasylate [33,34] of IBD patients has been related, in part, to the increased infiltration of neutrophils into the intestinal tissues [35]. Of relevance to our findings are observations that the metabolism of LTB$_4$ by omega-hydroxylase is altered in the colonic mucosa of IBD patients [36,37]. In particular, the decreased activity of the omega-hydroxylases suggested that the increased, persistent and recurrent inflammation that is characteristic of IBD may be the consequence of an inherent defect in the metabolism of LTB$_4$, leading to its enhanced accumulation and activity. It is to be noted however that the CYP4F3 enzyme is the major LTB$_4$ omega-hydroxylase [19,38] with higher detoxification potential as compared to CYP4F2. It would thus have been anticipated that variations in the *CYP4F3* gene were more likely to influence CD susceptibility. Our findings however indicate that the *CYP4F2* gene was more strongly associated with CD than *CYP4F3*. As the tag-SNPs we selected were of high frequency (>10%) it is possible that less frequent SNPs in the *CYP4F3* may be implicated in CD. For example SNP rs28371536 is a non-synonymous *CYP4F3* SNP of low frequency (2%) not investigated in our study. Certainly larger studies will be required to capture less frequent variation in the *CYP4F3* gene and to assess its influence in CD. On the other hand however, it can be speculated that the stronger associations with the *CYP4F2* gene may be related to observations that the enzyme is not only the major hepatic deactivator of LTB$_4$ but is also expressed in the small intestine [39] (although at lower levels compared to the liver) and hence would be expected to contribute to LTB$_4$ metabolism at the site of inflammation as well. This dual capacity may have contributed to the observed stronger associations. Certainly further studies are required to clarify the roles of both *CYP4F2* and *CYP4F3* genes in CD pathogenesis.

Based on reported observations of elevated levels of LTB$_4$ in IBD and CD patients, some studies have examined the expression of the enzymes/proteins involved in LTB$_4$ synthesis in IBD. In one study, Hendel et al (2002) [40] reported elevated trends in the levels of 5-LO mRNA when studying 21 CD patients and 12 healthy controls. More recently Jupp et al (2007) [18], in a comprehensive examination of LTB$_4$ synthesis pathway enzymes reported a 3-fold higher number of cells staining for 5-LO, a 7-fold higher number of cells staining for FLAP and a 4-fold higher number of cells staining for LTA$_4$H in colonic biopsies of patients with active IBD as compared to healthy controls. Although not withstanding corrections for multiple comparisons, nominal associations between the *ALOX5* gene (that codes for the 5-LO enzyme) were evident in our study. These observations highlight that an abnormal prevalence of enzymes that co-ordinate to synthesize LTB$_4$ may be intimately linked to tissue injury and inflammation in CD and that this pathway needs to be further investigated.

To our knowledge no previous candidate-gene study has examined associations between the *CYP4F2* gene and CD. Recently, Tello-Ruiz et al (2006) [41] screened variation across the 19p IBD6 locus for associations with IBD. The SNP panel however did not comprise variants in the *CYP4F2* gene. In the same study the authors examined 5 SNPs in the *CYP4F3* gene (including SNP rs1290617 that was part of our panel) but did not find associations with them. Support for a potential role for the *CYP4F2* and *CYP4F3* genes in IBD pathogenesis comes from observations by Curley et al (2006) [42] who found associations between the genes and celiac disease, a disease that bears an inflammatory phenotype similar to CD. On the other hand associations with CD for the three genes examined in this study were not noted in earlier GWA studies, at the genome-wide significance level implemented. However, in the recent GWA study on ulcerative colitis (UC) [43], strong associations between SNPs within the *PLA2G2E* (phospholipase A2, group 2E) locus were noted in a North American Caucasian cohort. The *PLA2G2E* gene codes for a secretory phospholipase A2 that releases arachidonic acid from the cell membrane. The enzyme has been shown to be involved in the synthesis of leucotrienes and participate in the inflammatory process [44]. Considering that UC and CD share pathogenetic features, the gene would be a prime candidate gene for study in CD susceptibility and is currently being investigated in our cohort.

It is interesting to note that of the *CYP4F2* associated SNPs, SNP rs2108622 is a non-synonymous coding SNP in exon 11 (M433V). eQTL analysis [45] indicated that the coding variation leads to significant alteration in mRNA expression (LOD score = 3.15, p-value = 0.00014). Similarly, SNP rs2074902 an intronic SNP is in perfect LD with SNP rs3093105, a non-synonymous coding SNP (W12G). Although eQTL data for rs3093105 was not available, using rs2074902 as a proxy indicated that the variation could alter mRNA expression significantly (LOD score = 2.905, p-value = 0.00025). Taken together these findings suggest that altered expression of the *CYP4F2* gene may be related to de-regulation of LTB$_4$ metabolism that in turn can modify the inflammatory responses.

In conclusion, our findings suggest that DNA variation in the metabolism of LTB$_4$ is associated with risk for CD in children. Larger studies to replicate findings in independent cohorts and functional studies to determine biological mechanisms are required. Furthermore studies to investigate other potential candidate genes in the pathway (viz. *FLAP*, *PLA2G2E*, *LTA4H*, *LTB4R1* etc.) need to be carried out. In addition, investigation of interactions between dietary consumption of fatty acids and PUFA pathway metabolic genes vis-à-vis risk for CD need to be pursued.

Supporting Information

Table S1 Primers used for genotyping the *ALOX5*, *CYP4F3* and *CYP4F2* SNPs.

Table S2 Associations between the *CYP4F2* gene and risk for CD in Canadian children.

Acknowledgments

We would like to thank Drs B. Willis and J. Jarvis for orthopaedic controls and A. Mack for facilitating the recruitment of these controls at the Ottawa (CHEO) study site. We also wish to thanks Dr's D. Sinnett, D. Labuda & M. Krajinovic for providing the adult DNA samples (controls).

Author Contributions

Conceived and designed the experiments: DKA IC. Performed the experiments: DKA IC AK. Analyzed the data: IC DKA. Wrote the paper: IC DKA. Participated in the recruitment of subjects: DRM DI EGS CD GG PL. Provided genetic epidemiology expertise: KM. Provided conceptual expertise in PUFA metabolism: EL.

References

1. Bernstein CN, Wajda A, Svenson LW, MacKenzie A, Koehoorn M, et al. (2006) The epidemiology of inflammatory bowel disease in Canada: a population-based study. Am J Gastroenterol 101: 1559–1568.
2. Lowe AM, Roy PO, Poulin M, Michel P, Bitton A, et al. (2009) Epidemiology of Crohn's disease in Quebec, Canada. Inflamm Bowel Dis 15: 429–435.
3. Kim SC, Ferry GD (2004) Inflammatory bowel diseases in pediatric and adolescent patients: clinical, therapeutic, and psychosocial considerations. Gastroenterology 126: 1550–1560.
4. Mamula P, Markowitz JE, Baldassano RN (2003) Inflammatory bowel disease in early childhood and adolescence: special considerations. Gastroenterol Clin North Am 32: 967–995.
5. Van IJ, Russell RK, Drummond HE, Aldhous MC, Round NK, et al. (2008) Definition of phenotypic characteristics of childhood-onset inflammatory bowel disease. Gastroenterology 135: 1114–1122.
6. Massey D, Parkes M (2007) Common pathways in Crohn's disease and other inflammatory diseases revealed by genomics. Gut 56: 1489–1492.
7. Barrett JC, Hansoul S, Nicolae DL, Cho JH, Duerr RH, et al. (2008) Genome-wide association defines more than 30 distinct susceptibility loci for Crohn's disease. Nat Genet 40: 955–962.
8. Kugathasan S, Baldassano RN, Bradfield JP, Sleiman PM, Imielinski M, et al. (2008) Loci on 20q13 and 21q22 are associated with pediatric-onset inflammatory bowel disease. Nat Genet 40: 1211–1215.
9. Imielinski M, Baldassano RN, Griffiths A, Russell RK, Annese V, et al. (2009) Common variants at five new loci associated with early-onset inflammatory bowel disease. Nat Genet 41: 1335–1340.
10. Amre DK, D'Souza S, Morgan K, Seidman G, Lambrette P, et al. (2007) Imbalances in dietary consumption of fatty acids, vegetables, and fruits are associated with risk for Crohn's disease in children. Am J Gastroenterol 102: 2016–2025.
11. Belluzzi A, Boschi S, Brignola C, Munarini A, Cariani G, et al. (2000) Polyunsaturated fatty acids and inflammatory bowel disease. Am J Clin Nutr 71: 339S–342S.
12. Calder PC (2006) n-3 polyunsaturated fatty acids, inflammation, and inflammatory diseases. Am J Clin Nutr 83: 1505S–1519S.
13. Amre DK, Seidman EG (2003) Etiopathogenesis of pediatric Crohn's disease. Biologic pathways based on interactions between genetic and environmental factors. Med Hypotheses 60: 344–350.
14. MacLean CH, Mojica WA, Newberry SJ, Pencharz J, Garland RH, et al. (2005) Systematic review of the effects of n−3 fatty acids in inflammatory bowel disease. Am J Clin Nutr 82: 611–619.
15. Kinsella JE, Lokesh B, Broughton S, Whelan J (1990) Dietary polyunsaturated fatty acids and eicosanoids: potential effects on the modulation of inflammatory and immune cells: an overview. Nutrition 6: 24–44.
16. Sharon P, Stenson WF (1984) Enhanced synthesis of leukotriene B4 by colonic mucosa in inflammatory bowel disease. Gastroenterology 86: 453–460.
17. Hawthorne AB, Boughton-Smith NK, Whittle BJ, Hawkey CJ (1992) Colorectal leukotriene B4 synthesis in vitro in inflammatory bowel disease: inhibition by the selective 5-lipoxygenase inhibitor BWA4C. Gut 33: 513–517.
18. Jupp J, Hillier K, Elliott DH, Fine DR, Bateman AC, et al. (2007) Colonic expression of leukotriene-pathway enzymes in inflammatory bowel diseases. Inflamm Bowel Dis 13: 537–546.
19. Hardwick JP (2008) Cytochrome P450 omega hydroxylase (CYP4) function in fatty acid metabolism and metabolic diseases. Biochem Pharmacol 75: 2263–2275.
20. Lennard-Jones JE (1989) Classification of inflammatory bowel disease. Scand J Gastroenterol Suppl 170: 2–6.
21. Sands BE (2004) From symptom to diagnosis: clinical distinctions among various forms of intestinal inflammation. Gastroenterology 126: 1518–1532.
22. Satsangi J, Silverberg MS, Vermeire S, Colombel JF (2006) The Montreal classification of inflammatory bowel disease: controversies, consensus, and implications. Gut 55: 749–753.
23. Amre DK, Mack DR, Morgan K, Israel D, Deslandres C, et al. (2010) Susceptibility loci reported in genome-wide association studies are associated

with Crohn's disease in Canadian children. Aliment Pharmacol Ther 31: 1186–1191.
24. Amre DK, Mack DR, Morgan K, Israel D, Deslandres C, et al. (2010) Association between genome-wide association studies reported SNPs and pediatric-onset Crohn's disease in Canadian children. Hum Genet 128: 131–135.
25. Amre DK, Mack DR, Morgan K, Krupoves A, Costea I, et al. (2009) Autophagy gene ATG16L1 but not IRGM is associated with Crohn's disease in Canadian children. Inflamm Bowel Dis 15: 501–507.
26. Amre DK, Mack DR, Morgan K, Israel D, Lambrette P, et al. (2009) Interleukin 10 (IL-10) gene variants and susceptibility for paediatric onset Crohn's disease. Aliment Pharmacol Ther 29: 1025–1031.
27. Amre DK, Mack DR, Israel D, Morgan K, Lambrette P, et al. (2008) Association between genetic variants in the IL-23R gene and early-onset Crohn's disease: results from a case-control and family-based study among Canadian children. Am J Gastroenterol 103: 615–620.
28. Amre DK, Mack DR, Morgan K, Fujiwara M, Israel D, et al. (2009) Investigation of reported associations between the 20q13 and 21q22 loci and pediatric-onset Crohn's disease in Canadian children. Am J Gastroenterol 104: 2824–2828.
29. Carlson CS, Eberle MA, Rieder MJ, Yi Q, Kruglyak L, et al. (2004) Selecting a maximally informative set of single-nucleotide polymorphisms for association analyses using linkage disequilibrium. Am J Hum Genet 74: 106–120.
30. Rioux JD, Silverberg MS, Daly MJ, Steinhart AH, McLeod RS, et al. (2000) Genomewide search in Canadian families with inflammatory bowel disease reveals two novel susceptibility loci. Am J Hum Genet 66: 1863–1870.
31. van Heel DA, Fisher SA, Kirby A, Daly MJ, Rioux JD, et al. (2004) Inflammatory bowel disease susceptibility loci defined by genome scan meta-analysis of 1952 affected relative pairs. Hum Mol Genet 13: 763–770.
32. Low JH, Williams FA, Yang X, Cullen S, Colley J, et al. (2004) Inflammatory bowel disease is linked to 19p13 and associated with ICAM-1. Inflamm Bowel Dis 10: 173–181.
33. Lauritsen K, Laursen LS, Bukhave K, Rask-Madsen J (1986) Effects of topical 5-aminosalicylic acid and prednisolone on prostaglandin E2 and leukotriene B4 levels determined by equilibrium in vivo dialysis of rectum in relapsing ulcerative colitis. Gastroenterology 91: 837–844.
34. Lauritsen K, Laursen LS, Bukhave K, Rask-Madsen J (1988) In vivo profiles of eicosanoids in ulcerative colitis, Crohn's colitis, and Clostridium difficile colitis. Gastroenterology 95: 11–17.
35. Lobos EA, Sharon P, Stenson WF (1987) Chemotactic activity in inflammatory bowel disease. Role of leukotriene B4. Dig Dis Sci 32: 1380–1388.
36. Ikehata A, Hiwatashi N, Kinouchi Y, Ito K, Yamazaki H, et al. (1993) Leukotriene B4 omega-hydroxylase activity in polymorphonuclear leukocytes from patients with inflammatory bowel disease. Prostaglandins Leukot Essent Fatty Acids 49: 489–494.
37. Ikehata A, Hiwatashi N, Kinouchi Y, Yamazaki H, Ito K, et al. (1995) Altered leukotriene B4 metabolism in colonic mucosa with inflammatory bowel disease. Scand J Gastroenterol 30: 44–49.
38. Kikuta Y, Kusunose E, Kusunose M (2002) Prostaglandin and leukotriene ω-hydroxylases. Prostaglandins Other Lipid Mediat 68–69: 345–362.
39. Hashizume T, Imaoka S, Hiroi T, Terauchi Y, Fujii T, et al. (2001) cDNA cloning and expression of a novel cytochrome p450 (CYP4F12) from human small intestine. Biochem Biophys Res Commun 280: 1135–1141.
40. Hendel J, Ahnfelt-Ronne I, Nielsen OH (2002) Expression of 5-lipoxygenase mRNA is unchanged in the colon of patients with active inflammatory bowel disease. Inflamm Res 51: 423–426.
41. Tello-Ruiz MK, Curley C, DelMonte T, Giallourakis C, Kirby A, et al. (2006) Haplotype-based association analysis of 56 functional candidate genes in the IBD6 locus on chromosome 19. Eur J Hum Genet 14: 780–790.
42. Curley CR, Monsuur AJ, Wapenaar MC, Rioux JD, Wijmenga C (2006) A functional candidate screen for coeliac disease genes. Eur J Hum Genet 14: 1215–1222.

5

Characterization of Changes in Serum Anti-Glycan Antibodies in Crohn's Disease

Florian Rieder[1,2,3]*, **Rocio Lopez**[4], **Andre Franke**[5], **Alexandra Wolf**[1], **Stephan Schleder**[1], **Andrea Dirmeier**[1], **Anja Schirbel**[2], **Philip Rosenstiel**[5], **Nir Dotan**[6], **Stefan Schreiber**[5], **Gerhard Rogler**[7], **Frank Klebl**[1]

1 Department of Internal Medicine I, University of Regensburg, Regensburg, Germany, **2** Department of Pathobiology, Lerner Research Institute, Cleveland Clinic Foundation, Cleveland, Ohio, United Sates of America, **3** Department of Gastroenterology, Cleveland Clinic Foundation, Cleveland, Ohio, United Sates of America, **4** Department of Quantitative Health Sciences, Cleveland Clinic Foundation, Cleveland, Ohio, United Sates of America, **5** Institute of Clinical Molecular Biology and Department of General Internal Medicine, Christian-Albrechts-University, Kiel, Germany, **6** Glycominds Ltd., Lod, Israel, **7** Departement of Internal Medicine, Clinic for Gastroenterology and Hepatology, University Hospital Zuerich, Zuerich, Switzerland

Abstract

Introduction: Anti-glycan antibodies are a promising tool for differential diagnosis and disease stratification of patients with Crohn's disease (CD). We longitudinally assessed level and status changes of anti-glycan antibodies over time in *individual* CD patients as well as determinants of this phenomenon.

Methods: 859 serum samples derived from a cohort of 253 inflammatory bowel disease (IBD) patients (207 CD, 46 ulcerative colitis (UC)) were tested for the presence of anti-laminarin (Anti-L), anti-chitin (Anti-C), anti-chitobioside (ACCA), anti-laminaribioside (ALCA), anti-mannobioside (AMCA) and anti-*Saccharomyces cerevisiae* (gASCA) antibodies by ELISA. All patients had at least two and up to eleven serum samples taken during the disease course.

Results: Median follow-up time for CD was 17.4 months (Interquartile range (IQR) 8.0, 31.6 months) and for UC 10.9 months (IQR 4.9, 21.0 months). In a subgroup of CD subjects marked changes in the overall immune response (quartile sum score) and levels of individual markers were observed over time. The marker status (positive versus negative) remained widely stable. Neither clinical phenotype nor NOD2 genotype was associated with the observed fluctuations. In a longitudinal analysis neither changes in disease activity nor CD behavior led to alterations in the levels of the glycan markers. The ability of the panel to discriminate CD from UC or its association with CD phenotypes remained stable during follow-up. In the serum of UC patients neither significant level nor status changes were observed.

Conclusions: While the levels of anti-glycan antibodies fluctuate in a subgroup of CD patients the antibody status is widely stable over time.

Editor: Jialin Charles Zheng, University of Nebraska Medical Center, United States of America

Funding: This study was supported by the German Ministry of Education and Research (BMBF) via the Kompetenznetz "Chronisch entzündliche Darmerkrankungen", the DFG Excellence Cluster Inflammation at Interfaces and by the Deutsche Forschungsgemeinschaft (DFG) to F.R. These funders had no role in study design, data collection and analysis, decision to publish, or preparation of the manuscript. Nir Dotan is employed by Glycominds Ltd. and was involved in study design and preparation of the manuscript.

Competing Interests: The authors have read the journal's policy and have the following conflicts: Dotan is an employee and shareholder of Glycominds Ltd., Lod, Israel.

* E-mail: florian.rieder@t-online.de

Introduction

The diagnosis of inflammatory bowel disease (IBD) and the differentiation between ulcerative colitis (UC) and Crohn's disease (CD) is currently based on the combination of clinical, laboratory, radiological, endoscopic and histopathologic criteria [1]. However, in about 15% of colitis patients a definitive diagnosis cannot be made, a disease category termed indeterminate colitis (IC). In addition, CD is characterized by the frequent occurrence of complicated disease behavior, defined as fistulae or stenoses, and the need for CD-related surgery in a high proportion of patients [2,3,4].

Serological markers linked to CD, such as anti-*Saccharomyces cerevisiae* (ASCA), anti-*Pseudomonas*-associated sequence I2 (anti-I2),

outer membrane porin C (OmpC) of *Escherichia coli* antibodies and antibodies against the bacterial flagellin cBir1 (Anti-cBir1) have been extensively investigated for diagnosis and disease stratification [5,6]. The most recently described serum markers directed against microbial antigens are anti-glycan-antibodies. A panel of antibodies consisting of anti-*Saccharomyces cerevisiae* antibodies (gASCA), anti-mannobioside carbohydrate antibodies (AMCA), anti-laminaribioside carbohydrate antibodies (ALCA), anti-chitobioside carbohydrate antibodies (ACCA), anti-laminarin carbohydrate antibody (Anti-L) and anti-chitin carbohydrate antibody (Anti-C) has been reported in several independent cohorts to show a high discriminatory capacity for CD versus UC and association with and prediction of complicated CD behavior [7,8,9,10,11,12,13].

Despite a large number of cross sectional studies and a growing number of prospective studies in patient cohorts examining the utility of anti-glycan antibodies and other serum markers for diagnosis, disease stratification and prediction [5,6,7,8,9,10,11,12,13,14,15] strikingly limited information is available on stability of antibody levels or antibody status (positive versus negative) over time. Most existing investigations determine stability of markers by facilitating one single sample per patient but this single-point cross-sectional study design makes claims about stability and potential influencing factors on level changes conflicting [7,9,16,17,18]. Whereas some data are available about level and status changes of serum markers over time in individual patients [11,14,19,20,21,22,23,24], all studies suffer from low patient numbers and/or short follow-up times. No publication exists assessing the stability of the novel anti-glycan antibodies in individual patients over time.

In contrast to this lack of information, knowledge in this field is crucial not only for interpreting existing studies but also for the design of future prospective trials that can ultimately lead to routine use of these biomarkers in clinical practice. The aim of this study was to fill these information gaps by I) defining the extent of level changes of anti-glycan antibodies in individual patients over time, II) interrogating potential associations of clinical factors and genotypes with marker fluctuations, III) performing a longitudinal analysis following marker levels correlated with distinct clinical events over time and IV) investigating, if the accuracy of the marker panel to differentiate UC from CD and association with complicated CD behavior changes over time.

Methods

Patient population

We performed a longitudinal cohort study among adult IBD patients. All IBD in- and outpatients seen at our tertiary referral center between 2000 and 2006 were considered for participation in the study. The diagnosis of CD and UC was made based on clinical, radiographic, endoscopic and histopathologic criteria according to Stange et al. [1,25].

Inclusion criterion for this study was the presence of more than one serum sample per individual IBD patient during the disease course. The samples were collected at arbitrary visits to our hospital. Clinical data including age at diagnosis, body mass index (BMI), gender, date of sample procurement, date and type of first complication and surgery, medication and disease location were obtained or updated, respectively, for each single visit and time point of sample procurement separately by the treating physician of the IBD unit. Collected data were transferred and stored in a secure coded anonymized database for analysis. In July 2007, all patient charts and the database were reviewed and updated for the data points mentioned above without knowledge of the antibody values. The treating IBD physician determined CD activity based on the criteria included in the Crohn's disease activity index (CDAI) at the time of the patient visit and patients were grouped in active (CDAI>150) and non-active disease (CDAI<150), without assigning a specific CDAI point value. This patient cohort represents a subgroup of the previously reported cross-sectional study [11].

Signed informed consent was obtained from all participants. The ethics committee of the University of Regensburg approved the study.

Serological analysis

After procurement of the blood samples the serum was separated by centrifugation and kept frozen at $-80°C$ until use. All sera were analyzed at the same time for the levels of gASCA

IgG, ALCA IgG, ACCA IgA, AMCA IgG, Anti-L IgA and Anti-C IgA in a blinded manner as previously described [11]. All assays were performed by ELISA following the manufacturer's conditions (Glycominds, Ltd; Lod, Israel). The optical density is directly proportional to the amount of bound antibody. Results were expressed as ELISA units (EU), which is a value relative to a calibration serum sample. The cut-off values were used as previously determined in a larger cross sectional analysis using ROC curves for 90% specificity of CD versus a large control group consisting of UC, other inflammatory GI-diseases, non-GI diseases and healthy controls [11]: ACCA 90 EU, Anti-L 120 EU, Anti-C 50 EU, ALCA 60 EU, AMCA 100 EU, gASCA 50 EU.

For the level of immune response of the serum-antibodies and for analysis of association with certain phenotypes quartile scores for each serologic marker were calculated, as previously described [7,9,11,19]. Briefly, for each antibody patients whose antibody levels were in the first, second, third and fourth quartile of the distribution were assigned a quartile score of 1, 2, 3 or 4, respectively. By adding individual quartile scores for each glycan antigen a semi-quantitative quartile sum score (QSS, range 6–24) representing the cumulative quantitative immune response towards all six antigens for each patient was obtained. In other words the QSS semiquantitatively depicts the overall serologic immune response taking into consideration the levels of all tested antibodies per sample. The QSS at the time of first sample procurement was used as a reference for the longitudinal follow-up analysis.

CRP was recorded as positive (values>0.5 mg/l) or negative (values<0.5 mg/l).

Determination of NOD2 genotypes of the IBD patients

Standardized TaqMan® SNP Genotyping Assays (Applied Biosystems, Foster City, USA) were used to determine the genotype of the three main CD-associated NOD2 variants SNP 8, 12 and 13 (rs2066844, rs2066845 and rs5743293). All processed data were written to and administered by a previously described database-driven laboratory information management system (LIMS) [26]. Duplicate or related samples were identified and excluded from the analyses, using algorithms implemented in the LIMS. All SNPs had a high call rate (> = 90% in cases and controls), were not monomorphic (minor allele frequency <1% in cases or controls), and did not deviate from Hardy-Weinberg equilibrium (HWE) in the control sample (PHWE>0.001).

Phenotypical characteristics of IBD patients

The IBD physician assessed the IBD patients for disease phenotype at arbitrary visits during the disease course. Patient demographics at time of first sample procurement can be seen in **Table 1**. For the purpose of this study complicated disease behavior in CD patients was defined as the occurrence of fistulae or stenoses before or during follow-up. We additionally distinguished internal penetrating from perianal fistulizing disease. Furthermore, we examined the need for CD-related surgery during the follow-up period. CD-related surgery included 23 patients that had surgeries other than bowel resection, 64 patients that had bowel resection only and 67 that had both types of surgeries during follow-up.

Statistical analysis

Descriptive statistics were computed for all variables. These include means, standard deviations and percentiles for continuous factors and frequencies for categorical variables. Lin's concordance correlation coefficients were estimated to assess correlation between first and maximal change samples. Associations of level

Table 1. Cohort Characteristics.

Factor	CD	UC
	(N = 207)	(N = 46)
Female, n (%)	103 (49.8)	18 (39.1)
Mean age at 1st sample (years) (SD)	35.3 (12.1)	38.0 (12.5)
Mean BMI (kg/m^2) (SD)	23.6 (5.1)	24.3 (4.7)
Mean age at diagnosis (years) (SD)	28.6 (11.9)	33.1 (12.6)*
Median disease duration at time of first sample (months) (P25, P75)	52.7 (9.2, 122.9)	40.9 (12.9, 97.6)
Median follow-up after first sample (months) (P25, P75)	17.4 (8.0, 31.6)	10.9 (4.9, 21.0)*
Location		
Ileum Involvement	178 (86.0)	----
Proctitis/Left Colon	----	11 (24.4)
Subtotal/Pancolitis	----	34 (75.6)
CRP>0.5 mg/l any time during FU‡	142 (69.3)	25 (54.4)
Behaviour (Montreal classification)⊺		
B1	40 (19.4)	---
B1p	20 (9.7)	---
B2	50 (24.3)	---
B2p	17 (8.3)	---
B3	48 (23.3)	---
B3p	31 (15.1)	---
IBD related surgery (%)	154 (74.4)	---
NOD2 Genotype†		
R702W C>T		
CC	1 (0.5)	0 (0.0)
CT	32 (17.0)	1 (2.3)
TT	155 (82.5)	42 (97.7)
G908R G>C		
CC	1 (0.5)	0 (0.0)
GC	12 (6.1)	2 (4.6)
GG	184 (93.4)	42 (95.5)
L1007fsinsC -/C		
C/C	7 (3.6)	0 (0.0)
-/C	43 (21.9)	3 (6.8)
-/-	146 (74.5)	41 (93.2)
All SNPs		
wt	107 (56.9)	37 (86.1)*
mut	81 (43.1)	6 (13.9)
Number of serology tests per subject		
2	76 (36.7)	29 (63.0)
3	56 (27.1)	6 (13.0)
4	26 (12.6)	5 (10.9)
≥5	49 (23.7)	6 (13.0)

BMI, body mass index; IBD, inflammatory bowel disease; CD: Crohn's disease; UC: Ulcerative colitis.
P25, P75: 25th and 75th percentiles; SD: standard deviation.
*p<0.05 versus other patient group.
‡2 CD patients did not have any CRP measures during follow-up.
⊺One patient did not have clinical information regarding the occurence of fistula.
†Complete NOD2 Genotype information was available for 188 CD and 43 UC patients.

and status changes with clinical phenotypes were evaluated using logistic regression models and adjustments for total follow-up time were done. To study changes in antibody levels, linear mixed models were built; time since diagnosis, use of immunosuppressants, active disease, occurrence of complication, and IBD-related surgery were included in the models. An unstructured covariance matrix was used to model within-subject correlation due to repeated measures. The sensitivity, specificity, positive and negative predictive values were estimated to assess whether the validity of each marker in diagnosing CD changed with repeated samples; subjects with at least 4 samples were included in this analysis. In addition, this same group of patients was used to study the association between antibody levels, positivity, number of positive markers and quartile group with Crohn's disease complications; Wilcoxon rank sum tests and Pearson's chi-square tests were used, as appropriate. A p<0.05 was considered statistically significant, unless otherwise stated. SAS version 9.2 software (The SAS Institute, Cary, NC) and R version 2.10.1 (The R Foundation for Statistical Computing, Vienna, Austria) were used for all analyses.

Results

20% of the sera were collected within six months, 30% within one year of diagnosis. The frequency of testing for the individual patients can be seen in **Table 1**. The median time between

sample procurements in the subjects was 6.2 months (Interquartile range (IQR) 3.5 months–12.2 months).

I) Definition of level and status changes over time

As not all samples were taken at time of diagnosis and follow-up times varied we first tested if these two criteria have an influence on our analysis. The magnitude of level changes in our IBD cohort was not dependent on the time from diagnosis to first sample procurement. In addition, there was no significant time-level association between subjects with a short or long follow-up period, indicating that the observed level changes are independent of the observation time (data not shown). This suggests that our cohort can be used for an analysis of fluctuations over time, despite not all samples being taken at the time of IBD diagnosis or with a fixed follow-up time.

Level changes in Crohn's disease. We next characterized the level changes of the glycan markers in patients with CD. We noted substantial changes of the overall immune response depicted by the QSS and of levels of all tested single serum markers in a subgroup of individual CD patients over time (**Figure 1** showing

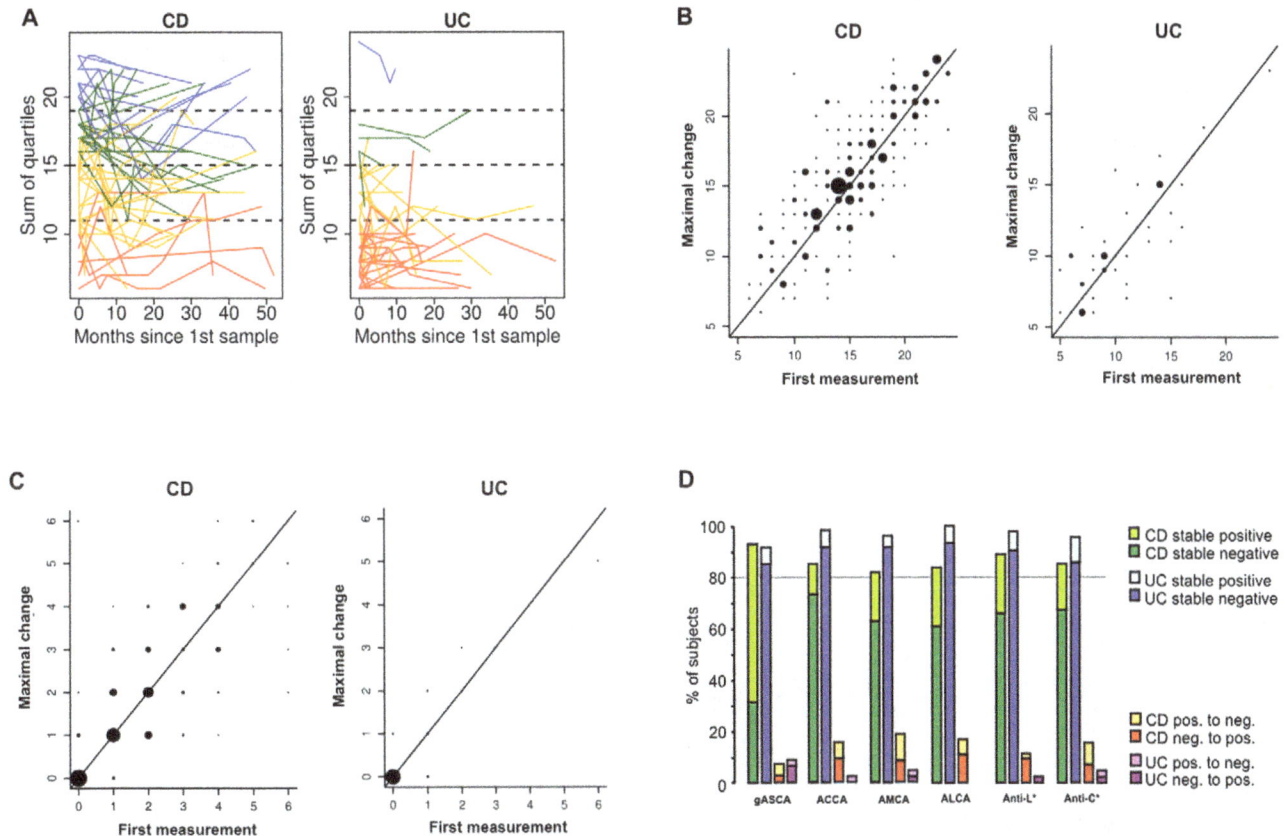

Figure 1. A. Changes in quartile sum score over time. Profile plots for changes in the quartile sum score (QSS) in individual Crohn's disease (CD) and Ulcerative colitis (UC) patients over time. The broken lines represent four equal sections of the QSS. The blue, green, yellow and red lines indicate patients starting in a certain section of the QSS. Depicted is a random set of 50 subjects per graph. B. Maximal changes in the quartile sum score. Scatter plots comparing the quartile sum score (QSS) of the first sample and the sample with the maximal changes in QSS during follow-up in Crohn's disease (CD) and Ulcerative colitis (UC) patients. The size of the dots represents the number of patients per datapoint. C. Maximal changes in number of positive markers. Scatter plots comparing the number of positive markers of the first sample and the sample with the maximal changes in quartile sum score during follow-up in Crohn's disease (CD) and Ulcerative colitis (UC) patients. The size of the dots represents the number of patients per datapoint. D. Stability in antibody status over time. First sample compared to sample with with the maximal changes in quartile sum score during follow-up in Crohn's disease (CD) and Ulcerative colitis (UC) patients. Values are presented as N (%) for changes in marker status. gASCA: anti-*Saccharomyces cerevisiae* antibodies, ACCA: anti-chitobioside carbohydrate IgA antibodies, ALCA: anti-laminaribioside carbohydrate IgG antibodies, AMCA: anti-mannobioside carbohydrate IgG antibodies, Anti-L: anti-laminarin carbohydrate antibody, Anti-C: anti-chitin carbohydrate antibody; pos.: positive, neg.: negative; *Anti-L and Anti-C were not available in all patients.

QSS for CD; **Figure S1** showing the levels of the individual markers in CD patients). To describe the magnitude of level changes in CD patients we first divided the QSS into four equal sections, assigned the CD subjects to a respective section and identified patients with changes of their QSS section over time (color coded in **Figure 1A**). Between 47.1% and 79% of the CD patients per section (versus 0% to 50% of the UC subjects; **Figure 1A**) changed their QSS section at least once during follow-up.

We next categorized the *average* fluctuation per individual patient by calculating the Z-scores (level changes in standard deviations (SD) from the per-patient mean) for all patients and samples. When taking into account the average Z-scores per patient, which includes all observed marker changes, we found while the absolute changes of the marker levels are more pronounced in CD versus UC the relative changes are comparable, which is true for the QSS and the levels of all single markers (**Table S1**).

To classify the *maximal* extent of level changes in individual CD patients over time we identified the samples with the maximal change in QSS (increase or decrease) compared to the first available sample per individual CD patient during follow-up. In other words we identified the two samples per individual patient with the maximal changes in serologic immune response to the tested glycan epitopes. The comparison of the first sample and the sample with the maximal QSS changes during follow-up can be seen in **Figure 1B**. We also assessed the *maximal* level changes for each individual antibody (**Table 2; Figure S2**). This further corroborated the finding of marked fluctuations in the overall immune response in a subgroup of CD patients. In CD patients the maximal Z-score per patient was 0.91 (SD 0.38) (versus UC 0.76 (SD 0.36)) again indicating that the relative level changes are comparable between CD and UC.

Taken together we show that on average across the whole CD cohort individual marker levels are rather stable, with however certain patients exhibiting stronger *average* and *maximal* fluctua-

tions. The relative level changes are comparable in CD versus UC, with stronger absolute changes in CD.

Status changes in Crohn's disease. A different way to assess stability in serologic markers is to use a dichotomic categorization - positive or negative for a respective antibody or if investigating a panel the number of positive markers. We therefore tested how often the levels of the single markers cross the respective cut-off values over time, changing their status from positive to negative or vice versa. In CD subjects in a median of 3.3% of the visits (IQR 0.0–11.1; minimum (min.) 0, maximum (max.) 50) any of the marker status changed compared to the previous consultation (versus UC with a median of 0% of the visits (IQR 0; min. 0, max. 16.7).

Considering the two samples per individual patient with the *maximal* changes in immune response during follow-up we next characterized the longitudinal CD patient samples for stability in marker status (positive versus negative for a respective antibody). We found a strikingly stable antibody status for both the total number of positive markers over time (**Figure 1C**) as well as for each single antibody (**Figure 1D**) per individual patient. Only between 7.3% (ASCA) and 18.3% (AMCA) of the CD patients changed the antibody status of an individual marker either from positive to negative or from negative to positive. This indicates while marked level changes occur in a subgroup of CD patients the antibody status is largely stable.

Level and status changes in ulcerative colitis. As partly stated above and in contrast to the serum of CD patients the absolute changes in the overall immune response and in the antibody status over time in UC patients were minute (**Table 2; Figure 1; Figure S3**). Only between 0% and 8.7% of the UC patients changed the antibody status of an individual marker during follow-up.

II) Association of level or status changes with clinical phenotypes

After defining the magnitude of level changes over time we aimed to assess clinical and genetic factors that are associated with

Table 2. Changes in antibody levels: First sample compared to sample with maximal change in sum of quartiles.

Marker	CD (N = 207)	UC (N = 46)
Absolute changes in levels, median (EU (P25, P75))		
gASCA	10.7 (4.1, 25.1)	2.8 (1.2, 9.6)
ACCA	14.4 (7.1, 25.8)	9.1 (3.3, 17.0)
AMCA	23.5 (8.8, 41.8)	11.8 (7.9, 21.9)
ALCA	8.5 (3.0, 16.6)	4.5 (1.8, 6.8)
Anti-L	21.5 (9.3, 41.1)	8.9 (5.3, 14.9)
Anti-C	8.0 (3.6, 16.8)	6.3 (3.3, 14.7)
Sum of quartiles	2.0 (1.0, 3.0)	1.0 (1.0, 3.0)
Absolute % changes from baseline (Median (P25, P75))		
gASCA	19.0 (6.1, 33.1)	17.7 (6.8, 35.3)
ACCA	26.7 (14.8, 45.5)	19.5 (7.1, 37.0)
AMCA	31.6 (13.7, 50.1)	21.2 (15.1, 39.0)
ALCA	21.8 (8.5, 39.8)	17.0 (7.7, 31.7)
Anti-L	26.7 (12.0, 57.2)	18.3 (12.3, 29.4)
Anti-C	24.5 (11.3, 39.2)	27.6 (13.8, 39.3)
Sum of quartiles	11.1 (5.6, 23.1)	13.8 (7.1, 25.0)

gASCA: anti-*Saccharomyces cerevisiae* antibodies, ACCA: anti-chitobioside carbohydrate IgA antibodies, ALCA: anti-laminaribioside carbohydrate IgG antibodies, AMCA: anti-mannobioside carbohydrate IgG antibodies, Anti-L: anti-laminarin carbohydrate antibody, Anti-C: anti-chitin carbohydrate antibody.
CD: Crohn's disease; UC: Ulcerative colitis; EU: ELISA units; P25, P75: 25th and 75th percentiles.

stronger versus weaker fluctuations in the serologic markers. This information is critical for identifying the subgroup of patients prone to more pronounced changes in their antibody levels during the disease course. As the absolute antibody levels and status in UC patients were highly stable over time we continued our analysis with the CD cohort only. At time of first sample procurement neither disease activity nor an elevated CRP were linked to increased or decreased QSS or levels or status of single markers.

We first tested the *average* fluctuation per individual patient using all samples over time. For this purpose a Z-score was calculated for each visit, averaged and associated with the above clinical phenotypes or NOD genotypes (**Tables S2 & S3**). We corrected for follow-up time and used a level of significance of p<0.01 to account for multiple testing. No phenotype or NOD2 genotype was associated with a higher magnitude of *average* fluctuations in the marker levels. The maximal difference in Z-score between the groups was 0.06 SD and cannot be considered clinically relevant.

To identify factors associated with *maximal* level fluctuations we divided our CD patients in two different groups based on the magnitude of *maximal* level changes in individual patients over time: "Non-level changers" (stable QSS over time, remaining within 0.5 standard deviations (SD) of the QSS in the initial sample) and "Any level changers" (increase or decrease >0.5 SD in QSS at any time during follow-up). These two groups were analyzed for association with certain clinical disease phenotypes and NOD2 genotypes (**Table S4**). To control for multiple testing we used a significance level of p<0.01 and the results were adjusted for follow-up time. We did not find any association between the magnitude of *maximal* level fluctuation in our cohort and any of the pheno- or NOD2 genotypes. We performed this analysis with considering only CD-patients with a minimal observation period of 12 months. Also here no association of pheno- or genotypes with fluctuations was found (data not shown).

The antibody levels in the first sample did not predict the degree of fluctuation of the markers at later time points in the disease course as revealed by a logistic regression analysis (data not shown). In other words the same degree of maximal level changes occurred in subjects during follow-up that had high, middle or low levels in the first sample. We additionally separated our cohort into two groups according to changes in marker status: "Non-status changers" (patients that did not change the number of positive markers during follow-up) and "Status changers" (patients that became positive or negative for one or more additional markers during follow-up). The distribution of subjects can be found in **Table S5**. We also assessed the groups for association with certain clinical disease phenotypes and NOD2 genotypes (**Table S6**). We accounted for multiple testing by using a significance level of p<0.01 and adjusted for follow-up time. No association of pheno- or genotypes with fluctuations was found, when considering the whole cohort but also when separately analyzing only CD patients with a minimum follow-up of 12 months (data not shown).

In summary, despite considering a broad range of clinical phenotypes and NOD2 genotypes no associations with *average* or *maximal* changes in marker levels and status over time could be found.

III) Level changes in individual patients over time – a longitudinal analysis

Even though a certain clinical phenotype or NOD2 genotype was not associated with stronger fluctuations *per se*, it is well likely that changes in CD behavior or treatment can lead to changes in the levels of the antibody markers over time. We therefore longitudinally analyzed our CD cohort for potential level changes

inflicted by clinical situations, namely the first occurrence of complicated CD-behavior, the first occurrence of CD-related surgery, the use of immunosuppressive medication or the onset of active disease. For this purpose repeated measures analysis was done using an unstructured covariance matrix to model within-subject correlation. The occurrence of first time complicated CD-behavior, first time CD-related surgery, active disease or the start of immunosuppressive medication did not influence the overall immune response or the levels of the individual markers. Pre-event antibody levels were not significantly different to post-event levels taking into consideration the above parameters (**Table 3** and **Figure 2** for the QSS; **Table S7** for the single markers). When looking at the use of corticosteroids separately we found a trend towards a decrease in the QSS (data not shown). Interestingly, overall the QSS mildly increased over time from diagnosis (0.13 points each year), which was due to a level increase in the IgA marker ACCA with a trend to increased levels for Anti-L and Anti-C (**Table 3**). This indicates a good model fit as this is a known phenomenon for antibodies of the IgA class.

IV) Clinical situations over time – a longitudinal analysis

The most important factor for the performance of the marker panel is, if the accuracy in clinical situations remains unchanged over time. We therefore tested, if the observed fluctuations in marker levels and status alter the capability of the glycan marker panel to differentiate between CD versus UC and their association with CD phenotypes. We used serum of the CD patients where at least four different samples were available during follow-up (n = 75). The expression of the glycan markers, the clinical phenotype and the overall immune response in this subpopulation was comparable to the total CD cohort (n = 207), indicating that no selection bias was present.

We assessed changes in the ability of the markers to differentiate CD *versus* UC (**Table 4**). We did not observe any significant changes in discriminatory capacity of the markers over time. We next investigated potential changes in association with CD phenotypes. 87.7% of the CD patients with at least four available samples already had a complication before sample procurement at first sample procurement, a proportion that increased to 90.8% (2nd sample), and 93.3% (3rd and 4th sample) during follow-up. 85% of the CD patients already underwent surgery once at time of first sample, which increased during follow-up to 90% for the other three time points. Also here an overall stable association pattern between the markers and clinical phenotypes was found. Independent of the time of sample procurement over the follow-up period the overall immune response, as depicted by the sum of

Table 3. Longitudinal analysis of level changes inflicted by clinical situations.

Factor	Sum of quartiles	
	Parameter Estimate (SE)	p-value
Months since diagnosis	0.011 (0.003)	*0.002*
Change in disease activity	−0.347 (0.443)	0.43
First occurrence of complicated CD behavior	0.021 (0.408)	0.96
First occurrence of CD-related surgery	−0.654 (0.999)	0.51
Use of immunosuppressants	0.410 (0.871)	0.64

SE: Standard error; CD: Crohn's disease.

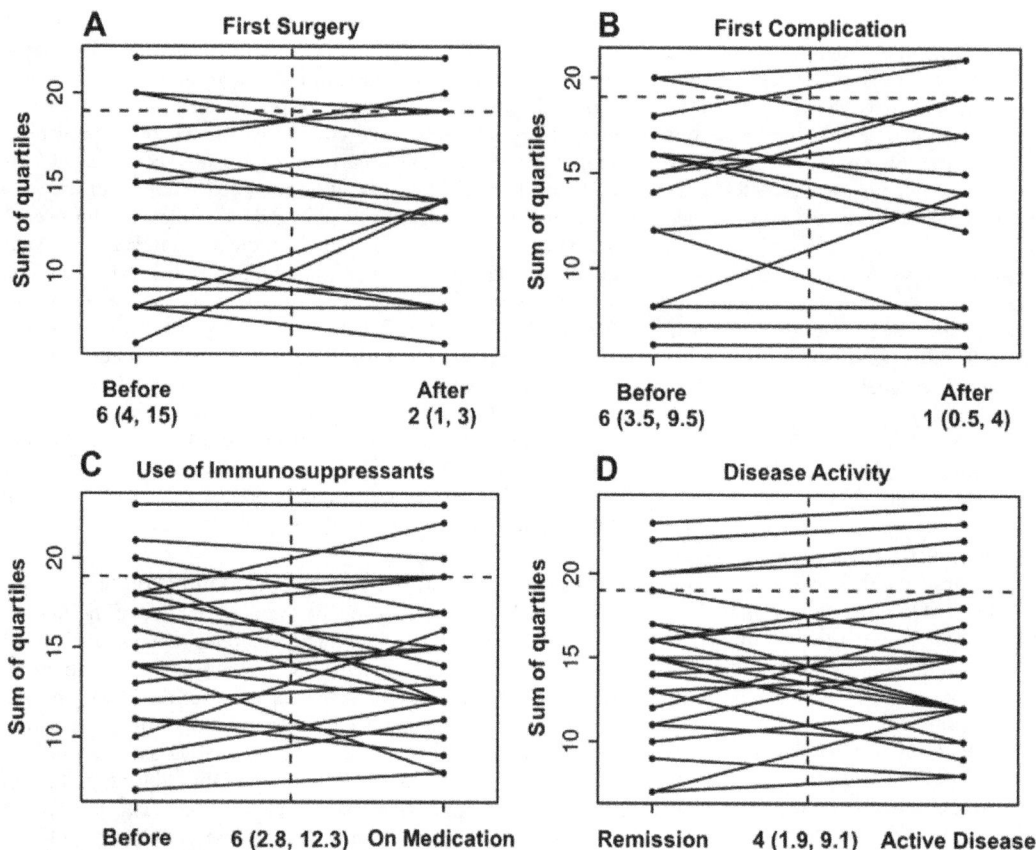

Figure 2. Change in the serum immune response in relation to clinical events. Change in antibody levels (quartile sum score) with (A) the first occurrence of Crohn's disease (CD)-related surgery (n = 17), (B) complications (fistulae or strictures; n = 16), (C) new intake of immunsuppressive medication (depicted is a random set of 25 patients out of total n = 152) or (D) onset of active disease (depicted is a random set of 25 patients out of total n = 124). Numbers relate to months before or after the event for A & B and months between the two samples for C & D (interquartile range (IQR)).

quartiles or the number of positive markers remained to be associated with ileal involvement, complicated CD behavior or CD-related surgery (**Table 5; Table S8** for all single markers).

Discussion

There is a growing interest in the use of anti-glycan antibodies as markers for differentiation and stratification of CD. Previous reports, including ours [7,8,9,10,11,13], suggest a potential use of these markers for discrimination between CD and UC as well as prediction of complicated CD behavior and CD-related surgery. Most information, however, is derived from cross-sectional studies [7,8,9,11,13], which should be interpreted with caution, because crucial information is missing about the stability of marker levels and status over time in individual patients, an open question we specifically addressed in our investigation.

We detected marked changes in the overall immune response (QSS) and levels of individual markers in a subgroup of CD subjects over time. The marker status (positive versus negative) remained widely stable. None of our tested clinical phenotypes or NOD2 genotypes was associated with stronger *average* or *maximal* changes in marker levels. In a longitudinal analysis with individual patients over time neither changes in disease activity, CD behavior or surgery, nor the intake of immunosuppressive medication led to changes in the QSS. The ability of the panel to discriminate CD *versus* UC or its association with CD location, behavior or surgery

remained stable during the follow-up time. In UC neither significant absolute level nor status changes were observed.

Incomplete and limited information is available on fluctuations in level and status of serum antibodies directed against microbial components and associated with CD over time. Most data derived from *cross-sectional single point studies* are controversial: In 32% of apparently healthy recruits of the Israeli Defence Forces, who were later diagnosed as having CD, levels of ASCA increased closer to the date of diagnosis [27]. Once diagnosis of CD was established disease duration did not seem to influence serological responses in several reports, investigating ASCA, OmpC, Anti-I2 and CBir1 [19,21]. In contrast to this, others found significant higher antibody responses against ASCA, AMCA, ACCA and OmpC associated with increased disease duration [7,9]. Oshitani et al. demonstrated lower ASCA titers in CD patients taking mesalazine compared to CD patients not taking mesalazine [17]. In contrary, Ruemmele et al. reported no difference in ASCA positivity with steroid and mesalazine treatment in a pediatric population. A decline in ASCA levels towards normal values had been observed post-surgically in CD [16]. Changes in disease activity did not seem to influence marker levels [9,11].

The information derived from *longitudinal studies* in individual patients over time is even scarcer and meaningful conclusions are difficult to make due to limited follow-up times or low patient numbers. Dotan et al. followed the serum levels of the glycan-markers anti-alpha-Rha, anti-alpha-GlcNAc and anti-cellotriose

Table 4. Validity of markers for differentiation of CD versus UC over time in individual patients.

Antibody	Sensitivity (%)	Specificity (%)	PPV (%)	NPV (%)
1st Sample				
gASCA	69.3	91.3	92.9	64.6
ACCA	24	91.3	81.8	42.4
AMCA	29.3	93.5	88	44.8
ALCA	34.7	95.7	92.9	47.3
Anti-L	28.4	93	87.5	43
Anti-C	36.5	88.4	84.4	44.7
2nd Sample				
gASCA	69.3	91.3	92.9	64.6
ACCA	17.3	91.3	76.5	40.4
AMCA	24	93.5	85.7	43
ALCA	29.3	95.7	91.7	45.4
Anti-L	28.4	93	87.5	43
Anti-C	25.7	88.4	79.2	40.9
3rd Sample				
gASCA	69.3	91.3	92.9	64.6
ACCA	18.7	91.3	77.8	40.8
AMCA	21.3	93.5	84.2	42.2
ALCA	33.3	95.7	92.6	46.8
Anti-L	33.3	93	89.3	44.4
Anti-C	20	88.4	75	38.8
4th Sample				
gASCA	70.7	91.3	93	65.6
ACCA	10.7	91.3	66.7	38.5
AMCA	17.3	93.5	81.3	41
ALCA	30.7	95.7	92	45.8
Anti-L	31.1	93	88.5	44
Anti-C	31.1	88.4	82.1	42.7

Includes 75 CD subjects with at least four samples per individual patient versus all 46 UC subjects.
PPV: positive predictive value, NPV: negative predictive value.
gASCA: anti-*Saccharomyces cerevisiae* antibodies, ACCA: anti-chitobioside carbohydrate IgA antibodies, ALCA: anti-laminaribioside carbohydrate IgG antibodies, AMCA: anti-mannobioside carbohydrate IgG antibodies, Anti-L: anti-laminarin carbohydrate antibody, Anti-C: anti-chitin carbohydrate antibody.

antibodies in seven healthy volunteers during the course of 13 weeks and found widely stable levels over time [28]. In a pediatric cohort (n = 61) with a mean follow-up time of 4.9 years and up to seven measurements during the CD course only 21 to 29.5% of the subjects changed ASCA status over time. Even though individual patients showed marked changes in titers the average levels across the total population showed little variability during follow-up [23].

Disease activity or relapse does not appear to influence marker levels in longitudinal studies [23,29]. ASCA was stable over time in relation to changes in CDAI, monitoring 26 CD patients before and after infliximab therapy for a median interval of 6.1 months [19]. Among patients who achieved complete remission through treatment with infliximab as evidenced by mucosal changes and healing, stability in anti-CBir1 expression was seen (n = 14) [21]. ASCA titers in CD patients taking mesalazine *versus* placebo for prophylaxis of postoperative relapse (n = 38) remained stable over

time [20]. However, ASCA levels decreased after two weeks of corticosteroid treatment (n = 25, follow-up 9 weeks) [20]. A decrease in ASCA levels after intestinal surgery with a later rise to preoperative levels within a few months was noted (n = 60) [22]. In contrast no significant changes in serological responses toward ASCA, Anti-I2 and Omp-C after small bowel surgery (n = 61 and 26) with or without fecal diversion (n = 14) was found [14,23,24].

Our study describes the dynamic change of anti-glycan antibodies in the to date largest cohort of CD patients with multiple samples collected during the disease course and scrutinizes detailed clinical information for each time point of sample procurement. Comparable studies but of smaller size have so far only been reported for ASCA [14,22,23].

We established that during the disease course significant fluctuations in marker levels occur in a subgroup of CD patients. The marker status, however, remained strikingly stable. Considering all markers a change in status occurred in only 3.3% of the visits per antibody. In an attempt to identify specific clinical phenotypes or genotypes that are associated with stronger level or status changes we included a wide range of phenotypes into our statistical analysis. Interestingly none of the clinical phenotypes was associated with level or status changes in antibodies over time. The immune response tended to decrease with intake of corticosteroids. This is in concordance with a previous report [20], but the effect was not noted when all immunosuppressive medications (including corticosteroids, azathioprine and methotrexate) were considered in the model. None of our patients received infliximab during the observation period.

The fact that our association analysis for disease phenotypes confirms the previously reported results from our larger cohort [11] underlines the appropriate power of our study to detect potential changes in marker levels and status, if they were present. In addition our longitudinal analysis detected a mild increase in the levels of the glycan IgA markers over time indicating a good model fit, because a rise in the serum titers of IgA antibodies over time is a known physiologic phenomenon. We see two possible explanations for our lack of association of phenotypes/phenotype changes with fluctuations: A clinical phenotype or genotype not considered in our model might lead to the observed changes. Alternatively our observation may reflect the natural fluctuation of the markers/immune response over time. This is supported by the finding of comparable results in *relative* changes of the marker levels (**Table 2**) with essentially identical Z-scores between CD and UC. UC is not associated with higher levels of anti glycan antibodies and, therefore, the absolute fluctuations are minute and not clinically relevant. The onset of level changes inflicted by clinical situation might be delayed, e.g. an increase in serologic glycan marker levels might lag behind an increase in disease activity and therefore would not be detected in our longitudinal analysis.

Determination of glycan markers in clinical practice may allow the differentiation between UC and CD, which could impact the type of therapy chosen for the respective disease. In addition, the ability to predict the progression from non-complicated to complicated disease and/or surgery with serum markers may classify patients into at-risk populations and influence the therapeutic management of patients with the goal of preventing the development of complications. One prerequisite for routine use is the stability of markers over time. The most important finding of our study is that despite the observed changes in the QSS the potency of the markers in clinical situations, namely discrimination between UC versus CD and association with CD phenotypes remained stable over time. Given the marker status stability over time in our study, association of marker positivity with CD and certain disease phenotypes are likely to be suitable as

Table 5. Validity of markers for association with disease phenotypes over time in individual patients.

Factor	Ileum Involvement (N = 67)	No Ileum Involvement (N = 8)	p-value	Complication (N = 65)	No Complication (N = 10)	p-value	Surgery (N = 60)	No Surgery (N = 15)	p-value
1st Sample									
Sum of quartiles	16.0 (13.5, 19.5)	10.0 (8.0, 14.0)	<*0.001*	17.0 (13.0, 20.0)	10.0 (8.0, 14.0)	<*0.001*	17.5 (14.0, 21.0)	14.0 (10.0, 16.0)	*0.003*
Number of positive markers	2.0 (1.0, 3.0)	0.0 (0.0, 1.0)	<*0.001*	2.0 (1.0, 4.0)	0.0 (0.0, 1.0)	<*0.001*	2.0 (1.0, 4.0)	1.0 (0.0, 2.0)	*0.002*
2nd Sample									
Sum of quartiles	15.5 (12.0, 19.0)	10.0 (8.0, 14.0)	<*0.001*	16.0 (12.0, 19.0)	10.0 (8.0, 13.0)	<*0.001*	16.5 (13.0, 19.5)	12.0 (12.0, 15.0)	*0.004*
Number of positive markers	2.0 (1.0, 3.0)	0.0 (0.0, 1.0)	<*0.001*	2.0 (1.0, 3.0)	0.0 (0.0, 1.0)	<*0.001*	2.0 (1.0, 3.0)	1.0 (0.0, 2.0)	*0.003*
3rd Sample									
Sum of quartiles	15.0 (12.0, 19.0)	10.0 (8.0, 14.0)	<*0.001*	15.0 (12.0, 19.0)	9.0 (7.0, 13.0)	<*0.001*	16.5 (13.0, 19.0)	11.0 (8.0, 15.0)	*0.004*
Number of positive markers	2.0 (1.0, 3.0)	0.0 (0.0, 1.0)	<*0.001*	2.0 (1.0, 3.0)	0.0 (0.0, 1.0)	<*0.001*	2.0 (1.0, 3.0)	1.0 (0.0, 2.0)	*0.006*
4th Sample									
Sum of quartiles	15.0 (12.0, 19.0)	10.0 (8.0, 14.0)	<*0.001*	15.0 (12.0, 19.0)	10.0 (8.0, 14.0)	<*0.001*	15.0 (13.0, 20.0)	13.0 (10.0, 16.0)	*0.02*
Number of positive markers	2.0 (1.0, 3.0)	0.0 (0.0, 1.0)	<*0.001*	2.0 (1.0, 3.0)	0.0 (0.0, 1.0)	<*0.001*	2.0 (1.0, 3.0)	1.0 (0.0, 2.0)	*0.025*

Includes 75 CD subjects with at least four samples per individual patient.
Sum of quartiles: Values presented are median (25th percentile, 75th percentile) and P-values correspond to Wilcoxon rank sum tests.
Antibody positivity: Values presented are N (%) and P-values correspond to Fisher's Exact test (F) and Pearson's chi-square tests otherwise.
Complication: fistula or stenosis.

a tool for differentiation and prediction of disease courses, independent of the time of sample procurement. Therefore, serial measurements of antibodies may not provide additional information for the evaluation of CD when considering the status of the markers. On the other hand the marked fluctuations in the QSS in a subgroup of CD patients suggests caution when using the overall immune response for the aforementioned clinical situations, namely diagnosis, differential diagnosis and disease stratification.

The strength of our study is its originality by being the first study investigating fluctuations in anti-glycan antibodies, the prospective follow-up design, blinded data abstraction, availability of up to 11 samples per patient and a longitudinal analysis paired with detailed clinical information. However, certain limitations apply: One has to keep in mind that our cohort is from a single university hospital, introducing possible referral bias. The first serum sample per patient was not in all cases taken close to diagnosis, which we corrected for in our statistical models. The follow-up samples were taken at arbitrary visits to our hospital and not in a fixed relation to certain events such as complications or surgery, information that was retrospectively added. Using this method, patients with a more severe disease course could be selected out, as only they have to come to a referral center for multiple treatments. The length of time in which immunosuppressive medication was taken by the patients before sample procurement is unknown to the authors, which is a limitation for our longitudinal model. We are aware of the potential presence of a subclinical complication at the time of sample procurement. One has to consider that this study does not aim at prediction of complicated CD courses with serology, but rather evaluates the fluctuations of the glycan markers longitudinally to assess, if and how already published cross sectional studies can be used for disease prediction. Even though this is the largest study of its kind ever reported, the overall number of patients is limited. A larger cohort would enable a more detailed analysis with respect to determinants of level changes.

In summary, our study indicates that anti-glycan antibody levels are changing in patients with CD whereas the status of the markers is stable over time. The observed fluctuations might be due to not yet identified clinical factors or genotypes or could represent natural changes in levels over time. Considering the follow-up time of our study we cannot recommend serial measurements, when considering the marker status and claim to use the overall immune response (QSS) with caution for disease stratification, due to strong fluctuations in a subgroup of CD subjects.

Supporting Information

Figure S1   Changes in the level of single markers over time. Profile plots for changes in the levels of single markers in individual Crohn's disease (CD) patients over time. The broken line represents the cut-off value for each individual marker. The red lines indicate patients starting above the cut-off value and the green lines indicate subjects starting below the cut-off values. Depicted is a random set of 50 subjects per graph. gASCA: anti-*Saccharomyces cerevisiae* antibodies, ACCA: anti-chitobioside carbohydrate IgA antibodies, ALCA: anti-laminaribioside carbohydrate IgG antibodies, AMCA: anti-mannobioside carbohydrate IgG antibodies, Anti-L: anti-laminarin carbohydrate antibody, Anti-C: anti-chitin carbohydrate antibody.

Figure S2   Maximal changes in levels of single markers in Crohn's disease. Scatter plot comparing the level of the first sample and the sample with the maximal changes in quartile sum score during follow-up for each individual marker in Crohn's disease (CD) patients. One dot represents one patient. gASCA: anti-*Saccharomyces cerevisiae* antibodies, ACCA: anti-chitobioside carbohydrate IgA antibodies, ALCA: anti-laminaribioside carbohydrate IgG antibodies, AMCA: anti-mannobioside carbohydrate

IgG antibodies, Anti-L: anti-laminarin carbohydrate antibody, Anti-C: anti-chitin carbohydrate antibody.

Figure S3 Maximal changes in levels of single markers in Ulcerative colitis. Scatter plot comparing the level of the first sample and the sample with the maximal changes in quartile sum score during follow-up for each individual marker in Ulcerative colitis (UC) subjects. One dot represents one patient. gASCA: anti-*Saccharomyces cerevisiae* antibodies, ACCA: anti-chitobioside carbohydrate IgA antibodies, ALCA: anti-laminaribioside carbohydrate IgG antibodies, AMCA: anti-mannobioside carbohydrate IgG antibodies, Anti-L: anti-laminarin carbohydrate antibody, Anti-C: anti-chitin carbohydrate antibody.

Table S1 Average of absolute standard deviations around the mean (Z-score).

Table S2 Average of absolute standard deviations around the mean (Z-score) and association with disease pheno- and NOD2 genotypes.

Table S3 Correlation coefficients of the Z-score with disease parameters.

Table S4 Association of clinical phenotypes and genotypes with maximal level changes.

Table S5 Number and distribution of CD subjects with antibody status changes.

Table S6 Assosiation of clinical phenotypes and genotypes with status changes.

Table S7 Longitudinal analysis of level changes inflicted by clinical situations.

Table S8 Validity of markers for association with disease phenotypes over time in individual patients.

Acknowledgments

We would like to thank the study nurses and physicians of the Department of Internal Medicine I and the Inflammatory Bowel Disease Research Group for their contribution to this work. This work is part of the medical thesis of Stephan Schleder, Alexandra Wolf and Florian Kamm.

Author Contributions

Conceived and designed the experiments: FR RL AF AW S. Schleder AD AS PR ND S. Schreiber GR FK. Performed the experiments: FR RL AF AW S. Schleder AD AS PR ND S. Schreiber GR FK. Analyzed the data: FR RL AF AW S. Schleder AD AS PR ND S. Schreiber GR FK. Contributed reagents/materials/analysis tools: FR RL AF AW S. Schleder AD AS PR ND S. Schreiber GR FK. Wrote the paper: FR RL AF AW S. Schleder AD AS PR ND S. Schreiber GR FK.

References

1. Stange EF, Travis SP, Vermeire S, Beglinger C, Kupcinkas L, et al. (2006) European evidence based consensus on the diagnosis and management of Crohn's disease: definitions and diagnosis. Gut 55 Suppl 1: i1–15.
2. Louis E, Collard A, Oger AF, Degroote E, Aboul Nasr El Yafi FA, et al. (2001) Behaviour of Crohn's disease according to the Vienna classification: changing pattern over the course of the disease. Gut 49: 777–782.
3. Farmer RG, Whelan G, Fazio VW (1985) Long-term follow-up of patients with Crohn's disease. Relationship between the clinical pattern and prognosis. Gastroenterology 88: 1818–1825.
4. Andres PG, Friedman LS (1999) Epidemiology and the natural course of inflammatory bowel disease. Gastroenterol Clin North Am 28: 255–281.
5. Devlin SM, Dubinsky MC (2008) Determination of serologic and genetic markers aid in the determination of the clinical course and severity of patients with IBD. Inflamm Bowel Dis 14: 125–128.
6. Targan SR (1999) The utility of ANCA and ASCA in inflammatory bowel disease. Inflamm Bowel Dis 5: 61–63.
7. Ferrante M, Henckaerts L, Joossens M, Pierik M, Joossens S, et al. (2007) New serological markers in inflammatory bowel disease are associated with complicated disease behaviour. Gut 56: 1394–1403.
8. Dotan I, Fishman S, Dgani Y, Schwartz M, Karban A, et al. (2006) Antibodies against laminaribioside and chitobioside are novel serologic markers in Crohn's disease. Gastroenterology 131: 366–378.
9. Papp M, Altorjay I, Dotan N, Palatka K, Foldi I, et al. (2008) New serological markers for inflammatory bowel disease are associated with earlier age at onset, complicated disease behavior, risk for surgery, and NOD2/CARD15 genotype in a Hungarian IBD cohort. Am J Gastroenterol 104: 1426–1434.
10. Rieder F, Schleder S, Wolf A, Dirmeier A, Strauch U, et al. (2010) Serum anti-glycan antibodies predict complicated Crohn's disease behavior: a cohort study. Inflamm Bowel Dis 16: 1367–1375.
11. Rieder F, Schleder S, Wolf A, Dirmeier A, Strauch U, et al. (2010) Association of the novel serologic anti-glycan antibodies anti-laminarin and anti-chitin with complicated Crohn's disease behavior. Inflamm Bowel Dis 16: 263–274.
12. Simondi D, Mengozzi G, Betteto S, Bonardi R, Ghignone RP, et al. (2008) Antiglycan antibodies as serological markers in the differential diagnosis of inflammatory bowel disease. Inflamm Bowel Dis 14: 645–651.
13. Seow CH, Stempak JM, Xu W, Lan H, Griffiths AM, et al. (2009) Novel anti-glycan antibodies related to inflammatory bowel disease diagnosis and phenotype. Am J Gastroenterol 104: 1426–1434.
14. Mow WS, Vasiliauskas EA, Lin YC, Fleshner PR, Papadakis KA, et al. (2004) Association of antibody responses to microbial antigens and complications of small bowel Crohn's disease. Gastroenterology 126: 414–424.
15. Dubinsky MC, Kugathasan S, Mei L, Picornell Y, Nebel J, et al. (2008) Increased Immune Reactivity Predicts Aggressive Complicating Crohn's Disease in Children. Clin Gastroenterol Hepatol 10: 1105–1111.
16. Ruemmele FM, Targan SR, Levy G, Dubinsky M, Braun J, et al. (1998) Diagnostic accuracy of serological assays in pediatric inflammatory bowel disease. Gastroenterology 115: 822–829.
17. Oshitani N, Hato F, Matsumoto T, Jinno Y, Sawa Y, et al. (2000) Decreased anti-Saccharomyces cerevisiae antibody titer by mesalazine in patients with Crohn's disease. J Gastroenterol Hepatol 15: 1400–1403.
18. Arnott ID, Landers CJ, Nimmo EJ, Drummond HE, Smith BK, et al. (2004) Sero-reactivity to microbial components in Crohn's disease is associated with disease severity and progression, but not NOD2/CARD15 genotype. Am J Gastroenterol 99: 2376–2384.
19. Landers CJ, Cohavy O, Misra R, Yang H, Lin YC, et al. (2002) Selected loss of tolerance evidenced by Crohn's disease-associated immune responses to auto- and microbial antigens. Gastroenterology 123: 689–699.
20. Teml A, Kratzer V, Schneider B, Lochs H, Norman GL, et al. (2003) Anti-Saccharomyces cerevisiae antibodies: a stable marker for Crohn's disease during steroid and 5-aminosalicylic acid treatment. Am J Gastroenterol 98: 2226–2231.
21. Targan SR, Landers CJ, Yang H, Lodes MJ, Cong Y, et al. (2005) Antibodies to CBir1 flagellin define a unique response that is associated independently with complicated Crohn's disease. Gastroenterology 128: 2020–2028.
22. Eser A, Papay P, Miehsler W, Dejaco C, Gangl A, et al. (2009) Impact of Intestinal Resection On and Prognostic Value of Anti-Saccharomyces Cerevisiae Serology in Patients with Crohn's Disease During Long-Term Follow-Up Gastroenterology 136: A-188.
23. Desir B, Amre DK, Lu SE, Ohman-Strickland P, Dubinsky M, et al. (2004) Utility of serum antibodies in determining clinical course in pediatric Crohn's disease. Clin Gastroenterol Hepatol 2: 139–146.
24. Spivak J, Landers CJ, Vasiliauskas EA, Abreu MT, Dubinsky MC, et al. (2006) Antibodies to I2 predict clinical response to fecal diversion in Crohn's disease. Inflamm Bowel Dis 12: 1122–1130.
25. Stange EF, Travis SP, Vermeire S, Reinisch W, Geboes K, et al. (2008) European evidence-based Consensus on the diagnosis and management of ulcerative colitis: Definitions and diagnosis. Journal of Crohn's and Colitis 2: 1–23.
26. Teuber M, Koch A, Manaster C, Wachter S, Hampe J, et al. (2005) Improving quality control and workflow management in high-throughput single-nucleotide polymorphism genotyping environments Journal of the Association for Laboratory Automation 2005: 43–47.
27. Israeli E, Grotto I, Gilburd B, Balicer RD, Goldin E, et al. (2005) Anti-Saccharomyces cerevisiae and antineutrophil cytoplasmic antibodies as predictors of inflammatory bowel disease. Gut 54: 1232–1236.

6

CD40: Novel Association with Crohn's Disease and Replication in Multiple Sclerosis Susceptibility

Fiona Blanco-Kelly[1][9], Fuencisla Matesanz[2,12][9], Antonio Alcina[2,12], María Teruel[2], Lina M. Díaz-Gallo[2], María Gómez-García[3], Miguel A. López-Nevot[4], Luis Rodrigo[5], Antonio Nieto[6], Carlos Cardeña[7], Guillermo Alcain[8], Manuel Díaz-Rubio[9], Emilio G. de la Concha[1,12], Oscar Fernandez[10,12], Rafael Arroyo[11,12], Javier Martín[2][9], Elena Urcelay[1,12*][9]

1 Department of Clinical Immunology, Hospital Clínico San Carlos, Madrid, Spain, 2 Instituto Parasitología y Biomedicina "López Neyra", C. S. I. C., Granada, Spain, 3 Servicio de Digestivo, Hospital Universitario Virgen de las Nieves, Granada, Spain, 4 Servicio de Inmunología, Hospital Universitario Virgen de las Nieves, Granada, Spain, 5 Servicio de Digestivo, Hospital Universitario Central de Asturias, Oviedo, Spain, 6 Servicio de Inmunología, Hospital Puerta del Mar, Cádiz, Spain, 7 Servicio de Digestivo, Hospital Clínico San Cecilio, Granada, Spain, 8 Servicio de Digestivo, Hospital Virgen de la Victoria, Málaga, Spain, 9 Digestive Department, Hospital Clínico San Carlos, Madrid, Spain, 10 Servicio de Neurología, Instituto de Neurociencias Clínicas, Hospital Carlos Haya, Málaga, Spain, 11 Multiple Sclerosis Unit, Neurology Department, Hospital Clínico San Carlos, Madrid, Spain, 12 Members of the Red Española de Esclerosis Múltiple (REEM), www.reem.es

Abstract

Background: A functional polymorphism located at −1 from the start codon of the *CD40* gene, rs1883832, was previously reported to disrupt a Kozak sequence essential for translation. It has been consistently associated with Graves' disease risk in populations of different ethnicity and genetic proxies of this variant evaluated in genome-wide association studies have shown evidence of an effect in rheumatoid arthritis and multiple sclerosis (MS) susceptibility. However, the protective allele associated with Graves' disease or rheumatoid arthritis has shown a risk role in MS, an effect that we aimed to replicate in the present work. We hypothesized that this functional polymorphism might also show an association with other complex autoimmune condition such as inflammatory bowel disease, given the CD40 overexpression previously observed in Crohn's disease (CD) lesions.

Methodology: Genotyping of rs1883832C>T was performed in 1564 MS, 1102 CD and 969 ulcerative colitis (UC) Spanish patients and in 2948 ethnically matched controls by TaqMan chemistry.

Principal Findings: The observed effect of the minor allele rs1883832T was replicated in our independent Spanish MS cohort [p=0.025; OR (95% CI)=1.12 (1.01–1.23)]. The frequency of the minor allele was also significantly higher in CD patients than in controls [p=0.002; OR (95% CI)=1.19 (1.06–1.33)]. This increased predisposition was not detected in UC patients [p=0.5; OR (95% CI)=1.04 (0.93–1.17)].

Conclusion: The impact of *CD40* rs1883832 on MS and CD risk points to a common signaling shared by these autoimmune conditions.

Editor: Francesc Palau, Instituto de Biomedicina de Valencia, CSIC, Spain

Funding: Elena Urcelay works for the "Fundación para la Investigación Biomédica-Hospital Clínico San Carlos". This work was supported by grants from: "Fundación Mutua Madrileña", "Fundación Ramón Areces", Junta de Andalucía-Feder P07-CVI-02551, Instituto de Salud Carlos III-Fondo Europeo de Desarrollo Regional (Feder) (PI081636, PI081676, PI070353 and RETICS-REEM RD07/0060) and Ministerio de Ciencia e Innovación-Feder (SAF2009-11491, SAF2006-00398). The funders had no role in study design, data collection and analysis, decision to publish, or preparation of the manuscript.

Competing Interests: The authors have declared that no competing interests exist.

* E-mail: eurcelay.hcsc@salud.madrid.org

[9] These authors contributed equally to this work.

Introduction

In the past three years genome-wide association studies have identified literally hundreds of genetic loci involved in the susceptibility conferred to complex inherited traits. Even though this scenario represents an extraordinary advance in complex disease genetics, the modest effect sizes of the common polymorphisms found associated explain only a small fraction of the heritability in most of these multifactorial conditions, suggesting that many more loci remain to be discovered. One of

the genes encoding a member of the tumor necrosis factor receptor family that plays a key role in adaptive immunity is *CD40* (MIM*109535) [1]. T-cell priming and B-cell activation can occur in the absence of the CD40/CD40-ligand costimulatory signal, but many immune functions are impaired without this interaction, underscoring its importance for an adequate immune response.

Candidate gene studies reported the association of a functional *CD40* polymorphism with Graves' disease; moreover, the association of this variant was replicated in populations of different ethnicity including Caucasians, Koreans, and Japanese [2–4]. This functional polymorphism, rs1883832, is located at -1 from the ATG within a Kozak sequence, a stretch of nucleotides essential for translation that is flanking the start codon in vertebrate genes [5]. The common allele of rs1883832 increased the translational efficiency of CD40 transcripts, resulting in 15–32% more CD40 protein than in the presence of the minor allele [6]. CD40 has been recently associated with rheumatoid arthritis through the meta-analysis of two genome-wide studies conducted in European populations [7]. The common allele frequency of a polymorphism located in the second intron of the CD40 gene, rs4810485 and which was in strong linkage disequilibrium with rs1883832 ($r^2 = 0.95$), was reduced in arthritic patients when compared to healthy controls. The broad functionality of CD40 on immune responses, coupled with its critical role in several experimental autoimmune conditions, such as collagen induced arthritis [8], experimental Graves' disease [9], experimental autoimmune encephalomyelitis (EAE), a model of multiple sclerosis (MS) [10], lupus nephritis [11] and type 1 diabetes [12] suggest its association with other immune-mediated diseases. However, no association has been detected with systemic lupus erythematosus [13] or with type 1 diabetes [14] and, therefore, it would be interesting to ascertain the diseases associated with the CD40 gene.

A recently performed genome-wide association study in MS identified two genetically equivalent polymorphisms ($r^2 = 1$) in the 5′ region of the CD40 gene in strong linkage disequilibrium with rs1883832C>T ($r^2 = 0.95$) [15]. Interestingly, the susceptibility allele described for Graves' disease or rheumatoid arthritis seemed to protect against MS, suggestive of a different molecular mechanism involved in the aetiology of these conditions. Our aim with the present study was to replicate this association with MS and to confirm the protective effect of the common C allele at position -1 of the CD40 gene.

Additionally, we pursued to test the effect of this polymorphism in inflammatory bowel disease. Antibodies blocking CD40 have been reported to dampen the severity of experimental colitis [16] and a CD40 overexpression in Crohn's disease lesions has been known for a decade [17]. Thus, we decided to focus attention on this component of the CD40/CD40-ligand costimulatory pathway and to investigate the association of the functional polymorphism of the CD40 gene in the two main clinical phenotypes of inflammatory bowel disease, Crohn's disease (CD) and ulcerative colitis (UC).

Materials and Methods

Spanish patients (1564 MS, 1102 CD and 969 UC) and 2948 ethnically matched controls, mostly blood donors and staff, were consecutively recruited from the following hospitals: H. Clínico S. Carlos (Madrid), H. Virgen Macarena (Sevilla), H. Carlos Haya

and H. Virgen de la Victoria (Málaga), H. Clínico S. Cecilio and H. Virgen de las Nieves (Granada), H. Puerta del Mar (Cádiz) and the Blood Bank (Granada). MS patients were diagnosed based on the Poser criteria [18] and 37% of patients carried the HLA DRB1*1501 allele. Most patients were relapsing remitting (79%), 19% secondary progressive and 2% primary progressive. Their mean age at MS onset was 30 ± 10 years. Diagnosis of IBD patients was based on standard clinical, radiologic, endoscopic and histologic criteria [19]. Some UC patients suffered from pancolitis (29%), extraintestinal manifestations (44%) or colectomy (27%). CD patients were classified according to the location of the lesions in ileal (L1, 40%), colonic (L2, 19%), ileocolonic (L3, 36%) and upper gastrointestinal tract (L4, 4%) and according to the disease behaviour in inflammatory (B1, 41%), stricturing (B2, 19%) and perforating (B3, 40%). Subjects were included in the study after informed consent. The Ethics Committee of the participant hospitals approved the study.

Genotyping of the samples was carried out with a pre-designed TaqMan Assay from Applied Biosystems in a 7900HT Fast Real-Time PCR system, under the conditions recommended by the manufacturer (Applied Biosystems, Foster City, CA, USA). Genotyping call-rate success was over 96% for all patient groups and controls.

The statistical analysis to compare allelic and genotypic distributions was performed using chi-square test or Fisher's exact test included in a standard statistical package (Epi Info v. 5; World Health Organization, Geneva, Switzerland) which was also used for statistical power calculations. Odds ratios (OR) and their 95% confidence intervals were estimated using the Cornfield method. Linkage disequilibrium was measured by r^2.

Results

Table 1 summarizes genotypic and allelic frequencies of the functional CD40 polymorphism rs1883832 in Spanish patients suffering from multiple sclerosis, Crohn's disease or ulcerative colitis and in ethnically-matched healthy controls. Results conformed to Hardy-Weinberg expectations. As shown, the minor allele frequency and the number of carriers of this minor allele were higher in both MS and CD patients than in controls. This increased susceptibility was not observed in UC patients. Being this result in MS a replication of the original finding, there is no need for correction. The significant result obtained in CD withstands Bonferroni's correction (x4).

No difference was observed in MS, CD and UC patients stratified by the well-known susceptibility factors HLA-DRB1* 1501, NOD2/CARD15 or HLA-DRB1*103, respectively (data not shown).

Table 1. Genotypic and allelic frequencies of the C/T$_{-1}$ polymorphism of the CD40 gene (p and OR values are shown for T allele and carriers of T allele).

rs1883832	MS n	%	CD n	%	UC n	%	Controls n	%	MS vs. controls p value	OR (95% CI)	CD vs. controls p value	OR (95% CI)	UC vs. controls p value	OR (95% CI)
TT	13	9	107	10	66	7	237	8						
TC	7	41	452	42	398	42	1098	38	0.018	1.16 (1.02–1.32)	0.002	1.24 (1.08–1.43)	0.13	1.12 (0.96–1.30)
CC	62	50	527	48	485	51	1562	54						
T	89	29	666	31	530	27	1572	27	0.025	1.12 (1.01–1.23)	0.002	1.19 (1.06–1.33)	0.5	1.04 (0.93–1.17)
C	9	71	1506	69	1368	73	4222	73						

Discussion

The CD40/CD40-ligand pathway is a key component of the pathophysiology of numerous autoimmune disorders [20]. Its contribution to autoimmunity could involve different processes. The physiological relevance of CD40/CD40-ligand in Th17-cell differentiation has been recently proven using a mouse model of experimental autoimmune encephalomyelitis and $Cd40^{-/-}$ mice were found to be protected from the disease [21]. Increased expression of the main cytokine produced by these T cells, IL-17, has been shown in immune and inflammatory diseases including rheumatoid arthritis, multiple sclerosis and inflammatory bowel diseases [22–25]. Moreover, the functional blockade of CD40 with a murine antibody effectively prevents clinical expression in an animal model of multiple sclerosis [26]. Indeed, the preclinical evaluation of a monoclonal antibody against CD40 has shown beneficial activities in an MS model when administered early in the disease development, as well as after the onset of brain inflammation [27]. As mentioned, two of the three most associated polymorphisms identified in a recent genome-wide association study in MS [15] are proxies of the functional polymorphism at −1 of the *CD40* gene. However, the minor allele of this variant that decreases the efficiency of CD40 translation led to an increased susceptibility towards the disease and we decided to replicate this effect of the *CD40* polymorphism in an independent MS cohort. Our present data validate the original finding and corroborate the association of the minor allele of this polymorphism in MS risk. Indeed, Buck *et al.* [28] observed a similar increase in minor allele frequency in patients when compared to controls (33% vs. 29%), although a limited statistical power prevented them from reaching the significance threshold.

Then, we aimed at addressing the influence of the functional polymorphism at −1 of the *CD40* gene in inflammatory bowel disease risk. Our data evidenced a parallel pattern of association of CD and MS, with the minor allele conferring susceptibility to both conditions. No significant effect of this polymorphism was detected in the other main subphenotype of inflammatory bowel diseases, UC, although the size of our collection would allow to detect the effect previously described for the minor allele in MS risk (OR = 1.18) with an 80% power ($\alpha = 0.05$). A pattern of CD susceptibility similar to the one herein described for the polymorphism at −1 in *CD40* was evidenced in the genome-wide study performed in CD by the Wellcome Trust Case Control Consortium

[29], where rs4810485 (proxy of rs1883832, $r^2 = 0.95$) was associated with CD [p=0.009; OR (95%CI)=1.14 (1.03–1.25)]. However, the significance threshold imposed in this type of whole-genome scans hampered the consideration of this signal as a CD susceptibility factor. Interestingly, in this WTCCC study, the minor allele revealed a borderline significant signal of opposite effect in rheumatoid arthritis [p=0.067; OR (95%CI)=0.91 (0.83–1.01)], in agreement with the meta-analysis recently published (OR=0.87, [7]). Therefore, the present data support the consideration of CD40 as a genuine risk factor for CD. Moreover, a significant difference between the allelic frequencies of this polymorphism in CD and UC patients is observed (p=0.027), concordantly with a recent study showing that only half of the known genes associated with CD are shared by UC [30].

As recently published by Zheng J et al. [31], CD8(+) Treg play important roles in the maintenance of immune tolerance. Adoptive transfer of these CD8(+) Treg in rodents or induction of CD8(+) Treg in humans can prevent or treat autoimmune diseases. CD8(+) T cell subsets could be induced from naive CD8(+) precursors in vitro by allogenic CD40-activated B cells. Moreover, the Tregs induced by CD40-B have greater suppressive capacity and are generated in larger numbers than those induced by immature dendritic cells [32]. Provided that the minor allele of the studied *CD40* variant decreases the efficiency of translation, this lower amount of CD40 would then result in a reduced induction of Treg, which would lead to a disruption of immune tolerance. Further research regarding the balance of effector and regulatory T cells will help to ascertain the pleiotropic action of CD40 signalling exerted on several immune-mediated diseases, and provide clues for the successful translation of new therapeutics.

Acknowledgments

The authors thank Carmen Martínez and M. Angel García for their expert technical assistance.

Author Contributions

Conceived and designed the experiments: FM EGdlC JM EU. Performed the experiments: FBK AA MT LMDG. Analyzed the data: FBK FM AA MT LMDG MGG MALN LR AN CC GA MDR OF RA JM EU. Contributed reagents/materials/analysis tools: EGdlC EU. Wrote the paper: EU. Revised a draft of the manuscript: FM JM. Diagnosed patients and collected samples: MGG MALN LR AN CC GA MDR OF RA.

References

1. Elgueta R, Benson MJ, de Vries VC, Wasiuk A, Guo Y, et al. (2009) Molecular mechanism and function of CD40/CD40L engagement in the immune system. In Immunol Rev. pp 152–72.
2. Tomer Y, Concepcion E, Greenberg DA (2002) A C/T single-nucleotide polymorphism in the region of the CD40 gene is associated with Graves' disease. Thyroid 12: 1129–35.
3. Ban Y, Tozaki T, Taniyama M, Tomita M (2006) Association of a C/T single-nucleotide polymorphism in the 5′ untranslated region of the CD40 gene with Graves' disease in Japanese. Thyroid 16: 443–6.
4. Kurylowicz A, Kula D, Ploski R, Skorka A, Jurecka-Lubieniecka B, et al. (2005) Association of CD40 gene polymorphism (C-1T) with susceptibility and phenotype of Graves' disease. Thyroid 15: 1119–24.
5. Kozak M (1987) At least six nucleotides preceding the AUG initiator codon enhance translation in mammalian cells. J Mol Biol 196: 947–50.
6. Jacobson EM, Concepcion E, Oashi T, Tomer Y (2005) A Graves' disease-associated Kozak sequence single-nucleotide polymorphism enhances the efficiency of CD40 gene translation: a case for translational pathophysiology. Endocrinology 146: 2684–91. Epub 2005 Feb 24.
7. Raychaudhuri S, Remmers EF, Lee AT, Hackett R, Guiducci C, et al. (2008) Common variants at CD40 and other loci confer risk of rheumatoid arthritis. Nat Genet 40: 1216–23. Epub 2008 Sep 14.
8. Durie FH, Fava RA, Foy TM, Aruffo A, Ledbetter JA, et al. (1993) Prevention of collagen-induced arthritis with an antibody to gp39, the ligand for CD40. Science 261: 1328–30.
9. Chen CR, Aliesky HA, Guo J, Rapoport B, McLachlan SM (2006) Blockade of costimulation between T cells and antigen-presenting cells: an approach to suppress murine Graves' disease induced by thyrotropin receptor-expressing adenovirus. Thyroid 16: 427–34.
10. Gerritse K, Laman JD, Noelle RJ, Aruffo A, Ledbetter JA, et al. (1996) CD40-CD40 ligand interactions in experimental allergic encephalomyelitis and multiple sclerosis. Proc Natl Acad Sci U S A 93: 2499–504.
11. Mohan C, Shi Y, Laman JD, Datta SK (1995) Interaction between CD40 and its ligand gp39 in the development of murine lupus nephritis. J Immunol 154: 1470–80.
12. Balasa B, Krahl T, Patstone G, Lee J, Tisch R, et al. (1997) CD40 ligand-CD40 interactions are necessary for the initiation of insulitis and diabetes in nonobese diabetic mice. J Immunol 159: 4620–7.
13. Chadha S, Miller K, Farwell L, Sacks S, Daly MJ, et al. (2006) Haplotype analysis of tumour necrosis factor receptor genes in 1p36: no evidence for association with systemic lupus erythematosus. Eur J Hum Genet 14: 69–78.
14. Cooper JD, Smyth DJ, Bailey R, Payne F, Downes K, et al. (2007) The candidate genes TAF5L, TCF7, PDCD1, IL6 and ICAM1 cannot be excluded from having effects in type 1 diabetes. BMC Med Genet 8: 71.
15. Australia and New Zealand Multiple Sclerosis Genetics Consortium (ANZgene) (2009) Genome-wide association study identifies new multiple sclerosis susceptibility loci on chromosomes 12 and 20. Nat Genet 41: 824–8. Epub 2009 Jun 14.

16. Gao D, Wagner AH, Fankhaenel S, Stojanovic T, Schweyer S, et al. (2005) CD40 antisense oligonucleotide inhibition of trinitrobenzene sulphonic acid induced rat colitis. Gut 54: 70–7.

17. Battaglia E, Biancone L, Resegotti A, Emanuelli G, Fronda GR, et al. (1999) Expression of CD40 and its ligand, CD40L, in intestinal lesions of Crohn's disease. Am J Gastroenterol 94: 3279–84.

18. Poser CM, Paty DW, Scheinberg L, McDonald WI, Davis FA, et al. (1983) New diagnostic criteria for multiple sclerosis: guidelines for research protocols. Ann Neurol 13: 227–31.

19. Lennard-Jones JE (1989) Classification of inflammatory bowel disease. Scand J Gastroenterol Suppl. 170: 2–6; discussion 16-9.

20. Peters AL, Stunz LL, Bishop GA (2009) CD40 and autoimmunity: The dark side of a great activator. Semin Immunol 10: 10.

21. Iezzi G, Sonderegger I, Ampenberger F, Schmitz N, Marsland BJ, et al. (2009) CD40-CD40L cross-talk integrates strong antigenic signals and microbial stimuli to induce development of IL-17-producing CD4+ T cells. Proc Natl Acad Sci U S A 106: 876–81. Epub 2009 Jan 9.

22. Chabaud M, Durand JM, Buchs N, Fossiez F, Page G, et al. (1999) Human interleukin-17: A T cell-derived proinflammatory cytokine produced by the rheumatoid synovium. Arthritis Rheum 42: 963–70.

23. Lock C, Hermans G, Pedotti R, Brendolan A, Schadt E, et al. (2002) Gene-microarray analysis of multiple sclerosis lesions yields new targets validated in autoimmune encephalomyelitis. Nat Med 8: 500–8.

24. Fujino S, Andoh A, Bamba S, Ogawa A, Hata K, et al. (2003) Increased expression of interleukin 17 in inflammatory bowel disease. Gut 52: 65–70.

25. Murugaiyan G, Mittal A, Weiner HL (2008) Increased osteopontin expression in dendritic cells amplifies IL-17 production by CD4+ T cells in experimental autoimmune encephalomyelitis and in multiple sclerosis. J Immunol 181: 7480–8.

26. Boon L, Brok HP, Bauer J, Ortiz-Buijsse A, Schellekens MM, et al. (2001) Prevention of experimental autoimmune encephalomyelitis in the common marmoset (Callithrix jacchus) using a chimeric antagonist monoclonal antibody against human CD40 is associated with altered B cell responses. J Immunol 167: 2942–9.

27. Hart BA, Hintzen RQ, Laman JD (2008) Preclinical assessment of therapeutic antibodies against human CD40 and human interleukin-12/23p40 in a nonhuman primate model of multiple sclerosis. Neurodegener Dis 5: 38–52.

28. Buck D, Kroner A, Rieckmann P, Maurer M, Wiendl H (2006) Analysis of the C/T(-1) single nucleotide polymorphism in the CD40 gene in multiple sclerosis. Tissue Antigens 68: 335–8.

29. Genome-wide association study of 14,000 cases of seven common diseases and 3,000 shared controls (2007). Nature 447: 661–78.

30. McGovern DP, Gardet A, Torkvist L, Goyette P, Essers J, et al. (2010) Genome-wide association identifies multiple ulcerative colitis susceptibility loci. Nature 42: 332–7. Epub 2010 Mar 14.

31. Zheng J, Liu Y, Qin G, Chan PL, Mao H, et al. (2009) Efficient induction and expansion of human alloantigen-specific CD8 regulatory T cells from naive precursors by CD40-activated B cells. J Immunol 183: 3742–50. Epub 2009 Aug 14.

32. Zheng J, Liu Y, Lau YL, Tu W (2010) CD40-activated B cells are more potent than immature dendritic cells to induce and expand CD4(+) regulatory T cells. Cell Mol Immunol 7: 44–50.

7

An Ileal Crohn's Disease Gene Signature based on Whole Human Genome Expression Profiles of Disease Unaffected Ileal Mucosal Biopsies

Tianyi Zhang[1], Bowen Song[1], Wei Zhu[1], Xiao Xu[2], Qing Qing Gong[3], Christopher Morando[3], Themistocles Dassopoulos[3], Rodney D. Newberry[3], Steven R. Hunt[4], Ellen Li[2,3]*

1 Department of Applied Mathematics and Statistics, Stony Brook University, Stony Brook, New York, United States of America, 2 Department of Medicine, Stony Brook University, Stony Brook, New York, United States of America, 3 Department of Medicine, Washington University-St. Louis School of Medicine, Saint Louis, Missouri, United States of America, 4 Department of Surgery, Washington University-St. Louis School of Medicine, Saint Louis, Missouri, United States of America

Abstract

Previous genome-wide expression studies have highlighted distinct gene expression patterns in inflammatory bowel disease (IBD) compared to control samples, but the interpretation of these studies has been limited by sample heterogeneity with respect to disease phenotype, disease activity, and anatomic sites. To further improve molecular classification of inflammatory bowel disease phenotypes we focused on a single anatomic site, the disease unaffected proximal ileal margin of resected ileum, and three phenotypes that were unlikely to overlap: ileal Crohn's disease (ileal CD), ulcerative colitis (UC), and control patients without IBD. Whole human genome (Agilent) expression profiling was conducted on two independent sets of disease-unaffected ileal samples collected from the proximal margin of resected ileum. Set 1 (47 ileal CD, 27 UC, and 25 Control non-IBD patients) was used as the training set and Set 2 was subsequently collected as an independent test set (10 ileal CD, 10 UC, and 10 control non-IBD patients). We compared the 17 gene signatures selected by four different feature-selection methods to distinguish ileal CD phenotype with non-CD phenotype. The four methods yielded different but overlapping solutions that were highly discriminating. All four of these methods selected FOLH1 as a common feature. This gene is an established biomarker for prostate cancer, but has not previously been associated with Crohn's disease. Immunohistochemical staining confirmed increased expression of FOLH1 in the ileal epithelium. These results provide evidence for convergent molecular abnormalities in the macroscopically disease unaffected proximal margin of resected ileum from ileal CD subjects.

Editor: Jacques Ravel, Institute for Genome Sciences - University of Maryland School of Medicine, United States of America

Funding: This work was supported partially by National Institutes of Health (NIH) grant UH2DK083994, the Crohn's and Colitis Foundation of America, the Simons Foundation, and by the Leona M. and Harry B. Helmsley charitable trust through the Sinai-Helmsley Alliance for Research Excellence (SHARE) Network and NIH grant R21HG005964. We acknowledge use of the Washington University Digestive Diseases Research Core Center Tissue Procurement Facility (P30 DK52574). The funders had no role in study design, data collection and analysis, decision to publish, or preparation of the manuscript.

Competing Interests: The authors have declared that no competing interests exist.

* E-mail: Ellen.Li@stonybrook.edu

Introduction

Transcriptomic analyses have highlighted differences in intestinal gene expression patterns between samples collected from patients with inflammatory bowel disease (IBD) compared to control patients without inflammatory bowel disease [1–11]. Differences in transcript levels, particularly those involved in inflammatory pathways, have been observed in macroscopically disease affected regions of the intestine compared to disease-unaffected regions of the intestine [6]. Molecular characterization of inflammatory bowel disease phenotypes based on transcriptomic analysis has been limited by sample heterogeneity with respect to disease phenotype, disease activity and anatomic sites. Most of the previous studies have focused on the colon, since this anatomic site is more easily accessible by colonoscopy.

We have previously examined genome wide expression profiles in the disease unaffected proximal margin of resected ileum collected from 4 patients with Crohn's disease of terminal ileum (ileal CD) undergoing initial ileocolic resection with that of 4 control non-IBD patients undergoing initial right hemicolectomy or total colectomy [8]. We have focused on the ileal CD phenotype and excluded subjects with Crohn's Colitis, sincethese two subphenotypes have distinct molecular characteristics [12]. Increased expression of candidate genes such as *MUC1*, *DUOX2* and *DMBT1* expression and decreased expression of *C4orf7* (follicular dendritic cell secreted peptide) was confirmed by reverse transcriptase polymerase chain reaction of 18 ileal CD and 9 control non-IBD samples. We found that these alterations in gene expression were independent of NOD2 genotype [8].

To better define the molecular characteristics of the ileal CD phenotype, we applied four different feature selection methods to select 17-gene signatures that would distinguish samples of the proximal disease unaffected proximal margin of ileum that were resected from individuals with ileal CD phenotype, from samples collected from non-CD phenotype (both non-IBD and ulcerative colitis patients) to a training set composed of 99 expression profiles. We then tested these features in an independently collected test set of 30 expression profiles.

Materials and Methods

Patients and Acquisition of Ileal Tissue Samples

This study was approved by the Washington University-St. Louis and Stony Brook University Institutional Review Boards. Ileal CD patients undergoing ileocolic resection, UC patients undergoing total colectomy and Control non-IBD patients undergoing either right hemicolectomy or total colectomy (for colon cancer, colonic adenomas, colonic inertia, diverticulosis and one case of a foreign body with perforation) were prospectively enrolled in a consecutive fashion by the Washington University Digestive Diseases Research Core Center Tissue Procurement Facility to donate surgically resected tissue samples between September 2005 and December 2010. A subset of 8 of the 99 expression profiles generated from samples collected between September 2005 and February 2010 in the training set were previously reported [8]. A subset of 81 of 99 expression profiles in the training set (Set 1) were previously reported in a study linking ileum associated microbial composition with cluster centroids corresponding to a cluster enriched in genes expressed in Paneth cells and two clusters enriched in genes associated with xenobiotic metabolism [11], [13]. The 30 expression profiles in the test set (Set 2) were collected from additional subjects recruited between February 2010 and December 2010. The diagnosis of CD or UC was based on the surgical pathological report for the surgical resection specimen, which was issued by the attending surgical pathologist assigned to the case. Patients who were unwilling or unable to give informed written consent were excluded. At least 4 ex-vivo biopsies were collected from the macroscopically disease-unaffected proximal margin of the freshly resected pathologic ileum specimens using Radial Jaw4 large-capacity biopsy forceps (Boston Scientific, Natick, MA) and placed immediately into RNAlater, an RNA stabilization solution, and stored at -80°C. The designation of *disease-unaffected* was based on the macroscopic appearance of the ileal mucosa and the surgical pathology report of adjacent ileal biopsies ("no histopathologic abnormality"). The clinical information and samples were collected as previously described [11], [13] and stripped of all identifying information and assigned both a patient code and sample code. All of the patients received intravenous antibiotic prophylaxis covering both aerobic and anerobic bacteria (e.g. ciprofloxacin and metronidazole, cefoxitin, cefotetan) within one hour of incision [14].

Microarray Analysis

Total RNA was extracted from the tissue samples using TRI Reagent® according to the manufacturer's recommendation, and RNA quality was assessed using an Agilent 2100 Bioanalyzer [8]. The test RNAs and a common reference ileal RNA were labeled with the Quick Amp Labeling Kit (Agilent No. 5190-0424) and the resulting probes were hybridized to Agilent Whole Human Genome Arrays (Agilent No. G4412A) as previously described [8], [9]. The pre-processing, filtering and normalization of the microarray data was conducted using the R package LIMMA [15], [16] Probes with all Genepix flags less than −100 were treated as absent and removed from the dataset. There were technical duplicates on three samples in the training set and two samples in the test set. For those samples, the log2 ratios for the technical duplicates were averaged prior to analysis. The data discussed in this publication have been deposited in NCBI's Gene Expression Omnibus and are accessible through GEO Series accession number GSE24287 (http://www.ncbi.nlm.nih.gov/geo/query/acc.cgi?acc = GSE24287).

Statistical Analysis

Two-class (ileal CD vs. non-CD) unpaired significance analysis of microarrays (SAM) was performed on 25,756 probes in the training set as previously described by Tusher *et al* [17] as an initial filtering step (>1.5 fold, <0.67 fold, FDR <0.05). SAM assigns a gene-specific t-test (q-value) based on changes in gene expression relative to the standard deviation of repeated measurements for that gene. Feature subset selection of 17-gene signatures was performed on the resulting 464 probes selected by SAM using the following four methods: Component-wise Boosting (Boosting) [18], Prediction Analysis of Microarrays (PAM) [19], Random Forest [20] and Least Absolute Shrinkage and Selection Operator (LASSO) [21]. In order to evaluate the four different feature selection methods, a majority vote [22] based on the median score of seven supervised machine learning tools, Boosting [18], PAM [19], Random Forest [20], LASSO [21], Support Vector Machine [23], Linear Discriminant Analysis [24], Naive Bayes [25]), was performed. The overall accuracy, sensitivity, specificity and area under the curves (AUC) were initially calculated based on the empirical receiver operating characteristic (ROC) curves [26]. The ROC curves were then smoothed to facilitate visual differentiation as previously described [27]. Partial correlation network analysis based on the joint sparse regression models [28] was further conducted to study the network relationship among the 17 gene signature selected by the boosting method.

Immunohistochemistry

Folate hydrolase 1 (FOLH1), also termed prostate specific membrane antigen (PSMA) [29], expression in formalin fixed paraffin embedded sections of the disease unaffected proximal margin of resected ileum from ileal CD patients and Control non-IBD patients, were stained using a monoclonal mouse anti-PSMA antibody (clone E6, catalog number N1611, DAKO) in the Washington University Digestive Diseases Research Core Center Morphology Core. Epitope retrieval was performed with the Diva DECLOAKER reagent (BIOCARE DV-2004) in a Biocare Decloaking chamber. Primary antibody was applied overnight at 4°C at a dilution of 1:500. Antigen antibody complexes were detected with biotinylated goat anti-mouse IgG (1:2000, Jackson Laboratories), then developed in diaminobenzimidine (Biocare Betazid DAB) and counterstained with hematoxylin. Negative control slides were incubated with isotype-matched immunoglobulin, and a prostatic adenocarcinoma specimen served as a positive control for staining with the anti-PSMA (FOLH1) antibody.

Results

Patient Characteristics in the Training and Test Sets (see Table 1)

The patients included in this study were predominantly white. As shown in Table 1, *C. difficile* was more prevalent among UC patients than ileal CD or control non-IBD patients [30], [31]. None of the control subjects were treated with5-ASA, immuno-modulators, and/or anti-TNFα biologics. However all of the patients received intravenous antibiotic prophylaxis that covered both aerobic and anaerobic bacteria within one hour prior to incision [14].

Two-Class Unpaired Significance Analysis of Microarrays (SAM) Comparing Ileal CD and Non-CD (UC and control non-IBD) Phenotypes (see Table S1)

Because a large amount of variability can be introduced in the fold change for low intensity signals, the threshold for gene filtering

Table 1. Patient characteristics associated with each disease phenotype in the training and test sets.

Training Set

Variables	Ileal CD (n = 47)	UC (n = 27)	Control (n = 25)
Gender (male)	43%	59%	32%
Race (white)	96%	100%	96%
Median Age (range) y	35 (20–75)	43 (17–64)	55 (18–84)
Current smoker	32%	10%	24%
Positive fecal *C. difficile* toxin	0%	30%	0%
Median BMI (range) kg/m^2	24 (16–38)	24 (18–43)	28 (20–38)
5-ASA	55%	63%	0%
Steroids	43%	67%	0%
Immunomodulators	45%	44%	0%
Anti-TNFα biologics			
Current (≤8 weeks of surgery)	28%	41%	0%
Past (>8 weeks of surgery)	8%	7%	0%
Never	64%	52%	0%

Test Set

Variables	Ileal CD (n = 10)	UC (n = 10)	Control (n = 10)
Gender (male)	40%	70%	40%
Race (white)	90%	90%	100%
Median Age (range) y	39 (19–58)	44 (16–62)	66 (21–77)
Current smoker	20%	20%	40%
Positive fecal *C. difficile* toxin	0%	30%	0%
Median BMI (range) kg/m^2	22 (19–39)	24 (20–33)	25 (20–36)
5-ASA	40%	80%	0%
Steroids	70%	100%	0%
Immunomodulators	40%	30%	0%
Anti-TNFα biologics			
Current (≤8 weeks of surgery)	40%	20%	0%
Past (>8 weeks of surgery)	0%	0%	0%
Never	60%	80%	0%

was selected to be twice the background, resulting in a total of 25,676 gene-probes [32]. Two-class unpaired SAM analysis comparing ileal CD with non-CD phenotype was performed as the initial filtering step, and identified 464 gene probes (see Table S1) that were differentially expressed (fold change ≥1.5 or ≤0.67, FDR <0.05) between ileal CD and Non-CD (UC and Control) samples [17]. In this training set of 99 microarrays, the mean *DMBT1* expression level was confirmed to be significantly increased, while that of *C4orf7* was confirmed to be significantly decreased in the disease unaffected proximal margin of ileum resected from ileal CD patients compared to nonIBD Control and UC patients [8]. We also observed that *MUC1* and *DUOX2* expression was increased relative to Control samples. However because *MUC1* and *DUOX2* expression was also increased in UC compared to nonIBD Control samples, these genes were not selected in this two-class unpaired SAM comparing ileal CD and non-CD (UC and Control).

Feature Subset Selection (see Table S2)

Four feature subset selection methods (Boosting [18], PAM [19], Random Forest (RF) [20], and LASSO [21]), were applied to

further select subsets of 17 gene probes or features that were useful for predicting the ileal CD phenotype. The union of the resulting four 17-gene signatures totaled 42 in number (see Table S2) because 26 of the features were selected by more than one method. Folate hydrolase 1 (*FOLH1*) gene was selected by all four feature selection methods. Three known genes, TLR4 interactor with leucine rich repeats (*TRIL*), Niemann-Pick disease, type C1, gene-like 1 (*NPC1L1*), and *C4orf7* also termed follicular dendritic cell secreted protein were selected by three of the four methods. Six known genes were selected by two of four methods, BCL2-associated X protein (*BAX*), cytochrome P 450, family 26, subfamily B, polypeptide 1 (*CYP26B1*), nephronectin (*NPNT*), protein phosphatase 1, regulatory (inhibitor) subunit 14A (*PPP1R14A*), family with sequence similarity129, member C (*FAM129C*) also termed B-cell novel protein 1 (*BCNP1*), cathelicidin antimicrobial peptide (*CAMP*), chemokine (C-C motif) ligand 23 (*CCL23*). We repeated our analysis using data excluding the *C. difficile* positive samples. *FOLH1* is still the only gene probe selected by all four feature selection methods and it is still ranked prominently by all four classifiers 2nd, 1,st, 1st and 4th by PAM, RF, LASSO and Boosting, respectively). In addition, ten out of 12 genes selected by two or more feature methods based on data without *C. difficile* positive samples overlap with those selected using data including the *C. difficile* positive samples. Meanwhile, the Bossting method still features the highest classification accuracy at 89.90% and 86.96% for data with and without the *C. difficile* positive samples, respectively. All these observations indicate that our method was not skewed by the *C. difficile* toxin factor.

Majority vote based on the median score of seven classifier tools (see Materials and Methods) was used to assess the accuracy associated with each feature subset for ileal CD phenotype in the training set via Jack-Knife (take-one-out) cross validation. The feature subset selected by the boosting method yielded the highest area under the curve (AUC) and overall accuracy (see Table 2). The smoothed receiver operating characteristic (ROC) curves for the seven classifiers as well as their majority vote based on the training data were comparable (see Figure 1). We then applied this 17 gene signature to an independent test set that was collected after the training set (see Figure 2, Table 3). As shown in Table S2, the polarity of the mean fold change for this 17 ileal gene signature was preserved in both the training and test set. Of note, errors in classification reflected misclassification of UC samples as ileal CD samples. The smoothed ROC curves are shown in Figure 2 in order to facilitate visual differentiation of the different classifiers. There was good agreement between the AUC for the empirical and smoothed ROC curves (see Table S3), indicating that the smoothed ROCs retained the key properties of the empirical ROCs.

FOLH1 is a "Hub" Gene by Partial Correlation Network Analysis

Partial correlation network analysis was conducted on the union of the features selected by the four methods using all 129 microarrays in both the training and test set to assess the coregulation of these 42 genes. As shown in Figure 3, the folate hydrolase 1 (*FOLH1*) gene was identified as a "hub" gene that has

significantly non-zero partial correlations to 12 of the other 16 gene biomarkers (see Figure 3). The *FOLH1* gene was originally identified as a prostate specific membrane antigen detected as upregulated in prostate carcinoma [33], however expression of *FOLH1* has since been observed in other tissues including the small intestine, particularly in the duodenal mucosa, the nervous system and the kidney [34]. Because *FOLH1* expression has been observed in neoplastic and nonneoplastic neovasculature [35], immunochemical localization of *FOLH1* was performed on the disease unaffected proximal margin of resected ileum from ileal CD and control non-IBD subjects. A representative micrograph is shown in Figure 4, which demonstrates that the more prominent staining in ileal CD samples was localized to the villous epithelium.

Discussion

In this study, we took a statistical approach to identify ileal gene biomarkers associated with ileal CD phenotype compared to non-CD (UC and control). Some of the genes (e.g. *DUOX2* and *MUC1*) that we noted previously to be upregulated in ileal CD with control non-IBD subjects were not selected in the current study because these genes were also upregulated in UC compared to control samples [8]. Feature selection is one of the most important issues in classification. In this study, four feature selection methods, (Boosting, PAM, Random Forest and LASSO), were applied to select subsets of 17 gene features. The four methods yielded different but overlapping solutions that were highly discriminating. Thus, feature selection with microarray data can lead to different solutions that are comparable with respect to prediction rates. Note that different underlying hypotheses are associated with each method in selecting features from an extremely large number of variables in the microarray datasets compared to the number of samples [36,37]. Combining different methods has been used as an approach to improve classification performance [38,39].

All four selection methods identified upregulation of *FOLH1* expression as predictive of the ileal CD phenotype compared to non-CD. *FOLH1* encodes a transmembrane glycoprotein that acts

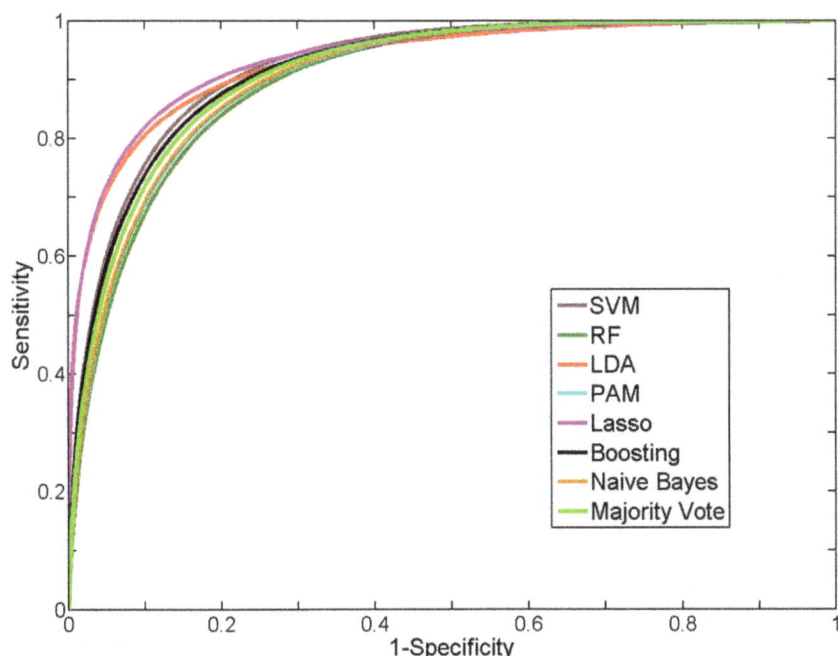

Figure 1. Receiver operating characteristic (ROC) curve for different classification methods on the training set.

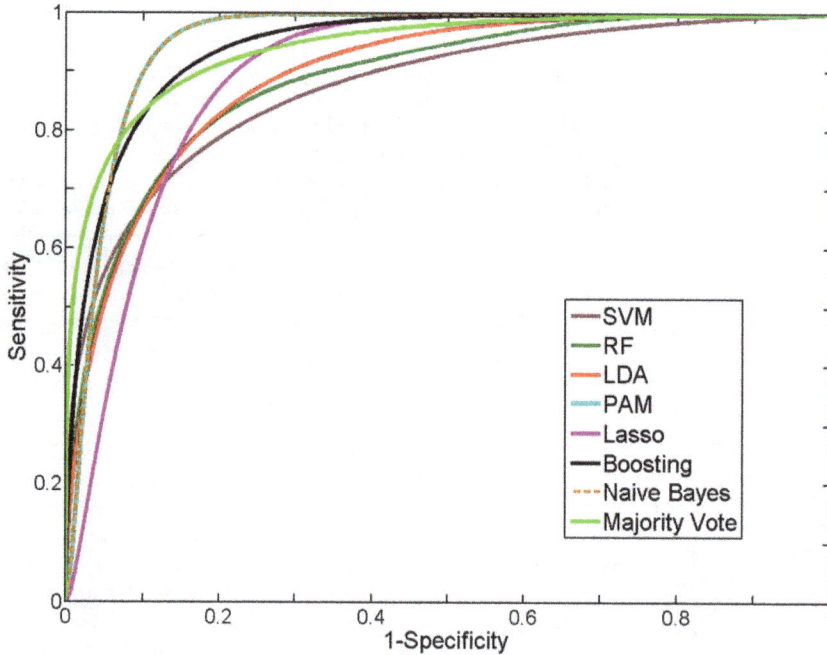

Figure 2. Receiver operating characteristic (ROC) curve for different classification methods on the test set.

as a glutamate carboxypeptidase on substrates including folate. Immunohistochemical staining localized more prominent expression of this gene in ileal CD samples to the villous epithelium [34]. Of the features selected by alternative feature selection methods (see Table 2), only *FOLH1B* clustered with *FOLH1* in the training dataset [11]. *FOLH1* is an established biomarker for prostate cancer, but has not been previously identified as a biomarker for Crohn's disease.

Three genes, *TRIL*, *NPCL1* and *C4orf7* were selected by three of four of the feature selection methods. *TRIL*, was recently identified as a novel component of the TLR4 complex and TLR3 complex [40], [41]. *TRIL* mRNA expression has been detected in the small intestine, as well as the central nervous system, lung, kidney and ovary. TRIL expression is upregulated in cell culture by lipopolysaccharide. The upregulation of *TRIL* expression could reflect altered host microbial interactions in macroscopically disease unaffected regions of the intestine in ileal CD patients. *NPC1L1* is required for intestinal uptake of cholesterol and plant

Table 2. Comparison of 17 ileal gene signatures selected by four different feature selection methods.

Methods	AUC	Accuracy
Boosting	**0.928**	**89.9%**
PAM	0.895	88.9%
Random forest	0.902	85.9%
LASSO	0.895	85.9%

Boosting [16], PAM) [17], random forest [18] and LASSO [19] were applied to the SAM filtered training microarray dataset to select 17 ileal gene signatures. The AUC and overall accuracy for each of the signatures were calculated based on the majority vote of 7 classifiers (Boosting, PAM, Random Forest, LASSO, Support Vector Machine, Linear Discriminant Analysis, and Naive Bayes), which is equivalently to the decision based on the median score using an usual probability threshold of 0.5 (see Materials and Methods).

Table 3. Classification results on the training and test sets.

Classification Method	Accuracy	Sensitivity	Specificity
Training Set			
Support Vector Machine (SVM)	90.9%	91.5%	90.4%
Random Forest (RF)	86.9%	87.2%	86.5%
Linear Discriminant Analysis (LDA)	90.9%	89.4%	92.3%
Predictive Analysis of Microarray (PAM)	88.9%	89.4%	88.5%
Lasso	91.9%	91.5%	92.3%
Boosting	88.9%	89.4%	88.5%
Naïve Bayes	88.9%	89.4%	88.5%
Majority Vote (Combined Classifiers)	***89.9%***	***91.5%***	***88.5%***
Test Set			
Support Vector Machine (SVM)	83.3%	80.0%	85.0%
Random Forest (RF)	73.3%	90.0%	65.0%
Linear Discriminant Analysis (LDA)	76.7%	80.0%	75.0%
Predictive Analysis of Microarray (PAM)	86.7%	100.0%	80.0%
Lasso	86.7%	80.0%	90.0%
Boosting	86.7%	90.0%	85.0%
Naïve Bayes	83.3%	100.0%	75.0%
Majority Vote (Combined Classifiers)	***80.0%***	***90.0%***	***75.0%***

The accuracy, sensitivity, specificity of the ileal gene signature selected by the boosting method [16] are calculated using Leaving-One-Out cross validation on the training and subsequently, direct classification of the test set based on the training set.

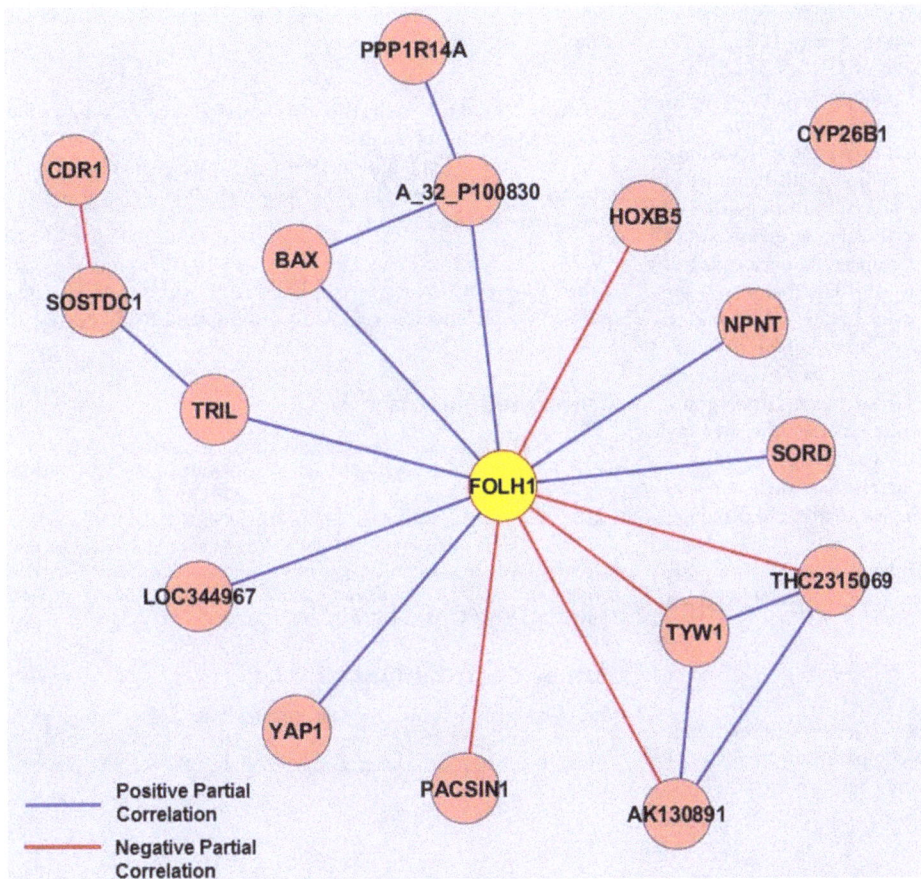

Figure 3. Partial correlation network among the 17 selected genes. FOLH1 is linked to multiple genes and serves as a hub gene. A red line between genes indicates a positive non-zero partial correlation and a blue line indicates a negative non-zero partial correlation.

sterols and is relatively abundant in the ileum [42], [43]. Upregulation of *NPC1L1* expression in ileal CD patients may also contribute to enhanced atherogenesis in Crohn's patients [44]. Partial correlation network analysis revealed that *FOLH1* has nonzero correlations with 12 of the other 16 genes in the signature.

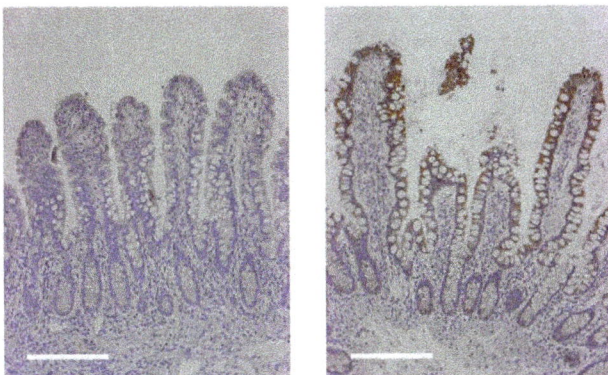

Figure 4. Immunohistochemical localization of FOLH1 in disease unaffected ileal mucosa from the proximal margin of resected ileum from an ileal CD subject (left panel) and a control non-IBD subject. The more prominent FOLH1 staining in the ileal CD sample is localized to the villous epithelium. Magnification is 100×. Bar is 200 μm.

The biological basis for the nonzero partial correlations between the "hub" gene, *FOLH* is not immediately apparent.

We have previously noted downregulation of *C4orf7* as well as other genes associated with organized lymphoid structures and/or B-cell function in ileal CD patients compared to non-IBD control patients [8]. This study indicates that downregulation of ileal *C4orf7* expression is also observed in ileal CD patients, when compared with UC patients.

Partial correlation network analysis revealed that *FOLH1* has nonzero correlations with 12 of the other 16 genes in the signature. The biological basis for the nonzero partial correlations between the "hub" gene, *FOLH* is not immediately apparent. Thus far, we have not detected association of the gene features listed above with alterations in microbial composition, but we are likely underpowered to detect such associations with only 81 samples with paired microbiome and microarray data [11]. We also noted that upregulation of *FOLH1* was observed in ileal CD samples regardless of NOD2 genotype [8].In this study we report the results of binary classification – ileal CD vs. non-CD. Our attempts to apply multiclassification to the data set yielded poor accuracy particularly between the UC and control non-IBD phenotypes. This may be partly because the number of UC samples and control non-IBD samples were both smaller than the number of ileal CD samples. Of note, the errors in the binary classification of ileal CD vs. non-CD reflected misclassification of two UC samples as ileal CD. In the original test set we had an additional sample from a subject with a pre-operative diagnosis of UC. However the post-operative diagnosis was changed to Crohn's colitis based on the pathological diagnosis of the resected specimen. Interestingly this discarded sample was classified as "ileal CD" based on the expression profile. While the ileal CD phenotype can be easily distinguished from ulcerative colitis based on imaging and endoscopic findings, it is more difficult to distinguish Crohn's colitis from ulcerative colitis even after pathological diagnosis of the resected colon [45]. Improving our ability to distinguish UC from Crohn's colitis at the time of the initial colon resection would improve clinical decision making with respect to performing a subsequent ileal pouch anal anastomosis [46]. For this reason we are continuing to follow our UC patients after colectomy to determine whether any of these patients are diagnosed subsequently as Crohn's disease. We also plan to begin analyzing disease unaffected ileal samples collected from patients undergoing colectomy for Crohn's colitis to determine whether there is any overlap in the ileal signature for ileal CD and Crohn's colitis.

In summary, we have identified potential biomarkers for ileal CD phenotype in the macroscopically disease unaffected proximal margin of resected ileum from ileal CD subjects. These results provide evidence for convergent molecular abnormalities in the macroscopically disease unaffected proximal margin of resected ileum from ileal CD subjects,

Supporting Information

Table S1 Differentially expressed gene probes selected by SAM. A. Upregulated probes in 47 ileal CD compared to 52 non-CD (UC and control non-IBD) samples (number of probes = 269). B.

Downregulated probes in 47 ileal CD compared to 52 non-CD samples (total number of probes = 195).

Table S2 Union of differentially expressed Agilent gene probes selected by four feature subset selection methods: Boosting, PAM, Random Forest (RF) and LASSO. A. Upregulated probes B. Downregulated probes The 17 genes selected by the boosting method are **bolded**.

Table S3 AUC values of empirical ROC curves, AUC values and 95% confidence interval (C.I.) of smoothed ROC curves.

Acknowledgments

The authors thank the patients who have generously contributed their blood, tissue and medical information to the Washington University Digestive Diseases Research Core Center (DDRCC) Tissue Procurement Facility. We also thank the faculty in the Division of Colon Rectal Surgery and the Division of Gastroenterology at Washington University for their help and support in recruiting patients. We thank Kymberly Carter for carrying out *FOLH1* immunohistochemical staining in the Washington University DDRCC Morphology Core.

Author Contributions

Conceived and designed the experiments: EL SH. Performed the experiments: QG CM EL. Analyzed the data: TZ BS WZ XX EL. Contributed reagents/materials/analysis tools: RN TD SH XX. Wrote the paper: TZ EL BS WZ.

References

1. Dieckgraefe B, Stenson W, Korzenik JR, Swanson PE, Harrington CA (2000) Analysis of mucosal gene expression in inflammatory bowel disease by parallel oligonucleotide arrays. Physiol Genomics 4: 1–11.
2. Lawrance IC, Fiocchi C, Chakravarti S (2001) Ulcerative colitis and Crohn's disease: distinctive gene expression profiles and novel susceptibility candidate genes. Hum Mol Genet 10: 445–456.
3. Langmann T, Moehle C, Mauerer R, Scharl M, Liebisch G, et al. (2004) Loss of detoxification in inflammatory bowel disease: dysregulation of pregnane X receptor target genes. Gastroenterology 2004; 127: 26–40.
4. Uthoff SM, Eichenberger MR, Lewis RK, Fox MP, Hamilton CJ, et al. (2001) Identification of candidate genes in ulcerative colitis and Crohn's disease using cDNA array technology. Int J Oncol 19: 803–810.
5. Dooley TP, Curto EV, Reddy SP, Davis RL, Lambert GW, et al. (2004) Regulation of gene expression in inflammatory bowel disease and correlation with IBD drugs: screening by DNA microarrays. Inflamm Bowel Dis 10: 1–14.
6. Wu F, Dassopoulos T, Cope L, Maitra A, Brant SR, et al. (2007) Genome-wide gene expression differences in Crohn's disease and ulcerative colitis from endoscopic pinch biopsies: insights into distinctive pathogenesis. Inflamm Bowel Dis 13: 807–821.
7. Noble CL, Abbas AR, Cornelius J, Lees CW, Ho GT, et al. (2008) Regional variation in gene expression in the healthy colon is dysregulated in ulcerative colitis. Gut 57: 1398–1405.
8. Hamm C, Reimers M, McCullough C, Gorbe EB, Lu J, et al. (2010) NOD2 status and human ileal gene expression. Inflamm Bowel Dis 16: 1649–1657.
9. Noble CL, Abbas AR, Lees CW, Cornelius J, Toy K, et al. (2010) Characterization of intestinal gene expression profiles in Crohn's disease by genome-wide microarray analysis. Inflamm Bowel Dis 16: 1717–1728.
10. Arijs I, De Hertogh G, Machiels K, Van Steen K, Lemaire K, et al. (2011) Mucosal gene expression of cell adhesion molecules, chemokines, and chemokine receptors in patients with inflammatory bowel disease before and after infliximab treatment. Am J Gastroenterol 106: 748–761.
11. Zhang T, DeSimone RA, Jiao X, Rohlf FJ, Zhu W, et al. (2012) Host genes related to Paneth cells and xenobiotic metabolism are associated with shifts in human ileum-associated microbial composition. PLoS ONE In press.
12. Hancock L, Beckly J, Geremia A, Cooney R, Cummings F, et al. (2008) Clinical and molecular characteristics of isolated colonic Crohn's disease. Inflamm Bowel Dis 14: 1667–1677.
13. Li E, Hamm CM, Gulati AS, Sartor RB, Chen H, et al. (2012) Inflammatory bowel diseases phenotype, *C. difficile* and NOD2 genotype are associated with shifts in human ileum associated microbial composition. PLoS ONE In press.
14. Nelson RL, Glenny AM, Song F (2009) Antimicrobial prophylaxis for colorectal surgery. Cochrane Database Syst Rev 1: CD001181.
15. Smyth GK, Speed TP (2003) Normalization of cDNA microarray data. Methods 31: 265–273.
16. Smyth GK (2005) Limma: linear models for microarray data. In Gentleman R, Carey V, Dudoit S, Irizarry R, Huber W, eds. Bioinformatics and Computational Biology Solutions using R and Bioconductor. New York: Springer. pp 397–420.
17. Tusher VG, Tibshirani R, Chu G (2001) Significance analysis of microarrays applied to the ionizing radiation response. Proc Natl Acad Sci USA 98: 5116–5121.
18. Bühlmann P, Yu B (2003) Boosting with the l2 loss: Regression and classification. JASA 98: 324–339.
19. Tibshirani R, Hastie T, Narasimhan B, Chu G (2002) Diagnosis of multiple cancer types by shrunken centroids of gene expression. Proc Natl Acad Sci U S A 99: 6567–6572.
20. Breiman L (2001) Random forests. Machine Learning 45: 5–32.
21. Young-Park M, Hastie T (2007) L1-regularization path algorithm for generalized linear models. Journal of the Royal Statistical Society B 69: 659–677.
22. Altmann A, Rosen-Zvi M, Prosperi M, Aharoni E, Neuvirth H, et al. (2008) Comparison of classifier fusion methods for predicting response to anti HIV-1 Therapy. PLoS ONE 3: e3470. doi:10.1371/journal.pone.0003470.
23. Statnikov A, Aliferis CF, Tsamardinos I, Hardin D, Levy S (2005) A comprehensive evaluation of multicategory classification methods for microarray gene expression cancer diagnosis. Bioinformatics 21: 631–643.
24. McLachlan GJ (1992) Discriminant Analysis and Statistical Pattern Recognition. New York: Wiley.
25. Langley P, Iba W, Thompson K An analysis of Bayesian classifier, Proc. Tenth National Conference on Artificial Intelligence. pp 223–228.
26. Bradley AP (1997) The use of the area under the ROC curve in the evaluation of machine learning algorithms. Pattern Recognition 30: 1145–1159.
27. Hanley JE (1988) The robustness of the "binormal" assumptions used in fitting ROC curves". Medical Decision Making 8: 197–203.
28. Peng J, Wang P, Zhou N, Zhu J (2009) Partial correlation estimation by joint sparse regression models. J Am Stat Assoc 104: 735–746.
29. Gong MC, Chang SS, Sadelain M, Bander NH, Heston WDH (1999) Prostate-specific membrane antigen (PSMA)-monoclonal antibodies in the treatment of prostate and other cancers. Cancer and Metastasis Reviews 18: 483–490.
30. Issa M, Vijaypal A, Graham MB, Beaulieu DB, Otterson MF, et al. (2007) Impact of Clostridium difficile on inflammatory bowel disease. Clin Gastroenterol Hepatol 5: 345–351.
31. Rodemann JF, Dubberke ER, Reske KA, Seo DH, Stone CD (2007) The incidence of Clostridium difficile infection in inflammatory bowel disease. Clin Gastroenterol Hepatol 5: 339–344.

32. Zahurak M, Parmigiani G, Yu W, Scharpf RB, Berman D, et al. (2007) Pre-processing Agilent microarray data. BMC Bioinformatics 8: 142.

33. Israeli RS, Powell CT, Corr JG, Fair WR, Heston WD (1994) Expression of the prostate specific membrane antigen. Cancer Res 54: 1807–1811.

34. Silver DA, Pellicer I, Fair WR, Heston WD, Cordon-Cardo C (1997) Prostate specific membrane antigen. Clin Cancer Res 3: 81–85.

35. Gordon IO, Tretiakova MS, Noffsinger AE, Hart J, Reuter VE, et al. (2008) Prostate-specific membrane antigen expression in regeneration and repair. Mol Pathol 21: 1421–1427.

36. Breiman L (2001) Statistical modeling: the two cultures (with discussion). Statistical Science 16: 199–203.

37. Harrell JFE (2001) Regression modeling strategies. Springer: New York.

38. Liu B, Cui Q, Jiang T, Ma S (2004) A combinational feature selection and ensemble neural network method for classification of gene expression data. BMC Bioinformatics 5: 136.

39. Saeys Y, Abeel T, Van de Peer Y (2008) Robust feature selection using ensemble feature selection techniques. In Proceedings of the 25th European Conference on Machine Learning and Knowledge Discovery in Databases, Part II. pp 313–325.

40. Carpenter S, Carlson T, Dellacasagrande J, Garcia A, Gibbons S, et al. (2009) TRIL, a functional component of the TLR4 signaling complex, highly expressed in brain. J Immunol 183: 3989–3995.

41. Carpenter S, Wochal P, Dunne A, O'Neill LA (2011) Toll-like receptor (TLR) 3 signaling requires the TLR4 interactor with leucine-rich repeats (TRIL). J Biol Chem 286: 38795–804.

42. Davis HR, Jr., Zhu LJ, Hoos LM, Tetzloff G, Maguire M, et al. (2004) Niemann-Pick C1 Like 1 (NPC1L1) is the intestinal phytosterol and cholesterol transporter and a key modulator of whole-body cholesterol homeostasis. J Biol Chem 279: 33586–33592.

43. Masson CJ, Plat J, Mensink RP, Namiot A, Kisielewski W, et al. (2010) Fatty acid- and cholesterol transporter protein expression along the human intestinal tract. PLoS ONE 5: e10380.

44. van Leuven SI, Hezemans R, Levels JH, Snoek S, Stokkers PC, et al. (2007) Enhanced atherogenesis and altered high density lipoprotein in patients with Crohn's disease. J Lipid Res 48: 2640–2646.

45. North American Society for Pediatric Gastroenterology, Hepatology, and Nutrition; Colitis Foundation of America, Bousvaros A, Antonioli DA, Colletti RB, et al. (2007) Differentiating ulcerative colitis from Crohn disease in children and young adults: report of a working group of the North American Society for Pediatric Gastroenterology, Hepatology, and Nutrition and the Crohn's and Colitis Foundation of America. J Pediatr Gastroenterol Nutr 44: 653–674.

46. Melton GB, Fazio VW, Kiran RP, He J, Lavery IC, et al. (2008) Long-term outcomes with ileal pouch-anal anastomosis and Crohn's disease: pouch retention and implications of delayed diagnosis. Ann Surg 248: 608–616.

8

Infliximab Induces Clonal Expansion of γδ-T Cells in Crohn's Disease: A Predictor of Lymphoma Risk?

Jens Kelsen[1]*, Anders Dige[1], Heinrich Schwindt[2], Francesco D'Amore[3], Finn S. Pedersen[2], Jørgen Agnholt[1], Lisbet A. Christensen[1], Jens F. Dahlerup[1], Christian L. Hvas[1]

1 Gastro-Immuno Research Laboratory (GIRL), Department of Medicine V, Aarhus University Hospital, Aarhus, Denmark, 2 Institute of Molecular Biology, Aarhus University, Aarhus, Denmark, 3 Department of Hematology, Aarhus University Hospital, Aarhus, Denmark

Abstract

Background: Concominant with the widespread use of combined immunotherapy in the management of Crohn's disease (CD), the incidence of hepato-splenic gamma-delta (γδ)-T cell lymphoma has increased sharply in CD patients. Malignant transformation of lymphocytes is believed to be a multistep process resulting in the selection of malignant γδ-T cell clones. We hypothesised that repeated infusion of anti-TNF-α agents may induce clonal selection and that concurrent treatment with immunomodulators further predisposes patients to γδ-T cell expansion.

Methodology/Principal Findings: We investigated dynamic changes in the γδ-T cells of patient with CD following treatment with infliximab (Remicade®; $n = 20$) or adalimumab (Humira®; $n = 26$) using flow cytometry. In patients with a high γδ-T cell level, the γδ-T cells were assessed for clonality. Of these 46 CD patients, 35 had a γδ-T cells level (mean 1.6%) comparable to healthy individuals (mean 2.2%), and 11 CD patients (24%) exhibited an increased level of γδ-T cells (5–15%). In the 18 patients also receiving thiopurines or methotrexate, the average baseline γδ-T cell level was 4.4%. In three male CD patients with a high baseline value, the γδ-T cell population increased dramatically following infliximab therapy. A fourth male patient also on infliximab monotherapy presented with 20% γδ-T cells, which increased to 25% shortly after treatment and was 36% between infusions. Clonality studies revealed an oligoclonal γδ-T cell pattern with dominant γδ-T cell clones. In support of our clinical findings, in vitro experiments showed a dose-dependent proliferative effect of anti-TNF-α agents on γδ-T cells.

Conclusion/Significance: CD patients treated with immunomodulators had constitutively high levels of γδ-T cells. Infliximab exacerbated clonal γδ-T cell expansion in vivo and induced γδ-T cell proliferation in vitro. Overall, young, male CD patients with high baseline γδ-T cell levels may be at an increased risk of developing malignant γδ-T cell lymphomas following treatment with anti-TNF-α agents.

Editor: Yehuda Shoenfeld, Sheba Medical Center, Israel

Funding: The study was supported by research funding from the Karen Elise Jensen Foundation, the Beckett Foundation, the Desiree and Niels Ydes Foundation, the Danish Colitis-Crohn Foundation, and the Toyota Foundation, Denmark. The funders had no role in study design, data collection and analysis, decision to publish, or preparation of the manuscript.

Competing Interests: The authors have read the journal's policy and have the following conflicts: Jørgen Agnholt is member of the Abbott Advisory Board, Denmark. Lisbet Ambrosius Christensen is a member of the MSD Advisory Board, Denmark. Anders Dige has received an unrestricted grant from Abbott. Abbott was not involved in the study design, collection, analysis and interpretation of data, writing of the paper, and/or decision to submit for publication.

* E-mail: jenskels@rm.dk

Introduction

T cells that express the γδ subunits of the T cell receptor link innate and adaptive immunity and have been implicated in the pathogenesis of autoimmune diseases, particularly Crohn's disease (CD) [1]. The frequency of γδ-T cells in the peripheral blood of healthy individuals ranges from 2–5%. However, higher γδ-T cell frequencies have been found in CD patients [2], and these increased levels have been reported to mirror disease activity, with higher levels in patients with active disease[3]. Hepatosplenic T cell lymphoma (HSTCL) is a rare and distinct peripheral T cell lymphoma that is nearly always γδ-T cell in origin[4]. HSTCL has been observed in patients receiving immunosuppressive treatment and in a disproportionately high number of young male CD patients [5–7].

To date, approximately 200 cases of HSTCL have been reported worldwide. Interestingly, of these cases, 28 cases were reported in patients with inflammatory bowel disease (IBD). With the exception of one case, the occurrence of anti-TNF-α treatment–associated HSTCL has only been reported in IBD patients [5,8]. Of these 28 cases, 22 patients had received infliximab in combination with a thiopurine analogue (azathioprine or 6-mercaptopurine) [9], 3 cases were associated with the use of infliximab followed by adalimumab. However, HSTCL was also reported to occur in patients receiving azathioprine monotherapy [10,11].

In a large study conducted by CESAME, where only 9% of the patients received anti-TNF-α therapy, evidence for a possible causal role of thiopurines in lymphomagenesis was reported; however, no cases of HTSCL were reported [12]. HSTCL incidence is very low, and clinical trials may not provide a follow-up period that is sufficiently long enough to detect overt lymphoma development in the studied cohorts. Thus, a causal link between thiopurine treatment and the possible increased risk of combining thiopurine treatment with anti-TNF-α agents has been difficult to establish[13]. Furthermore, it is unknown if there are differences in the risk associated with the various anti-TNF-α agents. As a result of the observed HSTCL cases, a stepdown to monotherapy has been advocated in young IBD patients [14]. However, the lymphoma risk apparently persists, as even a single exposure to infliximab appears to predispose patients to lymphoma development years later [15].

The malignant transformation of lymphocyte subsets in IBD patients is believed to be a multistep process resulting in the selection of γδ-T cell clones with a survival advantage [16]. In this context, we hypothesised that repeated treatment with anti-TNF-α antibodies in a standard maintenance regimen may contribute to this process and that concomitant thiopurine treatment may further promote γδ-T cell expansion. Therefore, we examined circulating γδ-T cells in patients with active CD before and after treatment with the anti-TNF-α antibodies infliximab (Remicade®) and adalimumab (Humira®). We confirmed the hypothesis raised by previous epidemiological studies that infliximab has a profound proliferative effect on γδ-T cells both in vivo and in vitro and that infliximab treatment results in the clonal expansion of γδ-T cells in specific CD patients. We hypothesise that markedly elevated γδ-T cell levels may identify CD patients prone to develop lymphoproliferative disease during anti-TNF-α therapy.

Materials and Methods

Patients and Healthy Volunteers

We examined 46 patients with active CD, diagnosed based on internationally accepted clinical, histopathological, and biochemical criteria [17]. The patient characteristics are listed in Tables S1 and 1, and clinical disease activity was estimated using the Harvey-Bradshaw Index (HBI) [18]. Systemic inflammation was evaluated using C-reactive protein levels; faecal calprotectin [19] was used to estimate mucosal inflammation. Treatment decisions were based on the combined evaluation of clinical, biochemical, and faecal disease markers. In total, twenty patients were treated with infliximab (Remicade®, Centocor; 5 mg/kg intravenously at days 0, 14, and 42), and 26 patients were treated with adalimumab (Humira®, Abbott). The adalimumab-treated patients received a

subcutaneous injection of 160 mg at week 0 and an injection of 80 mg at week 2. This was then followed by 40 mg maintenance injections every 2 weeks. Blood samples were obtained immediately before the administration of the anti-TNF-α agent and at days 1, 7, and 42 after the first treatment. One patient, number 47, was included post-hoc for further analyses and verification of our results. Sixteen healthy volunteers were recruited from the hospital staff to serve as controls. All participants provided written informed consent, and the study was approved by The Central Denmark Region Committee on Biomedical Research Ethics (j.no. 20040150).

Whole-blood Flow Cytometry

For flow cytometric staining, 100 μl of venous blood was incubated for 20 minutes at room temperature with the optimised amounts of the following fluorescent-conjugated antibodies: anti-αβ-TCR-FITC (clone WT-31), anti-Vδ2-PE (clone B6), anti-CD3-PerCP (clone SK7), anti-CD8-PE-Cy7 (clone RPA-T8), anti-γδ-TCR-APC (clone B1), and anti-CD4-APC-Cy7 (clone RPA-T4). All antibodies were from BD Biosciences (San Diego, CA). After 10 minutes, the red blood cells were lysed using 2 ml Pharm Lyse Buffer (BD Biosciences), and the samples were centrifuged for 5 minutes at $200 \times g$ at 20°C. The washed cells were resuspended in 200 μl phosphate-buffered saline (PBS) with 2% pooled human AB serum and 1% formaldehyde. Six-colour flow cytometry was performed within 4 hours on a FACSCanto flow cytometer (BD Biosciences). For each sample, 30,000 events in the forward/side scatter live lymphocyte gate were recorded. All γδ-T cell frequencies are out of total CD3+ T cells. The data were analysed using FACSDiva 5.1 Software (BD Biosciences).

Proliferation Assay

Peripheral blood mononuclear cells (PBMCs) were labelled with carboxyfluorescein succinimidyl ester (CFSE). The cells (1.5×10^6 cells/ml) were cultured in RPMI 1640 supplemented with 10% human AB serum, penicillin/streptomycin, and rIL-2 (200 IU/ml). Cells were cultured in the absence or presence of infliximab (0.1 or 1.0 μg/ml), adalimumab (0.1 or 1.0 μg/ml) or etanercept (1.0 μg/ml). Ustekinumab (1.0 μg/ml), an antibody against IL-12/23(p40), was used as a control. Recombinant human TNF-α (10 ng/ml) (Genzyme, Cambridge, MA) was added to selected wells. Proliferation was measured on day 5 using flow cytometry, as previously described [20].

Separation of γδ-T cells

PBMCs were isolated using Ficoll-Hypaque (GE Healthcare Bio-Sciences, Uppsala, Sweden) centrifugation, and γδ-T cells were purified using the TCRγ/δ T Cell Isolation Kit (Miltenyi Biotec, Bergisch Gladbach, Germany). Cell separation was performed on an AutoMACS Cell Separator, as recommended by the manufacturer. For all steps of the cell separation, we used PBS supplemented with 2 mM EDTA and 0.5% bovine serum albumin (BSA) (Sigma-Aldrich, Denmark). The purity of the γδ-T cells ranged between 90–95%.

Preparation of Genomic DNA and Total RNA

For fragment analysis, genomic DNA was extracted from 2 ml of EDTA-treated whole blood according to the manufacturer's instructions (NucleoSpin Blood L, Macherey-Nagel, Germany). DNA was dissolved in 5 mM Tris/HCl, pH 8.5. The quality of DNA was assessed by PCR amplification of three fragments (195 bp, 450 bp, and 650 bp) of the p53 gene. Combined extraction of mRNA and genomic DNA from enriched γδ-T cell

Table 1. Summarised baseline characteristics.

Variable	All	Infliximab	Adalimumab
n	46	20	26
Females, n (%)	22 (48%)	10 (50%)	12 (46%)
Age, median (range)	38 (19–67)	39 (19–61)	36 (20–67)
Smokers, n (%)	15 (33%)	5 (25%)	10 (39%)
Ileal disease, n (%)	28 (61%)	11 (55%)	17 (65%)
Colonic disease, n (%)	40 (87%)	17 (85%)	23 (89%)
Steroid, n (%)	5 (11%)	4 (20%)	1 (4%)
AZA/6MP, n (%)	15 (33%)	3 (15%)	12 (46%)
M, n (%)	3 (7%)	2 (10%)	1 (4%)
Previous infliximab, n (%)	19 (41%)	8 (40%)	11 (42%)
Previous adalimumab, n (%)	9 (20%)	1 (5%)	8 (31%)

fractions was performed according to the manufacturer's instructions (AllPrep DNA/RNA Mini Kit, Qiagen, Germany). The quality of the genomic DNA was verified using PCR, as described above, while mRNA quality was assessed using gel electrophoresis.

Multiplex PCR Assay

Identification of clonal populations with a specific T cell receptor delta (*TCRD*) rearrangement was performed according using the BIOMED-2 protocol [21], with slight modifications. PCR analysis of *TCRD* rearrangements was performed in a single tube with the *TCRD* primerset consisting of six Vδ and one Dδ2 (forward) primers or four Jδ and one Dδ3 primers (reverse) (Sigma Aldrich, St. Louis, MO, USA). Fluorescent labelling of the different Jδ and Dδ primers was done using HEX and 6FAM, respectively. The identification of clonal populations was performed by fragment analysis using a 3130xl genetic analyser and the Peak Scanner 1.0 Software (Applied Biosystems, Foster City, CA, USA). A clonal population was defined by the presence of a single peak or a predominant population. The fragment size was interpreted in accordance with the BIOMED-2 protocol. For all analyses, a second, confirmatory determination was performed.

DNA Heteroduplex Analysis

To verify the fragment analysis results, PCR products were denatured at 95°C for 5 minutes and then re-annealed at 4°C for 1 hour. Heteroduplex products were separated using 6% non-denaturating polyacrylamide electrophoresis in 0.5 × TBE-buffer, stained with 0.5 μg/ml ethidium bromide, and visualised using a UV-transilluminator.

Statistical analysis

Both parametric and non-parametric statistical tests were used. Unpaired bivariate comparisons of continuous variables were carried out using the Student's *t*-test. Dichotomous variables were compared using the χ^2 test. The mean and 95% confidence intervals (CI) are reported for continuous data. All correlations were evaluated using Spearman rho. A *p* value less than 0.05 was considered statistically significant. All statistical analyses were performed using SPSS 11.0 software.

Results

γδ-T cell Characteristics of CD Patients

We recruited 46 CD patients with an even distribution of gender and age (Tables S1 and 1). At the time of analysis, 20 patients were being treated with infliximab and 26 with adalimumab. In the latter group, 11 patients (42%) had previously received infliximab. Of the 46 CD patients, 35 (76%) had a γδ-T cell level comparable to the level found in healthy volunteers. CD patients had a mean frequency of 1.6% γδ-T cells of total CD3+ T cells, with values ranging from 1.3–2.0%. Similarly, healthy volunteers had a mean γδ-T cell frequency of 2.2% with values ranging from 1.7–2.8%. While no healthy volunteer had a γδ-T cell level above 5%, 11 CD patients (24%) exhibited a high baseline percentage of γδ-T cells, with frequencies ranging from 5% to 15% Of these 11 patients, all were non-smokers (*p* = 0.008, χ^2 test), and all had colonic inflammation (*p* = 0.14, χ^2 test). Of the 11 patients, 8 were males (*p* = 0.12, χ^2 test), and 7 were currently treated with azathioprine, 6-mercaptopurine, or methotrexate (*p* = 0.06, χ^2 test). The γδ-T cell levels were negatively correlated with age (*p* = 0.004, Spearman rho), with the highest γδ-T cell levels observed in young patients. In flow cytometric analysis we found a strong Vδ2 dominance within the γδ-T cell population (*p* = 0.005, Spearman rho) (Figure 1A). Interestingly, we found no

statistically significant associations between the γδ-T cell percentages and the disease activity markers (i.e., the Harvey-Bradshaw Index, faecal calprotectin, or C-reactive protein). This suggests that CD-mediated inflammation was not responsible for the observed changes in the γδ-T cell populations (Figure 1B).

In Vivo Clonal Expansion of γδ-T cells Induced by Infliximab

Subsequently, we investigated the dynamic changes in γδ-T cell populations during anti-TNF-α therapy. To be able to identify the direct effects and separate them from the secondary immunological effects, we examined changes in γδ-T cells at early points during anti-TNF-α therapy. The majority of CD patients exhibited only minor fluctuations in γδ-T cell frequency. However, in the subgroup of young male patients with high baseline γδ-T cells, we observed a dramatic increase following treatment; in fact, the percentage of γδ-T cells increased significantly within the first 24 hours after a single infliximab infusion (Figure 2).

In an attempt to confirm our findings that young male patients with a high baseline percentage of γδ-T cells appear to be prone to further γδ-T cell expansion during treatment with immunosuppressive drugs, we examined additional patients outside the original CD cohort. We identified a 33-year-old male CD patient (number 47) who had been treated with infliximab monotherapy at 8-week intervals for 9 years. He presented with an extraordinarily high baseline frequency of γδ-T cells (18–21% of all CD3+ T cells). These results were confirmed by three measurements performed between infliximab treatments over a 6-month period of stable clinical remission. From this high baseline frequency, the γδ-T cell population expanded to 25% 2 days after infliximab infusion and to 36% 3 months after treatment. Clonotypically, 90% of the γδ-T cells were Vδ2, suggesting the existence of a predominant γδ-T cell clone. Genescan analysis, as well as heteroduplex analysis, confirmed the monoclonal expansion of a γδ-T cell clone in the peripheral blood of this patient (Figure 3 A, B).

While the expansion of γδ-T cells was observed in CD patients treated with infliximab, no significant changes were observed in adalimumab-treated individuals. This finding was surprising, as the majority of patients in this group had received adalimumab in combination with additional immunosuppressive agents, such as thiopurines or methotrexate. One male CD patient with γδ-T cell expansion during maintenance therapy with infliximab and azathioprine was later shifted to adalimumab. Interestingly, unlike patients on continued infliximab treatment, we detected no further γδ-T cell expansion in this 'cross-over' patient following the change in therapy to adalimumab.

The Impact of Immunomodulators on γδ-T cells

In adalimumab-treated CD patients, the baseline level of γδ-T cells (mean 3.9%) was slightly higher than the baseline level in infliximab-treated CD patients (mean 2.7%) (*p* = 0.27, Student's *t*-test). This finding may, in part, be explained by the slightly higher frequency of patients treated with immunomodulators in the adalimumab group. In CD patients that received azathioprine, 6-mercaptopurine, or methotrexate, the baseline γδ-T cell represented an average of 4.4% of all T cells, with values ranging from 2.1–6.7%; these results were not significantly different from those found in CD patients not treated with immunomodulators (*p* = 0.17, Student's *t*-test). However, these values were masked by a subpopulation of CD patients with unusually high levels of γδ-T cells. Repeated blood sampling from this subgroup revealed persistently high percentages of γδ-T cells and we observed 8.5%

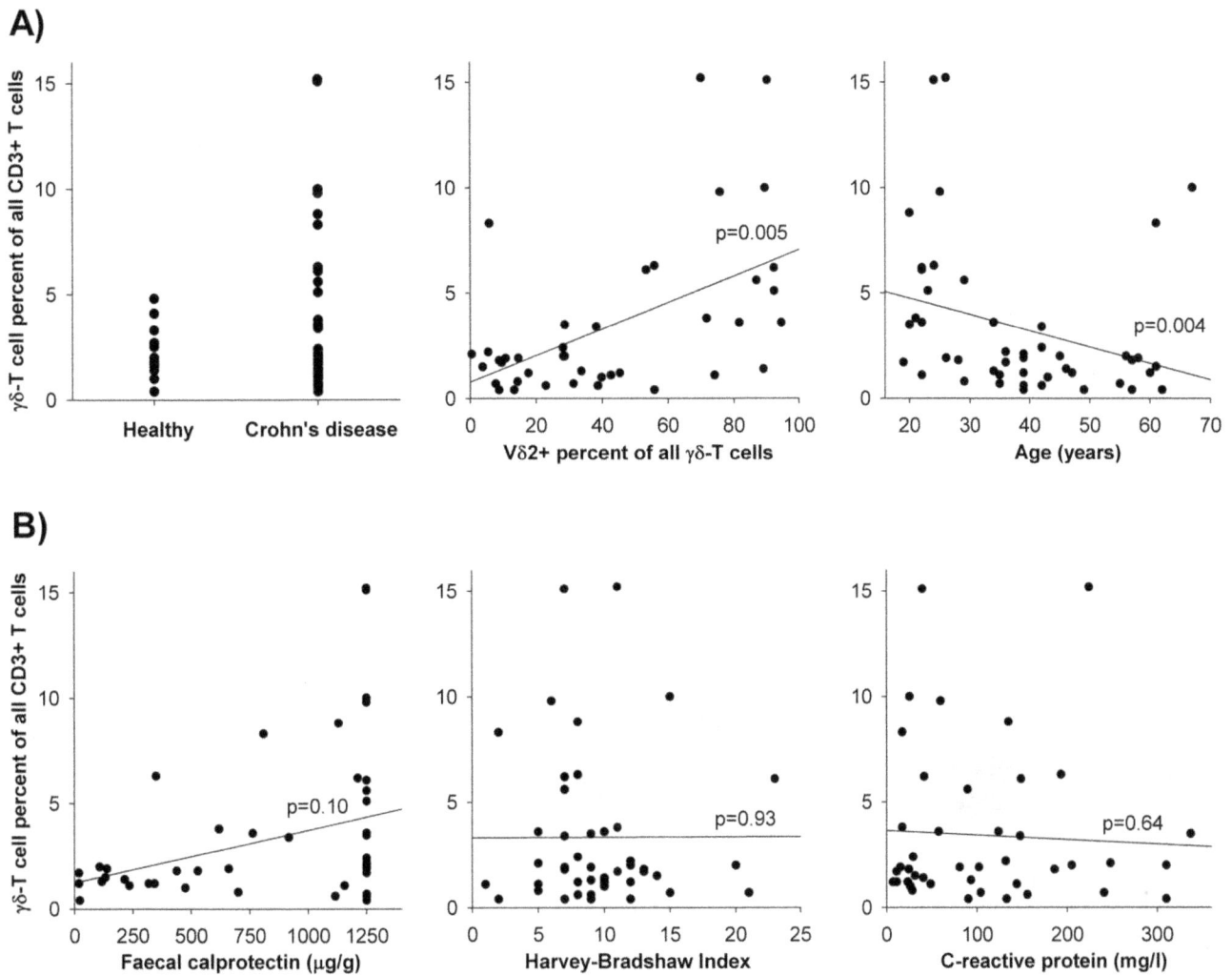

Figure 1. Baseline γδ-T cell characteristics in 46 CD patients. A) Of the 46 CD patients, 35 (76%) had a γδ-T cell level comparable to healthy volunteers, while 11 (24%) had a level ranging from 5 to 15% (left). The γδ-T cell level correlated with the expression of the Vδ2 subunit (middle), and the γδ-T cell levels correlated negatively with age (right). B) There were no statistically significant associations between γδ-T cell levels and markers of mucosal inflammation (faecal calprotectin), clinical disease activity (Harvey-Bradshaw Index), or systemic inflammation (C-reactive protein).

γδ-T cells in a patient (no. 8), receiving 6-mercaptopurine. Genescan analysis revealed a narrow oligoclonal γδ-T cell pattern with a dominant clone, which was confirmed by heteroduplex analysis (Figure 3 C, D). These results suggest that immunomodulators may induce proliferation and clonal selection of γδ-T cells.

In Vitro Proliferation of γδ-T cells Induced by Anti-TNF-α Agents

In order to discriminate between the direct effects of anti-TNF-α agents on γδ-T cells and the secondary, indirect effects that are mediated through the modulation of the inflammatory cytokine milieu in vivo, we examined the impact of anti-TNF-α agents on γδ-T cells in vitro. An in vitro analysis of the effects of infliximab, adalimumab, and the TNF-α receptor fusion protein etanercept on γδ-T cells would also allows us to exclude the possibility that the observed increases in circulating γδ-T cells was caused by a redistribution of the intestinal pool of γδ-T cells. When PBMCs from CD patients and healthy controls were cultured for 5 days, the anti-TNF-α agents induced the dose-dependent, selective proliferation of γδ-T cells in cultures supplemented with IL-2 (200 IU/ml). This proliferative effect was reversed by the addition

of recombinant TNF-α. Our findings with etanercept indicate that neutralisation of TNF-α in the culture medium, rather than the membrane-bound form of TNF-α, is involved (Figure 4). The induced proliferation was of the same magnitude for all anti-TNF-α agents. Proliferation was more pronounced in γδ-T cells compared to non-γδ-T cells, resulting in a relative increase in γδ-T cell frequency compared to other lymphocyte populations. Ustekinumab, an antibody against IL-12p40 that was used as a negative control did not affect the γδ-T cell frequency. Importantly, we observed a proliferative effect of anti-TNF-α agents on γδ-T cells from both CD patients and healthy controls, indicating that the proliferation of γδ-T cells in response to anti-TNF-α agents may not be restricted to CD patients.

Discussion

The clinical rationale for combined immunotherapy in the management of CD is well established and has been strengthened by the results of the recent SONIC study [22,23]. To date, the consensus is that the clinical benefits of immunomodulators outweigh the risk of lymphoma. Despite several case reports

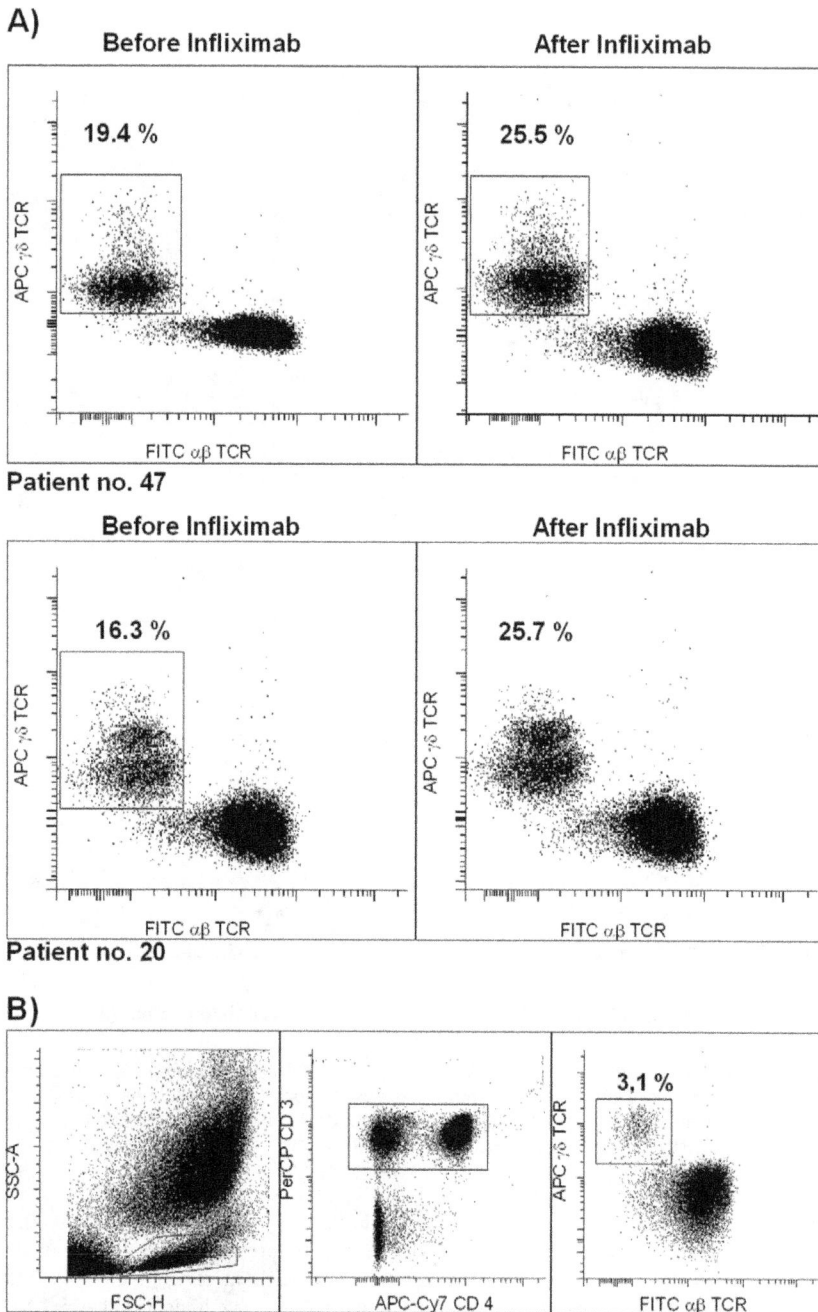

Figure 2. The γδ-T cell level of three CD patients who were treated with infliximab increased shortly after infliximab infusion. A) The results from two representative young male CD patients are shown. B) Illustration of the gating strategy. Using multicolour flow cytometry, γδ-T cells were identified by positive gating on live lymphocytes based on forward/side scatter (left panel), the selection of both CD4+ and CD4- cells among the CD3+ T cells (middle panel), and the separation of γδ-T cells from αβ-T cells (right panel).

detailing the development of HSTCL in CD patients, it has not been possible to determine if the anti-TNF-α agents played a primary role in the lymphomagenesis or if HSTCL should be regarded as the result of a clonal evolution within the more generalised chronic inflammatory processes that characterise IBD.

In the present study, we hypothesised that clonal γδ-T cell evolution, presumed to precede neoplastic transformation into HSTCL, may be promoted by the repeated administration of anti-TNF-α agents. In approximately 75% of CD patients, we observed a γδ-T cell frequency within the normal range (1–3% of all T cells).

However, in the remaining 25% of CD patients receiving immunomodulatory therapy, we observed a persistently high percentage of γδ-T cells; amongst these, young male patients appeared to be more prone to a clonal γδ-T cell expansion following repeated infliximab infusion. In addition, the analysis of *TCRD* rearrangements revealed a dominant clone in a female patient receiving monotherapy with 6-mercaptopurine, supporting the idea of stepwise clonal selection of γδ-T cells during combined immunotherapy.

These findings are difficult to interpret as being completely drug-induced as CD patients may have an increased number of

A) Genescan patient no. 47

size: 199,3bp
height: 3574

B) Heteroduplex analysis patient no. 47

200bp

100bp

Pt.no. 47   100 bp marker

C) Genescan patient no. 8

size: 184,6bp
height: 7120

D) Heteroduplex analysis patient no. 8

200bp

100bp

Pt.no 8   100 bp marker

E) Genescan healthy control

F) Heteroduplex analysis healthy control

200bp

100bp

Healthy control   100 bp marker

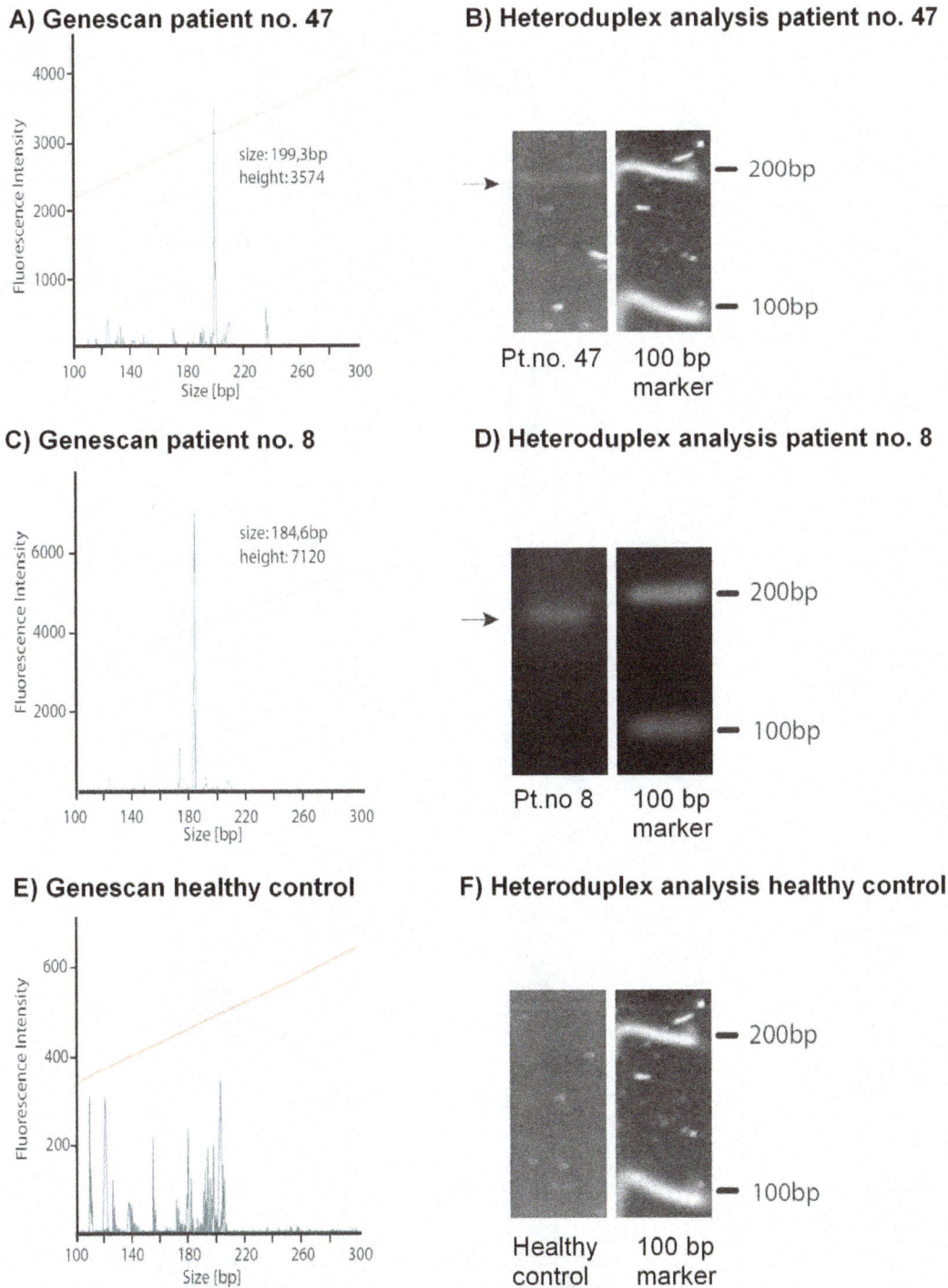

Figure 3. Analysis of *TCRD* rearrangement and heteroduplex analysis confirms the clonal expansion of γδ-T cells. For the fragment and heteroduplex analyses two representative examples of three CD patients are shown. A) Genescan analysis of patient number 47 shows a single monoclonal peak at 199 bp with a fluorescence intensity of 3574. B) Heteroduplex analysis of the same sample demonstrates a dominant band of approximately 200 bp. C) Genescan of patient number 8 shows a single monoclonal peak at 184 bp with a fluorescence intensity of 7120. D) Heteroduplex analysis of the same sample shows a very prominent band in the range of 180–190 bp. E) Genescan of a healthy control shows various polyclonal bands with different sizes and generally low fluorescence intensity. F) Heteroduplex analysis of the same sample resulted in a DNA smear with weak fluorescence intensity.

oligoclonal γδ-T cells caused by the chronic inflammation associated with this disease [2,3,24]. One explanation could be γδ-T cell recruitment from the inflamed intestinal mucosa, where γδ-T cells are abundant. However, new evidence challenges this hypothesis due to the lack of identical γδ-T cell clones in the intestinal mucosa and peripheral blood of CD patients [24]. Furthermore, a direct neoplastic effect on γδ-T cells cannot be ruled out. In fact, whether the chronic inflammation itself is

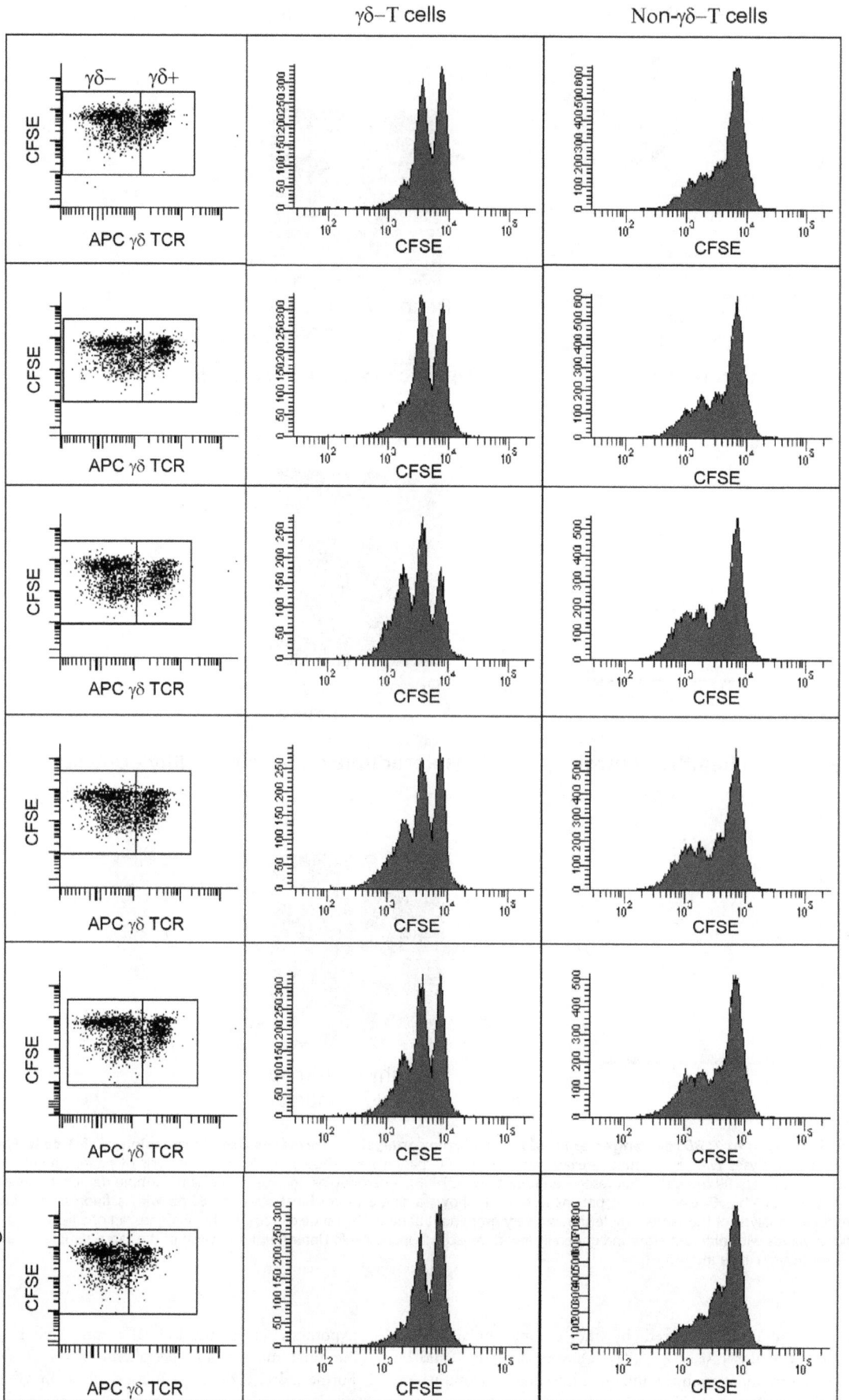

Figure 4. Anti-TNF-α agents promote the expansion of γδ-T cells in IL-2 stimulated PBMNC cultures. PBMCs were labelled with CFSE and were analysed by flow cytometry after 5 days of culture. γδ-T cells were stained with APC. The anti-TNF-α agents (infliximab, adalimumab, and etanercept) induced proliferation of γδ-T cells in vitro (middle panel), whereas the proliferation on non-γδ-T cells was negligible (right panel). In IL-2 - supplemented (200 IU/ml) PBMC cultures, infliximab (0.1 μg/ml or 1.0 μg/ml) induced a dose-dependent proliferation of γδ-T cells (middle panel). Etanercept induced proliferation of γδ-T cells in the same magnitude. The anti-IL-12p40 antibody ustekinumab had no effect on γδ-T cell proliferation in vitro. PBMCs from three CD patients and two healthy controls were analyzed.

responsible for the development of lymphoproliferative disorders in CD patients is still a matter of contention within the field [12]. Hence, the increased number of γδ-T cells in CD patients may simply reflect the degree of intestinal inflammation, and patients with refractory or uncontrolled inflammation may therefore be overrepresented in the group receiving thiopurines. However, in our study we did not find a significant correlation between the percentage of γδ-T cells and key inflammatory markers. Furthermore, inflammation certainly cannot explain the massive increase in γδ-T cells seen after infliximab treatment in cases where the disease activity index and systemic and intestinal inflammatory markers declined.

This study was focused on investigating the impact of immuno suppressive therapy on γδ-T cells and its possible role in lymphomagenesis thus allowing the identification of at risk patients. Our results indicate that γδ-T cells can be modulated by anti-TNF-α therapy in vitro, which may represent a first step to substantiate a causal role of infliximab in γδ-T cell malignancies. In this context, we measured changes in the frequency of γδ-T cells in the peripheral blood of CD patients as early as 24 hours after infliximab infusion. Three male patients showed a marked response, nearly doubling their number of γδ-T cells. The observed changes in γδ-T cells appeared robust compared with the minor changes we observed in other lymphocyte subpopulations [25]. In the light of the well-known preponderance of cases of HSTCL in males, it is noteworthy that our study only demonstrated high levels of γδ-T cell expansion in male CD patients. As a proof of concept, we analysed the peripheral blood of a CD patient who had undergone long-term treatment with infliximab (9 years). Interestingly, we found unusually high levels of γδ-T cells (on average 20% of all T cells), which increased further to 36% during the study period. Genescan analysis of *TCRD* rearrangements in cells from this patient showed a clonal expansion of γδ-T cells, which was confirmed by heteroduplex analysis. This finding, together with our in vitro data, suggests the infliximab-induced clonal expansion of γδ-T cells in the peripheral blood rather than a redistribution of the intestinal γδ-T cells. Furthermore, the expanded γδ-T cells were mainly of the Vδ2 subtype, and not δ-1, as one would expect if they were of mucosal origin [1]. However, we cannot yet say that this dominant clone actually represents a premalignant transformation as oligoclonal γδ-T cell populations are occasionally found in CD patients without the development of lymphomas [24]. Additionally, we do not have data confirming that the same γδ-T cell clone actually expanded as a direct consequence of repeated infliximab infusions. However, it is remarkable that the strongest increase in the proportion of γδ-T cells was seen in young males receiving infliximab.

The mechanisms underlying the action of thiopurines in the treatment of IBD are poorly understood [26]. The observed increased frequency of γδ-T cells following treatment with thiopurines may be a double-edged sword, as γδ-T cell expansion could represent a principal therapeutic mechanism in CD, while at the same time predisposing the patient to lymphoma. Gene expression profiling has recently established that γδ-T cell lymphomas have distinct molecular signatures [4]. In the future, various gene profiling strategies may be able to identify premalignant genetic lesions in CD patients receiving combined immunotherapy [27,28].

The proliferation of γδ-T cells in vivo was not seen in patients treated with adalimumab. We believe that this could be the result of the chosen observation window, dosage, or method of administration (subcutaneous *vs.* intravenous) rather than a genuine difference in intrinsic therapeutic mechanisms. Our in vitro data suggest that the γδ-T cell expansion is a dose-dependent effect of multiple anti-TNF-α reagents. However, a valid in vivo comparison of the drugs is difficult to undertake, as the conventional clinical algorithm dictates that most CD patients on adalimumab will have received infliximab earlier. It should be noted, however that lower doses of infliximab are recommended (3 vs. 5 mg/kg) in the treatment of rheumatoid arthritis, which might explain the single case of HSTCL that has been reported in patients with rheumatoid arthritis.

We present an example of how epidemiological data can be translated to the patient level and further to the in vitro level. Our results confirm earlier findings that the number of γδ-T cells is increased in a subgroup of CD patients; however, in our study, the increased γδ-T cell frequency was independent of disease activity. A subset of CD patients treated with thiopurines or methotrexate had an extremely high baseline frequency of γδ-T cells. These patients appear to have a lower threshold for expansion of γδ-T cells when treated with infliximab, which we found to be a potent inducer of γδ-T cells in vitro. Further studies are warranted to substantiate our observation that inflixmab may promote lymphomagenesis by the repeated clonal expansion of γδ-T cells.

Acknowledgments

The authors would like to thank Rikke Andersen for excellent technical assistance and Lars Iversen, Department of Dermatology, Aarhus University Hospital, for helpful advice regarding the in vitro studies.

Author Contributions

Conceived and designed the experiments: JK CLH. Performed the experiments: JK CLH AD HS FSP. Analyzed the data: JK CLH AD HS FD. Contributed reagents/materials/analysis tools: FSP FD LAC JA JFD. Wrote the paper: JK CLH FD JA JFD LAC. Recruited the patients: JA LAC JFD.

References

1. Beetz S, Wesch D, Marischen L, Welte S, Oberg HH, et al. (2008) Innate immune functions of human gammadelta T cells. Immunobiology 213: 173–182.

2. Soderstrom K, Bucht A, Halapi E, Gronberg A, Magnusson I, et al. (1996) Increased frequency of abnormal gamma delta T cells in blood of patients with inflammatory bowel diseases. J Immunol 156: 2331–2339.

3. Giacomelli R, Parzanese I, Frieri G, Passacantando A, Pizzuto F, et al. (1994) Increase of circulating gamma/delta T lymphocytes in the peripheral blood of patients affected by active inflammatory bowel disease. Clin Exp Immunol 98: 83–88.

4. Miyazaki K, Yamaguchi M, Imai H, Kobayashi T, Tamaru S, et al. (2009) Gene expression profiling of peripheral T-cell lymphoma including gammadelta T-cell lymphoma. Blood 113: 1071–1074.

5. Mackey AC, Green L, Liang LC, Dinndorf P, Avigan M (2007) Hepatosplenic T cell lymphoma associated with infliximab use in young patients treated for inflammatory bowel disease. J Pediatr Gastroenterol Nutr 44: 265–267.

6. Belhadj K, Reyes F, Farcet JP, Tilly H, Bastard C, et al. (2003) Hepatosplenic gammadelta T-cell lymphoma is a rare clinicopathologic entity with poor outcome: report on a series of 21 patients. Blood 102: 4261–4269.

7. Thayu M, Markowitz JE, Mamula P, Russo PA, Muinos WI, et al. (2005) Hepatosplenic T-cell lymphoma in an adolescent patient after immunomodulator and biologic therapy for Crohn disease. J Pediatr Gastroenterol Nutr 40: 220–222.

8. Mackey AC, Green L, Leptak C, Avigan M (2009) Hepatosplenic T cell lymphoma associated with infliximab use in young patients treated for inflammatory bowel disease: update. J Pediatr Gastroenterol Nutr 48: 386–388.

9. Ochenrider MG, Patterson DJ, Aboulafia DM (2010) Hepatosplenic T-cell lymphoma in a young man with Crohn's disease: case report and literature review. Clin Lymphoma Myeloma Leuk 10: 144–148.

10. Moran G, Dillon J, Green J (2009) Crohn's disease, hepatosplenic T-cell lymphoma and no biological therapy: are we barking up the wrong tree? Inflamm Bowel Dis 15: 1281–1282.

11. Navarro JT, Ribera JM, Mate JL, Granada I, Junca J, et al. (2003) Hepatosplenic T-gammadelta lymphoma in a patient with Crohn's disease treated with azathioprine. Leuk Lymphoma 44: 531–533.

12. Beaugerie L, Brousse N, Bouvier AM, Colombel JF, Lemann M, et al. (2009) Lymphoproliferative disorders in patients receiving thiopurines for inflammatory bowel disease: a prospective observational cohort study. Lancet 374: 1617–1625.

13. Rosh JR, Gross T, Mamula P, Griffiths A, Hyams J (2007) Hepatosplenic T-cell lymphoma in adolescents and young adults with Crohn's disease: a cautionary tale? Inflamm Bowel Dis 13: 1024–1030.

14. D'Haens G, Rutgeerts P (2009) Immunosuppression-associated lymphoma in IBD. Lancet 374: 1572–1573.

15. Shale M, Kanfer E, Panaccione R, Ghosh S (2008) Hepatosplenic T cell lymphoma in inflammatory bowel disease. Gut 57: 1639–1641.

16. Sokol H, Beaugerie L (2009) Inflammatory bowel disease and lymphoproliferative disorders: the dust is starting to settle. Gut 58: 1427–1436.

17. Stange EF, Travis SP, Vermeire S, Beglinger C, Kupcinkas L, et al. (2006) European evidence based consensus on the diagnosis and management of Crohn's disease: definitions and diagnosis. Gut 55 Suppl 1: i1–15.

18. Harvey RF, Bradshaw JM (1980) A simple index of Crohn's-disease activity. Lancet 1: 514.

19. Sipponen T, Savilahti E, Karkkainen P, Kolho KL, Nuutinen H, et al. (2008) Fecal calprotectin, lactoferrin, and endoscopic disease activity in monitoring anti-TNF-alpha therapy for Crohn's disease. Inflamm Bowel Dis 14: 1392–1398.

20. Dige A, Hvas CL, Kelsen J, Deleuran B, Dahlerup JF, et al. (2010) Ethylene-Diamine-Tetra-Acetate (EDTA) mimics the effect of regulatory T cells in suppression assays: a potential pitfall when using AutoMACS-separated cells. J Immunol Methods 353: 141–144.

21. van Dongen JJ, Langerak AW, Bruggemann M, Evans PA, Hummel M, et al. (2003) Design and standardization of PCR primers and protocols for detection of clonal immunoglobulin and T-cell receptor gene recombinations in suspect lymphoproliferations: report of the BIOMED-2 Concerted Action BMH4-CT98-3936. Leukemia 17: 2257–2317.

22. Prefontaine E, Sutherland LR, Macdonald JK, Cepoiu M (2009) Azathioprine or 6-mercaptopurine for maintenance of remission in Crohn's disease. Cochrane Database Syst Rev CD000067.

23. Colombel JF, Sandborn WJ, Reinisch W, Mantzaris GJ, Kornbluth A, et al. (2010) Infliximab, azathioprine, or combination therapy for Crohn's disease. N Engl J Med 362: 1383–1395.

24. Holtmeier W, Hennemann A, May E, Duchmann R, Caspary WF (2002) T cell receptor delta repertoire in inflamed and noninflamed colon of patients with IBD analyzed by CDR3 spectratyping. Am J Physiol Gastrointest Liver Physiol 282: G1024–G1034.

25. Hvas CL, Kelsen J, Agnholt J, Dige A, Christensen LA, et al. (2010) Discrete changes in circulating regulatory T cells during infliximab treatment of Crohn's disease. Autoimmunity 43: 325–333.

26. Atreya I, Neurath MF (2009) Understanding the delayed onset of action of azathioprine in IBD: are we there yet? Gut 58: 325–326.

27. Iqbal J, Liu Z, Deffenbacher K, Chan WC (2009) Gene expression profiling in lymphoma diagnosis and management. Best Pract Res Clin Haematol 22: 191–210.

28. Iqbal J, Weisenburger DD, Greiner TC, Vose JM, McKeithan T, et al. (2010) Molecular signatures to improve diagnosis in peripheral T-cell lymphoma and prognostication in angioimmunoblastic T-cell lymphoma. Blood 115: 1026–1036.

9

SNP-SNP Interactions Discovered by Logic Regression Explain Crohn's Disease Genetics

Irina Dinu[1,9], Surakameth Mahasirimongkol[2,9], Qi Liu[1], Hideki Yanai[2,3], Noha Sharaf Eldin[1], Erin Kreiter[1], Xuan Wu[1], Shahab Jabbari[1], Katsushi Tokunaga[2], Yutaka Yasui[1]*

1 School of Public Health, University of Alberta, Edmonton, Alberta, Canada, 2 Department of Human Genetics, School of International Health, Graduate School of Medicine, University of Tokyo, Tokyo, Japan, 3 Fukujuji Hospital, Japan Anti-Tuberculosis Association, Kiyose, Japan

Abstract

In genome-wide association studies (GWAS), the association between each single nucleotide polymorphism (SNP) and a phenotype is assessed statistically. To further explore genetic associations in GWAS, we considered two specific forms of biologically plausible SNP-SNP interactions, 'SNP intersection' and 'SNP union,' and analyzed the Crohn's Disease (CD) GWAS data of the Wellcome Trust Case Control Consortium for these interactions using a limited form of logic regression. We found strong evidence of CD-association for 195 genes, identifying novel susceptibility genes (e.g., *ISX, SLCO6A1, TMEM183A*) as well as confirming many previously identified susceptibility genes in CD GWAS (e.g., *IL23R, NOD2, CYLD, NKX2-3, IL12RB2, ATG16L1*). Notably, 37 of the 59 chromosomal locations indicated for CD-association by a meta-analysis of CD GWAS, involving over 22,000 cases and 29,000 controls, were represented in the 195 genes, as well as some chromosomal locations previously indicated only in linkage studies, but not in GWAS. We repeated the analysis with two smaller GWASs from the Database of Genotype and Phenotype (dbGaP): in spite of differences of populations and study power across the three datasets, we observed some consistencies across the three datasets. Notable examples included *TMEM183A* and *SLCO6A1* which exhibited strong evidence consistently in our WTCCC and both of the dbGaP SNP-SNP interaction analyses. Examining these specific forms of SNP interactions could identify additional genetic associations from GWAS. R codes, data examples, and a ReadMe file are available for download from our website: http://www.ualberta.ca/~yyasui/homepage.html.

Editor: Jan Wehkamp, Dr. Margarete Fischer-Bosch and University of Tübingen, Germany

Funding: This project was partially funded by an operating grant from the Canadian Institutes of Health Research to YY, ID, and SM, and by the Research Grants in the Natural Sciences (No. 30 in FY 2009) from the Mitsubishi Foundation to KT, YY, and YH. YY is supported by the Canada Research Chair Program, and YY, NSE, and EK are supported by the Alberta Innovates. NSE is supported by the Alberta Cancer Foundation. The funders had no role in study design, data collection and analysis, decision to publish, or preparation of the manuscript.

Competing Interests: The authors have declared that no competing interests exist.

* E-mail: yyasui@ualberta.ca

9 These authors contributed equally to this work.

Introduction

Analysis of genome-wide association studies (GWAS) often focuses on identifying individual single nucleotide polymorphisms (SNPs) that modify the risk of a phenotype, assuming the underlying association of an individual SNP without considering the involvement of any other SNPs. GWASs of Crohn's Disease (CD) have also focused largely on finding such *marginal* associations of individual SNPs, where the association of each SNP with CD risk is evaluated without considering other SNPs. If individual SNPs (or the regions tagged by them) are independently critical in the CD-risk-altering biological functions, this approach would be effective. This may be the case for the association between rs11209026 of the *IL23R* gene and CD risk, where the marginal association is quantified as an estimated odds ratio of 2.66[1]. The other SNPs that are statistically significantly associated with CD risk, however, show very weak associations with estimated odds ratios typically in the range of less than 1.5. In addition, the sum of such marginal associations is far from describing the estimated degree of genetic contributions to the risk of CD [1]. A possible explanation for this may be that an individual SNP (or a region

tagged by it) is not independently critical in the biological functions that affect the CD-risk: rather, interaction among multiple SNPs (or regions tagged by them) may *jointly* affect the CD-risk. Specifically, the following two forms of SNP-SNP interactions may be motivated biologically. One is the *SNP intersection* form using the set theory terminology, in which *all of* the SNPs in a set must take their respective high-risk genotypes for CD risk to be elevated, where one, or a subset, of the set is insufficient to influence CD-risk-altering biological functions. That is, an increase in the CD-risk requires all SNPs (i.e., SNP-A *and* SNP-B *and* ...) to take their respective high-risk genotypes. This form of interaction is similar to a set of sequential mutations that must accumulate before a cell transforms in the multistage carcinogenesis theory. The other form of SNP-SNP interaction that is biologically plausible is motivated by the notion of genetic heterogeneity. Specifically, CD risk may be elevated through multiple independent ways, each of which may be a SNP-intersection or an individual SNP (i.e., (SNP-A *and* SNP-B) *or* (SNP-C) each taking its respective high-risk genotype. This form of SNP-SNP interaction is referred to as a *SNP union*, also derived from the set theory terminology. Under a single or combination of SNP intersections and SNP unions, assessing the independent *marginal* effect of each individual SNP without considering these interaction forms will either fail to discover, or observe only weak, association between the individual SNP and the phenotype of interest.

To incorporate these specific forms of SNP-SNP interactions in GWAS data analysis, we propose using logic regression to search for sets of SNPs that are jointly associated with the phenotype of interest in the form of a single SNP intersection or union, or in combinations of thereof [2]. Logic regression is an innovative and powerful statistical learning technique that is used to model an outcome (e.g., the disease status in a case-control study) with intersections and/or unions of multiple potential predictors that are primarily binary, such as indicators of SNP genotypes (i.e., indicators of the minor-allele homozygous and indicators of the heterozygous and the minor-allele homozygous). As such, logic regression can select a model that may involve various intersections and/or unions of SNPs within a gene, or any set of SNPs (e.g., SNPs of genes in a certain biological pathway), that are associated with a phenotype. Logic regression has been applied successfully to a number of SNP data analyses *with selected candidate genes* [3–11]. To our knowledge, however, it has not been applied to GWAS analysis due to the considerable computational demands in searching for SNP intersection/union combinations among a large number of SNPs in GWASs.

Materials and Methods

Incorporating specific forms of SNP-SNP interactions in GWAS

Our logic-regression-based gene-level SNP-SNP-interaction analysis of GWAS data can be summarized as follows. Combinations of SNP intersections and unions can be expressed mathematically as Boolean combinations, such as $(X1 \wedge X2) \vee X3^c$, where "$\wedge$", "$\vee$", and "^{c}" represents intersection (AND), union (OR), and complement (NOT), and X's are indicators of SNP genotypes. The logic regression model takes the form:

$$logit(E[Y]) = \beta_0 + \beta_1 L_1 + \beta_2 L_2 + \ldots + \beta_p L_p$$

where Y is a binary phenotype, CD cases versus controls, β_0, β_1,... β_p are the parameters, and L_1, L_2, ..., L_p are Boolean combinations of genotype indicators of SNPs within a gene, also called logic trees. The logic trees are selected adaptively, using a Simulated Annealing algorithm, and based on deviance as the model fit measure [2]. Our logic-regression-based SNP-SNP interaction analysis uses genes with at least two genotyped SNPs. To reduce redundancy of logic trees that genotype indicators of SNPs within a gene can form, we removed SNPs within each gene sequentially, before logic regression, such that no pair of remaining SNPs within a gene had linkage disequilibrium ($r^2 \geq 0.8$). In each logic regression fit, we allowed a maximum of two Boolean combinations (Ls) of at most five indicators of SNP genotypes in total. Note that these constraints are necessary in GWAS because logic regression must search a large number of potential combinations, and therefore comes with a high computational cost. To correct for the inherent instability of the performance measure when searching a large space, we refit the logic regression 20 times, starting the algorithm with 20 different initial values: this process was applied to the original dataset as well as 20 datasets obtained by permutations of the case-control labels. Of the 20 results produced by the 20 starting values, we selected the best fit, measured by deviance.

Measure of evidence of association

Running logic regression for each gene in the original dataset, as well as their 20 case-control-label permuted datasets, yields an approximate Bayes Factor (BF) for each gene. The BF is approximated by the corresponding Likelihood Ratio in this case (which eliminates the need to specify priors, similar to the approximation used by Bayesian Information Criterion for BF), in the base-10 logarithm (equivalent to LOD Score), where the denominator is the median of 19 (log10) maximum likelihoods from the 19 permuted datasets (20 minus one because BF of a permuted dataset should not use its own BF in calculating the median of BF from the permuted datasets). An important feature of this approximate BF is that the denominator standardizes for the higher potential for genes with larger numbers of SNPs to overfit. We follow the Wellcome Trust Case Control Consortium (WTCCC) 's framework of using BF as the measure of evidence of the observed association between each gene and CD risk[12]. Specifically, suppose we have N genes to be investigated, of which 10 genes are assumed to be truly associated with CD risk. The prior odds for CD-risk association for any gene is therefore 10/(N-10). To make the posterior odds of CD-risk association for a gene to 10 (i.e., probability that the gene is associated with CD risk is 10/11, or approximately 0.91), a likelihood ratio for the association over no association (i.e., the BF under the same-size logic-regression model) has to be (N-10). Based on the number of genes we examined in the WTCCC dataset (13,106 after mapping), the WTCCC framework above specifies a BF of 4.12 as the threshold, above which there is strong evidence of association between the gene and CD risk. The P-value for each gene is calculated as the proportion of all permuted BF values of *all genes* larger than the gene's observed BF. This p-value calculation properly takes the multiple testing into account.

We checked if our BF-based hypothesis testing has a proper size (i.e. control over the false positive rate) by using a simulation study. We randomly chose 200 genes from Chromosome 1 (Chromosome 1 contains approximately 1,300 genes after mapping). We simulated a total of 50 null hypothesis datasets by shuffling case-control labels randomly and imposing an equal number of cases and controls in each dataset. We ran the logic-regression-based SNP-SNP interaction analysis and estimated p-value for each of the 200 genes in each of the 50 null datasets. The 10,000 p-values roughly followed a uniform distribution (data not shown), indicating that our testing procedure has a proper size and proper control over the false positive rate.

WTCCC and dbGaP Studies

We applied the logic-regression-based SNP-SNP interaction analysis method to the WTCCC's GWAS data comparing 2,005 CD cases to the 1,502 members of the British 1958 birth control cohort (58C) plus the 1,500 controls of the UK Blood Service sample: these used Affymetrix GeneChip Human Mapping 500K Array Sets [12]. We also repeated the analysis with two much smaller GWASs: the Database of Genotype and Phenotype (dbGaP) non-Jewish case-control GWAS data on 513 cases and 515 controls; and dbGaP Jewish case-control GWAS data on 300 cases and 432 controls. The dbGaP GWAS used the Illumina Sentrix HumanHap300 Genotyping BeadChip [13]. For exclusion of cases and controls from the WTCCC analysis, we followed the WTCCC's recommendations based on the sample call rates and evidence of recent non-European ancestry [12]. Specifically, 24 control subjects were excluded from the 1958 British birth cohort of controls, 42 control subjects were excluded from the UK Blood Service cohort of controls, and 257 CD cases were not used in the analysis. In the two dbGaP analyses, we removed subjects with sample call rates less than 95% (15 controls and 17 cases were excluded from the non-Jewish data, and three controls and nine cases were excluded from the Jewish data).

The genotype calls of the WTCCC were generated by the Chiamo calling algorithm. Following the WTCCC's recommendations, we only considered genotype calls with confidence score >0.9, and treated the rest of the calls as missing genotypes. SNPs with SNP call rates less than 95% were removed. We also removed SNPs based on their minor allele frequencies: the default minor allele frequency cutoff in the GenABEL R package was used (2.5/ N where N is the number of subjects), resulting in cutoffs of 0.05% for the WTCCC database and 0.3% for the Jewish and non-Jewish dbGaP databases. We used a cutoff of 0.2 for the Hardy-Weinberg Equilibrium (HWE) test's false discovery rates, based on controls. SNP-gene mapping files were retrieved from the OpenBioinformatics website (http://www.openbioinformatics.org/gengen/ tutorial_calculate_gsea.html#_Toc210887414).

We checked the homogeneity of the three populations, WTCCC, dbGaP non-Jewish and Jewish, by running Principal Component Analysis using the R package GenABEL [14]. We computed a matrix of genomic kinship between all pairs of subjects, based on the 22,498 SNPs common to the three datasets. More specifically, we calculated the average Identity-by-State (IBS) for the 6,400 subjects (4,684, 720, and 996 subjects from the WTCCC, dbGaP non-Jewish, and dbGaP Jewish studies, respectively), as the pairwise similarity measure. We then performed Principal Component Analysis based on the pairwise-similarity matrix of average IBS. A plot of the first two principal components, displayed in Figure S1, suggests that dbGaP Jewish population was genetically quite different from the WTCCC and the dbGaP non-Jewish populations, but the latter two populations also showed some appreciable between-population differences and within-population heterogeneity (Figure S1).

Results

There were 195 genes with strong evidence of association between the gene and CD risk in the logic-regression gene-level SNP-SNP-interaction analysis of the WTCCC GWAS data, 40 of which are listed in Table 1 (all are shown in Table S1). Notably, all nine regions of the genome showing strong evidence of association by the single-SNP analysis of WTCCC data[12], as well as seven out of the eight regions showing moderate evidence of association, were represented among the 195 genes. Thirty-seven (63%) of the 59 chromosomal locations, that were previously identified by a meta-analysis of single-SNP studies that involved over 22,000 cases and 29,000 controls [1], were included in the 195 genes. Also included in the 195 genes that showed strong evidence of association were three genes located in *IBD1* (Chr 16q12), two genes in *IBD2* (Chr 12q13), six genes in *IBD3* (Chr 6p21, HLA region), eight genes in *IBD5* (Chr 5q31-33), two genes in *IBD6* (Chr 19p13), and one gene in *IBD7* (Chr 1p36), well-established regions of chromosomes for CD risk: no gene in *IBD4* (Chr 14q11-12) was included, however. In addition, there were a number of chromosome regions that did not show strong or moderate evidence of association in the single-SNP analysis of WTCCC, but had three or more genes appearing among the 195 genes, namely, 1q32, 2q14, 8p12, 10q22, 10q26, 11p14, and 18q22. These are indicated by green highlighting in the tables. Furthermore, there are clusters corresponding to certain families of genes in the 195 genes. For example, genes associated with phosphoprotein phosphatase activity (e.g., *PPM1K, PPM1L, PPP2R2C, PTPN2*) showed strong evidence of association with CD risk, of which only *PTPN2* had been previously indicated.

Table 1. Forty genes with the strongest evidence for association with Crohn's Disease risk, with chromosomal locations, numbers of SNPs, approximate p-values, and Bayes factors.

Gene Name	Chromosome	#SNPs	p-value	C.BF
ISX	22q12	84	$<3.8\times10^{-6}$	148.5
SEMA6A*	5q23	152	$<3.8\times10^{-6}$	96.2
GTF3C4	9q34	4	$<3.8\times10^{-6}$	91.8
PTGFRN	1p13	15	$<3.8\times10^{-6}$	85.5
ADRA1B**	5q33	45	$<3.8\times10^{-6}$	82.3
MYLK3	16q11	2	$<3.8\times10^{-6}$	77.0
HTR3B	11q23	10	$<3.8\times10^{-6}$	75.7
RRP15	1q41	29	$<3.8\times10^{-6}$	75.4
RGL1	1q25	20	$<3.8\times10^{-6}$	69.9
SORBS1	10q23	46	$<3.8\times10^{-6}$	65.5
CALCOCO1	12q13	15	$<3.8\times10^{-6}$	57.9
TMEM156	4p14	13	$<3.8\times10^{-6}$	52.7
XRCC6BP1	12q14	38	$<3.8\times10^{-6}$	45.9
FXR1	3q28	7	$<3.8\times10^{-6}$	37.7
GARNL1	14q13	4	$<3.8\times10^{-6}$	34.9
GPR161*	1q24	7	$<3.8\times10^{-6}$	30.9
SORCS1**	10q23-q25	265	$<3.8\times10^{-6}$	30.6
SAC*	1q24	13	$<3.8\times10^{-6}$	28.4
LRP1B	2q21	241	$<3.8\times10^{-6}$	27.2
C18orf62	18q23	79	$<3.8\times10^{-6}$	25.9
CSRP1	1q32+	17	$<3.8\times10^{-6}$	24.2
POU6F2	7p14	58	$<3.8\times10^{-6}$	22.6
LEF1	4q23-q25	31	$<3.8\times10^{-6}$	22.3
SEL1L	14q31	170	$<3.8\times10^{-6}$	21.9
SVIP	11p14+	88	$<3.8\times10^{-6}$	21.7
VRK1	14q32	128	$<3.8\times10^{-6}$	19.3
GLRX3	10q26+	79	$<3.8\times10^{-6}$	18.4
ID4*	6p22	79	$<3.8\times10^{-6}$	15.3
CDH10	5p14	107	$<3.8\times10^{-6}$	14.9
NOD2**	16q21	5	$<3.8\times10^{-6}$	14.6
NHLRC1*	6p22	7	$<3.8\times10^{-6}$	14.0
FMN2	1q43	60	$<3.8\times10^{-6}$	14.0
IL23R**	1p31	11	$<3.8\times10^{-6}$	13.6
PTGER4**	5p13	46	$<3.8\times10^{-6}$	13.5
CTNNA3	10q22+	257	$<3.8\times10^{-6}$	13.3
PNPLA6	19p13	5	$<3.8\times10^{-6}$	13.0
FBXO15	18q22+	94	$<3.8\times10^{-6}$	12.5
ATG16L1**	2q37	7	$<3.8\times10^{-6}$	12.4
RTP2	3q27	4	$<3.8\times10^{-6}$	12.0
KCNIP4	4p15	154	$<3.8\times10-6$	11.8

indicates genes in the chromosomal locations where the WTCCC single-SNP analysis showed **strong evidence.
*indicates genes in the chromosomal locations where the WTCCC single-SNP analysis showed **moderate** evidence.
+indicates chromosomal locations are those with three or more genes in the 195 genes (see Table S1) showing strong evidence in our WTCCC logic-regression-based analysis, but without strong or moderate evidence in the single-SNP analysis of WTCCC.

Intestine Specific Homeobox (*ISX*) was the gene most strongly associated with CD risk in our WTCCC logic-regression-based analysis and represents a new CD susceptibility gene. Homeobox genes encode DNA-binding proteins, of which many are thought to be involved in early embryonic development. *ISX* is a transcription factor that regulates gene expression in the intestine [15]. The logic structure of *ISX* is shown in Table 2. Based on the genotypes of the SNPs in the two trees, the following three risk groups shown in Table 2 emerge: a reference risk group (1540 cases/2562 controls); a low risk group (1 cases/372 controls, estimated odds ratio 0.0045); and a high risk group (207 cases/2 controls, estimated odds ratio 172.2). Both the low and high risk groups are defined by uncommon variants with over 150-fold effect sizes. We confirmed the allele frequencies of these SNPs with the Hapmap CEU population as an informal check of the possibility of genotyping errors for the rare variants.

We note that using the WTCCC dataset for discovery and the dbGaP non-Jewish and Jewish datasets for replication is untenable, because of the observed population differences (Figure S1) and the difference in study power due to the large differences in sample sizes. Another disadvantage is the difference in genotyping platforms between these data sets, including their genotyping errors and genomic coverage. Nonetheless, we applied the same method of analysis to the dbGaP's non-Jewish and Jewish GWAS datasets. Since this analysis focused on the 195 genes with strong evidence of association with CD risk in the WTCCC analysis, the BF threshold for strong evidence for this stage of the analysis is 2.29. We applied this threshold to the larger BF of the two dbGaP GWAS analyses. Table 3 lists 17 genes that showed strong evidence for their CD-risk association in both stages of the analysis. Seven of the seventeen genes in Table 3 are located in regions of the genome that showed strong or moderate evidence of association with CD by the single-SNP analysis of WTCCC data [12]. Of the remaining ten genes, *TMEM183A* and *NEK2* are both located in Chromosome 1q32. Chromosome 1q32 has been shown to be associated with the risk of Ankylosing Spondylitis that is linked to CD [16]: this region was not identified by the single-SNP WTCCC or dbGaP analyses. A gene of organic anion transporter, *SLCO6A1*, showed strong evidence of association in all three GWASs, in spite of no previous implication of CD-risk association: this is significant in view of the known association of *SLC22A4* and *SLC22A5* (*IBD5*), genes of organic cation transporters, with CD risk [17]. In addition to *SLCO6A1*, three genes (*IL23R*, *NOD2*, and *TMEM183A*) showed consistently strong evidence across the three datasets.

Discussion

Our results illustrate the power of the logic-regression-based GWAS analysis in identifying specific forms of SNP-SNP interactions associated with a phenotype and explaining a greater extent of CD genetics. We found strong evidence of CD-Association with 195 genes including both previously identified loci through the single-SNP analysis, in addition to newly identified susceptibility genes.

In this paper, we reduced the computational demand of logic regression by limiting the search to SNP combinations within the same gene, and also by fixing the size of SNP combinations in the search. These strategies have a definite disadvantage: the search will not be comprehensive and true underlying SNP-SNP interactions that are more complex than the limited size under consideration will not be discovered. In view of the current practice of assessing the marginal effects of individual SNPs one at a time, however, we submit that the limited form of logic regression proposed here provides a clear advance over, and an alternative to, the individual-SNP analysis. It can search for more biologically-plausible forms of SNP effects (combination of SNP intersections and/or unions) with greater degrees of association indicated by appreciably larger values of odds ratios, although the search remains approximate due to the limited size.

Despite the limitation of our approach by the small fixed size of logic regression models, the successful discovery of CD susceptibility genes demonstrates the potential utility of the logic-regression-based SNP-SNP interaction analysis of GWAS in providing additional insights to the *marginal* single-SNP analysis approach of GWAS. Some of the genes (or their chromosomal regions) identified by our approach were previously identified only in linkage studies and not by GWAS: this also attests to the utility of the proposed approach.

False positive discoveries by GWAS in which a large number of SNPs are examined for association with a disease are a major concern. Any discoveries including those reported here have to be validated rigorously in further investigations for exclusion of false positive from population stratification and genotyping errors. The candidate gene approach is also a valid alternative to the data-driven approach of GWAS, whether driven by a functional or biological hypothesis or possibly following the potential discoveries of GWAS. The application of logic regression is less computationally involved in candidate-gene studies, compared to GWAS.

Proper phenotyping is a key for increasing the chance to identify susceptibility genes specific for a clinical phenotype of interest. A

Table 2. Logic structures, frequencies, and associated Crohn's Disease odds ratios of the *ISX* gene (p-value$<3.8\times10^{-6}$).

		rs9610191 TT	rs17778240 TT	rs17778240 TT	rs5999715AC	Logic-based Risk Groups		
	rs11089728CC							
Genotype Freq	Case N = 1748	797 (45.6%)	10 (0.6%)	466 (26.7%)	466 (26.7%)	214 (12.2%)		
	Cont N = 2936	1326 (45.2%)	18 (0.6%)	776 (26.4%)	776 (26.4%)	17 (0.6%)		
Logic 1	**AND (OR)**					**Frequency**		**Odds Ratio**
Logic 2				**AND**		**Case**	**Cont**	
Logic-based Risk Groups	Logic 1 = No			Logic 2 = No		1540	2562	1.0
	Logic 1 = Yes			Logic 2 = No		1	372	.0045
	Logic 1 = No			Logic 2 = Yes		2	0	172.2
	Logic 1 = Yes			Logic 2 = Yes		205	2	

Table 3. Seventeen genes with the strong evidence for association with Crohn's Disease risk in WTCCC and one or both of Non-Jewish and Jewish dbGap GWASs, with chromosomal locations, numbers of SNPs, approximate p-values, and Bayes factors.

GWAS Study Name		WTCCC			Non-Jewish dbGap			Jewish dbGap		
Sample Size (Cases/Controls)		(1748/2936)			(498/498)			(291/429)		
Gene Name	Chromosome	#SNPs	p-value	C.BF	#SNPs	p-value	C.BF	#SNPs	p-value	C.BF
IL23R**	1p31	11	$<3.8\times10^{-6}$	13.6	14	$<3.8\times10^{-6}$	9.3	18	1.4×10^{-3}	3.8
NOD2**	16q21	5	$<3.8\times10^{-6}$	14.6	4	2.9×10^{-5}	5.8	4	8.7×10^{-3}	2.8
TMEM183A	1q32+	10	7.6×10^{-5}	5.3	5	6.0×10^{-4}	4.3	5	1.9×10^{-3}	3.7
SLCO6A1	5q21	15	5.7×10^{-5}	5.4	11	4.7×10^{-4}	4.4	11	1.6×10^{-2}	2.4
PTGER4**	5p13	46	$<3.8\times10^{-6}$	13.5	50	1.6×10^{-4}	4.9	53	1.6×10^{-1}	0.9
CYLD**	16q12	30	$<3.8\times10^{-6}$	11.2	22	2.2×10^{-3}	3.6	21	1.1×10^{-1}	1.2
SOCS6	18q22+	111	3.4×10^{-5}	5.6	147	4.7×10^{-2}	1.8	145	1.5×10^{-2}	2.5
ACAD11	3q22	4	$<3.8\times10^{-6}$	6.2	5	3.7×10^{-1}	0.3	5	1.2×10^{-3}	3.9
CLSTN2	3q23	120	$<3.8\times10^{-6}$	6.3	100	4.0×10^{-4}	4.4	104	7.6×10^{-1}	−0.5
SOX11	2p25	194	$<3.8\times10^{-6}$	9.6	194	2.8×10^{-3}	3.4	188	3.0×10^{-1}	0.4
CEBPB	20q13	15	5.9×10^{-4}	4.2	27	2.2×10^{-1}	0.7	28	5.5×10^{-3}	3.1
C1orf141**	1p31	10	$<3.8\times10^{-6}$	10.3	6	4.1×10^{-3}	3.2	7	3.5×10^{-1}	0.3
NEK2	1q32-q41+	11	8.8×10^{-5}	5.1	13	4.0×10^{-1}	0.2	12	4.9×10^{-3}	3.1
NKX2-3**	10q24	14	7.6×10^{-6}	6.0	7	8.4×10^{-3}	2.8	7	2.9×10^{-1}	0.5
BSN**	3p21	4	$<3.8\times10^{-6}$	7.0	3	1.2×10^{-2}	2.6	3	7.0×10^{-1}	−0.4
RBMS3	3p24-p23	157	2.1×10^{-4}	4.7	177	8.8×10^{-1}	−0.8	175	6.9×10^{-3}	2.9
C10orf57	10q22+	6	6.3×10^{-4}	4.2	9	8.1×10^{-1}	−0.6	9	1.4×10^{-2}	2.5

indicates genes in the chromosomal locations where the WTCCC single-SNP analysis showed **strong evidence.
+indicates chromosomal locations are those with three or more genes in the 195 genes (see Table S1) showing strong evidence in our WTCCC logic-regression-based analysis, but without strong or moderate evidence in the single-SNP analysis of WTCCC.

recent paper on Crohn's disease [18] provided a good example on this point: it focused specifically on the small intestinal inflammation phenotype of the disease and showed that impairments in Wnt signalling and Paneth cell biology are pathophysiological hallmarks of this clinical phenotype.

Increasing attention has been paid recently to pathway-based analysis of GWAS [19]. Our approach can be extended from gene-level SNP-SNP interaction to pathway-level SNP-SNP interaction. This approach would be biologically appealing, as it uses sets of SNPs within the same pathway rather than within the same gene; however, the logic space to be explored in the pathway-level analysis is appreciably larger than in the gene-level counterpart. The search space may be restricted based on some biological criteria, such as restricting the search to non-synonymous coding variants. Such SNP-SNP interaction analysis at the pathway level could, however, provide further valuable insights into genetic interactions on the modification of phenotype risks.

Supporting Information

Table S1 One hundred and ninety five genes with the strongest evidence for association with Crohn's Disease risk, with chromosomal locations, numbers of SNPs, approximate p-values, and Bayes factors.

Figure S1 Principal components from the three datasets: WTCCC, Non-Jewish and Jewish subjects are represented by black circles, green pluses, and blue triangles, respectively.

Author Contributions

Conceived and designed the experiments: YY ID SM HY. Performed the experiments: YY QL ID SM. Analyzed the data: YY QL ID SM HY NSE EK XW SJ. Contributed reagents/materials/analysis tools: YY QL ID SM HY NSE EK XW. Wrote the paper: YY QL ID SM HY NSE EK XW KT.

References

1. Franke A, McGovern DPB, Barrett JC, Wang K, Radford-Smith GL, et al. (2010) Genome-wide meta-analysis increases to 71 the number of confirmed Crohn's disease susceptibility loci. Nat Genet 42: 1118–1125.
2. Ruczinski I, Kooperberg C, LeBlanc ML (2003) Logic Regression. Journal of Computational and Graphical Statistics 12 (3): 475–511.
3. Kooperberg C, Ruczinski I, LeBlanc ML, Hsu L (2001) Sequence analysis using logic regression. Genetic Epidemiology 21 Suppl 1: S626–S631.
4. Witte JS, Fijal BA (2001) Introduction: Analysis of Sequence Data and Population Structure. Genetic Epidemiology 21: 600–601.
5. Etzioni R, Falcon S, Gann PH, Kooperberg CL, Penson DF, et al. (2004) Prostate-specific antigen and free prostate-specific antigen in the early detection of prostate cancer: do combination tests improve detection? Cancer Epidemiol. Biomarkers Prev 13: 1640–1645.
6. Ruczinski I, Kooperberg C, LeBlanc M (2004) Exploring Interactions in High Dimensional Genomic Data: An Overview of Logic Regression, With Applications. Journal of Multivariate Analysis 90: 178–195.
7. Kooperberg C, Ruczinski I (2005) Identifying Interacting SNPs using Monte Carlo Logic Regression. Genetic Epidemiology 28(2): 157–170.
8. Andrew AS, Karagas MR, Nelson HH, Guarrera S, Polidoro S, et al. (2008) Dna repair polymorphisms modify bladder cancer risk: a multi-factor analytic strategy. Hum Hered 65(2): 105–118.

9. Harth V, Schafer M, Abel J, Maintz L, Maintz L, et al. (2008) Head and neck squamous-cell cancer and its association with polymorphic enzymes of xenobiotic metabolism and repair. J Toxicol Environ Health 71(13–14): 887–897.

10. Justenhoven C, Hamann U, Schubert F, Zapatka M, Zapatka M, et al. (2008) Breast cancer: a candidate gene approach across the estrogen metabolic pathway. Breast Cancer Res Treat 108(1): 137–149.

11. Suehiro Y, Wong CW, Chirieac LR, Kondo Y, Kondo Y, et al. (2008) Epigenetic-genetic interactions in the apc/wnt, ras/raf, and p53 pathways in colorectal carcinoma. Clin Cancer Res 14(9): 2560–2569.

12. WTCCC (2007) Genome-wide association study of 14,000 cases of seven common diseases and 3,000 shared controls. Nature 447: 661–678.

13. Duerr RH, Taylor KD, Brant SR, Rioux JD, Silverberg MS, et al. (2006) A genome-wide association study identifies IL23R as an inflammatory bowel disease gene. Science 314: 1461–1463.

14. Aulchenko YS, Ripke S, Isaacs A, van Duijn CM (2007) GenABEL: an R library for genome-wide association analysis. Bioinformatics 23 (10): 1294–1296.

15. Choi MY, Romer AI, Hu M, Lepourcelet M, Mechoor A, et al. (2006) A dynamic expression survey identifies transcription factors relevant in mouse digestive tract development. Development 133(20): 4119–4129.

16. Danoy P, Pryce K, Hadler J, Bradbury LA, Farrar C, et al. (2010) Association of Variants at 1q32 and STAT3 with Ankylosing Spondylitis Suggests Genetic Overlap with Crohn's Disease. PLoS Genet 6(12): e1001195.

17. Martinez A, Martin MC, Mendoza J, Taxonera C, Díaz-Rubio M, et al. (2006) Association of the organic cation transporter OCTN genes with Crohn's disease in the Spanish population. European Journal of Human Genetics 14: 222–226.

18. Koslowski MJ, Teltschik Z, Beisner J, Schaeffeler E, Wang G, et al. (2012) Association of a Functional Variant in the Wnt Co-Receptor LRP6 with Early Onset Ileal Crohn's Disease. PLoS Genetics. 8(2): e1002523. doi:10.1371/journal.pgen.1002523.

19. Wang K, Zhang H, Kugathasan S, Annese V, Bradfield JP, et al. (2009) Diverse Genome-wide Association Studies Associate the IL12/IL23 Pathway with Crohn Disease. The American Journal of Human Genetics 84: 399–405.

10

The *NOD2* Single Nucleotide Polymorphisms rs2066843 and rs2076756 are Novel and Common Crohn's Disease Susceptibility Gene Variants

Jürgen Glas[1,2,3◊], Julia Seiderer[1◊], Cornelia Tillack[1], Simone Pfennig[1], Florian Beigel[1], Matthias Jürgens[1,4], Torsten Olszak[1,5], Rüdiger P. Laubender[6], Maria Weidinger[1], Bertram Müller-Myhsok[7], Burkhard Göke[1], Thomas Ochsenkühn[1], Peter Lohse[8], Julia Diegelmann[1,2], Darina Czamara[7], Stephan Brand[1]*

1 Department of Medicine II - Grosshadern, Ludwig-Maximilians-University, Munich, Germany, 2 Department of Preventive Dentistry and Periodontology, Ludwig-Maximilians-University, Munich, Germany, 3 Department of Human Genetics, RWTH (Rheinisch-Westfälische Technische Hochschule), Aachen, Germany, 4 Division of Gastroenterology, University of Leuven, Leuven, Belgium, 5 Division of Gastroenterology, Hepatology and Endoscopy, Brigham and Women's Hospital, Harvard Medical School, Boston, Massachusetts, United States of America, 6 Institute of Medical Informatics, Biometry and Epidemiology (IBE), Ludwig-Maximilians-University, Munich, Germany, 7 Max-Planck-Institute of Psychiatry, Munich, Germany, 8 Institute of Clinical Chemistry - Grosshadern, Ludwig-Maximilians-University, Munich, Germany

Abstract

Background: The aims were to analyze two novel *NOD2* variants (rs2066843 and rs2076756) in a large cohort of patients with inflammatory bowel disease and to elucidate phenotypic consequences.

Methodology/Principal Findings: Genomic DNA from 2700 Caucasians including 812 patients with Crohn's disease (CD), 442 patients with ulcerative colitis (UC), and 1446 healthy controls was analyzed for the *NOD2* SNPs rs2066843 and rs2076756 and the three main CD-associated *NOD2* variants p.Arg702Trp (rs2066844), p.Gly908Arg (rs2066847), and p.Leu1007fsX1008 (rs2066847). Haplotype and genotype-phenotype analyses were performed. The SNPs rs2066843 (p = 3.01×10⁻⁵, OR 1.48, [95% CI 1.23-1.78]) and rs2076756 (p = 4.01×10⁻⁶; OR 1.54, [95% CI 1.28-1.86]) were significantly associated with CD but not with UC susceptibility. Haplotype analysis revealed a number of significant associations with CD susceptibility with omnibus p values <10⁻¹⁰. The SNPs rs2066843 and rs2076756 were in linkage disequilibrium with each other and with the three main CD-associated *NOD2* mutations (D'>0.9). However, in CD, SNPs rs2066843 and rs2076756 were more frequently observed than the other three common *NOD2* mutations (minor allele frequencies for rs2066843 and rs2076756: 0.390 and 0.380, respectively). In CD patients homozygous for these novel *NOD2* variants, genotype-phenotype analysis revealed higher rates of a penetrating phenotype (rs2076756: p = 0.015) and fistulas (rs2076756: p = 0.015) and significant associations with CD-related surgery (rs2076756: p = 0.003; rs2066843: p = 0.015). However, in multivariate analysis only disease localization (p<2×10⁻¹⁶) and behaviour (p = 0.02) were significantly associated with the need for surgery.

Conclusion/Significance: The *NOD2* variants rs2066843 and rs2076756 are novel and common CD susceptibility gene variants.

Editor: Manfred Kayser, Erasmus University Medical Center, Netherlands

Funding: J. Glas was supported by a grant from the Broad Medical Foundation (IBD-0126R2). J. Seiderer and J. Diegelmann were supported by grants from the Ludwig-Maximilians-University Munich (FoLe Nr. 422; Habilitationsstipendium, LMUExcellent to J.S. and Promotionsstipendium to J.D.); J. Seiderer was also supported by the Robert-Bosch-Foundation and the Else Kroener-Fresenius-Stiftung (81/08//EKMS08/01). T. Olszak was supported by a grant from the German Research Council (Deutsche Forschungsgemeinschaft, DFG). S. Brand was supported by grants from the DFG (BR 1912/5-1), the Else Kroener-Fresenius-Stiftung (Else Kroener Fresenius Memorial Stipendium 2005; P50/05/EKMS05/62 and the Else Kroener-Exzellenzstipendium 2010_EKES.32), by the Ludwig-Demling Grant 2007 from DCCV e.V., and by grants of Ludwig-Maximilians-University Munich (Excellence Initiative, Investment Funds 2008 and FoeFoLe program). The funders had no role in study design, data collection and analysis, decision to publish, or preparation of the manuscript.

Competing Interests: The authors have declared that no competing interests exist.

* E-mail: stephan.brand@med.uni-muenchen.de

◊ These authors contributed equally to this work.

Introduction

Crohn's disease (CD) and ulcerative colitis (UC) are chronic inflammatory bowel diseases (IBD) characterized by an exaggerated immune response of the intestinal mucosa and a dysfunctional epithelial barrier [1,2,3,4]. The identification of nucleotide-binding oligomerization domain 2 (*NOD2*, GeneID: 64127), also known as caspase recruitment domain-containing protein 15 (*CARD15*) as the first susceptibility gene in CD in 2001 [5,6] has provided significant new insights in the pathogenesis of IBD focusing on the genetic background of innate immune response and interaction with bacterial antigens [7,8,9,10]. Most recently, genome-wide association studies and subsequent replication studies have provided further insights into IBD pathogenesis by identification and confirmation of susceptibility genes such as the interleukin-23 receptor (*IL23R*) [11,12], *SLC22A4/5* [13] and *ATG16L1* [14] (autophagy-related 16-like 1) gene.

NOD2 represents a cytoplasmatic protein and functions mainly as a NF-κB pathway activating sensor for bacterial muramyl dipeptide (MDP) found in the cell wall of Gram-positive and Gram-negative bacteria [8,15,16,17]. In addition, NOD2 seems to be a negative regulator of Toll-like receptor 2-mediated T helper cell type 1 responses and modulates ileal expression of antimicrobial peptides such as alpha-defensins and the expression of proinflammatory cytokines and chemokines in the intestinal mucosa [18,19,20]. The identification of *NOD2* as a susceptibility gene for CD therefore suggests an important role of genetically determined enteric bacteria-host interactions and an inappropriate activation of the mucosal immune system in IBD. Large genotype-phenotype analyses by us [21,22] and others [23,24,25] also demonstrated a significant association of *NOD2* variants with ileal involvement, stricturing phenotype and early disease onset in CD patients.

The *NOD2* gene is located on chromosome 16q in the IBD1 locus and contains 11 constant exons and a twelfth alternatively spliced exon in the 5′-region. So far, three main *NOD2* variants, which include two amino acid substitutions, p.Arg702Trp encoded by exon 4, and p.Gly908Arg encoded by exon 8, and the frameshift mutation p.Leu1007fsX1008 located in exon 11, were identified to be overrepresented in CD patients. There is also evidence for further *NOD2* variants being involved in IBD pathogenesis as demonstrated by us [26] and others in recent association studies [18,19,20]. However, the extent of disease modification or phenotypic consequences of other *NOD2* variants such as the SNPs rs2066843 and rs2076756 have not been investigated so far.

We therefore genotyped 2700 individuals of Caucasian origin and performed a large and detailed genotype-phenotype analysis for the *NOD2* variants rs2066843 and rs2076756 analyzing the influence of these variants on the disease susceptibility and phenotype of patients with CD and UC.

Materials and Methods

Study population

The study population (n = 2700) was comprised of 1254 IBD patients of Caucasian origin including 812 patients with CD, 442 patients with UC, and 1446 healthy, unrelated controls. The patients were recruited in two cohorts; the discovery sample was recruited from the University Hospital Munich-Grosshadern and comprised 519 CD patients, 232 UC patients and 770 controls, while the replication cohort recruited from the University Hospitals Bochum and Munich-Innenstadt consisted of 293 CD patients, 210 UC patients and 676 controls. Patients with indeterminate colitis were excluded from the study. All individuals gave written, informed consent prior to the study. The study was approved by the local Ethics committee and adhered to the ethical principles for medical research involving human subjects of the Helsinki Declaration. Phenotypic parameters were collected blind to the results of the genotype analysis and included demographic and clinical data (behaviour and anatomic location of IBD, disease-related complications, surgical or immunosuppressive therapy). Two senior gastroenterologists analyzed data which were recorded by patient charts analysis and a detailed questionnaire based on an interview at time of enrolment. For the analysis of demographic and phenotypic data, the diagnosis of

CD and UC was related to established international guidelines based on endoscopic, radiological, and histopathological parameters [27]. CD patients were classified according to the Montreal classification [28] including age at diagnosis (A), location (L), and behaviour (B) of disease. In patients with UC, anatomic location was also assessed in accordance to the Montreal classification based on the criteria ulcerative proctitis (E1), left-sided UC (distal UC; E2), and extensive UC (pancolitis; E3). The clinical characteristics of the IBD study population are summarized in Table 1.

DNA extraction and NOD2 genotyping

Genomic DNA was isolated from peripheral blood leukocytes by standard procedures using the DNA blood mini kit from Qiagen (Hilden, Germany). Genotyping of the *NOD2* variants p.Arg702Trp (rs2066844), p.Gly908Arg (rs2066847), and p.Leu1007fsX1008 (rs2066847) were performed as described previously [26] (primer and probe sequences are available on request). The *NOD2* SNPs rs2066843 and rs2076756 were genotyped by PCR and melting curve analysis using a pair of fluorescence resonance energy transfer (FRET) probes, a sensor and an anchor probe, respectively, in a LightCycler 480 Instrument (Roche Diagnostics, Mannheim, Germany). The donor fluorescent molecule (fluorescein) at 3′-end of the sensor probe in case of rs2066843 or the anchor probe in case of rs2076756, respectively, is excited at its specific fluorescence excitation wavelength (533 nm) and the energy is transferred to the acceptor fluorescent molecule at the 5′-end of the anchor probe in case of rs2066843 (LightCycler Red 640) or the sensor probe in case of rs2076756 (LightCycler Red 670). The specific fluorescence signal emitted by the acceptor molecule is detected by the optical unit of the LightCycler 480 Instrument. The sensor probe is exactly matching to one allele of each SNP, whereas in the case of the other allele there is a mismatch resulting in a lower melting temperature. The total volume of the PCR was 5 μl containing 25 ng of genomic DNA, 1 x Light Cycler 480

Table 1. Demographic characteristics of the IBD study population.

	Crohn's disease n = 812	Ulcerative colitis n = 442	Controls n = 1446
Gender Male (%) Female (%)	49.0 51.0	48.1 51.9	63.1 36.9
Age (yrs) Mean ± SD Range	39.4±13.2 10-80	41.7±14.6 7-85	46.1±10.6 18-71
Body mass index Mean ± SD Range	23.1±4.1 13-40	23.9±4.2 15-41	
Age at diagnosis (yrs) Mean ± SD Range	27.5±11.5 7-71	32.1±13.5 9-81	
Disease duration (yrs) Mean ± SD Range	12.2±8.5 0-44	11.0±7.8 1-40	
Positive family history of IBD (%)	16.2	16.1	

Genotyping Master (Roche Diagnostics), 2.5 pmol of each primer and 0.75 pmol of each FRET probe (TIB MOLBIOL, Berlin, Germany). The PCR comprised an initial denaturation step (95°C for 10 min) and 45 cycles (95°C for 10 sec, primer annealing temperature as given in Supplemental Table S1 for 10 sec, 72°C for 15 sec). The melting curve analysis comprised an initial denaturation step (95°C for 1 min), a step rapidly lowering the temperature to 40°C and holding for 60 sec, and a heating step slowly (1 acquisition/°C) increasing the temperature up to 95°C and continuously measuring the fluorescence intensity. The results of melting curve analysis had been confirmed by analyzing samples representing all possible genotypes using sequence analysis. For sequencing, the total volume of the PCR was 100 µl containing 250 ng of genomic DNA, 1 x PCR-buffer (Qiagen, Hilden, Germany), a final MgCl$_2$ concentration of 1.5 mM, 0.5 mM of a dNTP-Mix (Sigma, Steinheim, Germany), 2.5 units of HotStar Plus Taq^{TM} DNA polymerase (Qiagen) and 10 pmol of each primer (TIB MOLBIOL, Berlin, Germany). The PCR used for sequencing comprised an initial denaturation step (95°C for 5 min), 35 cycles (denaturation at 94°C for 30 sec, primer annealing at 60°C for 30 sec, extension at 72°C for 30 sec) and a final extension step (72°C for 10 min). The PCR products were purified using the QIAquick PCR Purification Kit (Qiagen) and sequenced by a commercial sequencing company (Sequiserve, Vaterstetten, Germany). All sequences of primers and FRET probes and primer annealing temperatures used for genotyping and for sequence analysis are given in the supplementary data section (Supplemental Table S1 and S2). The results of the genotyping for the CD-associated *ATG16L1* variant rs2241880 (p.Thr300Ala) were available from a previous study [29].

Statistical analyses

Each genetic marker was tested for Hardy-Weinberg equilibrium in the control population. Fisher's exact test or χ^2 test for comparison between categorical variables were used where appropriate. Single-marker allelic tests were performed with Pearson's χ^2 test. Student's t-test was applied for quantitative variables. All tests were two-tailed and p-values <0.05 were considered significant. Odds ratios were calculated for the minor allele at each SNP. For evaluation of phenotypic consequences, we conducted a logistic regression analysis. Data were evaluated by using the SPSS 13.0 software (SPSS Inc., Chicago, IL, U.S.A.) and R-2.4.1. (http://cran.r-project.org). Haplotype analysis and calculation of linkage disequilibrium (LD) were conducted using PLINK (http://pngu.mgh.harvard.edu/~purcell/plink/).

Results

The novel NOD2 variants rs2066843 and rs2076756 are associated with susceptibility to CD but not to UC

In the controls, the genotype frequencies of the SNPs rs2066843 and rs2076756 were in agreement with the predicted Hardy-Weinberg equilibrium. Significant differences in the allele frequencies of the SNPs rs2066843 and rs2076756 were observed in CD patients but not in UC patients compared to healthy controls. As summarized in Table 2, the SNPs rs2066843 and rs2076756 were strongly associated with CD. In the group of CD patients, the frequency of the rarer T allele of the rs2066843 variant was 0.390, whereas in the controls it was 0.299 (p = 3.01×10^{-5}; OR 1.48, [95% CI 1.23-1.78]). The frequencies of the less common G allele of the rs2076756 variant were 0.390 in CD and 0.286 in the controls (p = 4.01×10^{-6}; OR 1.54, [95% CI 1.28-1.86]). In contrast to CD, no associations of both *NOD2* SNPs were observed in UC. The frequency of the rs2066843 T allele was 0.300 (p = 9.67×10^{-1}, OR 1.01 [95% CI 0.85-1.19]), while the frequency of the rs2076756 G allele was 0.270 (p = 3.74×10^{-1}, OR 1.09 [95% CI 0.94-1.27]). The association of the *NOD2* SNPs with CD susceptibility was found in both our initial discovery cohort from the University Hospital Munich-Grosshadern (Supplemental Table S3) and the replication cohort from the University Hospital Munich, Campus Innenstadt and from Ruhr-University Bochum (Supplemental Table S4). In this study, rs2066843 and rs2076756 were in LD in all studied subpopulations (CD, UC, healthy controls; Supplemental Tables S5, S6, S7).

To analyze for potential disease associations with certain NOD2 haplotypes, we performed a detailed haplotype analysis (Table 3 and Supplemental Table S8). As shown in Table 3, we demonstrated for a number of haplotypes significant associations with CD susceptibility, including several associations with omnibus p values of less than 10^{-10}. The strongest association of a haplotype including one of the SNPs rs2066843 or rs2076756 comprised of the NOD2 SNPs rs2066844-rs2066845-rs2066847-rs2076756 (omnibus p-value = 1.14×10^{-23}). In contrast, no significant associations were found with UC susceptibility (Supplemental Table S8).

Genotype-phenotype analysis of rs2066843 and rs2076756 NOD2 variants in CD patients

Since the three common *NOD2* variants p.Arg702Trp (rs2066844), p.Gly908Arg (rs2066847), and p.Leu1007fsX1008 (rs2066847) have been identified to be associated with a certain CD phenotype [21,22,23,24,30], we also performed a detailed

Table 2. Allele frequencies of the SNPs rs2066843 and rs2076756 in patients with Crohn's disease, ulcerative colitis and controls.

Gene marker	Minor allele	Crohn's disease n = 812			Ulcerative colitis n = 442			Controls n = 1446
		MAF	p value	OR [95% CI]	MAF	p value	OR [95% CI]	MAF
rs2066843	T	0.390	3.01×10^{-5}	1.48 [1.23–1.78]	0.300	9.67×10^{-1}	1.01 [0.85–1.19]	0.299
rs2076756	G	0.380	4.01×10^{-6}	1.54 [1.28–1.86]	0.270	3.74×10^{-1}	1.09 [0.94–1.27]	0.286
rs2066844 p.Arg702TrpT	0.089	1.43×10^{-6}	2.07 [1.53–2.79]	0.046	7.49×10^{-1}	0.92 [0.60–1.40]	0.050
rs2066845 p.Gly908ArgG	0.042	1.1×10^{-2}	1.72 [1.14–2.60]	0.022	1.00	0.94 [0.51–1.73]	0.024
rs2066847 p.Leu1007fsX1008	insC	0.121	1.88×10^{-14}	5.03 [3.54–7.15]	0.022	3.91×10^{-1}	0.76 [0.42–1.37]	0.028

Minor allele frequencies (MAF), allelic test *P*-values, and odds ratios (OR, shown for the minor allele) with 95% confidence intervals (CI) are depicted for both the CD and UC case-control cohorts.

Table 3. Haplotype analysis for *NOD2* SNPs in the CD patient cohort.

NOD2 haplotypes	p-value	OR	CI lower	CI upper
rs2066843-rs2066844	1.31×10^{-8}			
TT	1.34×10^{-5}	1.94	1.81	2.08
TC	3.09×10^{-4}	1.34	1.28	1.40
CC	1.72×10^{-8}	0.65	0.63	0.66
rs2066844-rs2066845	7.94×10^{-8}			
CC	3.25×10^{-3}	1.80	1.58	2.06
TG	3.80×10^{-6}	1.89	1.78	2.00
CG	1.08×10^{-8}	0.52	0.50	0.54
rs2066845-rs2066847	1.09×10^{-18}			
GC	6.88×10^{-17}	4.06	3.90	4.22
CX	6.67×10^{-3}	1.74	1.50	2.02
GX	4.38×10^{-20}	0.32	0.31	0.33
rs2066847-rs2076756	2.48×10^{-15}			
CG	2.88×10^{-14}	3.84	3.67	4.02
XG	3.31×10^{-1}	1.09	0.91	1.30
XA	2.35×10^{-9}	0.62	0.61	0.64
rs2066843-rs2066844-rs2066845	5.94×10^{-10}			
TCC	1.16×10^{-3}	1.90	1.69	2.14
TTG	8.40×10^{-7}	2.01	1.90	2.13
TCG	2.64×10^{-2}	1.21	1.12	1.31
CCG	9.68×10^{-10}	0.62	0.61	0.64
rs2066844-rs2066845-rs2066847	8.22×10^{-24}			
CGC	5.84×10^{-17}	4.07	3.91	4.23
CCX	1.08×10^{-2}	1.70	1.45	1.99
TGX	3.59×10^{-6}	1.89	1.78	2.00
CGX	4.19×10^{-26}	0.37	0.36	0.37
rs2066845-rs2066847-rs2076756	2.48×10^{-15}			
GCG	5.41×10^{-17}	4.09	3.93	4.25
CXG	1.04×10^{-3}	1.94	1.72	2.19
GXG	3.47×10^{-1}	0.92	0.76	1.11
GXA	3.89×10^{-12}	0.59	0.57	0.60
rs2066843-rs2066844-rs2066845-rs2066847	1.60×10^{-23}			
TCGC	4.10×10^{-17}	4.28	4.11	4.46
TCCX	1.18×10^{-3}	1.90	1.69	2.14
TTGX	8.51×10^{-7}	1.99	1.88	2.10
TCGX	2.32×10^{-5}	0.66	0.63	0.69
CCGX	8.57×10^{-13}	0.59	0.58	0.60
rs2066844-rs2066845-rs2066847-rs2076756	1.14×10^{-23}			
CGCG	5.20×10^{-17}	4.04	3.89	4.20
CCXG	1.10×10^{-3}	1.93	1.71	2.18
TGXG	4.75×10^{-7}	2.06	1.95	2.18
CGXG	1.24×10^{-5}	0.642	0.61	0.67
CGXA	7.82×10^{-13}	0.59		
rs2066843-rs2066844-rs2066845-rs2066847-rs2076756	1.43×10^{-21}			
TCGCG	6.33×10^{-17}	4.18	4.02	4.35
TCCXG	1.07×10^{-3}	1.93	1.71	2.18
TTGXG	6.00×10^{-7}	2.05	1.94	2.17
TCGXG	9.42×10^{-5}	0.67	0.64	0.71
TCGXA	6.48×10^{-2}	0.576	0.42	0.79
CCGXA	2.01×10^{-11}	0.61	0.60	0.63

Omnibus as well as individual p-values are presented.

genotype-phenotype correlation in IBD patients. In univariate analysis, CD patients homozygous for the SNP rs2066843 were found to have a lower body mass index (p = 0.039) and less colonic involvement (p = 0.041) compared to the wildtype patients and we observed also a trend towards a predominantly penetrating disease phenotype (B3) (p = 0.068; Table 4). In addition, a higher need for CD-related surgery in homozygous carriers of the SNP rs2066843 (p = 0.015) was observed compared to the wildtype group (Table 5).

Analyzing CD patients regarding the rs2076756 genotype status, a significant younger age at disease onset was observed in homozygous carriers (mean 25.8 ± 11.4 years) compared to wildtype patients (p = 0.023; Table 6). Similar to the analysis of SNP rs2066843, homozygous carriers of SNP rs2076756 had less colonic involvement than wildtype patients (p = 0.032) but showed a trend towards ileocolonic disease location (p = 0.058) and had a significant higher rate of penetrating disease phenotype (B3) (p = 0.015; Table 6). The significant association of SNP rs2076756 with a severe disease phenotype was also reflected by the significantly higher percentage of patients with CD-related surgery (p = 0.003) and internal fistulas (p = 0.015) in homozygous carriers of this SNP (Table 7). Moreover, there was also a trend towards stenotic complications (p = 0.067) in homozygous CD patients (Table 7). However, given the large number of associations investigated, most associations lost significance following Bonferroni correction.

Given the increased prevalence of the three common *NOD2* variants among carriers of the risk allele of rs2066843 and rs2076756 and previous reports demonstrating a severe phenotype in carriers of these three *NOD2* variants, we next investigated if the phenotypic effects of rs2066843 and rs2076756 were independent of the main three CD-associated *NOD2* variants p.Arg702Trp (rs2066844), p.Gly908Arg (rs2066847), and p.Leu1007fsX1008 (rs2066847). As shown in Table 8, there

were no significant differences regarding homozygous carriers of these SNPs when stratified for the presence and absence of the main three CD-associated *NOD2* variants and the significant phenotypic characteristics found in Tables 5, 6 and 7, suggesting that the CD-modifying effect of rs2066843 and rs2076756 is independent of the three main *NOD2* variants.

Analyzing potential therapeutic consequences such as need for surgery, we next conducted a logistic regression analysis with R, using the need for surgery as dependent variable, and the SNP genotype as independent variable, taking localization as well as behaviour as covariates. This revealed that disease localization has a significant influence on the need for surgery (p = 0.02). In addition, disease behaviour is significantly associated with the need for surgery (p = 2.0×10^{-16}, independently of localization). However, using the *NOD2* genotype status as further explanatory variable does not improve the model fit (F-test p = 0.36 rs2066843, p = 0.32 rs2076756).

In UC patients, the analysis revealed no significant associations of the SNPs rs2066843 and rs2076756 with phenotypic characteristics such as age, age a diagnosis, male-to-female-ratio, body mass index (BMI), family history, anatomic location and disease behaviour, use of immunosuppressive agents, or UC-related complications (data not shown).

No evidence for epistasis between NOD2 variants and the CD-associated ATG16L1 variant rs2241880 (p.Thr300Ala)

Very recent studies indicate that NOD2 recruits the autophagy protein ATG16L1 to the plasma membrane at the bacterial entry site [31]. In contrast, CD-associated mutants failed to recruit ATG16L1 to the plasma membrane and wrapping of invading bacteria by autophagosomes was impaired [31]. Moreover, dendritic cells from CD patients expressing

Table 4. Association between rs2066843 genotype and CD disease characteristics based on the Montreal classification [28].

rs2066843 genotype status	(1) CC n = 322	(2) CT n = 345	(3) TT n = 150	(1) vs. (2) p-value OR [95% CI]	(1) vs. (3) p-value OR [95% CI]	(1) vs. (2) + (3) p-value OR [95% CI]
Age at diagnosis	74/239 (31.0%)	81/237 (34.2%)	37/116 (31.9%)	0.494	0.903	0.591
≤16 years (A1)	150/239 (62.8%)	125/237 (52.7%)	69/116 (59.5%)	1.16 (0.79–1.70)	1.04 (0.65–1.68)	1.12 (0.79–1.59)
17–40 years (A2)	15/239 (6.2%)	31/237 (13.1%)	10/116 (8.6%)	0.033	0.562	0.062
>40 years (A3)				0.66 (0.46–0.95)	0.87 (0.55–1.37)	0.72 (0.52–1.01)
				0.013	0.507	0.032
				2.25 (1.18–4.28)	1.41 (0.61–3.24)	1.96 (1.06–3.63)
Location	32/244 (13.1%)	46/238 (19.3%)	12/120 (10.0%)	0.083	0.494	0.352
Terminal ileum (L1)	42/244 (17.2%)	33/238 (13.9%)	11/120 (9.2%)	1.59 (0.97–2.59)	0.74 (0.36–1.49)	1.28 (0.80–2.04)
Colon (L2)	166/244 (67.9%)	155/238 (65.1%)	93/120 (77.5%)	0.318	0.041	0.097
Ileocolon (L3)	4/244 (1.6%)	4/238 (1.7%)	4/120 (3.3%)	0.77 (0.47–1.27)	0.48 (0.24–0.98)	0.67 (0.43–1.07)
Upper GI (L4)	198/244 (81.1%)	201/238 (84.5%)	105/120 (87.5%)	0.501	0.066	0.788
Any ileal involvement (L1+L3)				0.88 (0.60–1.28)	1.62 (0.98–2.68)	1.06 (0.75–1.50)
				1.000	0.447	0.770
				1.03 (0.25–4.15)	2.07 (0.51–8.42)	1.37 (0.41–4.61)
				0.398	0.138	0.177
				1.26 (0.78–2.03)	1.63 (0.87–3.05)	1.37 (0.88–2.11)
Behaviour [1]	49/232 (21.1%)	61/233 (26.2%)	18/116 (15.5%)	0.230	0.249	0.684
Non-stricturing,Non-penetrat. (B1)	66/232 (28.4%)	64/233 (27.5%)	27/116 (23.3%)	1.32 (0.86–2.04)	0.69 (0.38–1.24)	1.09 (0.73–1.63)
Stricturing (B2)	117/232 (50.4%)	108/233 (46.3%)	71/116 (61.2%)	0.837	0.368	0.567
Penetrating (B3)				0.95 (0.63–1.43)	0.76 (0.45–1.28)	0.89 (0.61–1.29)
				0.404	0.068	0.866
				0.85 (0.59–1.22)	1.55 (0.98–2.44)	1.03 (0.74–1.44)

[1]Disease behaviour was defined according to the Montreal classification [28]. Stricturing disease phenotype was defined as presence of stenosis without penetrating disease. The diagnosis of stenosis was made surgically, endoscopically, or radiologically (using MR enteroclysis). For each variable, the number of patients included is given.

Table 5. Association between rs2066843 genotype and CD disease characteristics.

rs2066843 genotype status	(1) CC n=322	(2) CT n=345	(3) TT n=150	(1) vs. (2) p-value OR [95% CI]	(1) vs. (3) p-value OR [95% CI]	(1) vs. (2) + (3) p-value OR [95% CI]
Male sex	129/277 (46.6%)	153/289 (52.9%)	74/134 (55.2%)	0.131 1.29 (0.93–1.80)	0.115 1.41 (0.94–2.14)	0.075 1.33 (0.98–1.80)
Age at diagnosis (yrs) Mean ± SD Range	27.1±10.9 11–70	28.7±12.5 1–78	25.8±11.3 6–71	0.151	0.302	0.526
Disease duration (yrs) Mean ± SD Range	12.3±8.4 0–37	11.4±9.0 11–44	11.8±8.2 1–35	0.381	0.675	0.403
Body mass index (yrs) Mean ± SD Range	23.3±4.4 16–40	23.4±4.0 16–37	22.0±3.6 13–31	0.845	**0.039**	0.473
Use of immunosuppressive agents [2]	141/169 (83.4%)	135/175 (77.1%)	70/83 (84.3%)	0.176 0.67 (0.39–1.15)	1.000 1.07 (0.52–2.19)	0.316 0.77 (0.46–1.27)
Surgery because of CD [3]	113/221 (51.1%)	120/224 (53.6%)	76/116 (65.5%)	0.636 1.10 (0.76–1.60)	**0.015** 1.82 (1.14–2.89)	0.140 1.30 (0.93–1.83)
Fistulas	117/232 (50.4%)	108/233 (46.3%)	71/116 (61.2%)	0.404 0.85 (0.59–1.22)	0.068 1.55 (0.98–2.44)	0.866 1.03 (0.74–1.44)
Perianal fistulas	24/92 (26.1%)	18/90 (20.0%)	7/49 (14.3%)	0.212 1.41 (0.70–2.83)	0.079 2.12 (0.84–5.34)	0.096 1.61 (0.85–3.04)
Stenosis	140/229 (61.1%)	144/233 (61.8%)	80/115 (69.6%)	0.924 1.03 (0.71–1.50)	0.153 1.45 (0.90–2.34)	0.481 1.15 (0.81–1.62)

[2]Immunosuppressive agents included azathioprine, 6-mercaptopurine, 6-thioguanine, methotrexate, and/or infliximab.
[3]Only surgery related to CD-specific problems (e.g. fistulectomy, colectomy, ileostomy) was included. For each variable, the number of patients included is given.

CD-associated *NOD2* or *ATG16L1* risk variants are defective in autophagy induction, bacterial trafficking and antigen presentation [32]. We therefore hypothesized that there may be epistasis between CD-associated *NOD2* and *ATG16L1* variants regarding susceptibility to CD. However, as shown in Supplemental Table S9, none of the 5 CD-associated *NOD2* variants showed evidence for epistasis to the CD-associated *ATG16L1* variant rs2241880 (p.Thr300Ala).

Table 6. Association between rs2076756 genotype and CD disease characteristics based on the Montreal classification [28].

rs2076756 genotype status	(1) AA n=339	(2) AG n=334	(3) GG n=143	(1) vs. (2) p-value OR [95% CI]	(1) vs. (3) p-value OR [95% CI]	(1) vs. (2) + (3) p-value OR [95% CI]
Age at diagnosis ≤16 years (A1) 17–40 years (A2) >40 years (A3)	73/241(30.3%) 154/241(63.9%) 14/241 (5.8%)	75/233 (32.2%) 124/233 (53.2%) 34/233 (14.6%)	35/110 (31.8%) 66/110 (60.0%) 9/110 (8.2%)	0.692 1.09 (0.74–1.61) 0.020 0.64 (0.44–0.93) 0.002 2.77 (1.44–5.31)	0.804 1.07 (0.66–1.75) 0.552 0.85 (0.53–1.35) 0.486 1.44 (0.61–3.45)	0.717 1.09 (0.76–1.55) 0.041 0.70 (0.50–0.98) 0.007 2.32 (1.24–4.35)
Location Terminal ileum (L1) Colon (L2) Ileocolon (L3) Upper GI (L4) Ileocolonic Involvement	31/245 (12.7%) 41/245 (16.7%) 169/245 (70.0%) 4/245 (1.6%) 200/245 (81.6%)	45/235 (19.1%) 34/235 (14.5%) 152/235 (64.7%) 4/235 (1.7%) 197/235 (83.8%)	11/113 (9.7%) 9/113 (8.0%) 89/113 (78.8%) 4/113 (3.5%) 100/113 (88.5%)	0.061 1.63 (0.99–2.69) 0.531 0.84 (0.51–1.38) 0.333 0.82 (0.56–1.20) 1.000 1.04 (0.26–4.22) 0.548 1.17 (0.73–1.87)	0.483 0.74 (0.36–1.54) 0.032 0.43 (0.20–0.92) 0.058 1.67 (0.99–2.82) 0.268 2.21 (0.54–9.00) 0.123 1.73 (0.89–3.36)	0.289 1.32 (0.82–2.12) 0.151 0.70 (0.44–1.11) 1.000 1.01 (0.71–1.44) 0.769 1.48 (0.42–4.76) 0.258 1.31 (0.84–2.03)
Behaviour [1] Non-stricturing, Non-penetrat. (B1) Stricturing (B2) Penetrating (B3)	49/232 (21.1%) 67/232 (28.9%) 116/232 (50.0%)	64/231 (27.7%9 61/231 (26.4%) 106/231 (45.9%)	12/109 (11.0%) 27/109 (24.8%) 70/109 (64.2%)	0.106 1.43 (0.93–2.19) 0.604 0.88 (0.59–1.33) 0.403 0.85 (0.59–1.22)	0.023 0.46 (0.23–0.91) 0.516 0.81 (0.48–1.36) 0.015 1.79 (1.12–2.87)	0.758 1.07 (0.72–1.61) 0.444 0.86 (0.59–1.25) 0.733 1.07 (0.77–1.50)

Table 7. Association between rs2076756 genotype and CD disease characteristics.

rs2076756 genotype status	(1) AA n = 339	(2) AG n = 334	(3) GG n = 143	(1) vs. (2) p-value OR [95% CI]	(1) vs. (3) p-value OR [95% CI]	(1) vs. (2) + (3) p-value OR [95% CI]
Male sex	129/280 (46.1%)	152/283 (53.7%)	69/127 (54.3%)	0.077 1.36 (0.75–1.89)	0.135 1.39 (0.91–2.12)	**0.044** 1.37 (1.01–1.86)
Age at diagnosis (yr) Mean ± SD Range	26.8±10.5 11–70	29.2±12.7 1–78	25.8±11.4 6–71	**0.023**	0.465	0.157
Disease duration (yr) Mean ± SD Range	12.4±8.4 0–37	11.2±8.8 1–44	11.6±8.2 1–35	0.188	0.507	0.202
Body mass index (yr) Mean ± SD Range	23.4±10.5 11–70	23.2±4.0 16–37	22.3±3.7 13–31	0.691	0.074	0.309
Use of immunosuppressive agents [2]	147/174 (84.5%)	136/176 (77.3%)	65/80 (81.2%)	0.103 0.62 (0.36–1.07)	0.586 0.80 (0.40–1.59)	0.134 0.67 (0.40–1.11)
Surgery because of CD [3]	114/221 (51.6%)	120/222 (54.1%)	76/110 (69.1%)	0.635 1.10 (0.76–1.60)	**0.003** 2.10 (1.29–3.40)	0.097 1.35 (0.96–1.91)
Fistulas	116/232 (50.0%)	106/231 (45.9%)	70/109 (64.2%)	0.403 0.85 (0.59–1.22)	**0.015** 1.79 (1.12–2.87)	0.733 1.07 (0.77–1.50)
Perianal fistulas	21/95 (22.1%)	21/90 (23.3%)	5/47 (10.6%)	0.646 0.93 (0.47–1.86)	0.073 2.38 (0.84–6.79)	0.337 1.21 (0.64–2.31)
Stenosis	142/229 (62.0%)	139/230 (60.4%)	79/109 (72.5%)	0.774 0.94 (0.64–1.36)	0.067 1.61 (0.98–2.65)	0.595 1.10 (0.78–1.56)

For each variable, the number of patients included is given. Footnotes: see Table 4 and 5 for details.

Discussion

The identification of *NOD2* as the first CD susceptibility gene in 2001 represents a landmark finding that implicated bacterial recognition and innate immunity as key processes involved in the pathogenesis of CD. Since genotype-phenotype analyses of the *NOD2* variants p.Arg702Trp, p.Gly908Arg, and p.Leu1007fsX1008 have also provided strong evidence for the existence of a *NOD2*-related CD phenotype, these studies have not only changed our understanding of IBD pathogenesis but have also implications for clinical practice [21,22,23,25].

Table 8. Significant CD phenotype associations of rs2066843 and rs2076756 as shown in Tables 5, 6 and 7 stratified for the presence (*NOD2+*) or absence (*NOD2-*) of the three CD-associated *NOD2* mutations p.Arg702Trp (rs2066844), p.Gly908Arg (rs2066847), and p.Leu1007fsX1008 (rs2066847).

	NOD2+ n (%)	NOD2- n (%)	p value
rs2066843-TT carriers			
Surgery because of CD	65/95 (68.4%)	11/21 (52.4%)	0.206
	NOD2+ n (%)	NOD2- n (%)	
rs2076756-GG carriers			
Surgery because of CD	67/96 (69.8%)	9/14 (64.3%)	0.759
B3	63/96 (65.6%)	8/13 (61.5%)	0.765
Fistulas	63/96 (65.6%)	8/13 (61.5%)	0.765

Here, we investigated the two novel CD-associated *NOD2* variants rs2066843 and rs2076756 in a large German IBD patient cohort, confirming these *NOD2* variants as susceptibility gene variants for CD but not for UC. We could demonstrate a highly significant association of SNPs rs2066843 and rs2076756 with CD. The haplotype analysis revealed a number of significant associations with CD susceptibility, including several associations with omnibus p values of less than 10^{-10}.

In addition, for the first time, our genotype-phenotype analysis revealed a significant association of the SNPs rs2066843 and rs2076756 with phenotypic characteristics such as early disease onset, severe penetrating disease phenotype complicated by fistulas. Moreover, univariante analysis revealed a frequent need for CD-related surgery associated with SNPs rs2066843 and rs2076756 in CD patients. However, the two novel CD-associated NOD2 variants could not be identified as independent variables for the need for surgery in CD patients after logistic regression analysis, suggesting that ileal disease localization and a stricturing or penetrating phenotype are clinically more relevant predictors for the need for CD-related surgery than the NOD2 genotypes alone. In addition, the strength of the association of rs2066843 and rs2076756 with CD was less pronounced than that of the NOD2 variant rs2066847 (p.Leu1007fsX1008) which results in patients homozygous for this variant in a more severe phenotype [21,22] than found for rs2066843 and rs2076756 in this study. Early deep-sequencing studies of the NOD2 locus by the Hugot group also suggested that the NOD2 "gene-dosage" effect is more important in the CD phenotype development than the type of NOD2 mutation [25]. In the study by the Hugot group, patients with "double-dose" NOD2 mutations (homozygous or compound heterozygous) were characterized by a younger age at onset, a more frequent stricturing phenotype, and less frequent colonic involvement than were seen in those patients who had no mutation [25].

Although the phenotypic effects of rs2066843 and rs2076756 were independent of the presence of the three common *NOD2* variants p.Arg702Trp, p.Gly908Arg, and p.Leu1007fsX1008, the observed associations demonstrate similarities to the phenotype as previously shown to be related to the three common *NOD2* variants in our cohort [21,22]. The explorative character of our study has to be acknowledged. Given the large number of associations investigated, most associations would loose significance following Bonferroni correction. However, considering the size of our cohort and given that the highest percentages of carriers with ileocolonic involvement, stenoses, fistulas, and CD-related surgery were found without exception among the homozygous carriers of these two novel *NOD2* SNPs, an association with a severe CD phenotype is very likely. Moreover, this result has to be seen in the background of a study population of a tertiary referral center with a very high percentage of severe CD demonstrated by fistulas and stenoses and CD-related surgery in more than half of the study population regardless of the genotype. These phenotypic associations found in homozygous carriers of these SNPs were demonstrated with similar frequencies in the subgroup of CD patients with additional CD-associated *NOD2* mutations and in patients without these mutations, suggesting a specific disease-modifying effect of rs2066843 and rs2076756.

Our findings highlight the essential role of the *NOD2* region as CD susceptibility gene encoding a protein which acts as sensor for bacterial muramyl dipeptide (MDP) in the cell wall of Gram-positive and Gram-negative bacteria [8,15,16,17]. However, the exact mechanism how *NOD2* variants influence the intestinal inflammation is still under investigation. First, *NOD2* mutations are associated with diminished mucosal alpha-defensin expression in CD [33], although this finding is challenged by the results of a recent study [34], demonstrating that in ileal CD reduced alpha-defensin expression is the result of inflammation and not of *NOD2* mutation status. Second, there is evidence for an impaired dendritic cell function in CD patients with *NOD2* variants [35] and a loss of synergy between TLR9 and NOD2 in innate immune responses to CpG DNA [36]. Third, there might be cross-tolerization between NOD1 and NOD2 leading to increased recognition of both pathogenic and commensal bacteria in NOD2-deficient macrophages pre-exposed to microbial ligands [37]. Fourth, the study by Kobayashi et al. demontrated that *Nod2*-deficient mice are more susceptible to bacterial infection and thus Nod2 protein is a critical regulator of bacterial immunity within the intestine [38]. Finally, very recent evidence suggests that NOD1 and NOD2 are essential for recruitment of ATG16L1 during bacterial infection [31], which is impaired in patients with CD-associated *NOD* mutants [31]. We therefore analyzed CD-associated *NOD2* and *ATG16L1* variants for epistasis. However, we found no evidence for significant gene-gene interactions between these variants regarding CD susceptibility. This is in line with another large study demonstrating no epistasis for the three main CD-associated *NOD2* variants and *ATG16L1* [39], while another study found a weak gene-gene interaction between the *ATG16L1* variant rs2241880 and the three common CD-associated *NOD2* variants (p = 0.039) [14].

Despite the growing evidence for a strong genetic background in IBD by various genome-wide analyses and cohort studies [7,11,13,14,40,41,42,43,44], CD still remains a complex disorder modulated not only by susceptibility genes but also influenced by environmental factors. Moreover, there are genetic differences between different ethnic cohorts. For example, studies in Asian CD cohorts [45,46] could not show any evidence for a role of *NOD2* in CD susceptibility in Asian populations. Genetic counselling based on the *NOD2* genotype as well as the analysis of environmental risk factors could therefore benefit the individual at risk and change daily clinical practice.

Taken together, we conclude that the identification of the two novel *NOD2* variants rs2066843 and rs2076756 might have implications for the future risk assessment in CD patients, considering their high minor allele frequencies among Caucasian CD patients and the association with a severe disease phenotype. However, the association of these two *NOD2* variants with CD was less pronounced than that with rs2066847 (p.Leu1007fsX1008) which demonstrated even a more severe phenotypic effect than rs2066843 and rs2076756 in our previous studies [21,22]. So far, a major functional effect on the NF-κB pathway has only be shown for the p.Leu1007fsX1008 variant [6]. Therefore, further functional analyses of rs2066843 and rs2076756 as well as detailed genotype-phenotype analyses in very large cohorts including a comprehensive assessment of low frequency variants in the *NOD2* gene region are needed to clarify the contribution of these novel variants to the pathogenesis of CD. Currently, these two novel variants will not replace the other common CD-associated *NOD2* variants p.Arg702Trp (rs2066844), p.Gly908Arg (rs2066847), and p.Leu1007fsX1008 (rs2066847) when evaluating genetic risk factors in CD patients.

Supporting Information

Table S1 Primer sequences, FRET probe sequences and primer annealing temperatures used for genotyping of NOD2 variants rs2066843 and rs2076756. Note: FL: Fluorescein, LC640: Light-Cycler Red 640, LC670: LightCycler Red 670; the polymorphic position within the sensor probe is underlined. A phosphate is linked to the 3′-end of the acceptor probe to prevent elongation by the DNA polymerase in the PCR.

Table S2 Primer sequences used for sequence analysis of NOD2 variants rs2066843 and rs2076756.

Table S3 Allele frequencies of the SNPs rs2066843 and rs2076756 in patients with Crohn's disease (CD), ulcerative colitis (UC) and controls in the initial discovery cohort from the University Hospital Munich-Grosshadern. Minor allele frequencies (MAF), allelic test P-values, and odds ratios (OR, shown for the minor allele) with 95% confidence intervals (CI) are depicted for both the CD and UC case-control cohorts.

Table S4 Allele frequencies of the NOD2 SNPs in patients with Crohn's disease (CD), ulcerative colitis (UC) and controls from the replication cohort of the University Hospital Munich, Campus Innenstadt and Ruhr-University Bochum. Minor allele frequencies (MAF), allelic test P-values, and odds ratios (OR, shown for the minor allele) with 95% confidence intervals (CI) are depicted for both the CD and UC case-control cohorts.

Table S5 LD matrix for NOD2 SNPs in CD patients. Values are given as D'/r^2.

Table S6 LD matrix for NOD2 SNPs in UC patients. Values are given as D'/r^2.

Table S7 LD matrix for NOD2 SNPs in controls. Values are given as D'/r^2.

Table S8 Haplotype-analysis for NOD2 SNPs in the UC patient cohort. Only omnibus p-values are presented, given that none of these haplotypes showed significant disease association.

Table S9 Analysis for epistasis between SNPs rs2066843, rs2066843, rs2066844 (p.Arg702Trp), rs2066845 (p.Gly908Arg)

and rs2066847 (p.Leu1007fsX1008) in the NOD2 gene and the SNP rs2241880 = p.Thr300Ala within the ATG16L1 gene regarding CD susceptibility. *All p values given are uncorrected for multiple comparisons.

Author Contributions

Conceived and designed the experiments: JG SB. Performed the experiments: JG JS CT FB MW PL JD SB. Analyzed the data: JG SP MJ TO RPL BMM DC SB. Contributed reagents/materials/analysis tools: JG CT BG TO PL SB. Wrote the paper: JG JS SB.

References

1. Xavier RJ, Podolsky DK (2007) Unravelling the pathogenesis of inflammatory bowel disease. Nature 448: 427–434.
2. Podolsky DK (2002) Inflammatory bowel disease. N Engl J Med 347: 417–429.
3. Hanauer SB (2006) Inflammatory bowel disease: epidemiology, pathogenesis, and therapeutic opportunities. Inflamm Bowel Dis 12 Suppl 1: S3–9.
4. Brand S (2009) Crohn's disease: Th1, Th17 or both? The change of a paradigm: new immunological and genetic insights implicate Th17 cells in the pathogenesis of Crohn's disease. Gut 58: 1152–1167.
5. Hugot JP, Chamaillard M, Zouali H, Lesage S, Cezard JP, et al. (2001) Association of NOD2 leucine-rich repeat variants with susceptibility to Crohn's disease. Nature 411: 599–603.
6. Ogura Y, Bonen DK, Inohara N, Nicolae DL, Chen FF, et al. (2001) A frameshift mutation in NOD2 associated with susceptibility to Crohn's disease. Nature 411: 603–606.
7. Hugot JP (2006) CARD15/NOD2 mutations in Crohn's disease. Ann N Y Acad Sci 1072: 9–18.
8. Abreu MT (2005) Nod2 in normal and abnormal intestinal immune function. Gastroenterology 129: 1302–1304.
9. Kucharzik T, Maaser C, Lugering A, Kagnoff M, Mayer L, et al. (2006) Recent understanding of IBD pathogenesis: implications for future therapies. Inflamm Bowel Dis 12: 1068–1083.
10. Leon F, Smythies LE, Smith PD, Kelsall BL (2006) Involvement of dendritic cells in the pathogenesis of inflammatory bowel disease. Adv Exp Med Biol 579: 117–132.
11. Duerr RH, Taylor KD, Brant SR, Rioux JD, Silverberg MS, et al. (2006) A genome-wide association study identifies IL23R as an inflammatory bowel disease gene. Science 314: 1461–1463.
12. Glas J, Seiderer J, Wetzke M, Konrad A, Torok HP, et al. (2007) rs1004819 is the main disease-associated IL23R variant in German Crohn's disease patients: combined analysis of IL23R, CARD15, and OCTN1/2 variants. PLoS ONE 2: e819.
13. Torok HP, Glas J, Tonenchi L, Lohse P, Muller-Myhsok B, et al. (2005) Polymorphisms in the DLG5 and OCTN cation transporter genes in Crohn's disease. Gut 54: 1421–1427.
14. Hampe J, Franke A, Rosenstiel P, Till A, Teuber M, et al. (2007) A genome-wide association scan of nonsynonymous SNPs identifies a susceptibility variant for Crohn disease in ATG16L1. Nat Genet 39: 207–211.
15. Aldhous MC, Nimmo ER, Satsangi J (2003) NOD2/CARD15 and the Paneth cell: another piece in the genetic jigsaw of inflammatory bowel disease. Gut 52: 1533–1535.
16. Bonen DK, Ogura Y, Nicolae DL, Inohara N, Saab L, et al. (2003) Crohn's disease-associated NOD2 variants share a signaling defect in response to lipopolysaccharide and peptidoglycan. Gastroenterology 124: 140–146.
17. Girardin SE, Boneca IG, Viala J, Chamaillard M, Labigne A, et al. (2003) Nod2 is a general sensor of peptidoglycan through muramyl dipeptide (MDP) detection. J Biol Chem 278: 8869–8872.
18. Lakatos PL, Fischer S, Lakatos L, Gal I, Papp J (2006) Current concept on the pathogenesis of inflammatory bowel disease-crosstalk between genetic and microbial factors: pathogenic bacteria and altered bacterial sensing or changes in mucosal integrity take "toll"? World J Gastroenterol 12: 1829–1841.
19. Maeda S, Hsu LC, Liu H, Bankston LA, Iimura M, et al. (2005) Nod2 mutation in Crohn's disease potentiates NF-kappaB activity and IL-1beta processing. Science 307: 734–738.
20. Watanabe T, Kitani A, Murray PJ, Strober W (2004) NOD2 is a negative regulator of Toll-like receptor 2-mediated T helper type 1 responses. Nat Immunol 5: 800–808.
21. Seiderer J, Brand S, Herrmann KA, Schnitzler F, Hatz R, et al. (2006) Predictive value of the CARD15 variant 1007fs for the diagnosis of intestinal stenoses and the need for surgery in Crohn's disease in clinical practice: results of a prospective study. Inflamm Bowel Dis 12: 1114–1121.
22. Seiderer J, Schnitzler F, Brand S, Staudinger T, Pfennig S, et al. (2006) Homozygosity for the CARD15 frameshift mutation 1007fs is predictive of early

onset of Crohn's disease with ileal stenosis, entero-enteral fistulas, and frequent need for surgical intervention with high risk of re-stenosis. Scand J Gastroenterol 41: 1421–1432.
23. Economou M, Trikalinos TA, Loizou KT, Tsianos EV, Ioannidis JP (2004) Differential effects of NOD2 variants on Crohn's disease risk and phenotype in diverse populations: a metaanalysis. Am J Gastroenterol 99: 2393–2404.
24. Cuthbert AP, Fisher SA, Mirza MM, King K, Hampe J, et al. (2002) The contribution of NOD2 gene mutations to the risk and site of disease in inflammatory bowel disease. Gastroenterology 122: 867–874.
25. Lesage S, Zouali H, Cezard JP, Colombel JF, Belaiche J, et al. (2002) CARD15/NOD2 mutational analysis and genotype-phenotype correlation in 612 patients with inflammatory bowel disease. Am J Hum Genet 70: 845–857.
26. Schnitzler F, Brand S, Staudinger T, Pfennig S, Hofbauer K, et al. (2006) Eight novel CARD15 variants detected by DNA sequence analysis of the CARD15 gene in 111 patients with inflammatory bowel disease. Immunogenetics 58: 99–106.
27. Lennard-Jones JE (1989) Classification of inflammatory bowel disease. Scand J Gastroenterol Suppl 170: 2–6; discussion 16-19.
28. Silverberg MS, Satsangi J, Ahmad T, Arnott ID, Bernstein CN, et al. (2005) Toward an integrated clinical, molecular and serological classification of inflammatory bowel disease: Report of a Working Party of the 2005 Montreal World Congress of Gastroenterology. Can J Gastroenterol 19 Suppl A: 5–36.
29. Glas J, Konrad A, Schmechel S, Dambacher J, Seiderer J, et al. (2008) The ATG16L1 gene variants rs2241879 and rs2241880 (T300A) are strongly associated with susceptibility to Crohn's disease in the German population. Am J Gastroenterol 103: 682–691.
30. Alvarez-Lobos M, Arostegui JI, Sans M, Tassies D, Plaza S, et al. (2005) Crohn's disease patients carrying Nod2/CARD15 gene variants have an increased and early need for first surgery due to stricturing disease and higher rate of surgical recurrence. Ann Surg 242: 693–700.
31. Travassos LH, Carneiro LA, Ramjeet M, Hussey S, Kim YG, et al. (2010) Nod1 and Nod2 direct autophagy by recruiting ATG16L1 to the plasma membrane at the site of bacterial entry. Nat Immunol 11: 55–62.
32. Cooney R, Baker J, Brain O, Danis B, Pichulik T, et al. (2010) NOD2 stimulation induces autophagy in dendritic cells influencing bacterial handling and antigen presentation. Nat Med 16: 90–97.
33. Wehkamp J, Harder J, Weichenthal M, Schwab M, Schaffeler E, et al. (2004) NOD2 (CARD15) mutations in Crohn's disease are associated with diminished mucosal alpha-defensin expression. Gut 53: 1658–1664.
34. Simms LA, Doecke JD, Walsh MD, Huang N, Fowler EV, et al. (2008) Reduced alpha-defensin expression is associated with inflammation and not NOD2 mutation status in ileal Crohn's disease. Gut 57: 903–910.
35. Kramer M, Netea MG, de Jong DJ, Kullberg BJ, Adema GJ (2006) Impaired dendritic cell function in Crohn's disease patients with NOD2 3020insC mutation. J Leukoc Biol 79: 860–866.
36. van Heel DA, Ghosh S, Hunt KA, Mathew CG, Forbes A, et al. (2005) Synergy between TLR9 and NOD2 innate immune responses is lost in genetic Crohn's disease. Gut 54: 1553–1557.
37. Kim YG, Park JH, Daignault S, Fukase K, Nunez G (2008) Cross-tolerization between Nod1 and Nod2 signaling results in reduced refractoriness to bacterial infection in Nod2-deficient macrophages. J Immunol 181: 4340–4346.
38. Kobayashi KS, Chamaillard M, Ogura Y, Henegariu O, Inohara N, et al. (2005) Nod2-dependent regulation of innate and adaptive immunity in the intestinal tract. Science 307: 731–734.
39. Cummings JR, Cooney R, Pathan S, Anderson CA, Barrett JC, et al. (2007) Confirmation of the role of ATG16L1 as a Crohn's disease susceptibility gene. Inflamm Bowel Dis 13: 941–946.
40. Torok HP, Glas J, Tonenchi L, Bruennler G, Folwaczny M, et al. (2004) Crohn's disease is associated with a toll-like receptor-9 polymorphism. Gastroenterology 127: 365–366.
41. Baumgart DC, Carding SR (2007) Inflammatory bowel disease: cause and immunobiology. Lancet 369: 1627–1640.

42. Brand S, Staudinger T, Schnitzler F, Pfennig S, Hofbauer K, et al. (2005) The role of Toll-like receptor 4 Asp299Gly and Thr399Ile polymorphisms and CARD15/NOD2 mutations in the susceptibility and phenotype of Crohn's disease. Inflamm Bowel Dis 11: 645–652.

43. Cho J (2006) Genetic advances in inflammatory bowel disease. Curr Treat Options Gastroenterol 9: 191–200.

44. Dambacher J, Staudinger T, Seiderer J, Sisic Z, Schnitzler F, et al. (2007) Macrophage migration inhibitory factor (MIF) -173G/C promoter polymor-phism influences upper gastrointestinal tract involvement and disease activity in patients with Crohn's disease. Inflamm Bowel Dis 13: 71–82.

45. Yamazaki K, Takazoe M, Tanaka T, Ichimori T, Saito S, et al. (2004) Association analysis of SLC22A4, SLC22A5 and DLG5 in Japanese patients with Crohn disease. J Hum Genet 49: 664–668.

46. Wang YF, Zhang H, Ouyang Q (2007) Clinical manifestations of inflammatory bowel disease: East and West differences. J Dig Dis 8: 121–127.

11

Exome Sequencing Identifies *DLG1* as a Novel Gene for Potential Susceptibility to Crohn's Disease in a Chinese Family Study

Shufang Xu[1❂], **Feng Zhou**[1,2❂], **Jinsheng Tao**[3❂], **Lu Song**[1], **Siew Chien NG**[4], **Xiaobing Wang**[1], **Liping Chen**[1,2], **Fengming Yi**[1], **Zhihua Ran**[5], **Rui Zhou**[2], **Bing Xia**[1,2*]

1 Department of Gastroenterology, Zhongnan Hospital of Wuhan University School of Medicine, Wuhan, People's Republic of China, 2 Hubei Clinical Center and Key Laboratory for Intestinal and Colorectal Diseases, and Hubei Key Laboratory of Immune Related Diseases, Wuhan, People's Republic of China, 3 BGI-Shenzhen, Bei Shan Industrial Zone, Yantian District, Shenzhen, People's Republic of China, 4 Institute of Digestive Disease, Department of Medicine and Therapeutics, Li Ka Shing Institute of Health Sciences, The Chinese University of Hong Kong, Hong Kong, People's Republic of China, 5 Department of Gastroenterology, Renji Hospital, Shanghai Institute of Digestive Disease, Shanghai Jiao Tong University School of Medicine, Shanghai, People's Republic of China

Abstract

Background: Genetic variants make some contributions to inflammatory bowel disease (IBD), including Crohn's disease (CD) and ulcerative colitis (UC). More than 100 susceptibility loci were identified in Western IBD studies, but susceptibility gene has not been found in Chinese IBD patients till now. Sequencing of individuals with an IBD family history is a powerful approach toward our understanding of the genetics and pathogenesis of IBD. The aim of this study, which focuses on a Han Chinese CD family, is to identify high-risk variants and potentially novel loci using whole exome sequencing technique.

Methods: Exome sequence data from 4 individuals belonging to a same family were analyzed using bioinformatics methods to narrow down the variants associated with CD. The potential risk genes were further analyzed by genotyping and Sanger sequencing in family members, additional 401 healthy controls (HC), 278 sporadic CD patients, 123 UC cases, a pair of monozygotic CD twins and another Chinese CD family.

Results: From the CD family in which the father and daughter were affected, we identified a novel single nucleotide variant (SNV) c.374T>C (p.I125T) in exon 4 of discs large homolog 1 (*DLG1*), a gene has been reported to play mutiple roles in cell proliferation, T cell polarity and T cell receptor signaling. After genotyping among case and controls, a PLINK analysis showed the variant was of significance ($P<0.05$). 4 CD patients of the other Chinese family bore another non-synonymous variant c.833G>A (p.R278Q) in exon 9 of *DLG1*.

Conclusions: We have discovered novel genetic variants in the coding regions of *DLG1* gene, the results support that *DLG1* is a novel potential susceptibility gene for CD in Chinese patients.

Editor: Deyu Fang, Northwestern University Feinberg School of Medicine, United States of America

Funding: The study was supported by the Hubei Clinical Center and Key Laboratory of Intestinal and Colorectal Diseases, the Natural Science Foundation of China (No. 81070280) and a grant from the Ministry of Public Health of China (201002020). The funders had no role in study design, data collection and analysis, decision to publish, or preparation of the manuscript.

Competing Interests: The authors have declared that no competing interests exist.

* Email: bingxia@aliyun.com

❂ These authors contributed equally to this work.

Introduction

Crohn's disease (CD) and ulcerative colitis (UC) are classified as chronic, idiopathic inflammatory bowel diseases (IBD) [1,2]. Familial aggregation, high concordance in twins and a higher prevalence of the disease in a certain ethnic population imply a strong genetic influence on the risk of disease development [3,4]. Identifying the genetic loci or rare detrimental mutations in different populations or families with the disease will help elucidate the pathogenesis of these complex traits and facilitate the development of more targeted therapy.

It is now widely recognized that common variants shown in GWAS can explain only relatively modest proportions of risk for diseases. Numerous functional and deleterious variants in the population are at frequencies of 0.5 to 5% that are too low to be detected by GWAS [5,6]. As predisposing variants will present at a much higher frequency in the affected relatives of an index case, family studies may facilitate the detection of the 'missing heritability' not identified by GWAS [7]. Exome sequencing, which is a technique that focuses on the protein-coding portion of the genome, is not limited by the detailed and complete pedigree data that are necessary for classical linkage analysis and can be performed on only a few patients for the detection of causal mutations [8,9].

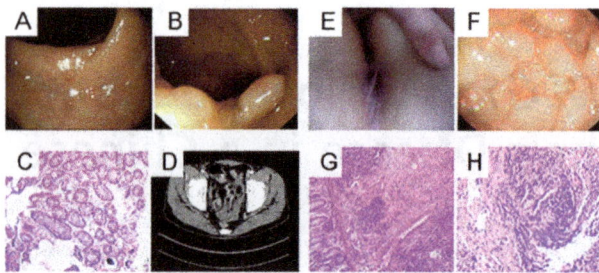

Figure 1. Clinical characteristics of two patients in Chinese CD family A. The index patient in the family, the father (Panels A to D) had evidence of mucous membrane granulation, polypoid proliferation and hyperemia in his colonoscopy, as shown in Panels A and B. Panel C shows the patient's pathological findings of chronic intestinal inflammation. Panel D shows the thickening of the ileum wall by small intestine computed tomography enterography (CTE). The daughter in the family is another Patient (Panels E to H). Panel E shows her anal fistula at disease onset. Endoscopy showed intestinal poly-ulcers in Panel F. A biopsy showed non-specific granulomatous inflammation, as shown in Panel G, and the higher magnification of the pathology shown in Panel H reveals negative acid-fast staining granulomas. All of the images were collected in March 2012 in Zhongnan Hospital of Wuhan University.

Researchers have successfully identified a causal hemizygous mutation in the XIAP gene [10] and novel compound heterozygous mutations in interleukin-10 receptor 1 (IL-10R1) [11], using exome sequencing in children presenting with very early-onset and intractable IBD. The sequencing of eight pediatric IBD patients' exomes revealed various profiles of specific variants with a limited number in each case [12].

Numerous candidate genes for Western IBD patients have been shown, but causality for specific variants in Chinese IBD patients is largely absent. In this study, we applied whole exome sequencing to 4 individuals belonging to a same family (Family A) to discover novel deleterious genetic variants associated with IBD and then validated these findings in other 10 family members of Family A, 401 healthy controls (HC), 278 subjects with sporadic CD, 123 subjects with UC, a pair of monozygotic twins and another Han Chinese CD family (Family B).

Materials and Methods

Patients and Controls

The familial patients included in this study were selected from the Hubei Clinical Center & Key Lab of Intestinal & Colorectal Diseases. Written informed consent was obtained from all subjects and the next of kin on behalf of the children enrolled in the study. This study was approved by the ethics committee of the Zhongnan Hospital of Wuhan University as part of the human subjects' protocol to study the genetics of IBD in humans. The CD patients

and HC were all unrelated subjects of Chinese descent and born to non-consanguineous parents. The ancestry of the patients and control individuals was assessed by self-report and appearance. Phenotypic data were acquired from a review of medical records, phone interviews and photographs. A combination of symptom assessment, laboratory and radiological examinations and endoscopy with histology was applied to make the diagnosis.

For whole exome sequencing, we selected a Han Chinese family (Family A) including a daughter and a father both affected with CD from Hubei province. In this family, the father is the proband, the proband's unaffected mother and wife were taken as exome sequencing controls. The father, who was diagnosed with CD at the age of 31 years in 1999 with terminal ileitis and proctitis, was treated with oral prednisolone and aminosalicylic acid (5-ASA). Small intestine computed tomography enterography (CTE) showed a thickened ileum wall in 2012.

The affected daughter developed CD at the age of 16 years in 2012, with high fever, diarrhea, oral ulcers and an anal fistula. Endoscopy showed upper digestive tract ulcers, aphthous ulcers at the ileocecal junction and colitis involving the rectum, sigmoid colon, descending colon and transverse colon. A biopsy showed non-specific granulomatous inflammation and staining was negative for acid-fast bacilli. She was finally diagnosed with CD and was treated with an intravenous injection of corticosteroids, 5-ASA, immunosuppressants and infliximab for severe refractory disease. She is now in remission with azathioprine and 5-ASA (the supporting data are provided in Fig. 1).

An additional 10 healthy members' blood DNA samples from family A were also taken as Sanger sequencing controls to validate the co-segregation of the mutations in the CD family.

In addition, 278 sporadic CD and 123 sporadic UC patients were enrolled from the Inflammatory Bowel Disease Center of Zhongnan Hospital of Wuhan University (131 CD, 76 UC), Renji Hospital of Shanghai Jiaotong University School of Medicine (40 CD) and the Institute of Digestive Disease of The Chinese University of Hong Kong (107 CD, 47 UC) from January 2001 to December 2012; 401 HC were from Wuhan, China (Table 1).

Moreover, we collected 25 young and intractable CD cases (Table 2), including a pair of monozygotic twins (Patient ID in Table 2: 24 and 25) and 23 cases selected from 131 sporadic CD patients of Hubei province. Another CD family (family B) was also from Wuhan city.

DNA Extraction

Genomic DNA was extracted from EDTA-anticoagulated peripheral venous blood samples using a QIAamp DNA Blood Midi Kit (Qiagen, Germany) according to the manufacturer's instructions.

Whole Exome Sequencing and Variant Detection

Using an E210 ultrasonicator (Covaris, MA, USA), the genomic DNA samples were randomly fragmented into 250–300 bp

Table 1. Characteristics of 401 sporadic inflammatory bowel disease (IBD) patients and 401 healthy controls.

Index	CD 278	UC 123	HC
Male (n=)	176	72	239
Female (n=)	102	51	162
Average age (years)	32.25±13.38	35.40±10.63	36.42±12.42

Table 2. Data of 25 young and intractable CD patients.

Patient ID	Age at diagnosis (year)	Sex	Disease location	Treatment					Surgery
				Diagnostic anti-TB	Aminosalicylates	Corticosteroids	Immunosuppressive agentes	Biological agentes	
1	25	Female	Terminal ileum	NO	YES	NO	NO	NO	YES
2	15	Male	Terminal ileum	NO	YES	YES	NO	YES	NO
3	24	Male	Terminal ileum	NO	YES	NO	YES	NO	NO
4	34	Male	Terminal ileum and ascending colon	YES	YES	NO	YES	NO	YES
5	16	Male	Terminal ileum and sigmoid colon	YES	YES	YES	YES	YES	NO
6	14	Male	Terminal ileum	YES	YES	NO	YES	YES	NO
7	19	Female	Terminal ileum and right sided colon	NO	YES	YES	YES	YES	YES
8	17	Male	Terminal ileum and descending colon	YES	YES	YES	YES	NO	NO
9	21	Male	Small intestine	NO	YES	YES	YES	NO	NO
10	20	Male	Terminal ileum and right sided colon	YES	YES	YES	YES	YES	YES
11	24	Female	Terminal ileum	NO	YES	NO	NO	YES	NO
12	21	Male	Terminal ileum	YES	YES	YES	YES	YES	NO
13	22	Female	Terminal ileum and sigmoid colon	YES	YES	YES	YES	YES	NO
14	23	Male	Terminal ileum and right sided colon	NO	YES	YES	YES	YES	NO
15	23	Male	Small intestine	NO	YES	YES	YES	YES	NO
16	17	Male	Terminal ileum and right sided colon	NO	YES	YES	YES	YES	NO
17	13	Female	Terminal ileum and ascending colon	YES	YES	YES	YES	YES	YES
18	24	Female	Terminal ileum	NO	YES	YES	YES	YES	NO
19	25	Male	Terminal ileum and ascending colon	NO	YES	YES	YES	YES	YES
20	11	Male	Terminal ileum and right sided colon	YES	YES	YES	YES	YES	YES
21	21	Female	Terminal ileum and ascending colon	YES	YES	YES	YES	NO	NO
22	14	Female	Terminal ileum and right sided colon	NO	YES	YES	YES	NO	YES
23	11	Male	Terminal ileum and right sided colon	YES	YES	YES	YES	YES	YES

Table 2. Cont.

Patient ID	Age at diagnosis (year)	Sex	Disease location	Treatment					
				Diagnostic anti-TB	Aminosalicylates	Corticosteroids	Immunosuppressive agentes	Biological agents	Surgery
24	26	Male	Terminal ileum	NO	YES	YES	YES	NO	YES
25	29	Male	Terminal ileum	NO	YES	YES	YES	YES	YES

TB: tuberculosis.

fragments and subjected to library preparation according to NimbleGen's standard protocol. Target region enrichment was performed for the shotgun libraries using the NimbleGen SeqCap EZ custom design kit (NimbleGen, Madison, WI, USA), which consisted of SeqCap EZ Human Exome Library v2.0 and a continuous region covering the MHC genes. The enriched shotgun libraries were sequenced using the Hiseq2000 platform, and 90-bp paired-end reads were generated. Raw image data and base calling were processed by Illumina Pipeline software version 1.7 with the default parameters. Quality control for the reads was performed by discarding adaptor-containing reads and low-quality reads. For SNP calling, SOAP aligner [13] was used to align the reads to the human reference genome (hg19), and SOAP snp [14] was then used to assemble the consensus sequence and call SNPs. As another quality control, low-quality SNPs satisfying one of the four following criteria were discarded: (i) genotype quality<20; (ii) total reads covering the variant site<4; (iii) estimated copy number >2; (iv) distance from the nearest SNP<5 bp (except for SNPs present in dbSNP). For indel calling, high-quality reads were aligned to the human reference genome using BWA (version 0.5.9-r16) [15]. GATK Indel Realigner was used to realign reads around insertion/deletion sites, and then small indels were called using the IndelGenotyperV2 tool from GATK (version v1.0.4705) [16,17]. Indels were called as heterozygous and homozygous if indel-supporting reads consisted of 30–70% and >70% of the total reads, respectively. SNP and indel detection was performed only for the targeted regions and flanking regions within 200 bp of the targeted regions.

Variant Annotation and Prioritization

The detected variants were annotated based on four databases, including NCBI CCDS, RefSeq, Ensembl and Encode (http://genome.ucsc.edu/ENCODE/). Exclusion steps were taken to help identify candidate mutations. Variants falling within intergenic, intronic and untranslated regions and synonymous substitutions were excluded; variants documented in 4 public genetic variant databases, including dbSNP132, 1000 Genomes, HapMap and YH (http://yh.genomics.org.cn/), with an allele frequency >0.5% (except for YH) were rejected; and variants shared by 2 exome sequenced cases and absent from 2 exome sequenced controls were kept. Additionally, we used the following criteria to evaluate and prioritize the candidate genes: (i) SIFT (http://sift.bii.a-star.edu.sg/), MutationTaster (http://www.mutationtaster.org/), Poly-Phen-2 (http://genetics.bwh.harvard.edu/pph2/index.shtml) and PMut (http://mmb.pcb.ub.es/PMut/) were used to predict whether single amino acid changes in genes would alter the protein function; (ii) the conservation of candidate mutations was analyzed by evaluating the GERP score (http://snp.gs.washington.edu/SeattleSeqAnnotation137/); (iii) the candidate mutations' total frequency of occurrence in the EVS (http://evs.gs.washington.edu/EVS/) and the BGI in-house database was analyzed and (iii) the tissue distributions and functions were analyzed using the online tools BioGPS (http://biogps.org/), Entrez Gene (http://www.ncbi.nlm.nih.gov/gene) and Proteinatlas (http://www.proteinatlas.org/).

As a final step, we compared and prioritized the remaining candidate genes using 4 internet tools: GeneDistiller2 (http://www.genedistiller.org/), SUSPECTS (http://www.genetics.med.ed.ac.uk/suspects/index.shtml), ToppGene (http://toppgene.cchmc.org/) and Endeavour (http://www.esat.kuleuven.be/endeavour). To prioritize the SNVs and genes, we chose 20 reported CD susceptibility genes (*NOD2, ATG16L1, STAT3, IL23R, IL10R2, IL10R1, JAK2, ICOSLG, CDKAL1, MST1,*

Table 3. The PCR primers of 22 candidate SNPs by Sanger Sequencing.

SNP_ID	Gene	F-primer sequences (5'-3')	R-primer sequences (5'-3')
chr17_55183450	AKAP1	TCAGAGTCCTCGGGCATT	CTGCTACATACTCTTCCTCC
chr20_30232655	COX4I2	ACAGTCCTTGGGGTCTAA	CCACTGCTTCTTCTCATAG
chr9_110249480	KLF4	AGTCCCGCCGCTCCATTA	TCTTTGGCTTGGGCTCCT
chr1_26368197	SLC30A2	ACTGCCTTATTCTGAACTGT	GAAGCATAATCCTCACCC
chr7_73279329	WBSCR28	GAGAATCGCCCGAAACC	CCAGGCACTGAGCAAGG
chr9_125582872	PDCL	GATTCTTGTTGTGCCTCAG	TTCCTGGTGAACTGACTGC
chr6_90418252	MDN1	AACCTCTTCCCCATCAT	TCCAACACCCCACAACT
chr20_420894	TBC1D20	GACCTGACACCTGCCTTTC	ACCCAGCATTTCCCAACT
chr9_2717768	KCNV2	CCACAGCCAGGAGGAAA	CTCGTAGTCGTCGCACA
chr16_20492206	ACSM2A	CAGGGCAGGGGATTTAG	TTGCTGGATCGTATGGTAGTT
chr15_41275952	INO80	AGCCAAAGCAGCCTCAAC	GGAATCAGGACCTTACCC
chr6_168366533	MLLT4	GAAGCAGGAGGCTGAGAA	TTGAGGTAGGAGGCGTTT
chr3_196921405	DLG1	GGTAAGAAATGAGCAATCAATATTCAG	GGGCGAACCTACATGAAAGAATA
chr1_1470881	TMEM240	GACGCCTCCGAGAACTACTTTG	ACAGCTTGGGCAGCCAGGTC
chr16_16170185	ABCC1	AACCCGTGGCTGATGTC	TGTCCAAGGCTGCTGTA
chr15_39885853	THBS1	TGGGTGCTGAGGATGTC	TGGTGATGCTGGGAACT
chr10_116225553	ABLIM1	TTCCTTGGCAGTGTTTG	GGAAATGTTTAGTCGTTGA
chr7_98602860	TRRAP	TTTCCCGTGACAGTTCG	CTCTTGGTGGTCTCCTTT
chr6_152536152	SYNE1	TTGGCTTTTCGCTATTC	ACCTTGACTGCGGACTT
chr14_21860964	CHD8	GCCCAAGGTAACAAACAG	CCAGGAGTCAATGAGGGA
chr7_99160120	ZNF655	TATGGGCTTTATTCCGTAG	CGGAGAAGACGATGTGAA
chr7_87051466	ABCB4	ATCCAAGTGGGCGTTTT	TGAATGTCTGCTGAGGG

PTGER4, IRGM, TNFSF15, ZNF365, NKX2-3, PTPN2, PTPN22, IL12B, XIAP and *ITLN1*) as the training set.

Validation Phase

All shared SNVs of the two affected individuals were verified for all members acquired from family A to detect co-segregation, by direct polymerase chain reaction (PCR) amplification followed by Sanger sequencing (PCR primers are listed in Table 3, Invitrogen). The sequencing reactions were conducted on an ABI 3730XL DNA Analyzer.

Genotyping was conducted by the MassARRAY (MALDI-TOF MS) method using the SEQUENOM System (Sequenom, Inc.) to screen the candidate genes in an additional 401 HC individuals (278 sporadic CD patients and 123 UC cases), and the data were analyzed using TYPER 4.0 software. The primer sequences for genotyping were designed and synthesized using Primer 5.0 software (PCR primer sequences are listed in Table 4, and the primers were synthesized by Invitrogen). To further study the genes (*DLG1* and *PDCL*) that we identified through the series of steps listed above, we applied PCR amplification followed by Sanger sequencing to examine all of the exons of *DLG1* and *PDCL* in 25 young and intractable CD cases (the PCR primer sequences are listed in Table 5).

SPSS17.0 statistical software was used for statistical analysis, the measurement data were expressed as means +/− standard deviation (SD). PLINK was performed on analysis of genotype data. P values<0.05 were considered as significant.

Results

Whole Exome Sequencing of the CD Family

Whole exome sequencing was performed on DNA extracted from the peripheral blood of 4 members of Family A using next-generation sequencing technology. As shown in Table 6, we obtained at least 88.5 million reads that mapped to the target region for each exome, more than 98.5% of the target region was covered and the mean depth of the target region was 128.64×, 148.90×, 202.26× and 158.25×. The summary statistics of the total quality-passing SNPs and indels are all listed in Table 6.

Bioinformatic Analysis Identifies 22 Candidate Genes

In total, 82 variants shared by the 2 cases remained through the exclusion of 4 public genetic databases (the procedures are shown in Table 7), and no reported IBD single nucleotide variant was found. After performing filtering steps for gene function and mutation prediction, we obtained 22 candidate genes (Table 8). Using 4 internet tools, we acquired the top 6 genes from the 22 candidates: *THBS1, KLF4, SYNE1, CHD8, PDCL* and *DLG1*. These genes were the most likely to be the genetic cause of the 2 affected patients.

Sanger Sequencing and Genotyping Combined with Bioinformatic Analyses Identifies DLG1 as a Potential Susceptibility Gene

Sanger sequencing confirmed the presence of the 22 mutations in the affected father and daughter. 10 healthy members of family A were sequenced to test for these variants. We found that one

Table 4. The primers of the 22 candidate SNPs for the MassARRAY method.

SNP_ID	Gene	F-primer sequences (5′-3′)	R-primer sequences (5′-3′)
chr17_55183450	AKAP1	ACGTTGGATGAGAGGGCAAGAGAGACAGGT	ACGTTGGATGACAGAGCTTCTTCAAGCACC
chr20_30232655	COX4I2	ACGTTGGATGAGCGCATGCTGGACATGAAG	ACGTTGGATGCTGCTTCTTCTCATAGTCCC
chr9_110249480	KLF4	ACGTTGGATGTCTTTGGCTTGGGCTCCTCT	ACGTTGGATGATGATGCTCACCCCACCT
chr1_26368197	SLC30A2	ACGTTGGATGAACCTTGACCATCCTGAGAG	ACGTTGGATGAAGAGCAAAAAGGGAGCCAC
chr7_73279329	WBSCR28	ACGTTGGATGTGATGGCTGACGGTTGTCTC	ACGTTGGATGGGAGCAGGAAATTATAGAGG
chr9_125582872	PDCL	ACGTTGGATGTGACTCTGAAGGAGTTTGCC	ACGTTGGATGATTCGCTGCTTCCGGTACTG
chr6_90418252	MDN1	ACGTTGGATGTTTGATGGACTTTGACCCAC	ACGTTGGATGTGCAGCTGATTCTAAAAGGG
chr20_420894	TBC1D20	ACGTTGGATGATGGGTGATGGTGAACCCAG	ACGTTGGATGACCCACTGATGCCGATTTAC
chr9_2717768	KCNV2	ACGTTGGATGAGCCATGCTCAAACAGAGTG	ACGTTGGATGCCTCATTCTCCGTCGTGTTC
chr16_20492206	ACSM2A	ACGTTGGATGGGTAGAGAATGCACTGATGG	ACGTTGGATGACGGGGTCTGGGCTGCTGAT
chr15_41275952	INO80	ACGTTGGATGACAACCAAACCAGTGCTGGG	ACGTTGGATGGTCTCAGATACCGTGAATGG
chr6_168366533	MLLT4	ACGTTGGATGAGACAGCACGACGAGGCGG	ACGTTGGATGTAGTCCCGGGGAAGCGGAG
chr3_196921405	DLG1	ACGTTGGATGGAACCAATTCTGGACCTATC	ACGTTGGATGGGATGAAGATACACCTCCTC
chr1_1470881	TMEM240	ACGTTGGATGAGCCGCCTGACCGCCCCTGT	ACGTTGGATGTGCACAGCTTGGGCAGCCAG
chr16_16170185	ABCC1	ACGTTGGATGTGTCCCTGACATGTCTCTGT	ACGTTGGATGTGAATGTGGCATTCCTCACG
chr15_39885853	THBS1	ACGTTGGATGTGGCGAGCACCTGCGGAAC	ACGTTGGATGTCCAGGGCTTTGCTTCTTAC
chr10_116225553	ABLIM1	ACGTTGGATGTGTACACAGGGGAGTTGATG	ACGTTGGATGAGGATGTTCGGGATCGGATG
chr7_98602860	TRRAP	ACGTTGGATGTGCAACACACGCTCCTCTC	ACGTTGGATGTGGCAAGATCTACCCATACC
chr6_152536152	SYNE1	ACGTTGGATGCTTCCTTCTAGGGACAGATG	ACGTTGGATGGGGTAACCTATATCCAAGCTC
chr14_21860964	CHD8	ACGTTGGATGCACAGCTAGTACTCAGACTC	ACGTTGGATGCGAGGTCAATACGGTTTATC
chr7_99160120	ZNF655	ACGTTGGATGGATAAACCGAATAATAAGG	ACGTTGGATGACCTCTACAGAGAAGTGATG
chr7_87051466	ABCB4	ACGTTGGATGGCAGAAGTGCAACATATTCTC	ACGTTGGATGACCTACCTGAAGGAAGAAAG

family member carried the variant in the *KLF4* gene. The other 21 mutations absent in healthy family members showed co-segregation.

The genotyping of the 22 SNVs indicated that 8 variants in *THBS1*, *SYNE1*, *CHD8*, *TMEM240*, *AKAP1*, *COX4I2*, *ZNF655* and *KCNV2* were positive in 401 HC, whereas the other 14 variants were negative. We again focused on the 6 top candidate genes (*THBS1*, *KLF4*, *SYNE1*, *CHD8*, *PDCL* and *DLG1*) identified through the prioritization analysis. In contrast to *THBS1*, *KLF4*, *SYNE1* and *CHD8*, none of the 401 HC was found to carry *PDCL* or *DLG1* mutations. Subsequent genotyping of 22 SNVs in 401 sporadic IBD cases indicated that one female CD patient aged 21 years carried a mutation in *DLG1* (Table 9), and no patients had variation in *PDCL*. A PLINK analysis showed the variant in *DLG1* was of significance ($P<0.05$).

By examining all of the exons of *PDCL* and *DLG1* in 25 young and intractable CD patients, we found two cases (Table 2, Patient ID are 3 and 4) who carried another variant in *DLG1* (Figure 2, exon 9, c.833G>A, p.R278Q). We traced Patient 3, 4 and their families, and found that two cousin sisters (Cases CJ2 and CJ3) and one brother (Case CJ4) of Patient 4 who were unexpectedly found to have ulcers in the terminal ileum by endoscopy, and a biopsy showed non-specific chronic inflammation. After being treated with 5-ASA and azathioprine, four affected cases in this family have almost achieved their colonic mucosal healing. Cases CJ2, CJ3 and CJ4 were all found to be carriers of mutation R278Q (c.833G>A) by Sanger sequencing, and the family was called family B. We found 4 unaffected carriers (CJ5, CJ6, CJ7 and CJ8) of this variant after sequencing the other 15 members of family B,

and these individuals will be followed up. CJ5 received a diagnosis of rheumatic heart disease with arthritis. The variants and carriers of *DLG1* are listed in Table 9. Neither of the monozygotic CD twins carried any mutation in all 3 exons of *PDCL* or in all 25 exons of *DLG1*.

Bioinformatics analyses were used to dissect the two non-synonymous mutations of *DLG1* found in the study described above. MutationTaster showed that the variant in *DLG1* (Figure 2, c.374T>C, p.I125T) was likely to be disease-causing. We compared the SNV sequence of species at different evolutionary distances by GERP and found that the amino acid substitution of *DLG1* was highly conserved. Regarding another variant of *DLG1* (Figure 2, exon 9, c.833G>A, p.R278Q), the PMut analysis of the mutation indicated that it is pathological (http://mmb.pcb.ub.es/PMut/), and the prediction from PolyPhen-2 was that the mutation was most likely damaging; however, the MutationTaster analysis indicated polymorphism, and SIFT predicted the mutation to be tolerated.

Discussion

Rare and low-frequency variants might have substantial effect sizes in complex disorders such as IBD [18]. A main goal of human genetic studies is to identify uncommon variants that play important roles in pathogenesis and reveal the familial transmission of diseases [6,8]. Furthermore, uncommon alleles shared by affected individuals in a family are more prone to familial clustering of disease than common alleles carried in a population.

In this study, we applied whole exome sequencing to anatomize the genetic background of a Chinese family with CD and

Table 5. The PCR primers of all exons of *DLG1* and *PDCL*.

Primer ID	F-primer sequences (5'-3')	R-primer sequences (5'-3')	Annealing temperature (°C)
DLG1			
Exon 1	CCGACTTCTGTCTGTTCTT	GGACCGTGCTGTCTCAT	54
Exon 2	CTCCTCCGTTTTCTAATG	GTTACCGAATGCCTCAG	51.5
Exon 3	GTTAAGTAGTTTGCCTGAACTTGTAGC	CAGATGAAGCCTTGTTGAGGTCT	62
Exon 4	GGTAAGAAATGAGCAATCAATATTCAG	GGGCGAACCTACATGAAAGAATA	55.5
Exon 5	TTTATCTTTATGGCACAGC	AAATGGCAAATCCTGACT	51.5
Exon 6	TTCTGTTTGGTGCTGGAG	GGTCTTCGCATTTGTATC	55.5
Exon 7	CAGAGAAGGATCGGAGGTTGA	GTAAATGGAAACTCTTGGGACTATC	58.8
Exon 8	CCTCCAGAACAAGTCCA	GTATTTATCCCTTATCCAGTC	51.5
Exon 9	TGTTCCTTTTGCTGGCCCTT	ATGACTGCACCACTGGACTC	63
Exon 10	TTCGTAACTCTAGGAGCAGCTGT	CTGTGCATACAAGCCCTCAAC	61
Exon 11	AGACTGGGAGAATAGGAGG	TCACTAATGGCATCACAAC	55.5
Exon 12	TTGAGACTAACCTGGGCAACAT	AAGGACAATTTACCAAGCCTCAA C	61
Exon 13	CTTCTAAGTAGGGGCAGTG	AATAGGTCCAGTGAAAATAAC	54
Exon 14	CAGTAGGCGTGAGAATGTGGC	GCCTGGGCAGTAAGAGTGGA	63
Exon 15	GATTACTGCTGTCTGATGC	GCCTCCTTTGCTACTATG	55.5
Exon 16	TCAATATAACTTACCATTGGATTACAATC	AGTACTATTACCTGTAGTTGCCATGCT	57
Exon 17	TTAAACTCAGAAATGGTGCCTCA	GGTCTGTGAAATGGGTGCTTG	61
Exon 18	AGGTATAAATGAACTATGCTGTCTGAA	CCTTGAAGACAATTAGCAACCTG	58.8
Exon 19	AGTTTGTCCCCTTTGCC	TCAGAATCCCTCCACCC	55.5
Exon 20	AAATAAAGGAGTAGCACATAGC	GAAAGAAGTGGGATAAACAG	54
Exon 21	CATCTTTGGTTGATGGTAGAGTGAG	AGAAAGGACAATAATATGGAGGATG	58.8
Exon 22	ATCCATCCTCCATATTATTGTCCT	ACCCGGCCCTTATCTCCT	57
Exon 23	TTTCATTTCCTATCTAAAGTTTGCTG	ATGGTTCTGCCTCACATTCTGT	57
Exon 24	TGTGTCATCTCTCCTTTGCCA	GAGCCGAGTCATACCATTGC	62
Exon 25	CTATGGGATTGTACCCAGTTTCC	GGTCAGGCCATTCCATCTTC	57
PDCL			
Exon 1	TGTCCTGGAAATTGTAGGATCTCA	GACTAGGTTACCTCTGAAAGTGGGA	60.5
Exon 2	ATGTTGGGCATTAGCTTGGC	TTTGACAGGGCTCTATGATTTCTC	60.5
Exon 3-1	TCAAGTGATCCGCTCGTCT	AGCTTCAAGGTCCACAGCA	60.5
Exon 3-2	GCCAGCAGTCAGTTCACCAG	TTTGACAGGGCTCTATGATTTCTC	60.5

Table 6. Summary of original exome sequencing data of four familial individuals.

Exome Capture Statistics	Daughter	Father	Grandmother	Mother
Target region (bp)	48959543	49062223	48959543	48959543
Raw reads	243896508	204592452	253503938	192147514
Raw data yield (Mb)	21951	18413	22815	17293
Reads mapped to genome	204193470	145810600	202993882	156292035
Reads mapped to target region[2]	88581652	101995817	138982919	108872112
Data mapped to target region (Mb)	6298.25	7305.56	9902.46	7748.06
Mean depth of target region (X)	128.64	148.90	202.26	158.25
Coverage of target region (%)	98.77	98.56	98.81	98.75
Average read length (bp)	89.87	89.84	89.78	89.85
Total quality-passing SNPs	116950	114204	119780	117371
Total quality-passing indels	7442	7361	7773	7500

Table 7. Filtration of SNPs/Indels.

Individual ID	Grandmother	Mother	Daughter	Father
Total SNPs and indels	173991+7773	172848+7500	172005+7442	173055+7361
Quality-passing SNPs and indels	119780+7773	117371+7500	116950+7442	114204+7361
Protein-disrupting SNPs and indels (PDSI)	14553+1369	14345+1314	14581+1280	14547+1294
PDSI after filtering against dbSNP	2144+382	2138+366	2108+348	2129+359
PDSI after filtering against dbSNP+1000 Genomes	1459+220	1498+221	1469+189	1448+208
PDSI after filtering against dbSNP+1000 Genomes+HapMap	1457+220	1497+221	1467+189	1446+208
PDSI after filtering against dbSNP+1000 Genomes+HapMap+YH	1420+220	1460+221	1438+189	1413+208
PDSI after filtering against dbSNP+1000 Genomes+HapMap+YH+inhouse data and fitting a dominant model (**shared by two cases**)	0	0	82+0	
Filtered candidate genes			**22**	
Sanger sequence for validation			**22**	

successfully identified genetic variants in the coding regions of the *DLG1* gene that may be associated with increased risk of CD. We first identified a novel SNV c.374T>C (p.I125T) in exon 4 of *DLG1* through whole exome sequencing and bioinformatic analysis. In subsequent validation studies, we also identified 4 CD patients of another Han Chinese family harbored the variant c.833G>A. Altogether these data suggest that *DLG1* is a susceptible gene for CD.

DLG1 encodes a multi-domain scaffolding protein, which may have a role in septate junction formation, signal transduction, cell proliferation, synaptogenesis and lymphocyte activation (http://www.ncbi.nlm.nih.gov/gene/). The DLG1 protein is composed of an N-terminal L27b oligomerization domain, a proline-rich domain (PRD), three PDZ (PSD-95, Dlg and ZO-1) domains, an SH3 (Src Homology 3) domain and a catalytically inactive GUK (GUanylate Kinase) domain. During antigen recognition, these modular domains allow DLG1 to co-localize with synaptic actin, translocate into sphingolipid-rich microdomains within the IS and associate with Lck, ZAP-70, Vav, WASp Ezrin and p38 [19]. *DLG1* has been shown to play roles in T cell polarity and T cell receptor signal specificity [20,21], and be involved in the generation of memory T cells [22]. The loss of *DLG1* leads to increased invasion in response to pro-tumorigenic cytokines, such as IL-6 and TNF-α [23,24].

In accord with the suggested autoimmune nature of CD, strong evidence has implicated T cells and T-cell migration to the gut in initiating and perpetuating the intestinal inflammatory process and tissue destruction [25,26]. Anti-cytokine agents are therefore likely to be useful in the treatment of IBD [27,28]. After intravenous injection with six cycles of infliximab, the affected daughter in Family A has almost achieved mucosal healing of her colonic disease and was likely to have a better prognosis than those *DLG1* mutation carriers who did not accept infliximab treatments in our study. It was corroborative evidence that *DLG1* was causative for the CD patients of the two Chinese families.

Complex human disease is a large collection of individually rare, even private variants [29]. A single locus can harbor both common variants of weak effect and rare variants of strong effect [30]. The results of our study of two CD families indicated genetic heterogeneity and susceptibility. We analyzed family A using an autosomal dominant model, and several factors were important to the success of this study.

First, according to the database at our center [31], although the incidence of CD and UC is still low, the number of cases and severity of disease are increasing in China [32,33], which provides the appropriate conditions to recruit patients for the subsequent validations.

Second, a stepwise approach was taken to help narrow down the list of genetic variants responsible for this disease. For the genetic susceptibility of CD, despite the success of GWAS in identifying significantly associated loci [34], the currently identified variants are estimated to account for less than a quarter of the predicted heritability [35]. Uncommon alleles may be maintained at a lower frequency in the population through negative selection, and it is not possible to create a complete catalog in the general population [36]. Therefore, rare causal variants are not likely to be found in public SNP databases and control exomes [37]. We did not find mutations in any reported susceptibility genes that were shared by the affected father and daughter, which suggested that other variants may be associated with CD in these 2 individuals. To predict the impact of nonsynonymous variants, we applied 4 popular methods (PolyPhen2, SIFT, MutationTaster and PMut) [38,39]. However, none of these methods was perfectly sensitive or specific. Regarding the mutation c.374T>C, SIFT and MutationTaster predicted it to be tolerated and disease causing, respectively. Different prediction algorithms used different information, and each had its own relative merits. It is thought to be better to use predictions from multiple algorithms rather than relying on a single one [40,41]. We also used several different bioinformatic methods to filter and prioritize the SNVs and genes to increase the robustness of the analysis results.

Finally, to confirm the results and identify the susceptibility gene, we used genotyping and Sanger sequencing methods for validation. Traditional Sanger sequencing is the gold standard for mutation detection [9]. We were able to narrow the scope to only a few genes through these steps. By scanning all exons of *DLG1* and *PDCL*, a nonsynonymous variant c.833G>A of *DLG1* was found in family B, thus confirming that *DLG1* is a gene whose mutation is associated with high risk.

Some limitations must be addressed. First, IBD patients with family history are rare among Han Chinese. In this family study, there were only two affected members, so the size of the pedigree was small. Second, the patients studied did not have an onset as early as those were previous reported in Caucasian population [42,43]. Third, because of genetic heterogeneity, the variants

Table 8. List of 22 candidate genes and mutations prediction.

NO	Chromosome	Position	Reference	Gene name	Codons	SIFT Prediction	MutationTaster Prediction	ConsScore GERP
1	chr6	90418252	C	MDN1	GAC7861CAC	DAMAGING	polymorphism	2.23
2	chr14	21860964	C	CHD8	CGT5636CAT	DAMAGING	disease causing	5.34
3	chr9	125582872	T	PDCL	GAT398GGT	DAMAGING	disease causing	5.47
4	chr17	55183450	G	AKAP1	GTG625ATG	DAMAGING	polymorphism	4.22
5	chr15	39985853	G	THBS1	GGA3251GAA	DAMAGING	disease causing	5.78
6	chr16	16170185	G	ABCC1	GGG1915TGG	DAMAGING	disease causing	4.11
7	chr1	1470881	G	TMEM240	TCG380TTG	DAMAGING	disease causing	3.37
8	chr7	73279329	C	WBSCR28	CAG79AAG	DAMAGING	polymorphism	4.43
9	chr9	2717768	C	KCNV2	TCC29TGC	DAMAGING	disease causing	4.45
10	chr7	99160120	A	ZNF655	–	–	–	3.92
11	chr15	41275952	G	INO80	–	–	–	2.69
12	chr10	116225553	G	ABLIM1	CGG1345TGG	DAMAGING	disease causing	3.37
13	chr1	26368197	T	SLC30A2	ATG685GTG	DAMAGING	disease causing	5.6
14	chr20	30232655	T	COX4I2	GTG464GCG	DAMAGING	disease causing	4.38
15	chr6	167570520	G	GPR31	ACG800ATG	DAMAGING	polymorphism	2.65
16	chr6	168366533	G	MLLT4	GGA4993AGA	DAMAGING	disease causing	5.03
27	chr16	2049206	C	ACSM2A	ACG1472ATG	DAMAGING	polymorphism	3.26
18	chr20	420894	C	TBC1D20	GTG766ATG	DAMAGING	disease causing	5.65
19	chr9	110249480	G	KLF4	–	–	–	3.45
20	chr3	196921405	A	DLG1	ATC374ACC	TOLERATED	disease causing	5.17
21	chr6	152536152	C	SYNE1	CGT22022CAT	TOLERATED	disease causing	5.07
22	chr7	87051466	T	ABCB	ATT2287GTT	TOLERATED	polymorphism	4.85

Table 9. Distributions of rare variants in the *DLG1* gene.

Patient ID	Gender	Age (years)	Nucleotide change	Amino acid change	Chromosome Position	Exon	Sequencing method
CD Family A							
Father(diagnosed)	Male	44	c.374T>C	p.I125T	chr3_196921405	4	Exome
Daughter(diagnosed)	Female	16	c.374T>C	p.I125T	chr3_196921405	4	Exome
Mother(unaffected)	Female	42	–	–	–	–	Exome
Grandma(unaffected)	Female	81	–	–	–	–	Exome
CD Family B							
Case 1(diagnosed)	Male	39	c.833G>A	p.R278Q	chr3_196865242	9	Direct PCR sequencing
Case 2(diagnosed)	Male	42	c.833G>A	p.R278Q	chr3_196865242	9	Direct PCR sequencing
Case 3(diagnosed)	Female	32	c.833G>A	p.R278Q	chr3_196865242	9	Direct PCR sequencing
Case 4(diagnosed)	Female	24	c.833G>A	p.R278Q	chr3_196865242	9	Direct PCR sequencing
CJ 5(undiagnosed)	Female	56	c.833G>A	p.R278Q	chr3_196865242	9	Direct PCR sequencing
CJ 6(undiagnosed)	Female	6	c.833G>A	p.R278Q	chr3_196865242	9	Direct PCR sequencing
CJ 7(undiagnosed)	Female	6	c.833G>A	p.R278Q	chr3_196865242	9	Direct PCR sequencing
CJ 8(undiagnosed))	Male	7	c.833G>A	p.R278Q	chr3_196865242	9	Direct PCR sequencing

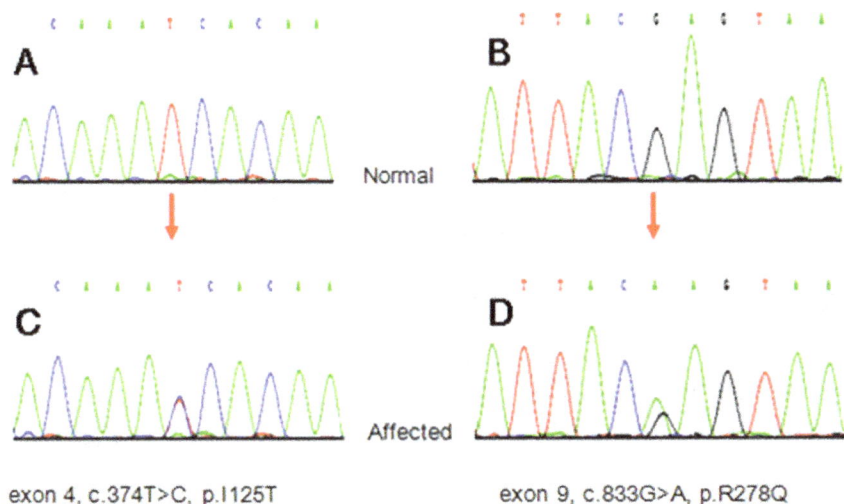

Figure 2. Chromatogram of *DLG1* gene mutations. The Sanger sequence traces from normal human controls are shown in panel A and B; the mutations were heterozygous at the corresponding locus (orange arrows indicating) in panel C and D.

appear to be present only in a subset of CD patients, and were not carried by the pair of monozygotic twins studied. Furthermore, in complex diseases, a central problem is that each variant only makes a small contribution to the disorder [44]. Other candidate genes discovered by us, such as *THBS1*, *KLF4*, *SYNE1*, *CHD8* and *PDCL*, may also contribute to CD. However, variation in these genes must be identified in more cases and controls. Additionally, considering that the variant was also present in the unaffected individuals of family B, other disease-causing factors lying outside of our set of candidate genes may also exist [45]. Finally, functional analyses are needed to elucidate the biological role of this gene in CD susceptibility.

In conclusion, we report the discovery of coding region variants in *DLG1* in human CD through whole exome sequencing and bioinformatic analysis and identify *DLG1* as a potential susceptibility gene for CD in the Chinese population. Our study also demonstrates that whole exome sequencing is an efficient and cost-effective genetic strategy. Bioinformatic approaches are likely to become useful tools for the discovery of genes and to provide important guidance for finding rare variants in a complex disorder. Finding different, rare and pathogenic mutations in the

same gene in unrelated individuals with the same phenotype provides important support for our study. However, confirmation of *DLG1*'s involvement in CD pathogenesis still requires validation in further functional experiments and clinical trials. Personalized medicine is also anticipated to be developed based on definite biological processes and molecular causes.

Acknowledgments

The authors would like to thank the patients with IBD and the healthy controls who volunteered to participate in this study. The works of whole exome sequencing and MassARRAY genotyping were performed in BGI-Shenzhen. We thank editors in American Journal Experts for the valuable contribution to edit and revise the manuscript.

Author Contributions

Conceived and designed the experiments: BX SFX RZ LPC. Wrote the paper: SFX FZ. Clinic data extraction: SCNG RZ LPC FMY ZHR. DNA collection and quality assessment: SFX LS XBW. Bioinformatics and statistical analysis: JST.

References

1. Van Assche G, Dignass A, Panes J, Beaugerie L, Karagiannis J, et al. (2010) The second European evidence-based Consensus on the diagnosis and management of Crohn's disease: Definitions and diagnosis. J Crohns Colitis 4: 7–27.
2. Mowat C, Cole A, Windsor A, Ahmad T, Arnott I, et al. (2011) Guidelines for the management of inflammatory bowel disease in adults. Gut 60: 571–607.
3. Freeman HJ (2002) Familial Crohn's disease in single or multiple first-degree relatives. J Clin Gastroenterol 35: 9–13.
4. Brant SR (2011) Update on the heritability of inflammatory bowel disease: the importance of twin studies. Inflamm Bowel Dis 17: 1–5.
5. Majewski J, Schwartzentruber J, Lalonde E, Montpetit A, Jabado N (2011) What can exome sequencing do for you? J Med Genet 48: 580–589.
6. Teer JK, Mullikin JC (2010) Exome sequencing: the sweet spot before whole genomes. Hum Mol Genet 19: R145–151.
7. Manolio TA, Collins FS, Cox NJ, Goldstein DB, Hindorff LA, et al. (2009) Finding the missing heritability of complex diseases. Nature 461: 747–753.
8. Nazarian A, Sichtig H, Riva A (2012) Knowledge-Based Method for Association Studies on Complex Diseases. PLoS One 7: e44162.
9. Gilissen C, Hoischen A, Brunner HG, Veltman JA (2012) Disease gene identification strategies for exome sequencing. Eur J Hum Genet 20: 490–497.
10. Worthey EA, Mayer AN, Syverson GD, Helbling D, Bonacci BB, et al. (2011) Making a definitive diagnosis: Successful clinical application of whole exome

sequencing in a child with intractable inflammatory bowel disease. Genet Med 13: 255–262.
11. Mao H, Yang W, Lee PP, Ho MH, Yang J, et al. (2012) Exome sequencing identifies novel compound heterozygous mutations of IL-10 receptor 1 in neonatal-onset Crohn's disease. Genes Immun 13: 437–442.
12. Christodoulou K, Wiskin AE, Gibson J, Tapper W, Willis C, et al. (2013) Next generation exome sequencing of paediatric inflammatory bowel disease patients identifies rare and novel variants in candidate genes. Gut 62: 977–984.
13. Li R, Yu C, Li Y, Lam TW, Yiu SM, et al. (2009) SOAP2: an improved ultrafast tool for short read alignment. Bioinformatics 25: 1966–1967.
14. Li R, Li Y, Fang X, Yang H, Wang J, et al. (2009) SNP detection for massively parallel whole-genome resequencing. Genome Re Li R, Li Y, Fang X, Yang H, Wang J, search 19: 1124–1132.
15. Li H, Durbin R (2010) Fast and accurate long-read alignment with Burrows-Wheeler transform. Bioinformatics 26: 589–595.
16. McKenna A, Hanna M, Banks E, Sivachenko A, Cibulskis K, et al. (2010) The genome analysis toolkit: a MapReduc framework for analyzing next-generation DNA sequencing data. Genome Research 20: 1297–1303.
17. Wang J, Wang W, Li R, Li Y, Tian G, et al. (2008) The diploid genome sequence of an Asian individual. Nature 456: 60–65.

18. Cho JH, Brant SR (2011) Recent insights into the genetics of inflammatory bowel disease. Gastroenterology 140: 1704–1712.

19. O'Neill AK, Gallegos LL, Justilien V, Garcia EL, Leitges M, et al. (2011) Protein kinase Cα promotes cell migration through a PDZ-dependent interaction with its novel substrate discs large homolog 1 (DLG1). J Biol Chem 286: 43559–43568.

20. Humphries LA, Shaffer MH, Sacirbegovic F, Tomassian T, McMahon KA, et al. (2012) Characterization of in vivo Dlg1 deletion on T cell development and function. PLoS One 7: e45276.

21. Xavier R, Rabizadeh S, Ishiguro K, Andre N, Ortiz JB, et al. (2004) Discs large (Dlg1) complexes in lymphocyte activation. J Cell Biol 166: 173–178.

22. Gmyrek GB, Graham DB, Sandoval GJ, Blaufuss GS, Akilesh HM, et al. (2013) Polarity gene discs large homolog 1 regulates the generation of memory T cells. Eur J Immunol 43: 1185–1194.

23. Chatterjee S, Seifried L, Feigin ME, Gibbons DL, Scuoppo C, et al. (2012) Dysregulation of cell polarity proteins synergize with oncogenes or the microenvironment to induce invasive behavior in epithelial cells. PLoS One 7: e34343.

24. Surena AL, de Faria GP, Studler JM, Peiretti F, Pidoux M, et al. (2009) DLG1/SAP97 modulates transforming growth factor alpha bioavailability. Biochim Biophys Acta 1793: 264–272.

25. Strober W, Fuss IJ (2011) Proinflammatory cytokines in the pathogenesis of inflammatory bowel diseases. Gastroenterology 140: 1756–1767.

26. MacDonald TT, Monteleone I, Fantini MC, Monteleone G. (2011) Regulation of homeostasis and inflammation in the intestine. Gastroenterology 140: 1768–1775.

27. Plevy SE, Targan SR (2011) Future therapeutic approaches for inflammatory bowel diseases. Gastroenterology 140: 1838–1846.

28. Danese S (2012) New therapies for inflammatory bowel disease: from the bench to the bedside. Gut 61: 918–932.

29. McClellan J, King MC (2010) Genetic heterogeneity in human disease. Cell 141: 210–217.

30. Altshuler D, Daly MJ, Lander ES (2008) Genetic mapping in human disease. Science 322: 881–888.

31. Zhao J, Ng SC, Lei Y, Yi F, Li J, et al. (2013) First Prospective, Population-Based Inflammatory Bowel Disease Incidence Study in Mainland of China: The Emergence of "Western" Disease. Inflamm Bowel Dis 19: 1839–1845.

32. Ng SC, Tang W, Ching JY, Wong M, Chow CM, et al. (2013) Incidence and Phenotype of Inflammatory Bowel Disease Based on Results From the Asia-Pacific Crohn's and Colitis Epidemiology Study. Gastroenterology 145: 158–165.

33. Yi F, Chen M, Huang M, Li J, Zhao J, et al. (2012) The trend in newly diagnosed Crohn's disease and extraintestinal manifestations of Crohn's disease in central China: a retrospective study of a single center. Eur J Gastroenterol Hepatol 24: 1424–1429.

34. Franke A, McGovern DP, Barrett JC, Wang K, Radford-Smith GL, et al. (2010) Genome-wide meta-analysis increases to 71 the number of confirmed Crohn's disease susceptibility loci. Nat Genet 42: 1118–1125.

35. Clarke AJ, Cooper DN (2010) GWAS: heritability missing in action? Eur J Hum Genet 18: 859–861.

36. Gibson G. (2012) Rare and common variants: twenty arguments. Nat Rev Genet 13: 135–145.

37. Tennessen JA, Bigham AW, O'Connor TD, Fu W, Kenny EE, et al. (2012) Evolution and functional impact of rare coding variation from deep sequencing of human exomes. Science 337: 64–69.

38. Ng PC, Henikoff S (2003) SIFT: predicting amino acid changes that affect protein function. Nucleic Acids Res 31: 3812–3814.

39. Schwarz JM, Rödelsperger C, Schuelke M, Seelow D (2010) MutationTaster evaluates disease-causing potential of sequence alterations. Nat Methods 7: 575–576.

40. Liu X, Jian X, Boerwinkle E (2011) dbNSFP: a lightweight database of human nonsynonymous SNPs and their functional predictions. Hum Mutat 32: 894–899.

41. Brunham LR, Hayden MR (2013) Hunting human disease genes: lessons from the past, challenges for the future. Hum Genet 132: 603–617.

42. Glocker EO, Frede N, Perro M, Sebire N, Elawad M, et al. (2010) Infant colitis–it's in the genes. Lancet 376: 1272.

43. Glocker EO, Kotlarz D, Boztug K, Gertz EM, Schäffer AA, et al. (2009) Inflammatory bowel disease and mutations affecting the interleukin-10 receptor. N Engl J Med 361: 2033–2045.

44. Kevin J, Mitchell (2012) What is complex about complex disorders? Genome Biol 13: 237.

45. Gibson G. (2009) Decanalization and the origin of complex disease. Nat Rev Genet 10: 134–140.

12

GLP2-2G-XTEN: A Pharmaceutical Protein with Improved Serum Half-Life and Efficacy in a Rat Crohn's Disease Model

Susan E. Alters*, Bryant McLaughlin, Benjamin Spink, Tigran Lachinyan, Chia-wei Wang, Vladimir Podust, Volker Schellenberger, Willem P. C. Stemmer

Amunix Inc., Mountain View, California, United States of America

Abstract

Objectives: Glucagon-like peptide 2 (GLP2) is an intestinal growth factor that has been shown to stimulate intestinal growth and reduce disease severity in preclinical models of short bowel syndrome and inflammatory bowel disease. Teduglutide, a recombinant human GLP2 variant (GLP2-2G), has increased half-life and stability as compared to the native GLP2 peptide, but still requires twice daily dosing in preclinical models and daily dosing in the clinic. The goal of this study was to produce and characterize the preclinical pharmacokinetic and therapeutic properties of GLP2-2G-XTEN, a novel, long-acting form of GLP2-2G.

Methodology and Results: A GLP2-2G-XTEN fusion protein with extended exposure profile was produced by genetic fusion of GLP2-2G peptide to XTEN, a long, unstructured, non-repetitive, hydrophilic sequence of amino acids. The serum half-life of GLP2-2G-XTEN in mice, rats and monkeys was 34, 38 and 120 hours, respectively. Intestinotrophic effects were demonstrated in normal rats, where GLP2-2G-XTEN administration resulted in a significant increase in both small intestine weight and length. Efficacy of the GLP2-2G-XTEN protein was compared to that of GLP2-2G peptide in a rat Crohn's disease model, indomethacin-induced inflammation. Prophylactic administration of GLP2-2G-XTEN significantly increased the length, reduced the number of trans-ulcerations and adhesions, and reduced the TNFα content of the small intestine. GLP2-2G-XTEN demonstrated greater *in vivo* potency as compared to GLP2-2G peptide, and improvement in histopathology supported the GLP2-2G-XTEN treatment effects.

Conclusions and Significance: GLP2-2G-XTEN is intestinotrophic and demonstrates efficacy in a rat Crohn's disease model requiring a lower molar dose and less frequent dosing relative to GLP2-2G peptide. Allometric scaling based on pharmacokinetics from mouse, rat and monkey projects a human half-life of 240 hours. These improvements in preclinical pharmacokinetics and dosing indicate that GLP2-2G-XTEN may offer a superior therapeutic benefit for treatment of gastrointestinal diseases including Crohn's disease.

Editor: Partha Mukhopadhyay, National Institutes of Health, United States of America

Funding: The project was supported by funding from Amunix, Inc. Employees of Amunix had a primary role in the design, data collection and analysis, decision to publish, and preparation of the manuscript. No current external funding sources for this study.

Competing Interests: All authors are employed by or have an ownership interest in Amunix, Inc. The project was supported by funding from Amunix, Inc. There are no patents, products in development or marketed products to declare.

* E-mail: salters@amunix.com

Introduction

Glucagon-like peptide 2 (GLP2) is a 33 amino acid peptide derived from the post-translational processing of glucagon. First identified by Drucker [1], GLP2 is secreted from the enteroendocrine L cells of the small intestine and colon in response to nutritional stimulation. A specific gastrointestinal growth factor, GLP2 has been shown to increase the ability of the intestine to digest and absorb nutrients. In addition, it was found to possess potent intestinotrophic properties as well as significant reparative activity for the mucosal epithelium of the small and large intestine [2]. These features indicate that the GLP2 receptor is an attractive target for development of treatment interventions to promote intestinal adaptation and repair.

Teduglutide (NPS Pharmaceuticals) is a recombinant human GLP2 variant with a stabilizing alanine to glycine substitution at the second amino acid residue (GLP2-2G). Preclinical studies have shown that GLP2, or GLP2-2G injection, causes an increase in intestinal length and weight, villus height, crypt depth and crypt cell proliferation in both normal rodents and during intestinal adaptation in surgical models of short bowel syndrome [1–7]. Clinical studies have confirmed the significant enterotrophic effects [8–11]. Teduglutide is pending approval by the US FDA and has received a recommendation for approval by the European Medicines Agency as treatment for short bowel syndrome.

GLP2 therapy may also be beneficial for treatment of other gastrointestinal diseases involving malabsorption, inflammation, or mucosal damage of the small intestine, including Crohn's disease.

Mucosal GLP2 concentrations are reduced in areas of colonic inflammation in mice with inflammatory bowel disease [12], and treatment with GLP2 or GLP2-2G has been shown to reduce inflammation and severity of disease in a variety of relevant models. These include indomethacin-induced enteritis [13], HLA-B27 [14], DSS- induced ulcerative colitis [15,16], and TNBS-induced colitis [17]. In these models GLP2 or GLP2-2G reduced mucosal damage, crypt cell apoptosis, intestinal lesions, inflammation, and mucosal cytokine production including TNFα, IL-1β, and IFNγ.

Given the enterotrophic and anti-inflammatory effects of GLP2 in preclinical models, and the preferential location of GLP2 receptors within the areas of intestine most affected by Crohn's disease [18], a clinical trial of Teduglutide in Crohn's disease was undertaken. While further study is necessary, results from this study revealed that Teduglutide may be an effective therapy for inducing mucosal healing in patients with moderate to severe Crohn's disease. In this pilot study, subjects received once or twice daily injections (dependent on body weight); the frequent injections were said to contribute to injection site reactions and high subject withdrawal rate, and it was suggested that future trials use a formulation that allows for less frequent injections [19]. Therefore, additional GLP2 therapeutics with better pharmacokinetic properties are needed.

Native GLP2 has a short half-life in human circulation of about seven minutes due to rapid proteolytic degradation by dipeptidyl peptidase IV (DPPIV) [20] as well as removal from circulation by kidney filtration. Both the intact and DPPIV cleaved forms are subject to renal clearance [21]. Teduglutide, the GLP2-2G variant, has increased resistance to DPPIV, and shows a modest increase in half-life to 3–5 hours in healthy humans [22].

In this study, we show that the GLP2-2G peptide genetically fused to XTEN yields a therapeutically active fusion protein with a greatly improved half-life and lower dose requirement in a rat Crohn's disease model. XTEN is a long, unstructured, non-repetitive, hydrophilic sequence of amino acids [23,24]. Fusion of XTEN to the C-terminus of GLP2-2G increases the hydrodynamic radius of the peptide, reducing glomerular filtration and increasing half-life. GLP2-2G-XTEN may offer a pharmacokinetic and therapeutic advantage over native GLP2-2G peptide for treatment of inflammatory bowel disease, including Crohn's disease.

Materials and Methods

GLP2-2G-XTEN Sequence

<u>HGDGSFSDEMNTILDNLAARDFINWLIQTKITDGG</u>-SPAGSPTSTEEGTSESATPESGPGTSTEPSEGSAPG-SPAGSPTSTEEGTSTEPSEGSAPGTSTEPSEGSAPGTSE-SATPESGPGSEPATSGSETPGSEPATSGSETPGSPAGSPT-STEEGTSESATPESGPGTSTEPSEGSAPGTSTEPSEGSAPG-SPAGSPTSTEEGTSTEPSEGSAPGTSTEPSEGSAPGTSE-SATPESGPGTSTEPSEGSAPGTSESATPESGPGSEPATSG-SETPGTSTEPSEGSAPGTSTEPSEGSAPGTSESAT-PESGPGTSESATPESGPGSPAGSPTSTEEGTSESAT-PESGPGSEPATSGSETPGTSESATPESGPGTSTEPSEG-SAPGTSTEPSEGSAPGTSTEPSEGSAPGTSTEPSEGSAPGT-STEPSEGSAPGTSTEPSEGSAPGSPAGSPTSTEEGTSTEP-SEGSAPGTSESATPESGPGSEPATSGSETPGTSESAT-PESGPGSEPATSGSETPGTSESATPESGPGTSTEPSEG-SAPGTSESATPESGPGSPAGSPTSTEEGSPAGSPTSTEEG-SPAGSPTSTEEGTSESATPESGPGTSTEPSEGSAPGTSE-SATPESGPGSEPATSGSETPGTSESATPESGPGSEPATSG-SETPGTSESATPESGPGTSTEPSEGSAPGSPAGSPT-

STEEGTSESATPESGPGSEPATSGSETPGTSESATPESGPG-SPAGSPTSTEEGSPAGSPTSTEEGTSTEPSEGSAPGTSE-SATPESGPGTSESATPESGPGTSESATPESGPGSEPATSG-SETPGSEPATSGSETPGSPAGSPTSTEEGTSTEPSEG-SAPGTSTEPSEGSAPGSEPATSGSETPGTSESATPESGPGT-STEPSEGSAPG.

GLP2-2G Gene Construction and Expression

GLP2-2G-XTEN gene construction was performed as previously described [25]. The final construct comprised the gene encoding the cellulose binding domain (CBD) from *Clostridium thermocellum* (accession #ABN54273), a tobacco etch virus (TEV) protease recognition site (ENLYFQ), the GLP2-2G sequence, and an 864 amino acid XTEN sequence under control of a T7 promoter. The removal of CBD from GLP2-2G-XTEN is mediated by the TEV protease, which is co-expressed on the same plasmid but from a separate operon using the constitutive GroE promoter. The host strain for expression, AmE025, was derived from W3110 (Yale CGSC #4474) in which the *fhuA* gene was deleted by P1 transduction from strain JW0146-2 (Yale CGSC #8416) and the lambda DE3 prophage was integrated onto the chromosome using a λDE3 lysogenization kit (EMD Chemicals USA #69734). GLP2-2G-XTEN was expressed in a 5L glass jacketed fermentation vessel with a B. Braun Biostat B controller, with an initial growth temperature of 37°C, followed by a reduction to 26°C upon addition of IPTG at 20 hours run time. After a total fermentation run time of 45 hours the culture was harvested by centrifugation, yielding cell pellets ~1 kg in wet weight. The pellets were stored frozen at −80°C until purification was initiated.

GLP2-2G-XTEN Purification

The *E. coli* cell pellet was re-suspended in 20 mM Tri-HCl pH 7.5, 50 mM NaCl and lysed by homogenization. The resulting cell lysate was heat coagulated at 85°C for 10 minutes, rapidly cooled to 10°C and clarified by centrifugation. The supernatant was collected and stored at 4°C for purification. GLP2-2G-XTEN protein was purified to homogeneity out of the clarified, heat-treated lysate using three bind and elute chromatography steps, two anion exchange and one hydrophobic interaction, run on an AKTA FPLC system. The final material was formulated using diafiltration in 20 mM Tris-HCl pH 7.5, 135 mM NaCl, sterile filtered using a 0.22 micron filter, and frozen at −80°C until further use. Overall purification yield was approximately 30%.

Analytical Size Exclusion Chromatography

Analytical size exclusion chromatography (SEC) was performed using a BioSep-SEC-s4000, 7.8 × 600 mm HPLC column (Phenomenex) connected to an LC2010 integrated HPLC system equipped with an autosampler and a UV/VIS detector (Shimadzu). The system and the column were equilibrated in 50 mM NaPO$_4$ pH 6.5, 300 mM NaCl at a flow rate of 0.5 mL/min at ambient temperature. For column performance, a SEC column check standard (Phenomenex, AL0-3042) was used. For sample analysis, 20 µL of 1 mg/mL purified GLP2-2G-XTEN was injected and the absorbance at 214 nm was monitored for 75 min.

ESI-MS

200 µg of purified GLP2-2G-XTEN protein was desalted by solid phase extraction using Extract-Clean C18 column (Discovery Sciences). Desalted protein solution in 0.1% formic acid, 50% acetonitrile was infused at 4 µl/min into a QSTAR XL mass spectrometer (AB Sciex). Multi-charge TOF spectrum was

acquired in 800–1400 amu range. Zero-charge spectrum was obtained by Bayesian reconstruction in 10–100 kDa range.

Peptide

Human GLP2-2G peptide (HGDGSFSDEMNTILDN-LAARDFINWLIQTKITD) was purchased from American Peptide (catalog # - 304076). The purity was greater than 95% as confirmed by HPLC and MS.

Potency Assay – GPCR

Sample analysis was performed by Millipore's GPCRProfiler® service using Millipore's cloned human GLP-2 Receptor - expressing cell line made in the Chem-11 host (Millipore catalog #HTS164C) and their standard assay conditions. Calcium flux was monitored in real-time by FLIPR analysis after addition of serial dilutions of GLP2-2G-XTEN and GLP2-2G. Calcium flux was monitored in real-time by FLIPR analysis after addition of serial dilutions of GLP2-2G-XTEN and GLP2-2G. Eight and four replicates of the assay were performed on GLP2-2G-XTEN and GLP2-2G, respectively. After baseline corrections were applied, percentage activation relative to the Millpore reference agonist Emax were calculated. Then, dose response curves and EC50 values were generated and calculated using GraphPad Prism (Sigmoidal Dose Response).

Animal Ethics Statement

Animal welfare for these studies was in compliance with the U.S. Department of Agriculture's (USDA) Animal Welfare Act (9 CFR Parts 1, 2 and 3). The Guide for the Care and Use of Laboratory Animals, Institute of Laboratory Animal Resources, National Academy Press, Washington, D.C., was followed. The contract facilities performing this work maintain an Animal Welfare Assurance statement with the National Institutes of Health, Office of Laboratory Animal Welfare. In order to ensure compliance, all protocols were approved by the Institutional Animal Care and Use Committee (IACUC) of each contract facility before the initiation of treatment. No procedures or test articles were used that would cause more than momentary pain or distress to the animals. Detailed protocols, in-life summaries, and study reports are on file at Amunix, Inc.

Monkeys completed a quarantine and acclimation period and only healthy animals were selected for study. All monkeys were housed individually in stainless steel cages and provided environmental enrichment during the study. Fluorescent lighting was provided via an automatic timer for approximately 12 hours per day. Food and water was available ad libitum. Temperature and humidity was monitored and recorded daily and maintained to the maximum extent possible between 64 to 84°F and 30 to 70%, respectively.

Pharmacokinetics

Pharmacokinetic studies in mice were performed using female C57BL/6 mice dosed subcutaneously (3 mice per time point) with 25 nmol/kg (2 mg/kg) GLP2-2G-XTEN. Plasma samples were collected at pre-dose and at selected time points over 120 hours in heparinized collection tubes. Pharmacokinetic studies in rats were done using catheterized female Wistar rats (3 rats per group) dosed subcutaneously with 25 nmol/kg and 200 nmol/kg GLP2-2G-XTEN. Plasma samples were collected at pre-dose and at selected time points over 168 hours in heparinized collection tubes.

The pharmacokinetics of GLP2-2G-XTEN after intravenous and subcutaneous injection was determined in male cynomolgus monkeys. Monkeys (6 per group) were dosed with 25 nmol/kg

GLP2-2G-XTEN by intravenous or subcutaneous administration using a cross-over study design. Plasma samples were taken pre-dose and at selected time points post-dose up to 21 days (504 hours) following injection in heparinized collection tubes.

ELISA for Pharmacokinetic Experiments

A quantitative sandwich enzyme-linked immunosorption assay (ELISA) technique was developed to measure GLP2-2G-XTEN in mouse, rat and cynomolgus monkey plasma. In the assay, standards, controls and test samples were incubated with mouse anti-XTEN monoclonal antibody (ProSci, 4D9G3) which was immobilized on a microtiter plate at a concentration of 8 μg/mL. After incubation, unbound material was washed away and GLP2-2G-XTEN was detected using biotinylated rabbit polyclonal to human GLP2 antibody (Phoenix Pharmaceuticals, B-G-028) at a 1:20,000 dilution, followed by streptavidin-HRP (Pierce, 21130) at 0.1 μg/mL, and visualized with a TMB peroxidase substrate (Immunochemistry Technologies, SUB1). The assay has a range of 480–0.47 ng/mL in 3% plasma.

Analysis of Pharmacokinetic Experiments

Pharmacokinetic curves were analyzed by fitting a non-compartmental model to the profile from each animal. The resulting pharmacokinetic parameters were averaged for the final results. Bioavailability was determined by dividing the area under the curve (AUC_∞) from the subcutaneous administration and the AUC_∞ from the intravenous administration on a per animal basis. The results were averaged for the final data. Analysis was performed using Phoenix WinNonLin software (Pharsight, Cary NC).

Rat Intestinotrophic Studies

Small intestine growth in rats was measured as a primary pharmacodynamic endpoint. GLP2-2G peptide, GLP2-2G-XTEN or vehicle was administered via subcutaneous injection into male Sprague-Dawley rats weighing 200–220 grams (10–12 rats per group). GLP2-2G peptide was dosed using the previously published regimen of 12.5 nmol/kg (0.05 mg/kg) twice daily for 12 days. GLP2-2G-XTEN was dosed at 25 nmol/kg once daily for 12 days. After sacrifice, a midline incision was made, the small intestines were removed, stretched to their maximum length and the length recorded. The fecal material was flushed from the lumen and the small intestinal wet weight recorded.

Indomethacin-induced Inflammation

Male Wistar rats (180–220 grams) were weighed and randomized into treatment groups of ten rats each to ensure balance for average body weight across the treatment groups. Using a prophylactic study design, rats were injected subcutaneously with vehicle, GLP2-2G peptide (12.5 nmol/kg twice per day) or GLP2-2G-XTEN (25 nmol/kg once daily, 25 nmol/kg every other day for a total of three doses, or 75 nmol/kg once, as indicated), starting three days prior to indomethacin administration on day −3. Rats were fasted for 12 hours before receiving the first subcutaneous injection of freshly prepared indomethacin (7 mg/kg) on day 0; a second injection of indomethacin was administered 24 hours later on day 1. For the remainder of the experiment rats had unlimited access to food and water. Rats were euthanized 24 hours after receiving the second dose of indomethacin on day 2.

Disease readouts for the indomethacin model were performed as follows: 24 hours after the last indomethacin injection, rats were injected intravenously with 1 mL 1% Evan's Blue dye. Thirty minutes later rats were anesthetized and exsanguinated. A midline incision was made in the abdomen and the rats were scored for the presence of adhesions. The small intestine was removed and the length recorded. The intestinal lumen was flushed with sterile 0.9% sodium chloride for injection and the length of the ulcerated area recorded. The intestines were gently blotted to remove excess fluid and weighed. The small intestine was scored for adhesions and trans-ulcerations using the following scoring system: Adhesions: none = 0, mild = 1, moderate = 2, severe = 3; transmural ulceration: none = 0, few = 1, multiple = 2, continuous = 3.

Histopathology

Rat small intestine samples consisted of a 3 cm section of proximal jejunum and a 3 cm section of mid-jejunum collected 15 cm and 30 cm from the pylorus, respectively. Samples were fixed in 10% neutral buffered formalin. Samples were trimmed into multiple sections without bias toward lesion presence or absence. These sections were placed in cassettes, embedded in paraffin, microtomed at approximately 4 microns thickness, and stained with hematoxylin and eosin (H&E). The slides were evaluated microscopically by a board certified veterinary pathologist and scored for villous height as well as infiltration/inflammation, mucosal atrophy, villi/crypt appearance, abscesses/ulceration. A 1 to 4 severity grading scale was used, where 1 = minimal, 2 = mild, 3 = moderate, 4 = marked/severe, reflecting the combination of the cellular reactions seen histopathologically.

Statistics

Parametric variables (small intestine length, small intestine weight, TNFα levels) were compared using an ANOVA with a Tukey-Kramer post hoc test for individual pairwise comparisons using an overall alpha of 0.05. Non-parametric variables (adhesion score, ulceration score) were compared with the vehicle control using a Mann Whitney U test with a Bonferroni correction for the p-value to create an overall alpha of 0.05. Calculations were performed using JMP or Excel as appropriate.

Results

Expression, Purification and G-protein Coupled Receptor Assay

GLP2-2G-XTEN was expressed in *Escherichia coli* and purified to homogeneity (Figure 1; see Methods). Expression titers of 3–4 g/L were achieved for multiple batches with final purification yields of ~30%. ESI-MS analysis of purified GLP2-2G-XTEN (calculated MW 83,144 Da) showed experimental molecular weight of 83,142 Da, with an accuracy of 24 ppm (Figure 1A). The only detectable impurity was a species lacking the N-terminal histidine, experimental molecular weight 83,003 Da (Figure 1A). Characterization of GLP2-2G-XTEN preparations by SDS-PAGE and size exclusion chromatography further indicates that the protein is homogeneous and non-aggregated in solution (Figure 1B and 1C). In a potency assay, based on calcium flux in a GLP-2 receptor expressing cell line, the purified protein and unmodified GLP2-2G were found to have EC50 values of 380 nM and 7 nM, respectively, indicating GLP2-2G-XTEN retains 2% of the potency (on a molar basis) as GLP2-2G peptide (Figure 1D).

Pharmacokinetics

To assess the pharmacokinetics of GLP2-2G-XTEN, studies were performed in mice, rats and monkeys (Table 1). In all three species, animals were dosed subcutaneously with GLP2-2G-XTEN at 25 nmol/kg. Plasma levels of GLP2-2G-XTEN were determined at various time points using a sandwich ELISA with antibodies specific for the GLP2 and XTEN portions of the protein. The resulting pharmacokinetic curves were fit to a non-compartmental pharmacokinetic model and the terminal half-life of GLP2-2G-XTEN in mice, rats and monkey was determined to be 34, 38 and 120 hours respectively. In addition, the pharmacokinetic profile of GLP2-2G-XTEN after single subcutaneous administration to rats at 25 nmol/kg and 200 nmol/kg was dose proportional with the Cmax and AUC increasing in an approximately linear manner.

To determine the bioavailability of GLP2-2G-XTEN after subcutaneous injection, the pharmacokinetics of the protein was studied in cynomolgus monkeys after intravenous and subcutaneous administration of 25 nmol/kg GLP2-2G-XTEN (Figure 2). The bioavailability was 96% demonstrating that GLP2-2G-XTEN is rapidly and near completely absorbed after subcutaneous administration.

Rat Intestinotrophic Study

Intestinotrophic effects were assessed in normal rats administered GLP2-2G peptide and GLP2-2G–XTEN at doses previously shown to be efficacious in preclinical studies using GLP2-2G peptide [13]. Treatment with GLP2-2G peptide for 12 days (12.5 nmol/kg/dose using the standard twice daily dosing regimen) resulted in a significant increase in small intestine weight of 24% (Figure 3). There were no significant effects on small intestine length. Administration of equal molar GLP2-2G-XTEN over the 12 day study (25 nmol/kg/dose, once daily) resulted in a similar significant increase in small intestine weight of 31%. In contrast to the results seen with GLP2-2G peptide, the small intestine of GLP2-2G-XTEN treated rats showed a significant increase in length of 9% (10 cm), and was visibly thicker than the tissues from vehicle-treated control animals.

Indomethacin-induced Disease Model

GLP2-2G peptide has been studied in indomethacin-induced enteritis, a model for Crohn's disease [13]. Indomethacin-induced disease was characterized by a significant reduction in weight gain relative to the non-diseased animals (Figure 4A). This reduction was accompanied by clinical signs including pale color, indicating possible anemia, poor body tone and discharge at the nose, indicative of distress, and black feces, indicative of occult blood. GLP2-2G peptide was administered twice a day for five days at 12.5 nmol/kg/dose (total dose of 125 nmol/kg), a dose regimen that demonstrated an intestinotrophic effect on small intestine weight and was shown to be effective at ameliorating symptoms in previous indomethacin-induced inflammation studies. For comparison, the efficacy of GLP2-2G-XTEN, was initially investigated using an equal molar dose (total dose of 125 nmol/kg) to that of GLP2-2G peptide over the course of the study. GLP2-2G-XTEN was administered once daily; GLP2-2G peptide was administered twice daily.

Administration of prophylactic GLP2-2G-XTEN starting three days prior to disease induction and continuing until the end of the study had a significant impact on the change in body weight; rats treated with GLP2-2G-XTEN showed a two-fold increase in net body weight gain versus vehicle treated diseased rats (Figure 4A). In contrast, treatment with GLP2-2G peptide had no significant effect on the change in body weight throughout the duration of the study.

As shown in Figure 4B–D, the small intestine of vehicle treated rats was severely damaged within 24 hours following the second indomethacin injection; it was significantly shorter in the vehicle treated diseased rats than in the non-diseased rats (56.9 vs.96.3 cm; Figure 4B) and 96% of the length of the small

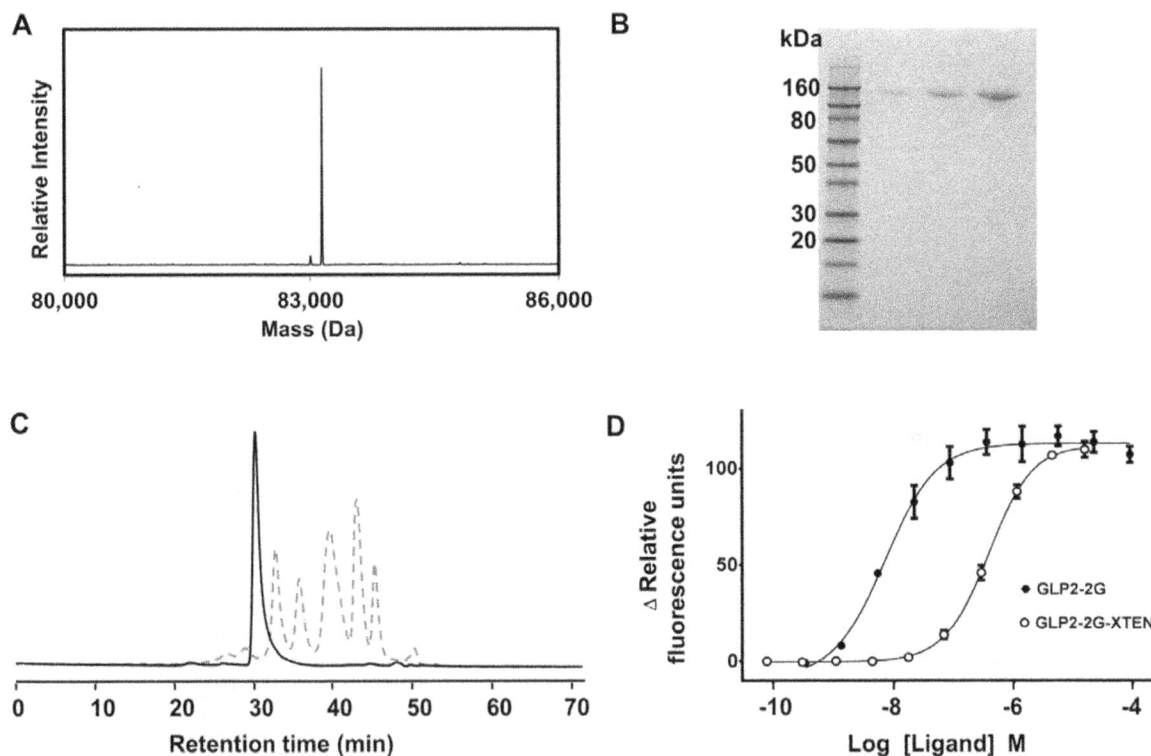

Figure 1. *In vitro* **characterization of purified GLP2-2G-XTEN protein.** A) ESI-MS analysis, major peak 83,142 Da – full length intact GLP2-2G-XTEN; minor peak 83,003 Da – des-His GLP2-2G-XTEN. B) non-reducing SDS-PAGE. Lane 1: molecular weight markers, lanes 2–4: 2 µg, 5 µg and 10 µg of GLP2-2G-XTEN, respectively. C) Size exclusion HPLC analysis. Solid curve: GLP2-2G-XTEN, 20 µg; dashed curve: molecular weights standard, which includes thyroglobulin 670 kDa, IgG 156 kDa, BSA 66 kDa, ovalbumin 45 kDa, myoglobin 17 kDa. D) Potency GPCR assay of GLP2-2G EC50 = 7 nM (95% confidence interval 4 nM to 12 nM) and GLP2-2G-XTEN EC50 = 380 nM (95% confidence interval 330 nM to 430 nM).

intestine was ulcerated. Examination revealed severe adhesions and trans-ulcerations (2.8 and 2.6 respectively out of a maximum score of 3). GLP2-2G-XTEN treatment resulted in a significant increase in small intestine length as compared to both vehicle-treated and peptide-treated rats, the small intestine length was close to that of normal, non-diseased rats. In addition, the ulceration and adhesion scores of GLP2-2G-XTEN treated rats also reverted back to normal, non-disease levels. In GLP2-2G peptide-treated rats, the small intestine was also significantly longer and less ulcerated than in the untreated diseased rats and GLP2-2G treatment resulted in a significant improvement in both adhesions and ulcerations although the levels did not return to those seen in normal, non-diseased rats.

Having documented GLP2-2G-XTEN intestinotrophic properties as well as protective effects on the small intestine mucosal epithelium, we next examined the anti-inflammatory potential of

the molecule. Inflammation of the small intestine was determined by measuring the TNFα content by ELISA. As expected due to the inflammatory nature of the model, there was an approximately 50-fold increase in the TNFα content of small intestine in the vehicle treated indomethacin-induced diseased rats (~3700 pg/g tissue) relative to the normal non-diseased tissue (~80 pg/g tissue). Both GLP2-2G peptide and GLP2-2G-XTEN treatment significantly reduced the TNFα content of the diseased small intestine (Figure 4E), indicating an anti-inflammatory effect.

To assess the *in vivo* potency of GLP2-2G-XTEN, dose ranging studies (Figure 5, 6, 7) were performed comparing lower doses of GLP2-2G-XTEN (total dose of 125 nmol/kg down to 7.5 nmol/kg administered as 5, 3, or 1 dose over the five day study) to the standard twice daily dose of GLP2-2G peptide (125 nmol/kg total dose administered as 10 doses). There was a clear dose-response to GLP2-2G-XTEN treatment (Figure 5). Furthermore, a single dose

Table 1. Pharmacokinetic data for GLP2-2G-XTEN in mouse, rat and cynomolgus monkey.

Species	Route	Dose (nmol/kg)	T 1/2 (hour)	Cmax (ng/mL)	AUC∞ (hr*ng/mL)	Vd (mL/kg)	Clearance (mL/hr)
Mouse	SC	25	34	11,000	720,000	140	0.07
Rat	SC	25	38	6,900	530,000	210	0.80
Cyno	SC	25	120	20,000	3,400,000	110	2.0
Cyno	IV	25	110	62,000	3,700,000	90	1.9

A

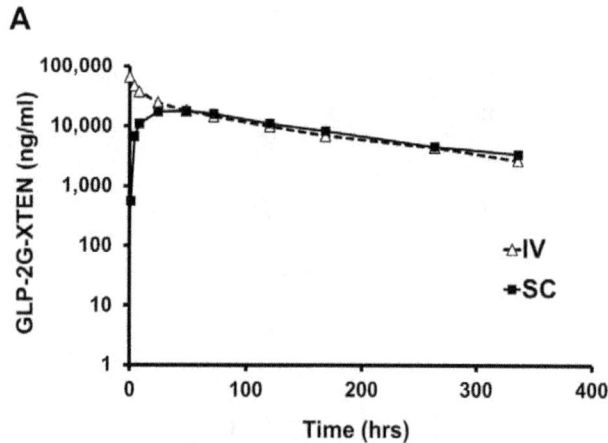

Figure 2. Pharmacokinetics of GLP2-2G-XTEN in cynomolgous monkeys. GLP2-2G-XTEN plasma concentration is shown following 25 nmol/kg administration via intravenous (triangle) or subcutaneous (square) route. Three animals were dosed by each route of administration. Data points are the average ± s.d. of three animals per time point.

of 75 nmol/kg GLP2-2G-XTEN administered once on day −3 resulted in a significant reduction in adhesions and ulcerations, comparable to results seen using ten doses of GLP2-2G peptide at a total dose of 125 nmol/kg.

Histopathological analysis confirmed the GLP2-2G-XTEN treatment effects (Figure 6). Compared to normal rats, the ileum and jejunum of diseased rats showed severe mucosal atrophy, perforated ulcers, and chronic peritonitis; the villi appeared stunted and atrophied (Figure 6A). Treatment with GLP2-2G peptide (125 nmol/kg, ten doses, not shown), GLP2-2G-XTEN (125 nmol/kg, five doses, Figure 6B), and even low dose GLP2-2G-XTEN (75 nmol/kg, Figure 6C–D) showed a reduction in mucosal atrophy, ulceration, and infiltration as compared to untreated diseased rats; the villi appeared normal.

Quantitative histopathology was performed on a subset of samples. The increase in small intestine length of the GLP2-2G-XTEN-treated diseased rats as compared to vehicle-treated diseased rats (Figure 7A) correlated with a significant increase in villi height (Figure 7B). Both high (125 nmol/kg) and low (75 nmol/kg) dose GLP2-2G-XTEN-treated groups showed a significant increase in villi height; the increase in villi height seen in peptide treated rats was not significant. There was also a significant decrease in mucosal atrophy as both high and low dose GLP2-2G-XTEN-treated rats showed a significantly lower mucosal atrophy score than vehicle-treated diseased rats (Figure 7C). Although there was a trend showing a reduction in mucosal ulceration and mixed cell infiltrate following GLP2-2G-XTEN and GLP2-2G peptide treatment, these results were not significant for any of the three treatment groups.

Discussion

Crohn's disease is a chronic immune-related disorder of the gastrointestinal tract whose symptoms, including diarrhea, abdominal pain, weight loss and other complications, may lead to surgery, disability and increased mortality [19,26]. There is no cure for Crohn's disease and current therapy, targeted only toward the inflammatory component of the disease rather than providing for mucosal protection and healing, is not sufficient. These anti-inflammatory therapies, including an antibody to TNFα, show

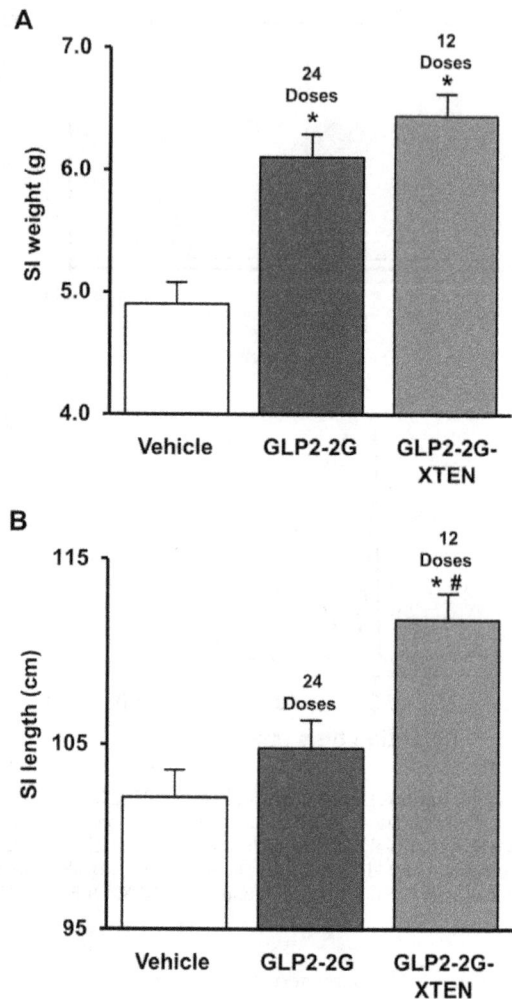

A

B

Figure 3. Intestinotrophic effects of GLP2-2G peptide and GLP2-2G-XTEN. Small intestine weight A) and length B) in normal rats following treatment with a total dose of 300 nmol/kg GLP2-2G peptide or GLP2-2G-XTEN. Data shown are from day 12 following SC injection of GLP2-2G peptide (12.5 nmol/kg per injection; twice per day for 12 days) and GLP2-2G-XTEN (25 nmol/kg per injection; once per day for 12 days). Data are means and SE, n = 10 per group. * P<0.05 compared to vehicle-treated rats, # P<0.05 compared to GLP2-2G peptide treated rats.

remission rates of only 26–38%, an increase of only 4.5–24% over placebo [27–31]. Therapy with agents targeting the GLP2 receptor provide for mucosal healing and repair and may increase the response rate in patients with Crohn's disease. A pilot study revealed that Teduglutide induces mucosal healing and may be an effective therapy for patients with Crohn's disease [19]. However, this pilot study also indicated that GLP2 therapeutics with better pharmacokinetic properties would be useful because the need for daily injections of Teduglutide led to a high withdrawal rate and placebo response.

The current study provides evidence that GLP2-2G-XTEN is a long-acting enterotrophic GLP2 receptor agonist that has increased *in vivo* exposure. GLP2-2G-XTEN increases the small intestine length and weight in normal rats and reduces the damage to the small intestine seen in a rat model of Crohn's disease. Due to increased *in vivo* exposure, GLP2-2G-XTEN shows comparable therapeutic effects, including an increase in small intestine length, and a decrease in adhesions and ulcerations, when used at 60% of

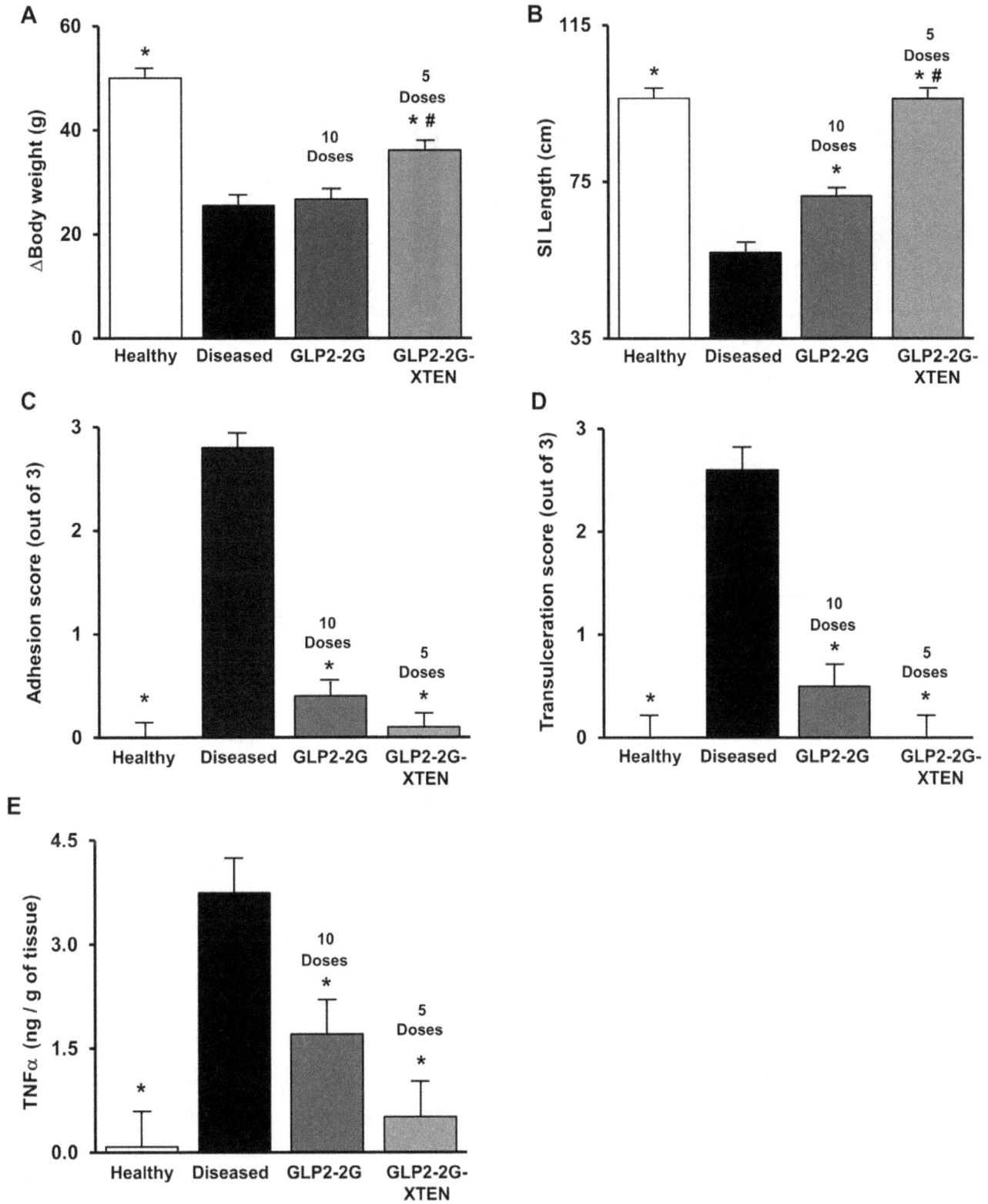

Figure 4. Efficacy of equal molar GLP2-2G-XTEN and GLP2-2G peptide in rat indomethacin-induced disease model. Data shown are A) change in body weight from day −3 through day 2, B) small intestine length, C) small intestine adhesion score, D) small intestine trans-ulceration score and E) small intestine TNFα concentration. Open bars are healthy rats treated with vehicle; colored bars are indomethacin-induced diseased rats treated with vehicle, GLP2-2G peptide (12.5 nmol/kg per injection; twice per day for 5 days) or GLP2-2G-XTEN (25 nmol/kg once per day for 5 days) as indicated. Compounds were dosed starting three days prior to first indomethacin injection (Day −3) and data shown are from the time of sacrifice on Day 2 (24 hours post second indomethacin injection). Data are means and SE, n = 10 per group. * P<0.05 compared to diseased, vehicle-treated rats, # P<0.05 compared to diseased GLP2-2G peptide treated rats.

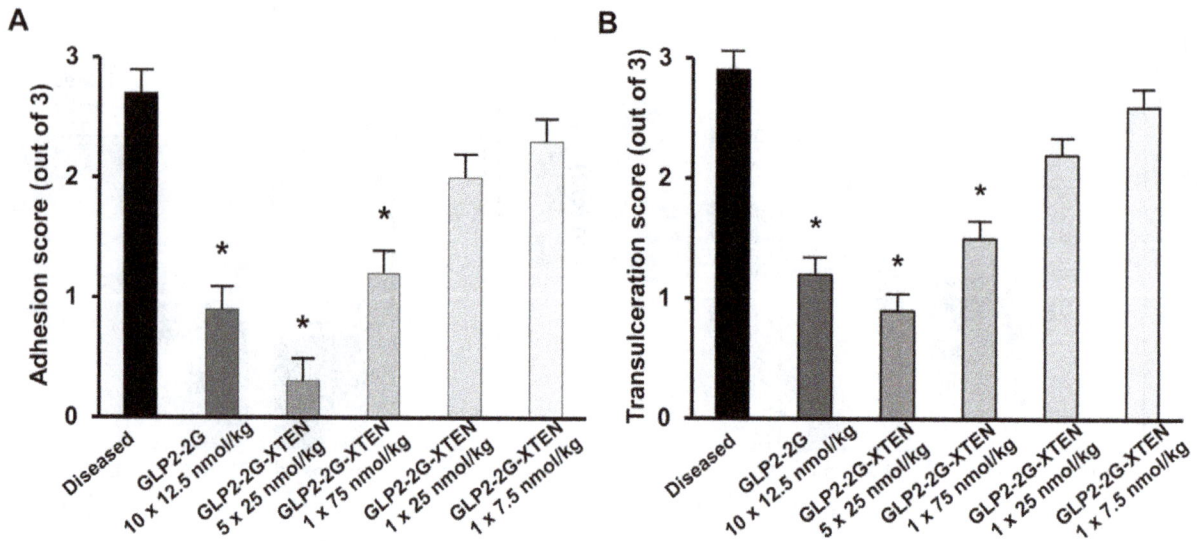

Figure 5. Efficacy of low dose GLP2-2G-XTEN treatment in rat indomethacin-induced disease model. Data shown are effects on A) small intestine adhesions and B) small intestine trans-ulcerations. Treatment with GLP2-2G peptide (12.5 nmol/kg per injection; twice per day for 5 days) or GLP2-2G-XTEN (25 nmol/kg once daily or only once at the indicated doses) was initiated on Day −3 and sacrifice is on Day 2. Data are means and SE, n = 10 per group. * P<0.05 compared to diseased, vehicle-treated rats.

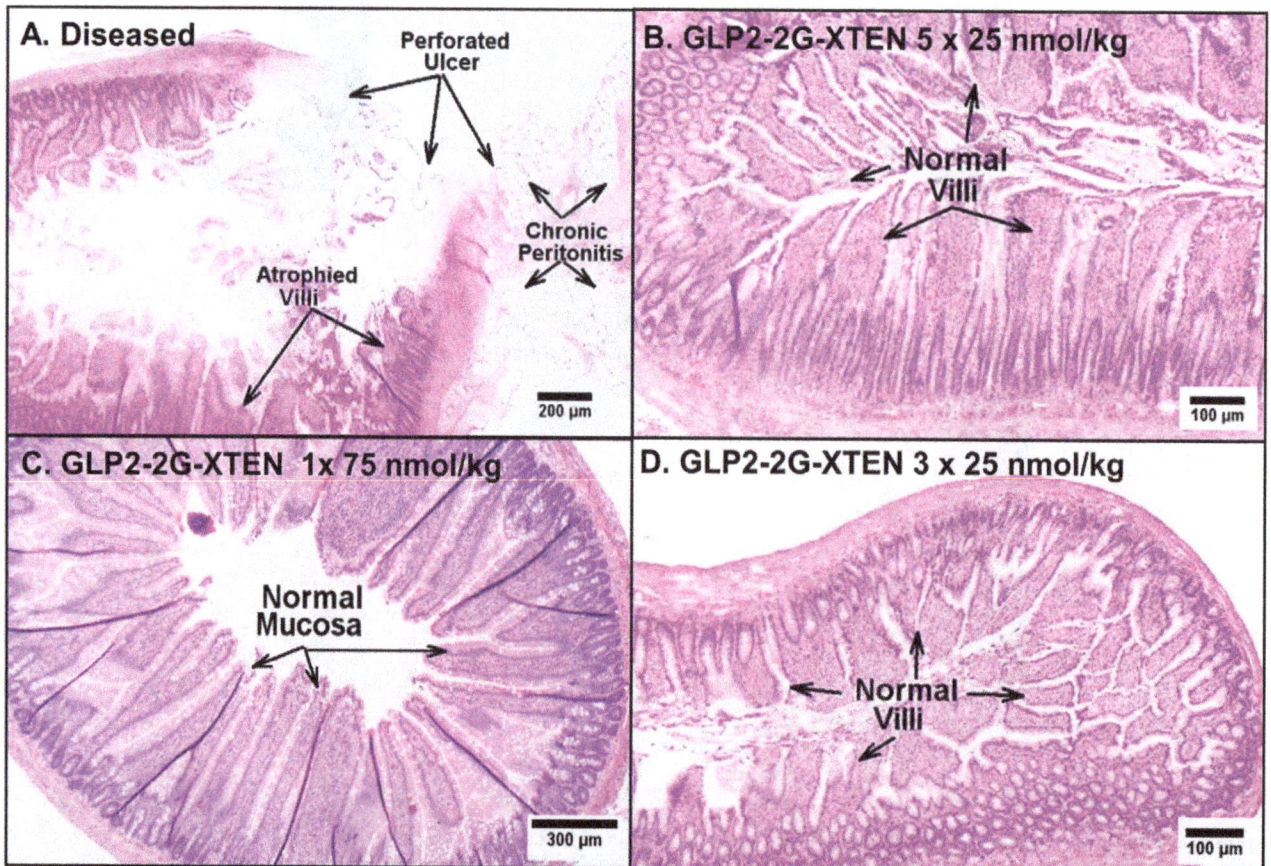

Figure 6. GLP2-2G-XTEN administration improves small intestine histopathology in the indomethacin-induced rat disease model. A) Hematoxylin and eosin staining of jejunum sections from A) diseased, vehicle-treated rats, B) diseased, GLP2-2G-XTEN high dose treated rats (125 nmol/kg total dose divided into five daily 25 nmol/kg doses), C) diseased, GLP2-2G-XTEN low dose treated rats (75 nmol/kg total dose given once on day −3) and D) diseased, GLP2-2G-XTEN low dose treated rats (divided into three 25 nmol/kg doses on day −3, −1 and 1).

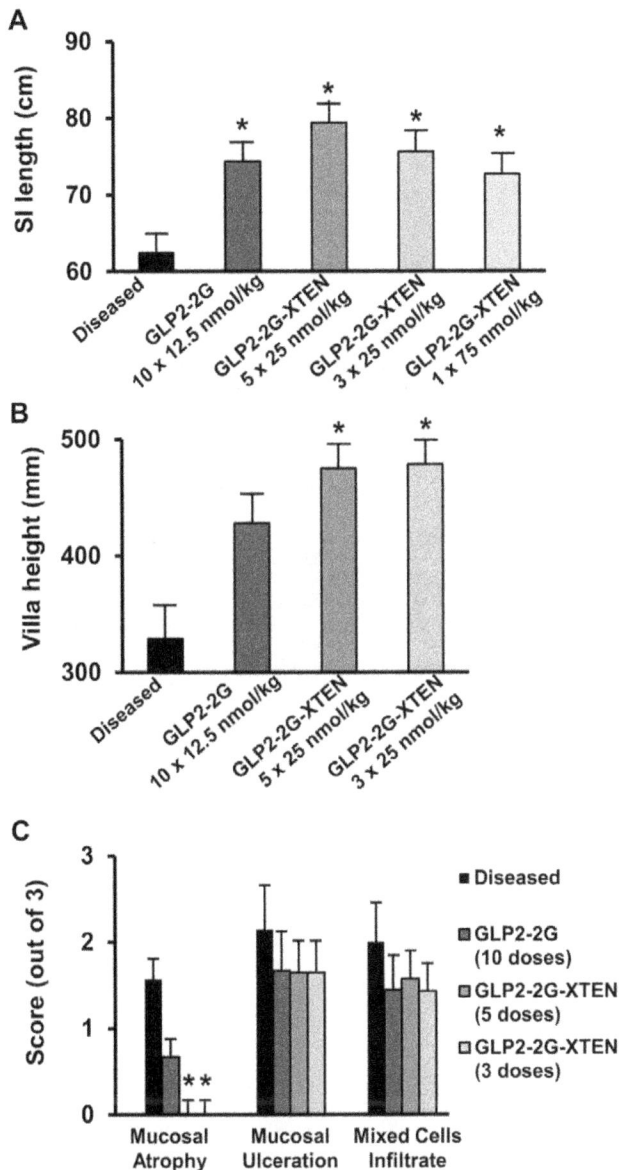

Figure 7. Treatment effects on small intestine length correlate with small intestine histopathology. A) Small intestine length B) villi height and C) mucosal atrophy, ulceration, infiltration measurements from diseased, vehicle-treated, GLP2-2G peptide-treated, and GLP2-2G-XTEN-treated rats. Quantitative histopathology was not performed on GLP2-2G-XTEN 75 nmol/kg single dose group.

the total dose of GLP2-2G peptide. Furthermore, GLP2-2G-XTEN dosed once at 75 nmol/kg or three times at 25 nmol/kg is as effective as GLP2-2G peptide dosed ten times at 12.5 nmol/kg.

While it remains to be seen how the improvement in total molar dose and dosing frequency seen in a preclinical model of Crohn's disease translates into the required clinical dose, the allometric scaling of GLP2-2G-XTEN half-life from three species reveals a projected human half-life of 240 hours (Figure 8). The robustness of this projection is bolstered by scaling the clearance (Cl) and volume of distributions (Vd) from the three species and calculating the terminal half-life (T½) using the relationship $T\frac{1}{2} = 0.693 \times Vd/Cl$ [32]. This results in a projection of 230 hours, in good agreement with the allometric scaling projection. Similar methodology was used to project the human half-life of the

Ex4-XTEN fusion by Schellenberger et al [23]. The projection from the preclinical data was a human half-life of 139 hours, which is comparable to the actual half-life that was observed in the human trials (Diartis Pharmaceuticals, Inc., 2012 American Diabetes Association presentation). Therefore, the 240 hour projection is considered a reasonable estimate of anticipated human performance backed by a verified methodology.

This projected terminal half-life opens the possibility of monthly dosing intervals in humans, as the drug would pass through about three half-lives in a month. The peak to trough ratio is expected to be low, limiting safety concerns from the highest plasma concentrations, and hopefully increasing efficacy through a flatter, more even, exposure profile. The volume of distribution is greatly reduced compared to the unfused GLP2-2G peptide with the GLP2-2G-XTEN fusion being limited to approximately two times blood volume (Table 1) as is seen consistently with multiple XTEN fusions [23,24]. Concentration of GLP2-2G-XTEN in the plasma implies a lower total dose requirement; however, because the volume of distribution is larger than blood volume, it also demonstrates that XTEN fusions are capable of penetrating into other peripheral tissues to reach sites of action.

In summary, our results demonstrate that prophylactic administration of GLP2-2G-XTEN, a long-acting GLP2 receptor agonist, increases small intestine length and reduces the severity of disease in a rat Crohn's disease model. GLP2-2G-XTEN has increased *in vivo* exposure and requires a lower molar dose and less frequent dosing as compared with GLP2-2G peptide. Allometric scaling based on pharmacokinetics from mouse, rat and monkey projects a human half-life of 240 hours. GLP2-2G-XTEN may

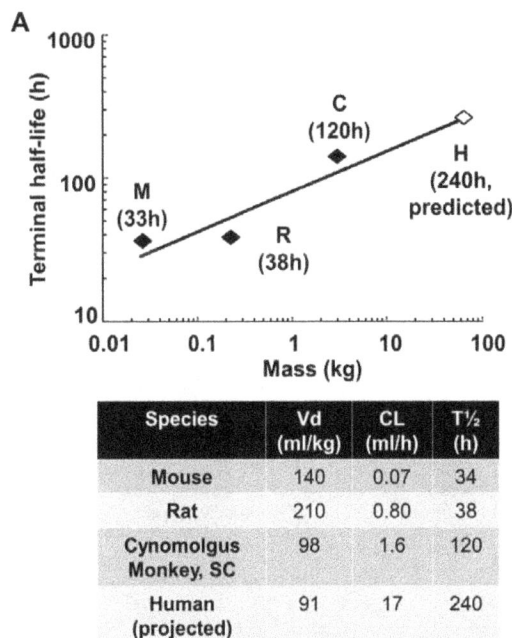

Species	Vd (ml/kg)	CL (ml/h)	T½ (h)
Mouse	140	0.07	34
Rat	210	0.80	38
Cynomolgus Monkey, SC	98	1.6	120
Human (projected)	91	17	240

Figure 8. Allometric scaling human projection based on mouse, rat and monkey pharmacokinetic data. Allometric scaling was performed by fitting a linear regression model with the log of animal mass as the X variable and log of terminal half-life as the Y variable. The resulting linear model was extrapolated to a 70 kg human to produce a predicted value. The terminal half-life in humans can also be estimated using the predicted values for clearance (Cl) and volume of distribution (Vd) in the formula $T\frac{1}{2} = 0.693 \times Vd/Cl$. Applying this formula yields a predicted terminal half-life of 240 hours in humans, which agrees with the linear extrapolation.

offer superior pharmacokinetics and a therapeutic benefit for treatment of gastrointestinal diseases involving malabsorption, inflammation or mucosal damage of the small intestine, including Crohn's disease.

Acknowledgments

The authors would like to thank Darlene Horton, Bryan Lawlis, Kirk Hayenga and Jerry Beers for their contributions to this program, Amanda Hartman for a critical review of the manuscript, and Stephen Voglewede for technical assistance.

Author Contributions

Conceived and designed the experiments: SEA BM BS VS WPCS. Performed the experiments: BM TL CW VP. Analyzed the data: SEA BM BS TL VP. Wrote the paper: SEA BM.

References

1. Drucker DJ, Erlich P, Asa SL, Brubaker PL (1996) Induction of intestinal epithelial proliferation by glucagon-like peptide 2. Proc Natl Acad Sci U S A 93: 7911–7916.
2. Brubaker PL, Izzo A, Hill M, Drucker DJ (1997) Intestinal function in mice with small bowel growth induced by glucagon-like peptide-2. Am J Physiol 272: E1050–1058.
3. Tsai CH, Hill M, Asa SL, Brubaker PL, Drucker DJ (1997) Intestinal growth-promoting properties of glucagon-like peptide-2 in mice. Am J Physiol 273: E77–84.
4. Drucker DJ, DeForest L, Brubaker PL (1997) Intestinal response to growth factors administered alone or in combination with human [Gly2]glucagon-like peptide 2. Am J Physiol 273: G1252–1262.
5. Martin GR, Wallace LE, Hartmann B, Holst JJ, Demchyshyn L, et al. (2005) Nutrient-stimulated GLP-2 release and crypt cell proliferation in experimental short bowel syndrome. Am J Physiol Gastrointest Liver Physiol 288: G431–438.
6. Martin GR, Wallace LE, Sigalet DL (2004) Glucagon-like peptide-2 induces intestinal adaptation in parenterally fed rats with short bowel syndrome. Am J Physiol Gastrointest Liver Physiol 286: G964–972.
7. Scott CE, Abdullah LH, Davis CW (1998) Ca2+ and protein kinase C activation of mucin granule exocytosis in permeabilized SPOC1 cells. Am J Physiol 275: C285–292.
8. Jeppesen PB, Hartmann B, Thulesen J, Graff J, Lohmann J, et al. (2001) Glucagon-like peptide 2 improves nutrient absorption and nutritional status in short-bowel patients with no colon. Gastroenterology 120: 806–815.
9. Jeppesen PB, Sanguinetti EL, Buchman A, Howard L, Scolapio JS, et al. (2005) Teduglutide (ALX-0600), a dipeptidyl peptidase IV resistant glucagon-like peptide 2 analogue, improves intestinal function in short bowel syndrome patients. Gut 54: 1224–1231.
10. Jeppesen PB, Lund P, Gottschalck IB, Nielsen HB, Holst JJ, et al. (2009) Short bowel patients treated for two years with glucagon-like Peptide 2: effects on intestinal morphology and absorption, renal function, bone and body composition, and muscle function. Gastroenterol Res Pract 2009: 616054.
11. Jeppesen PB, Gilroy R, Pertkiewicz M, Allard JP, Messing B, et al. (2011) Randomised placebo-controlled trial of teduglutide in reducing parenteral nutrition and/or intravenous fluid requirements in patients with short bowel syndrome. Gut 60: 902–914.
12. Schmidt PT, Hartmann B, Bregenholt S, Hoist JJ, Claesson MH (2000) Deficiency of the intestinal growth factor, glucagon-like peptide 2, in the colon of SCID mice with inflammatory bowel disease induced by transplantation of CD4+ T cells. Scand J Gastroenterol 35: 522–527.
13. Boushey RP, Yusta B, Drucker DJ (1999) Glucagon-like peptide 2 decreases mortality and reduces the severity of indomethacin-induced murine enteritis. Am J Physiol 277: E937–947.
14. Alavi K, Schwartz MZ, Palazzo JP, Prasad R (2000) Treatment of inflammatory bowel disease in a rodent model with the intestinal growth factor glucagon-like peptide-2. J Pediatr Surg 35: 847–851.
15. Drucker DJ, Yusta B, Boushey RP, DeForest L, Brubaker PL (1999) Human [Gly2]GLP-2 reduces the severity of colonic injury in a murine model of experimental colitis. Am J Physiol 276: G79–91.
16. L'Heureux MC, Brubaker PL (2003) Glucagon-like peptide-2 and common therapeutics in a murine model of ulcerative colitis. J Pharmacol Exp Ther 306: 347–354.
17. Sigalet DL, Wallace LE, Holst JJ, Martin GR, Kaji T, et al. (2007) Enteric neural pathways mediate the anti-inflammatory actions of glucagon-like peptide 2. Am J Physiol Gastrointest Liver Physiol 293: G211–221.
18. Yusta B, Huang L, Munroe D, Wolff G, Fantaske R, et al. (2000) Enteroendocrine localization of GLP-2 receptor expression in humans and rodents. Gastroenterology 119: 744–755.
19. Buchman AL, Katz S, Fang JC, Bernstein CN, Abou-Assi SG (2010) Teduglutide, a novel mucosally active analog of glucagon-like peptide-2 (GLP-2) for the treatment of moderate to severe Crohn's disease. Inflamm Bowel Dis 16: 962–973.
20. Hartmann B, Harr MB, Jeppesen PB, Wojdemann M, Deacon CF, et al. (2000) In vivo and in vitro degradation of glucagon-like peptide-2 in humans. J Clin Endocrinol Metab 85: 2884–2888.
21. Tavares W, Drucker DJ, Brubaker PL (2000) Enzymatic- and renal-dependent catabolism of the intestinotropic hormone glucagon-like peptide-2 in rats. Am J Physiol Endocrinol Metab 278: E134–139.
22. Marier JF, Beliveau M, Mouksassi MS, Shaw P, Cyran J, et al. (2008) Pharmacokinetics, safety, and tolerability of teduglutide, a glucagon-like peptide-2 (GLP-2) analog, following multiple ascending subcutaneous administrations in healthy subjects. J Clin Pharmacol 48: 1289–1299.
23. Schellenberger V, Wang CW, Geething NC, Spink BJ, Campbell A, et al. (2009) A recombinant polypeptide extends the in vivo half-life of peptides and proteins in a tunable manner. Nat Biotechnol 27: 1186–1190.
24. Cleland JL, Geething NC, Moore JA, Rogers BC, Spink BJ, et al. (2012) A novel long-acting human growth hormone fusion protein (vrs-317): enhanced in vivo potency and half-life. J Pharm Sci.
25. Geething NC, To W, Spink BJ, Scholle MD, Wang CW, et al. (2010) Gcg-XTEN: an improved glucagon capable of preventing hypoglycemia without increasing baseline blood glucose. PLoS One 5: e10175.
26. Lichtenstein GR, Yan S, Bala M, Hanauer S (2004) Remission in patients with Crohn's disease is associated with improvement in employment and quality of life and a decrease in hospitalizations and surgeries. Am J Gastroenterol 99: 91–96.
27. Sandborn WJ, Colombel JF, Enns R, Feagan BG, Hanauer SB, et al. (2005) Natalizumab induction and maintenance therapy for Crohn's disease. N Engl J Med 353: 1912–1925.
28. Hanauer SB, Sandborn WJ, Rutgeerts P, Fedorak RN, Lukas M, et al. (2006) Human anti-tumor necrosis factor monoclonal antibody (adalimumab) in Crohn's disease: the CLASSIC-I trial. Gastroenterology 130: 323–333; quiz 591.
29. Targan SR, Feagan BG, Fedorak RN, Lashner BA, Panaccione R, et al. (2007) Natalizumab for the treatment of active Crohn's disease: results of the ENCORE Trial. Gastroenterology 132: 1672–1683.
30. Sandborn WJ, Feagan BG, Stoinov S, Honiball PJ, Rutgeerts P, et al. (2007) Certolizumab pegol for the treatment of Crohn's disease. N Engl J Med 357: 228–238.
31. Targan SR, Hanauer SB, van Deventer SJ, Mayer L, Present DH, et al. (1997) A short-term study of chimeric monoclonal antibody cA2 to tumor necrosis factor alpha for Crohn's disease. Crohn's Disease cA2 Study Group. N Engl J Med 337: 1029–1035.
32. Mahmood I (2007) Application of allometric principles for the prediction of pharmacokinetics in human and veterinary drug development. Adv Drug Deliv Rev 59: 1177–1192.

13

The Functional −765G→C Polymorphism of the COX-2 Gene May Reduce the Risk of Developing Crohn's Disease

Hilbert S. de Vries[1]*, Rene H. M. te Morsche[1], Martijn G. H. van Oijen[1,3], Iris D. Nagtegaal[2], Wilbert H. M. Peters[1], Dirk J. de Jong[1]

1 Department of Gastroenterology and Hepatology, Radboud University Nijmegen Medical Center, Nijmegen, The Netherlands, **2** Department of Pathology, Radboud University Nijmegen Medical Center, Nijmegen, The Netherlands, **3** Department of Gastroenterology and Hepatology, University Medical Center Utrecht, Utrecht, The Netherlands

Abstract

Background: Cyclooxygenase-2 (COX-2) is a key enzyme involved in the conversion of arachidonic acid into prostaglandins. COX-2 is mainly induced at sites of inflammation in response to proinflammatory cytokines such as interleukin-1α/β, interferon-γ and tumor necrosis factor-α produced by inflammatory cells.

Aim: The aim of this study was to investigate the possible modulating effect of the functional COX-2 polymorphisms −1195 A→G and −765G→C on the risk for development of inflammatory bowel disease (IBD) in a Dutch population.

Methods: Genomic DNA of 525 patients with Crohn's disease (CD), 211 patients with ulcerative colitis (UC) and 973 healthy controls was genotyped for the −1195 A→G (rs689466) and −765G→C (rs20417) polymorphisms. Distribution of genotypes in patients and controls were compared and genotype-phenotype interactions were investigated.

Results: The genotype distribution of the −1195A→G polymorphism was not different between the patients with CD or UC and the control group. The −765GG genotype was more prevalent in CD patients compared to controls with an OR of 1.33 (95%CI 1.04–1.69, p<0.05). The −765GC and −765CC genotype carriers showed a tendency to be less frequent in patients with CD compared to controls, with ORs of 0.78 (95%CI: 0.61–1.00) and 0.49 (95%CI 0.22–1.08), respectively. Combining homozygous and heterozygous patients with the −765C allele showed a reduced risk for developing CD, with an OR of 0.75 (95%CI: 0.59–0.96). In the context of this, the $G_{-1195}G_{-765}$/$A_{-1195}C_{-765}$ diplotype was significantly less common in patients with CD compared to controls, with an OR of 0.62 (95%CI: 0.39–0.98). For UC however, such an effect was not observed. No correlation was found between COX-2 diplotypes and clinical characteristics of IBD.

Conclusions: The −765G→C polymorphism was associated with a reduced risk for developing Crohn's disease in a Dutch population.

Editor: Stefan Bereswill, Charité-University Medicine Berlin, Germany

Funding: The authors have no support or funding to report.

Competing Interests: The authors have declared that no competing interests exist.

* E-mail: h.devries@mdl.umcn.nl

Introduction

Inflammatory bowel disease (IBD) is an idiopathic, chronic, relapsing auto inflammatory disorder of the gastro-intestinal tract. The two major types of IBD are Crohn's disease (CD) and ulcerative colitis (UC). Genetic, immunological and environmental factors are thought to play a role in the pathogenesis of IBD [1]. A dysregulated immune response against the intestinal microbiota in genetic susceptible individuals has been heavily implicated in the pathogenesis of inflammatory bowel disease [2]. Therefore, genes involved in inflammatory responses are under investigation to look for variants predisposing to IBD.

Cyclooxygenase (COX) is a modifier gene and key enzyme in the conversion of free arachidonic acid into prostaglandins and is involved in the regulation of inflammatory processes through its products, mainly prostaglandin E_2 (PGE_2) [3]. The COX family consists of two main isozymes: COX-1 and COX-2. COX-1 is constitutively expressed in most cell types, including the mucosal compartment of the gastrointestinal tract, and is important for maintaining mucosal integrity, mucosal defence and regulation of the mucosal blood flow [4,5]. Being very low expressed in the normal gut mucosa, COX-2 expression can be induced by mitogenic and proinflammatory stimuli [5,6].

The relevance of COX-2 in the pathogenesis of IBD has been demonstrated; increased expression of COX-2 has been observed in colonic epithelial cells, the myenteric plexus and in the medial layer of arteries from patients with active IBD [7–9]. In addition, a relationship between endoscopic activity of IBD and mucosal COX-2 mRNA levels was noticed [10]. Although COX-2 is involved in the regulation of inflammatory processes, it also seems

Table 1. Clinical characteristics of patients with Crohn's disease (n = 525).

Characteristics (%)	
Age at diagnosis	27.1±10.7
Family history of IBD*	75/272 (27.6)
Disease localization	
Ileal	187 (35.6)
Colonic	127 (24.2)
Ileocolonic	211 (40.2)
Isolated upper disease+	36 (6.9)
Disease behaviour CD	
Non stricturing, non penetrating	176 (33.5)
Stricturing	89 (17.0)
Penetrating	260 (49.5)
Extra-intestinal disease*	161/491 (32.8)
Peri-anal disease*	180/509 (35.4)
Surgery	320 (61.0)

+Patients could be classified as having disease localisation in the upper gastrointestinal tract next to ileal, colonic or ileocolonic localisation.
*Note that data of patients are missing.

Table 2. Clinical characteristics of patients with Ulcerative Colitis (n = 211).

Characteristics (%)	
Age at diagnosis	32.9±12.7
Disease localization*	
Proctitis	13/203 (6.4)
Left sided	70/203 (34.5)
Extended/pancolitis	120/203 (59.1)
Surgery	59 (28.0)

*Note that data of 8 patients are missing.

to play a physiological role in the defence of the gastric mucosa, as well as in the maintenance of gastric mucosal integrity when other defence mechanisms are impaired or COX-1 activity is latent [3,5]. Moreover, COX-2 seems to be a major contributor to the processes that lead to resolution of inflammation [11]. In line with this, the use of non-steroidal anti-inflammatory drugs (NSAIDs) in patients with IBD, may be associated with exacerbation of the underlying IBD and gastrointestinal-related complications [12–14]. Overall, these findings suggest that COX-2 has a dual role by both initiation as well as resolution of inflammation.

Functional polymorphisms in the *COX-2* promoter, being $-765G{\rightarrow}C$ (rs20417) and $-1195A{\rightarrow}G$ (rs689466), may alter the enzyme function of COX-2 by differential regulation of COX-2 expression [15]. Recently, a study by Østergaard et al. reported an association of the $-765G{\rightarrow}C$ polymorphism with IBD in a Danish population [16]. Another study from a previous relatively small sample size study performed in the Netherlands however, showed no association between these two polymorphisms and IBD [17]. We therefore investigated the *COX-2* -1195 $A{\rightarrow}G$ and $-765G{\rightarrow}C$ polymorphisms in relation to the development and clinical severity of IBD in a phenotypically well characterized and relatively large IBD cohort of Dutch origin and hypothesized that carriers of the -1195 $A{\rightarrow}G$ and/or $-765G{\rightarrow}C$ polymorphisms might be at risk for developing IBD.

Materials and Methods

Patients and controls

This case-control study included 736 patients with inflammatory bowel disease (39% men, mean age 45.0±13.9 years), being 525 patients with Crohn's disease (35% men, mean age 44.5±13.9) and 211 patients with ulcerative colitis (48% men, mean age 46.1±14.0) and 973 disease-free controls (43% men, mean age 47.2±16.6 years). All patients were of Dutch origin and were recruited from the outpatient clinic of the Radboud University Nijmegen Medical Center, the Netherlands. Controls were recruited from the Nijmegen area by advertisement in local

papers. The clinical characteristics of the patients are summarized in Tables 1 and 2. Diagnosis of inflammatory bowel disease was based on accepted clinical, endoscopic, radiological and histological findings [18]. Clinical data of the patients were retrieved by retrospective collection from patients' clinical charts. Phenotypes of the patients were described according to age of onset, necessity of surgery, family history of IBD, the occurrence of extra-intestinal manifestations and maximum extent of disease according to the Vienna [19] and Montreal [20] classifications for Crohn's disease and ulcerative colitis respectively.

Information on development of dysplasia and colorectal cancer (CRC) in our patient cohort was retrieved using PALGA, the nationwide network and registry of histopathology and cytopathology in the Netherlands [21].

The ethical committee of region Nijmegen and Arnhem reviewed and approved the protocol under number CWOM-nr 9804-0100. Verbal informed consent was obtained from each patient before study participation in agreement with the approval and all samples were anonymized. Since research data were collected anonymously, at least verbal informed consent was needed according to national regulations. Therefore, no written informed consent procedure was introduced at time of data collection.

Genotyping

Whole blood from patients and healthy controls was obtained by venapuncture in sterile vacutainer tubes, anti-coagulated with EDTA and stored at −20°C until use. DNA from patients and controls was isolated from whole blood using the Pure Gene DNA isolation kit, according to the instructions of the manufacturer (Gentra Systems, Minneapolis, MN) and stored at 4°C. Genotypes of the *COX-2* $-1195A{\rightarrow}G$ polymorphism was determined by polymerase chain reaction (PCR)-based restriction fragment length polymorphism assays, as described by Zhang *et al* [15]. The *COX-2* $-765G{\rightarrow}C$ polymorphism was determined by a dual-color discrimination assay using the iCycler iQ Multicolour Real-Time Detection System (Bio-Rad Laboratories, Hercules, CA), as described by Peters *et al* [22].

Statistical analysis

Baseline and clinical characteristics were analysed with standard descriptive statistics. The observed genotype frequencies were tested for deviation from the Hardy-Weinberg equilibrium. Estimates of linkage disequilibrium (LD) between SNPs were determined by calculating pair-wise D′ and r^2 statistics in unrelated individuals, using Haploview. Differences in $-1195A{\rightarrow}G$ and $-765G{\rightarrow}C$ genotype distributions between the patient and control groups were determined by Chi-square analysis. Odds ratios (ORs) with 95%

Table 3. Distribution of the COX-2 −1195 and −765 genotypes and corresponding ORs in patients with IBD, CD or UC versus controls.

Genotype COX-2	All patients with IBD (n = 736)			Patients with Crohn's disease (n = 525)			Patients with Ulcerative Colitis (n = 211)+			Controls
	Number (%)	OR (95% CI)	p-value	Number (%)	OR (95% CI)	p-value	Number (%)	OR (95% CI)	p-value	n = 973 (%)
−1195AA	476 (64.7)	Reference	-	339 (64.6)	Reference	-	137 (64.9)	Reference	-	618 (63.5)
−1195GA	221 (30.0)	0.91 (0.74–1.12)	0.38	159 (30.3)	0.92 (0.73–1.16)	0.48	62 (29.4)	0.89 (0.64–1.23)	0.48	315 (32.4)
−1195GG	39 (5.3)	1.27 (0.80–2.00)	0.31	27 (5.1)	1.23 (0.74–2.04)	0.42	12 (5.7)	1.35 (0.69–2.65)	0.38	40 (4.1)
−765GG	535 (73.2)	Reference	-	394 (75.0)	Reference	-	141 (68.4)	Reference	-	675 (69.4)
−765GC	179 (24.5)	0.84 (0.67–1.04)	0.11	123 (23.4)	0.78 (0.61–1.00)	0.05	56 (27.2)	0.99 (0.71–1.40)	0.97	270 (27.7)
−765CC	17 (2.3)	0.77 (0.42–1.41)	0.39	8 (1.5)	0.49 (0.22–1.08)	0.07	9 (4.4)	1.53 (0.71–3.33)	0.27	28 (2.9)

+In the ulcerative colitis group, there are some missing data (n = 5) due to unsuccessful PCR for the −765 G→C polymorphism.
OR = Odds ratio; CI = confidence interval.

confidence interval (95% CI) were calculated for genotypes associated with predicted normal versus predicted altered enzyme activities (variant genotypes) between IBD patients and controls. These analyses were also applied for testing of either UC or CD with the control group. Based on the two polymorphisms investigated, a diplotype analysis was performed. Diplotypes were compared with regard to phenotypical characteristics and comparisons were given as ORs with 95% CI. Additionally, we investigated in patients with IBD whether the $-1195A{\rightarrow}G$ and $-765G{\rightarrow}C$ polymorphisms were associated with development of mucosal dysplasia or colon cancer. Data analysis was performed using SPSS software (Version 16.0, SPSS, Chicago, IL, USA). A p-value of <0.05 was used as a criterion for statistical significance.

Results

In this study 736 patients with inflammatory bowel disease, 525 patients with Crohn's disease and 211 patients with ulcerative colitis as well as 973 healthy controls were included. No statistical significant differences were observed between patients with IBD and controls regarding age and gender. However when the CD or UC patient groups were compared to controls separately, significant more females were present in the group with Crohn's disease (p<0.01).

Distribution of the -1195 and -765 COX-2 genotypes in both patient and control groups fitted the Hardy Weinberg equilibrium; for the -1195 genotypes, p-values of p = 0.14, p = 0.17 and p = 0.99, for the patients with Crohn's disease, ulcerative colitis and controls were found; whereas corresponding p-values for the -765 genotypes were p = 0.64, p = 0.26 and p = 0.87, respectively. As been reported before by others [15,17,23], both SNPs were found to be in strong linkage disequilibrium ($D' = 1$, $r^2 = 0.05$).

Genotype distribution and association with inflammatory bowel disease

The distribution of the -1195 and -765 COX-2 genotypes as found in patients with IBD and controls is given in Table 3. The -1195 genotype distribution was not different between the patients with Crohn's disease, ulcerative colitis, or all IBD patients taken together in comparison with the control group. However, the -765 genotype distribution showed a tendency towards a significant difference between patients with Crohn's disease and controls, with the $-765GC$ and $-765CC$ genotypes being less prevalent in patients, with ORs of 0.78 (95%CI 0.61–1.00,

p<0.05) and 0.49 (95%CI 0.22–1.08) respectively and the $-765GG$ genotype being more prevalent in patients (OR 1.33, 95%CI 1.04–1.69, p<0.05). No differences were found between patients with ulcerative colitis and controls. Combining homozygous ($-765CC$) and heterozygous ($-765GC$) patients bearing the $-765C$ allele, showed a reduced risk for developing Crohn's disease in this group (OR = 0.75, 95%CI 0.59–0.96, p<0.05).

The effects of the two COX-2 polymorphisms were then studied in the context of diplotypes. Six diplotypes were identified, with the $A_{-1195}G_{-765}/A_{-1195}G_{-765}$ diplotype being the most prevalent in both patients and controls (Table 4). The $G_{-1195}G_{-765}/A_{-1195}C_{-765}$ diplotype was significantly less frequent in patients with Crohn's disease compared to controls with an OR of 0.62 (95%CI: 0.39–0.98, p<0.05).

Correlation of the COX-2 diplotypes with clinical characteristics of IBD patients

Additionally, clinical characteristics of patients with Crohn's disease and ulcerative colitis were studied in the context of diplotypes in which the most common $A_{-1195}G_{-765}/A_{-1195}G_{-765}$ diplotype served as reference. No significant association between the COX-2 diplotypes and clinical characteristics of either Crohn's disease or ulcerative colitis was found (Tables 5 and 6). When data were corrected for age and gender, no significant changes in data were observed.

COX-2 polymorphisms and the risk for developing dysplasia and colon cancer in patients with inflammatory bowel disease

The PALGA search regarding dysplasia and colon cancer in our IBD cohort demonstrated that 29 patients (15 patients with CD and 14 patients with UC) developed mucosal dysplasia, which is regarded as a pre-malignant phase of CRC. Furthermore, in the CD cohort 7 patients with CRC were identified; 4 having the $A_{-1195}G_{-765}/A_{-1195}G_{-765}$ diplotype and 3 having the $G_{-1195}G_{-765}/A_{-1195}G_{-765}$ diplotype. In the UC cohort, no patients were identified who developed CRC. When tested, no association was found between the COX-2 diplotypes and the development of colonic dysplasia or cancer (Tables 5 and 6).

Discussion

This study was performed to determine the possible modulating effect of the COX-2 -1195 $A{\rightarrow}G$ and $-765G{\rightarrow}C$ polymorphisms

Table 4. *COX-2* diplotype distribution and corresponding ORs in patients with IBD, CD or UC versus controls.

Diplotype COX-2	All patients			Crohn's disease			Ulcerative colitis			Controls
	n = 731 (%)	OR (95% CI)	p-value	n = 525 (%)	OR (95%CI)	p-value	n = 206 (%)	OR (95%CI)	p-value	n = 973 (%)
$A_{-1195}G_{-765}$/ $A_{-1195}G_{-765}$	322 (43.8)	Reference	-	237 (45.1)	Reference	-	85 (40.3)	Reference	-	395 (40.6)
$G_{-1195}G_{-765}$/ $A_{-1195}G_{-765}$	174 (23.6)	0.90 (0.70–1.15)	0.38	130 (24.8)	0.91 (0.70–1.19)	0.49	44 (20.9)	0.86 (0.58–1.28)	0.45	238 (24.5)
$A_{-1195}G_{-765}$/ $A_{-1195}C_{-765}$	133 (18.1)	0.84 (0.65–1.10)	0.20	94 (17.9)	0.81 (0.60–1.08)	0.15	39 (18.5)	0.93 (0.62–1.42)	0.75	194 (19.9)
$G_{-1195}G_{-765}$/ $A_{-1195}C_{-765}$	46 (6.5)	0.72 (0.49–1.07)	0.11	29 (5.5)	0.62 (0.39–0.98)	0.04	17 (8.1)	1.01 (0.57–1.80)	0.97	78 (8.0)
$G_{-1195}G_{-765}$/ $G_{-1195}G_{-765}$	39 (5.3)	1.20 (0.75–1.90)	0.45	27 (5.1)	1.13 (0.67–1.88)	0.65	12 (5.7)	1.39 (0.70–2.77)	0.34	40 (4.1)
$A_{-1195}C_{-765}$/ $A_{-1195}C_{-765}$	17 (2.3)	0.75 (0.40–1.39)	0.35	8 (1.5)	0.48 (0.21–1.06)	0.06	9 (4.3)	1.49 (0.68–3.28)	0.32	28 (2.9)

OR = Odds ratio; CI = confidence interval.

on the risk of developing inflammatory bowel disease. Carriers of the −765C allele showed a reduced risk for developing CD. This result suggests that the −765G→C change induces an altered enzyme expression and enzyme activity with potential anti-inflammatory consequences.

Studies regarding the functional consequences of the −765G→C polymorphism in the *COX-2* promoter are conflicting. Therefore, the (physiological) consequences of our findings are difficult to interpret. First of all, the −765C-containing COX-2 promoter was reported to drive lower reporter gene expression in vitro compared to the −765G-containing counterpart [15,24]. Furthermore, serum prostaglandin E$_2$ (PGE$_2$) concentrations of renal transplant recipients patients with the GG genotype were significantly higher than PGE$_2$ concentrations from patients with the C allele [25]. Subsequent work from Zhang and coworkers showed that the −765G→C polymorphism creates a binding site for nucleophosmin (NPM) and phosphorylated nucleophosmin (p-NPM), which acts as an inhibitor of COX-2 transcription [26]. The −1195 A→G polymorphism creates a c-MYB binding site, which can activate COX-2 expression, and displays a higher promoter activity [15].

In normal colorectal mucosa COX-2 expression is enhanced in patients with IBD when compared to subjects with normal colonoscopy [27]. Taken together in light of our results, this would imply that low levels of COX-2 are associated with an reduced risk for developing CD. In vitro however, when cells were treated with smoking condensate, the −765C-containing promoter exerted a significantly higher reporter gene expression compared to the −765G-containing counterpart [26]. Besides this, Szczeklik and co-workers reported an increased production of prostaglandin E$_2$ and D$_2$ (PGE$_2$ and PGD$_2$) by monocytes obtained from female patients with asthma who were homozygous for the −765C variant of the COX-2 gene [28,29]. In the context of IBD, PGE$_2$ appears to play a dual role. In IBD, PGE$_2$ production is increased [30] and in an experimental model of IBD high levels of PGE$_2$ exacerbate inflammation [31]. On the other hand, PGE$_2$ signaling is required for suppressing colitis symptoms and protecting mucosal damage by maintaining the integrity of the epithelial intestinal wall, presumably through the enhancement of epithelial survival and regeneration [32]. Furthermore, PGE$_2$ has been

recently identified to promote naive T cell differentiation to IL-17 – producing T helper (Th17) cells, a subset of T helper cells which have been implicated as potent effector cells in IBD [33].

Several limitations of our study should be noticed. First of all we were not able to retrieve the smoking status of our patients and controls, as Zhao et al. [26] demonstrated an effect of smoking on the expression of the −765G→C polymorphism. Secondly, the effect of the COX-2 −1195 A→G and −765G→C polymorphisms on colonic mucosal COX-2 expression and/or PGE$_2$ production in patients with IBD is unknown. However regardless of these data, the functional consequences of PGE$_2$ in IBD still remains conflicting as pointed out above.

The results of our study are in conflict with a Danish case control study by Østergaard et al. who identified that carriers of the homozygous −765CC variant had a relatively high risk for developing CD as well as UC, with an OR of 2.78 (95%CI = 1.33–5.88, p = 0.006) and 2.63 (95%CI = 1.35–5.26, p = 0.005) respectively [16]. The −765CC variant however is very rare in our population of IBD patients (n = 17, 2.3%) and controls (n = 28, 2.9%) as is the case in another Dutch study by Cox et al. in which (2.4%) of the patients and (2.4%) of the controls had this variant [17]. In the study of Cox et al., no significant association between the −1195 A→G and −765G→C polymorphisms and IBD was found, although the number of patients with IBD involved (n = 291) was rather small. However, a recent subsequent study from the Danish group of Østergaard and co-workers extended the original data with data from Scottish IBD patients and showed no association any more with the −765G→C polymorphism and development of IBD [34]. The differences between our results and the Danish and Scottish findings could be attributed to the fact that the genetical contribution to the etiology of IBD in the northern part of Europe differs from central Europe. Mutations in the three common CD-associated variants of CARD15, R702W, G908R and 1007fsinsC, are relatively rare in Northern countries including Denmark and Scotland, while the mutation frequencies are relatively high in Central Europe [35].

As stated before, patients with IBD show increased expression of COX-2 in the gastrointestinal tract [7,8,10,27]. This increased expression of COX-2 has also been observed in gastrointestinal adenocarcinomas and in UC-associated neoplasia [36,37]. Addi-

Table 5. Diplotype-phenotype correlations in patients with Crohn's disease.

	AG/AG*	GG/AG	Odds ratio (95%CI)	p-value	AG/AC	Odds ratio (95%CI)	p-value	GG/AC	Odds ratio (95%CI)	p-value	GG/GG	Odds ratio (95%CI)	p-value	AC/AC	Odds ratio (95%CI)	p-value
Disease localization (n=525)																
Ileal	83	51	Reference	-	34	Reference	-	8	Reference	-	8	Reference	-	3	Reference	-
Colonic	63	26	0.67 (0.38–1.19)	0.17	23	0.89 (0.48–1.66)	0.72	8	1.32 (0.47–3.70)	0.60	6	0.99 (0.33–2.99)	0.98	1	0.44 (0.05–4.32)	0.47
Ileocolonic	91	53	0.95 (0.58–1.54)	0.83	37	0.99 (0.57–1.73)	0.98	13	1.48 (0.59–3.76)	0.41	13	1.48 (0.59–3.76)	0.41	4	1.22 (0.26–5.60)	0.80
Isolated upper disease+	18	7	0.63 (0.25–1.62)	0.34	8	1.09 (0.43–2.73)	0.86	2	1.15 (0.23–5.89)	0.86	1	0.58 (0.07–4.90)	0.61	0	-	0.42
Disease behavior (n=525)																
Non stricturing/penetrating	75	44	Reference	-	37	Reference	-	10	Reference	-	8	Reference	-	2	Reference	-
Stricturing	43	18	0.71 (0.37–1.39)	0.32	14	0.66 (0.32–1.36)	0.26	8	1.40 (0.51–3.80)	0.51	4	0.87 (0.25–3.07)	0.83	2	1.74 (0.24–12.83)	0.58
Penetrating	119	68	0.97 (0.61–1.57)	0.91	43	0.73 (0.43–1.24)	0.25	11	0.69 (0.28–1.71)	0.43	15	1.18 (0.48–2.92)	0.72	4	1.26 (0.23–7.05)	0.79
Surgery	146	87	1.26 (0.81–1.98)	0.31	50	0.71 (0.44–1.15)	0.16	16	0.77 (0.35–1.67)	0.50	17	1.06 (0.47–2.42)	0.89	4	0.62 (0.15–2.55)	0.51
Extra-intestinal (n=491)	77	32	0.69 (0.43–1.13)	0.14	37	1.39 (0.84–2.30)	0.21	8	0.80 (0.34–1.92)	0.62	6	0.64 (0.24–1.67)	0.36	1	0.27 (0.03–2.26)	0.20
Family history of IBD (n=272)	36	18	0.82 (0.43–1.59)	0.57	14	1.08 (0.52–2.26)	0.84	2	0.62 (0.13–3.05)	0.55	3	0.67 (0.18–2.56)	0.56	2	1.65 (0.26–10.28)	0.59
Dysplasia	7	4	1.04 (0.30–3.63)	0.95	1	0.35 (0.04–2.91)	0.31	1	1.17 (0.14–9.89)	0.88	2	2.63 (0.52–13.35)	0.23	0	-	0.62
Colon cancer	4	3	0.73 (0.16–3.30)	0.68	0	-	0.21	0	-	0.21	0	-	0.48	0	-	0.71

Diplotype-phenotype correlations in patients with Crohn's disease in which the AG/AG diplotype served as reference.
+Patients could be classified as having disease localisation in the upper gastrointestinal tract next to ileal, colonic or ileocolonic localisation.
*For full notation see Table 4.

Table 6. Diplotype-phenotype correlations in patients with ulcerative colitis.

	AG/AG#	GG/AG	Odds ratio (95%CI)	p-value	AG/AC	Odds ratio (95%CI)	p-value	GG/AC	Odds ratio (95%CI)	p-value	GG/GG	Odds ratio (95%CI)	p-value	AC/AC	Odds ratio (95%CI)	p-value
Disease localization (n=198)																
Proctitis	6	2	Reference	-	2	Reference	-	2	Reference	-	1	Reference	-	0	Reference	-
Left sided	27	13	1.44 (0.26–8.16)	0.676	15	1.67 (0.30–9.31)	0.558	7	0.78 (0.13–4.72)	0.784	3	0.67 (0.06–7.57)	0.742	4	-	0.351
Pancolitis	46	28	1.83 (0.35–9.68)	0.474	21	1.37 (0.26–7.36)	0.713	8	0.52 (0.09–3.06)	0.465	8	1.04 (0.11–9.86)	0.970	5	-	0.422
Surgery (n=206)	24	11	0.85 (0.37–1.94)	0.695	11	1.00 (0.43–2.32)	0.997	8	2.26 (0.78–6.54)	0.127	2	0.51 (0.10–2.49)	0.397	2	0.73 (0.14–3.75)	0.701
Dysplasia (n=211)	5	3	1.17 (0.27–5.14)	0.835	2	0.87 (0.16–4.67)	0.866	0	-	0.305	1	1.46 (0.16–13.63)	0.741	2	4.57 (0.75–28.01)	0.076

Diplotype-phenotype correlations in patients with ulcerative colitis in which AG/AG served as reference.
#For full notation see Table 4.

tionally, the $COX\text{-}2 - 1195\ A{\to}G$ and $-765G{\to}C$ polymorphisms were demonstrated to influence the expression of COX-2 and confer a risk for developing (adeno)carcinomas in the gastrointestinal tract [15,38,39]. Chronic intestinal inflammation-associated colorectal carcinogenesis is thought to occur via a stepwise progression beginning with epithelial hyperplasia, leading to various grades of dysplasia, adenoma, and then to adenocarcinoma [40]. We investigated whether or not an association could be found between the $COX\text{-}2$ polymorphisms and dysplasia or CRC in patients with IBD. Due to the restricted number of patients who developed dysplasia or CRC, no differences could be observed.

In conclusion, subjects with the $-765C$ allele showed a reduced risk for developing CD. No correlation could be found between the $COX\text{-}2$ diplotypes and clinical characteristics of IBD patients and the development of colonic dysplasia or cancer. Further studies are required to confirm the association we found and efforts should be made to unravel the role of COX-2 and its derived prostaglandins in the pathogenesis of IBD.

Author Contributions

Conceived and designed the experiments: HdV DJJ WHMP. Performed the experiments: RHMM. Analyzed the data: HdV MGHO. Contributed reagents/materials/analysis tools: IDN. Wrote the paper: HdV.

References

1. Xavier RJ, Podolsky DK (2007) Unravelling the pathogenesis of inflammatory bowel disease. Nature 448: 427–34.
2. Sartor RB (2008) Microbial influences in inflammatory bowel diseases. Gastroenterology 134: 577–94.
3. Warner TD, Mitchell JA (2004) Cyclooxygenases: new forms, new inhibitors, and lessons from the clinic. Faseb Journal 18: 790–804.
4. Martin GR, Wallace JL (2006) Gastrointestinal inflammation: A central component of mucosal defense and repair. Exp Biol Med 231: 130–137.
5. Fornai M, Antonioli L, Colucci R, Bernardini N, Ghisu N, et al. (2010) Emerging role of cyclooxygenase isoforms in the control of gastrointestinal neuromuscular functions. Pharmacol Therapeut 125: 62–78.
6. Trifan OC, Hla T (2003) Cyclooxygenase-2 modulates cellular growth and promotes tumorigenesis. J Cell Mol Med 7: 207–222.
7. Singer II, Kawka DW, Schloemann S, Tessner T, Riehl T, et al. (1998) Cyclooxygenase 2 is induced in colonic epithelial cells in inflammatory bowel disease. Gastroenterology 115: 297–306.
8. Roberts PJ, Morgan K, Miller R, Hunter JO, Middleton SJ (2001) Neuronal COX-2 expression in human myenteric plexus in active inflammatory bowel disease. Gut 48: 468–472.
9. Tabernero A, Reimund JM, Chasserot S, Muller CD, Andriantsitohaina R (2003) Cyclooxygenase-2 expression and role of vasoconstrictor prostanoids in small mesenteric arteries from patients with Crohn's disease. Circulation 107: 1407–1410.
10. Hendel J, Nielsen OH (1997) Expression of cyclooxygenase-2 mRNA in active inflammatory bowel disease. Am J Gastroenterol 92: 1170–1173.
11. Wallace JL (2006) COX-2: A pivotal enzyme in mucosal protection and resolution of inflammation. Thescientificworldjournal 6: 577–588.
12. Matuk R, Crawford J, Abreu MT, Targan SR, Vasiliauskas EA, et al. (2004) The spectrum of gastrointestinal toxicity and effect on disease activity of selective cyclooxygenase-2 inhibitors in patients with inflammatory bowel disease. Inflamm Bowel Dis 10: 352–356.
13. Takeuchi K, Smale S, Premchand P, Maiden L, Sherwood R, et al. (2006) Prevalence and mechanism of nonsteroidal anti-inflammatory drug-induced clinical relapse in patients with inflammatory bowel disease. Clin Gastroenterol H 4: 196–202.
14. Biancone L, Tosti C, Geremia A, Fina D, Petruzziello C, et al. (2004) Rofecoxib and early relapse of inflammatory bowel disease: an open-label trial. Aliment Pharm Ther 19: 755–764.
15. Zhang XM, Miao XP, Tan W, Ning BT, Liu ZH, et al. (2005) Identification of functional genetic variants in cyclooxygenase-2 and their association with risk of esophageal cancer. Gastroenterology 129: 565–576.
16. Ostergaard M, Ernst A, Labouriau R, Dagiliene E, Krarup HB, et al. (2009) Cyclooxygenase-2, multidrug resistance 1, and breast cancer resistance protein gene polymorphisms and inflammatory bowel disease in the Danish population. Scand J Gastroentero 44: 65–73.
17. Cox DG, Crusius JB, Peeters PH, Bueno-de-Mesquita HB, Pena AS, et al. (2005) Haplotype of prostaglandin synthase 2/cyclooxygenase 2 is involved in the susceptibility to inflammatory bowel disease. World J Gastroenterol 2005 11: 6003–6008.
18. Podolsky DK (2002) Inflammatory bowel disease. New Engl J Med 347: 417–429.
19. Gasche C, Scholmerich J, Brynskov J, D'Haens G, Hanauer SB, et al. (2000) A simple classification of Crohn's disease: Report of the Working Party for the world congresses of gastroenterology, Vienna 1998. Inflamm Bowel Dis 6: 8–15.
20. Silverberg MS, Satsangi J, Ahmad T, Arnott IDR, Bernstein CN, et al. (2005) Toward an integrated clinical, molecular and serological classification of inflammatory bowel disease: Report of a Working Party of the 2005 Montreal World Congress of Gastroenterology. Can J Gastroenterol 19: 5A–36A.
21. Casparie M, Tiebosch ATMG, Burger G, Blauwgeers H, van de Pol A, et al. (2007) Pathology databanking and biobanking in The Netherlands, a central role for PALGA, the nationwide histopathology and cytopathology data network and archive. Cell Oncol 29: 19–24.
22. Peters WHM, Lacko M, Morsche RHMT, Voogd AC, Ophuis MBO, et al. (2009) Cox-2 Polymorphisms and the Risk for Head and Neck Cancer in White Patients. Head Neck 31: 938–943.
23. Rudock ME, Liu Y, Ziegler JT, Allen SG, Lehtinen AB, et al. (2009) Association of polymorphisms in cyclooxygenase (COX)-2 with coronary and carotid calcium in the Diabetes Heart Study. Atherosclerosis 203: 459–465.
24. Papafili A, Hill MR, Brull DJ, McAnulty RJ, Marshall RP, et al. (2002) Common promoter variant in cyclooxygenase-2 represses gene expression - Evidence of role in acute-phase inflammatory response. Arterioscl Throm Vas 22: 1631–1636.
25. Courivaud C, Bamoulid J, Loupy A, Deschamps M, Ferrand C, et al. (2009) Influence of Cyclooxygenase-2 (COX-2) Gene Promoter Polymorphism-765 on Graft Loss After Renal Transplantation. Am J Transplant 9: 2752–2757.
26. Zhao D, Xu DK, Zhang XM, Wang L, Tan W, et al. (2009) Interaction of Cyclooxygenase-2 Variants and Smoking in Pancreatic Cancer: A Possible Role of Nucleophosmin. Gastroenterology 136: 1659–1668.
27. Mariani F, Sena P, Marzona L, Riccio M, Fano R, et al. (2009) Cyclooxygenase-2 and Hypoxia-Inducible Factor-1 alpha protein expression is related to inflammation, and up-regulated since the early steps of colorectal carcinogenesis. Cancer Lett 279: 221–229.
28. Szczeklik W, Sanak M, Szczeklik A (2004) Functional effects and gender association of COX-2 gene polymorphism G(−765)C in bronchial asthma. J Allergy Clin Immun 114: 248–253.
29. Sanak M, Szczeklik W, Szczeklik A (2005) Association of COX-2 gene haplotypes with prostaglandins production in bronchial asthma. J Allergy Clin Immun 116: 221–223.
30. Carty E, De Brabander M, Feakins RM, Rampton DS (2000) Measurement of in vivo rectal mucosal cytokine and eicosanoid production in ulcerative colitis using filter paper. Gut 46: 487–492.
31. Sheibanie AF, Yen JH, Khayrullina T, Emig F, Zhang M, et al. (2007) The proinflammatory effect of prostaglandin E-2 in experimental inflammatory bowel disease is mediated through the IL-23 -> IL-17 axis. Journal Immunol 178: 8138–8147.
32. Jiang GL, Nieves A, Im WB, Old DW, Dinh DT, et al. (2007) The prevention of colitis by E prostanoid receptor 4 agonist through enhancement of epithelium survival and regeneration. J Pharmacol Exp Ther 320: 22–8.
33. Boniface K, Bak-Jensen KS, Li Y, Blumenschein WM, McGeachy MJ, et al. (2009) Prostaglandin E2 regulates Th17 cell differentiation and function through cyclic AMP and EP2/EP4 receptor signaling. J Exp Med 206: 535–548.
34. Andersen V, Nimmo E, Krarup HB, Drummond H, Christensen J, Ho GT, et al. Cyclooxygenase-2 (COX-2) polymorphisms and risk of inflammatory bowel disease in a Scottish and Danish case-control study. Inflamm Bowel Dis. In press.
35. Hugot JP, Zaccaria I, Cavanaugh J, Yang HY, Vermeire S, et al. (2007) Prevalence of CARD15/NOD2 mutations in Caucasian healthy people. Am J Gastroenterol 102: 1259–1267.
36. Hasegawa K, Ichikawa W, Fujita T, Ohno R, Okusa T, et al. (2001) Expression of cyclooxygenase-2 (COX-2) mRNA in human colorectal adenomas. Eur J Cancer 37: 1469–1474.
37. Agoff SN, Brentnall TA, Crispin DA, Taylor SL, Raaka S, et al. (2000) The role of cyclooxygenase 2 in ulcerative colitis-associated neoplasia. Am J Pathol 157: 737–745.
38. Hoff JH, te Morsche RH, Roelofs HM, van der Logt EM, Nagengast FM, et al. (2009) COX-2 polymorphisms −765G{\to}C and −1195A{\to}G and colorectal cancer risk. World J Gastroenterol 15: 4561–4565.
39. Tan W, Wu JX, Zhang XM, Guo YL, Liu JN, et al. (2007) Associations of functional polymorphisms in cyclooxygenase-2 and platelet 12-lipoxygenase with risk of occurrence and advanced disease status of colorectal cancer. Carcinogenesis 28: 1197–1201.
40. Westbrook AM, Szakmary A, Schiestl RH (2010) Mechanisms of intestinal inflammation and development of associated cancers: Lessons learned from mouse models. Mutat Res 705: 40–59.

14

Extreme Evolutionary Disparities Seen in Positive Selection across Seven Complex Diseases

Erik Corona[1,2], Joel T. Dudley[1,2], Atul J. Butte[1,2]*

1 Lucile Packard Children's Hospital, Stanford, California, United States of America, **2** Department of Pediatrics, Stanford University School of Medicine, Stanford, California, United States of America

Abstract

Positive selection is known to occur when the environment that an organism inhabits is suddenly altered, as is the case across recent human history. Genome-wide association studies (GWASs) have successfully illuminated disease-associated variation. However, whether human evolution is heading towards or away from disease susceptibility in general remains an open question. The genetic-basis of common complex disease may partially be caused by positive selection events, which simultaneously increased fitness and susceptibility to disease. We analyze seven diseases studied by the Wellcome Trust Case Control Consortium to compare evidence for selection at every locus associated with disease. We take a large set of the most strongly associated SNPs in each GWA study in order to capture more hidden associations at the cost of introducing false positives into our analysis. We then search for signs of positive selection in this inclusive set of SNPs. There are striking differences between the seven studied diseases. We find alleles increasing susceptibility to Type 1 Diabetes (T1D), Rheumatoid Arthritis (RA), and Crohn's Disease (CD) underwent recent positive selection. There is more selection in alleles increasing, rather than decreasing, susceptibility to T1D. In the 80 SNPs most associated with T1D (p-value $<7.01\times10^{-5}$) showing strong signs of positive selection, 58 alleles associated with disease susceptibility show signs of positive selection, while only 22 associated with disease protection show signs of positive selection. Alleles increasing susceptibility to RA are under selection as well. In contrast, selection in SNPs associated with CD favors protective alleles. These results inform the current understanding of disease etiology, shed light on potential benefits associated with the genetic-basis of disease, and aid in the efforts to identify causal genetic factors underlying complex disease.

Editor: John Hawks, University of Wisconsin, United States of America

Funding: This work was supported by the Lucile Packard Foundation for Children's Health, the Hewlett Packard Foundation, the Armin and Linda Miller Fellowship Fund, the National Library of Medicine (T15 LM 007033), the National Institute of General Medical Sciences (R01 GM079719), a National Science Foundation Graduate Research Fellowship, and the Howard Hughes Medical Institute. These funders had no role in study design, data collection and analysis, decision to publish, or preparation of the manuscript. The commercial funder provided funds for hardware equipment and unrestricted funds for research. No commercial organization had any role in the research design, implementation, or findings.

Competing Interests: No patents or products in development are pending related to this work.

* E-mail: abutte@stanford.edu

Introduction

Humans have gone from existing solely in Africa to inhabiting every continent on Earth [1]. More recently, humans have begun cultivating specialized food-crop, domesticating animals, and living in towns and cities. Such environmental changes are known to alter common genetic variation via the positive selection of advantageous mutations [2]. As many populations were exposed to new food sources, diseases, and cultural lifestyles, positive selection likely played a major role in shaping the genetic architecture. A positive selection event represents a net gain of fitness, and there is room for the simultaneous selection of harmful mutations if they are linked to a relatively strongly beneficial mutation [3]. This can occur when a locus is in linkage disequilibrium (LD) with a beneficial mutation. Alternatively, the beneficial mutation may simultaneously harbor a harmful component [4]. Positive selection may occur as long as the benefits outweigh the harm. Therefore, increased susceptibility to disease may accompany a fitness-increasing mutation introduced by positive selection.

Complex diseases contain many distinct associations across the human genome that contribute only slightly to the absolute risk of

disease [5]. These disease-associated mutations may undergo positive selection if they are simultaneously associated with relatively strongly beneficial traits. For example, the sickle cell mutation in the *Hemoglobin-B* (*HBB*) gene was found to be the target of positive selection due to its properties related to malaria resistance, despite its simultaneous role in introducing sickle cell disease [3]. It has also been recently shown that the variants in the antiviral response gene *IFIH1* associated with protection against enterovirus infection simultaneously increase susceptibility to Type 1 Diabetes (T1D) [6]. In this case, the benefits of having variants of the *IFIH1* gene that increase susceptibility to T1D depend on the prevalence of enterovirus infection. Having *IFIH1* gene variants increasing susceptibility to T1D may be considered advantageous and undergo positive selection if the probability of being exposed to the virus were high.

Rheumatoid Arthritis (RA) can be detected in human skeletal remains, and likely originated from the Americas and spread to Europe after the pre-Columbian era ended, possibly by a microorganism or allergen that is a necessary trigger for the disease [7]. This paves the way for selection to proceed strongly for potential benefits associated with the genetic-basis of RA. Prior to exposure to microorganisms or allergens required for the onset of RA, there would be no disadvantage to having mutations associated with RA in European populations. Ultimately, the cumulative contribution of such mutations with low effect sizes may play a large role in causing the disease.

It is currently unknown how much of the genetic-basis of complex disease originates from genetic mutations driven to prevalence by positive selection pressures. Blekhman *et al.* demonstrated that coding positions within disease associated genes underlying a number of complex human diseases are more rapidly evolving than coding regions of genes not associated with disease [8]. This suggests that evolutionary changes and natural selection may play a role in regions associated with complex disease.

We define a risk/susceptibility allele as the allele associated with more disease cases in the GWAS data used for our study, while the protective allele is necessarily present more often in healthy controls. Finding positively selected risk-associated alleles in complex human disease is challenging. It is easiest to learn more about the origins and history of disease when a mutation simultaneously confers a selective advantage while increasing susceptibility to disease in the same environment. It becomes more challenging when the risk-associated allele may falsely appear to be the target of selection if it is linked to a very advantageous allele due to linkage disequilibrium. To fully explain the origins of such risk-associated alleles, the nearby target of positive selection must first be identified.

An allele increasing susceptibility to disease in today's environment may have increased fitness only in an alternative environmental context [9], which makes it difficult to determine how (now absent) fitness-increasing properties can fully explain the history and origins of disease. While it is well established that more strongly deleterious mutations exhibit evolutionary profiles that differ from more neutral forms of variation in the human genome, it has been challenging to assess how much of a role natural selection has played in weakly deleterious mutations [10]. In previous studies excluding non-coding SNPs, it was shown that SNPs within complex disease associated genes are likely to be undergoing positive selection [11] [8], even in diseases having little impact on fitness [12]. If weakly deleterious mutations rise to prevalence via the positive selection of separate fitness increasing traits, we expect to find positive selection within relatively weakly deleterious mutations.

The first steps in addressing the issue of positive selection in complex diseases (including Crohn's Disease, Type 1, and Type 2 Diabetes) were taken in a study that scanned specific disease associated SNPs for positive selection [10]. This study examined an exclusive set of associated SNPs to avoid false associations, but excludes many hidden associations found in moderate association p-values. Consequently, while positive selection was found in individual SNPs, the search for positive selection of the overall genetic-basis of the each disease was inconclusive. A more thorough approach with positive selection detection methods proven to be more sensitive is warranted. Other approaches employing evolutionary analysis to characterize the genetic basis of disease are not applicable to complex disease. For example, selective pressures acting on specific conserved codon positions are used to predict deleterious mutations in human disease genes [13]. While evolutionary analysis of coding SNPs (cSNPs) within conserved amino acid sequences is informative most often for monogenic and Mendelian diseases, the same approach holds less utility in the analysis of complex, polygenic disorders due to association of many low-risk non-coding SNPs.

Modern approaches that incorporate haplotype structure have more power to detect recent positive selection [14], making them ideal for finding evidence of selection among complex diseases that have only recently emerged in the human genome. Detecting positive selection in loci associated with complex disease informs on the evolutionary history of disease and narrows down the search for positively selected components, possibly exposing the presence of unknown advantageous functions associated with the genetic basis of such diseases. These methods also indicate whether selection is acting on the major or minor allele.

It has been shown that different diseases can share association to the same SNPs, and that while one allele increases disease risk for one disease, the other allele may decrease disease risk for another [15]. By extending this principle, it is possible to determine whether selecting for protection against a disease also selects for increased risk for a separate disease.

Previous studies have focused on explaining the evolutionary role of the most highly selected genes in the human genome [14], [16], genes leading to monogenic disorders [17], or searching for selection within a handful of candidate genes [18], [19]. This study explores the role of selection across all SNPs moderately (p-value <0.05) associated with seven complex diseases characterized by the Wellcome Trust Case Control Consortium (WTCCC) within the context of population-based evolutionary histories [20]. In particular, this study investigates i) the relative patterns of positive selection across the WTCCC disease panel, ii) differences in positive selection signal strength in risk and protective alleles of disease-associated SNPs, and iii) proposes a method for identifying regions of interest likely to be strongly associated with disease despite modest association p-values from GWA studies. Insights into the selective pressures acting on disease-associated SNPs inferred from GWA studies offer a novel perspective that promises to augment the biological interpretation of the results and potentially serve as a complementary method for prioritizing disease-associated SNPs for follow-up validation studies. The overall aim of this study is to find evidence of positive selection within the genetic-basis of complex disease.

Results

The Wellcome Trust Case Control Consortium (WTCCC) only identified twenty-four independent loci associated with the seven diseases at p $<5\times10^{-7}$; however, we expected there to be many additional associated loci likely hidden among SNPs with moderate p-values of association. Therefore, the association p-value threshold of 0.005 was used throughout this study in order to capture a larger proportion of these hidden associations, and any SNP with a p-value below this threshold is referred to as "associated". We expect an increasing proportion of false associations as the p-value threshold is increased. Every allele of each associated SNP was evaluated for positive selection using both the integrated Haplotype Score (iHS) [14] and Long Range Haplotype (LRH) [21] methods, and was normalized with respect to the allele frequency and the ancestral or derived allele state (see Methods). Normalizing procedures are performed on all positive selection scores before any data analysis takes place. A different distribution of positive selection scores using both iHS and LRH is observed when the data is partitioned into distinct allele frequency scores as well as ancestral or derived allele states. This occurs because higher frequency alleles are older and their surrounding regions have had more time to undergo recombination, which makes it harder to detect positive selection. Likewise, ancestral alleles are older and have more recombination in the surrounding region. We also control for linkage disequilibrium by partitioning the entire genome into haplotype blocks and only including the SNP most strongly associated with disease in our analysis prior to any data analysis. This avoids the problem of measuring the same positive selection event twice (see Methods).

The number of SNPs moderately associated with each of the seven studied diseases is shown in Table 1. Out of the 1896 SNPs with moderate association with Type 1 Diabetes (T1D; p-values <0.005), there are 80 SNPs with strong evidence for selection, defined as having an absolute iHS score over 2.2. Calculating iHS values for each SNP yields two scores, one for each allele [14]. It is thus possible to further divide SNPs into those where selection is stronger for the allele increasing susceptibility to disease (i.e. the risk allele) and those in which selection favors the other "protective" allele. As shown in Table 1, we found surprising asymmetry in the selection of protective alleles compared to risk-associated alleles for certain diseases. We expect the same number of risk and protective alleles to be selected under the neutral model; in contrast to this, 58 alleles associated with increased risk of T1D exhibit selection, compared to 22 for protective alleles, revealing an asymmetrical distribution (binomial test p-value 7.01×10^{-5} against the null hypothesis of equal likelihood of risk and protective alleles to show stronger positive selection).

Crohn's Disease (CD) shares this asymmetrical distribution in the opposite direction, with 34 of 47 associated and positively selected SNPs exhibiting selection towards protective alleles (binomial test p-value 3.09×10^{-3}). Bipolar Disorder (BD), like CD, also shows asymmetry in selecting for protective alleles, with 18 out of 22 alleles showing stronger selection for the protective allele. The findings in Table 1 were reproduced using the LRH test to detect positive selection yielding results matching very closely (see Table S1).

Figure 1 shows the cumulative mean positive iHS selection score for SNPs at or stronger than threshold p-values of association, for all seven diseases. Interestingly, we find the strongest selected SNPs are found among the most significantly associated SNPs for T1D (Fig. 1a). Rheumatoid Arthritis (RA) also shows a concentration of high selection scores within the most significantly associated SNPs, as does Type 2 Diabetes.

The gray regions in Figure 1 represent neutral selection, made up of 1000 simulated control diseases having a random distribution of positive selection scores across SNPs with low p-values of association. In order to create each neutral control disease, all sets of SNPs from each of the 7 diseases were combined. From this combined set of SNPs, 86,972 SNPs were randomly drawn (matching the size of the data set for an LD

controlled WTCCC disease). Each individual control disease then undergoes a random permutation of all of its positive selection scores, thereby producing a random distribution of positive selection scores in SNPs having low association p-values.

While Table 1 shows that three diseases show bias towards selection of risk-associated alleles or protective alleles, it does not show whether the selection itself is stronger among the risk associated alleles or protective alleles. Figures 1b and 1c show that the asymmetry of evidence for positive selection in risk and protective alleles shown in Table 1 is present within the most significantly associated SNPs.

Surprisingly, T1D shows the strongest selection pressure for its risk-associated alleles (Figure 1b), compared to the other six diseases and compared to its protective alleles (Figure 1c). RA and Type 2 Diabetes (T2D) also show strong selective pressure for both its risk-associated and protective alleles, but this selection is symmetrical, consistent with the results in Table 1. Table 1 shows that selection in CD more frequently acts on protective alleles; consistent with this, Figures 1b and 1c show that among protective alleles, there is a very strong signal of positive selection compared to risk-associated CD alleles (which show no deviation from the gray neutral region).

Analyzing GWA studies in the context of selection can complement and augment the standard p-value of association and aid in the identification and characterization of causal loci for follow-up validation studies. Figure 2 places the SNPs on chromosome 6 associated with T1D within their evolutionary context. Deviations from the gray control region are observed in favor of susceptibility alleles in two regions, one in the HLA region and another towards the right side of the figure. T1D SNPs show more selection for risk than for protective alleles in the HLA region (left peak in Fig. 2). Another peak of selection is seen within a region with the positively selected SNP rs6917204 in linkage disequilibrium with the moderately T1D-associated SNP rs7760387. Many true associations are likely hidden among those SNPs with moderate p-values of association produced in GWA studies. Since selection is exclusively detectable in risk alleles within some moderately associated regions, it may be reasonable to up-weight the importance of these kinds of SNPs for follow-up deep sequencing and functional validation.

An inclusive list of all genes containing associated SNPs showing signs of recent positive selection is included in Table S2. In order to produce an inclusive list of associated SNPs that are likely

Table 1. Analysis of selection within risk-associated and protective alleles.

Disease	Number of SNPs associated with disease with p <0.005	Number of SNPs associated with disease with p <0.005 and |iHS| >2.2	Risk Allele Is More Selected	Protective Allele is More Selected	Binomial Test p-value
T1D	1896	80 (4.22%)	58	22	7.01×10^{-5}
T2D	1632	42 (2.57%)	16	26	0.16
CD	1658	47 (2.83%)	13	34	3.09×10^{-3}
CAD	1583	37 (2.34%)	21	16	0.51
RA	1695	48 (2.83%)	27	21	0.47
HT	1578	33 (2.09%)	17	16	1.00
BD	869	22 (2.53%)	4	18	4.34×10^{-3}

Type 1 Diabetes risk alleles show significantly more selection than protective alleles, while Crohn's Disease and Bipolar Disorder show the opposite trend. We considered the set of moderately associated SNPs (p-value <0.005) across seven diseases studied by the Wellcome Trust Case Control Consortium. In Type 1 Diabetes, Crohn's Disease, and Bipolar Disorder, we see significant bias towards strong selection (defined as having an absolute iHS score >2.2) among these moderately associated SNPs. Each SNP represents a risk allele (allele increases susceptibility to disease) and a protective allele (the other allele). Among moderately selected SNPs associated with Type 1 Diabetes, 58 are SNPs in which the risk allele shows more selection, and only 22 are SNPs in which the protective allele shows more selection, showing that risk alleles are more likely to have undergone positive selection (p-value $= 7.01 \times 10^{-5}$).

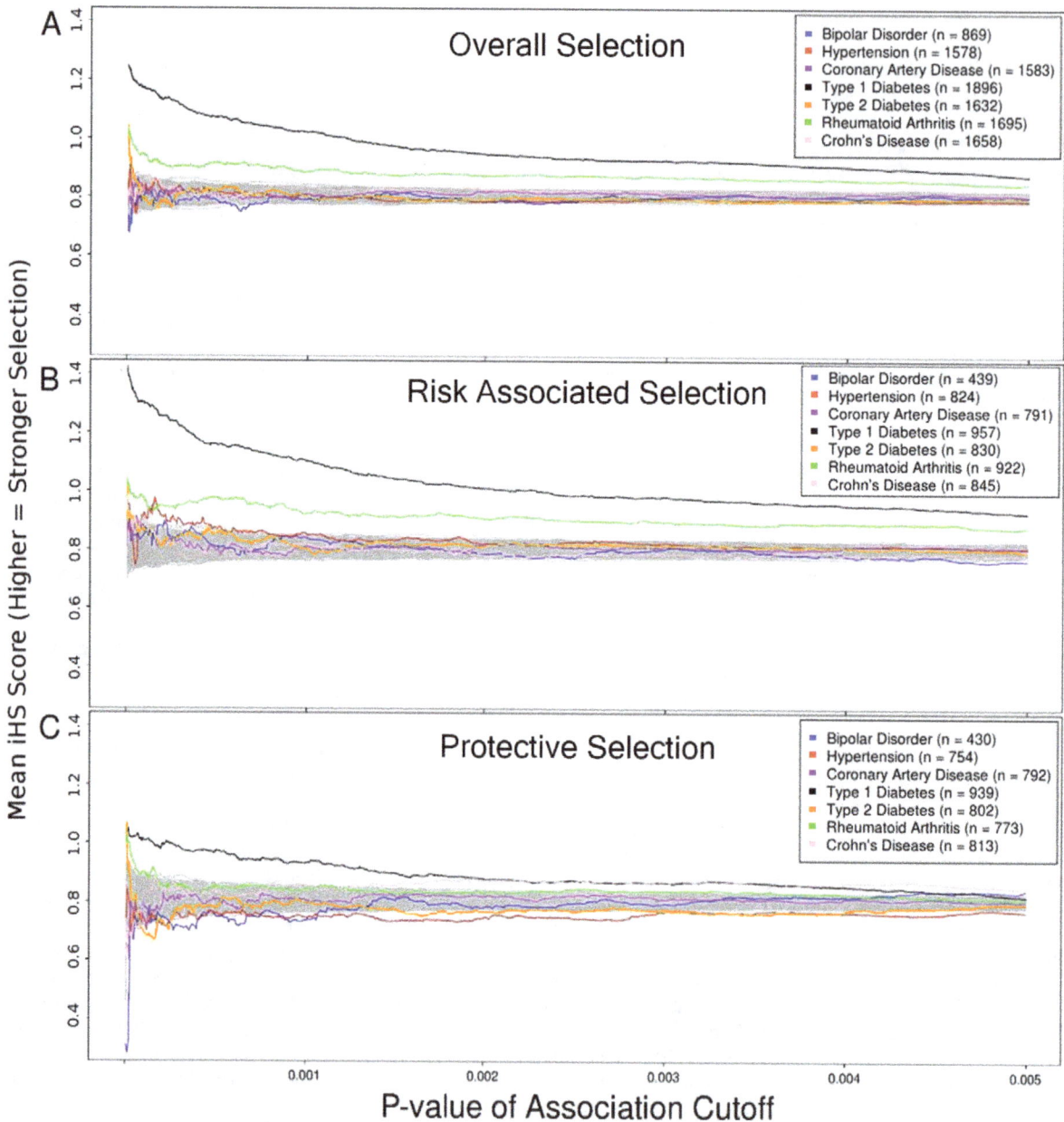

Figure 1. Selection in 7 WTCCC diseases. Comparison of selection pressures reveals stark heterogeneity across the 7 diseases studied. The x-axis represents the p-value of association cutoff used for each disease when calculating the mean iHS score (y-axis). Figure 1a shows Type 1 Diabetes and Rheumatoid Arthritis have strong evidence of positive selection. Type 2 Diabetes shows signs of positive selection only in the most strongly associated SNPs (left side of figure). Figures 1b and 1c expose differences in selection of risk-associated and protective alleles. Crohn's Disease shows stronger positive selection of protective alleles versus risk alleles. Like Type 1 Diabetes, Hypertension shows stronger selection for risk alleles. The gray regions represent a neutral random region used as a control, created by randomizing the data (see Methods).

undergoing positive selection, a p-value of association cutoff of 0.005 is maintained. In addition to meeting this threshold, all SNPs in Table S2 have an absolute iHS score above 1.645 *and* an LRH score below 0.05, representing SNPs that pass the top 95th percentile for both iHS and LRH. Two missense mutations show up in this list for T1D, including *MOGS* (in SNP rs1063588), which encodes the first enzyme in the N-linked oligosaccharide processing pathway. A second SNP (rs1525791) within the *POU6F2* gene shows up for four different diseases: T1D, T2D, CD, and BD. The selected allele in this SNP represents the risk-associated allele for all four diseases. Table S3 shows all selected SNPs appearing in more than one disease.

Discussion

Consistent with previous studies, we find positive selection is acting on loci associated with complex disease, when viewed from the perspective of Genome-Wide Association Studies (Fig. 1). While one might expect positive selection to eradicate risk-associated mutations and favor protective variants, like we find for CD (Table 1), we also surprisingly find the strongest selection working in favor of risk-associated alleles in both T1D and RA (Fig. 1b and Table 1).

It may be the case that some risk alleles are positively selected individually or as components of an abstract biological function

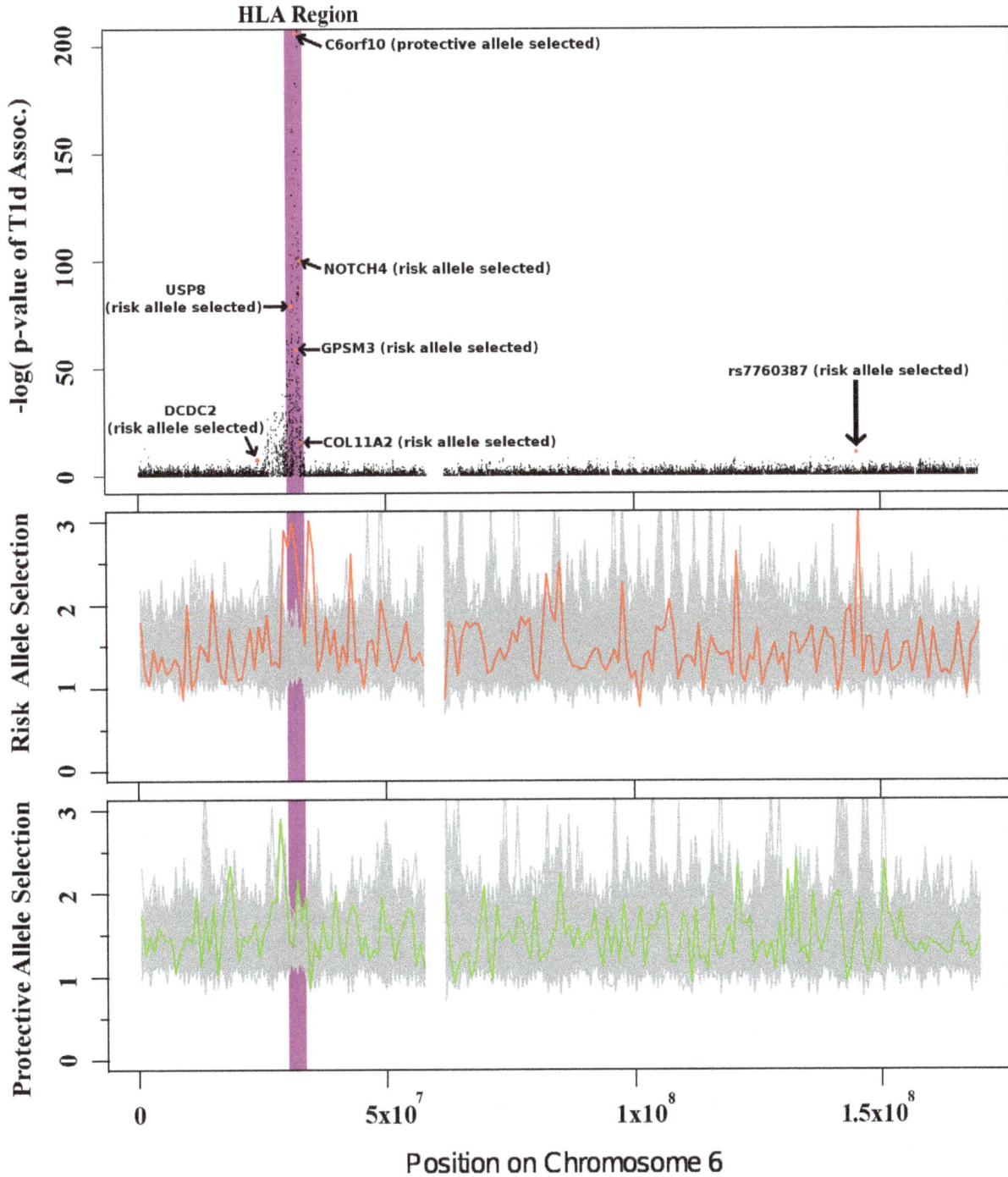

Figure 2. Selection of Type 1 Diabetes risk associated alleles in chromosome 6. Selection of associated alleles in chromosome six indicates that selection occurs more often on risk associated alleles versus protective alleles. The y-axis in the top plot represents how strongly each SNP is associated with Type 1 Diabetes. The y-axis in the bottom two plots represent how confident we can be that susceptibility alleles and protective alleles have been selected in each chromosomal region. The HLA (purple) region contains the strongest signs of positive selection for susceptibility alleles, yet the signal is within the neutral region for protective alleles. The second peak on the right side of the figure shows selection favors risk alleles in a region only moderately associated with the disease. Such asymmetry in selecting for risk-associated alleles suggests that SNPs in this region are more likely to be associated with the disease than the p-values suggest. Similar scans for regions moderately associated with diseases containing mutually exclusive selection of risk or protective disease alleles could be used to find novel associations. The gray regions in the bottom two graphs represent random neutral regions produced by randomizing the data (see Materials and Methods S1 for details).

due to a presently unknown benefit they confer on the host. This implies that there may be hidden benefits associated with some of the RA and T1D positively selected risk alleles. Positive selection in favor of risk alleles may occur if these alleles lead to an advantageous trait in an alternative environmental context (e.g. protection from pathogens). It is worth mentioning that there must be some reason why the ancestral allele characterized ancient populations in the first place in the cases where the derived allele shows strong signs of positive selection. There are many possible explanations for this. Possibilities include genetic drift driving a benign mutation to fixation in ancient populations, only to have this benign mutation become deleterious relative to a different allele in a modern environment. Another possibility is that an ancient environment may have also caused the ancestral allele to undergo positive selection, only for a modern environment to induce the ancestral allele to undergo negative selection.

There is recent evidence suggesting that protection from pathogens helps explains why positive selection has occurred for T1D susceptibility alleles. Rare variants in the antiviral response gene *IFIH1* have recently been shown to be protective against T1D [6]. The protective alleles are functionally deleterious to *IFIH1*, effectively reducing the ability to mediate an immune response against enterovirus infection. Recent immunological studies of beta cells in patients recently diagnosed with T1D have shown an abundance of enteroviral capsid proteins in the islet cells of affected patients, whereas the protein is found to be scarce among the beta cells of healthy controls [22]. It is plausible that signatures of recent positive selection in T1D and other autoimmune diseases are due to an overactive immune system driven at least in part by an adaptive immune response to viruses. Due to the evolutionary trajectory of T1D favoring susceptibility alleles and the severe effect on fitness in afflicted individuals, we would expect that this evolutionary event would have happened recently in human evolution. While T1D is rapidly fatal without insulin therapy, there was likely a net selective pressure favoring intense immune responses to enterovirus, even with T1D as an occasional consequence.

RA has been found to originate from Native American populations from the Green River region in west central Kentucky. There are verified cases of RA in this population as far back as 6,500 years ago. No signs of RA were found in 63 archaeological sites bordering the original area in central Kentucky, where it was originally found [7]. Yet, there is documented spread in America over time. The first evidence of RA outside the original "catchment" area occurs in western Ohio about 1,100 to 800 years ago. At the same time, virtually no incidence of RA in other parts of the world has been found towards the end of the pre-Columbian era in 1785. This suggests that some environmental factor, perhaps a microorganism or allergen, might play a critical role in the cause of RA [7]. Our analysis reveals that there is a huge disparity in positive selection scores between alleles increasing and decreasing susceptibility to RA. Susceptibility alleles show very strong signs of positive selection, while alleles decreasing susceptibility are nearly devoid of any signs of positive selection (Fig. 1b–1c). The history of RA helps explain why susceptibility alleles show signs of positive selection in European-derived populations (Fig. 1). Since RA was non-existent in these populations during the pre-Columbian era, there were probably no disadvantages to selecting for the genetic-basis of RA. Indeed, there may have been many benefits associated with selecting for RA susceptibility alleles. Tuberculosis is responsible for millions of deaths worldwide in recent human history, with one in four deaths caused by tuberculosis in Western Europe in the 19th century alone. It is suspected that this disease has historically acted as a powerful selective force. There is a stark correlation between populations having higher incidence of tuberculosis also having lower incidence of RA, and vice versa. It has been speculated that genetic variants enhancing resistance to tuberculosis underwent positive selection and provide the genetic basis for RA susceptibility today [9]. Our analysis is completely compatible with this theory, since we produce evidence that RA susceptibility alleles have undergone positive selection. In addition,

tumor necrosis factor inhibitors alleviate symptoms of RA while simultaneously increasing the risk of infection from tuberculosis, *Myobacterium marinum tenosynovitis*, fungal infection, and other opportunistic infections [23], [24], [25], [26], [27]. It is clear that factors increasing susceptibility to RA also decrease susceptibility to infectious disease. RA and T1D are known to share associated variants [28], [29]. This may partially explain why there is a small, but detectable signal of positive selection in alleles decreasing susceptibility for RA. The evolutionary history of RA is unique in that a precise date of introduction of RA into European-derived populations has been established. We have shown that strong positive selection of RA susceptibility alleles is observed, most likely due to altered ability to fight infectious disease without increasing the risk of RA itself until the pre-Columbian era ended.

Not much is known about the history of Crohn's Disease (CD) as it does not leave unambiguous signs in skeletal remains, as is the case with RA. It is known that the incidence of CD increased during the 19th century in industrialized countries. The rate of CD increases as under-developed countries become more industrialized (e.g. Japan and Brazil) [30]. Many bacteria are implicated in CD, including anaerobic organisms, paratuberculosis, Boeck's sarcoid, and mycobacteria. *Mycobacterial paratuberculosis* infection of the terminal ileum in cattle (Johne's disease) resembles also closely resembles Crohn's disease, which has suggested possible bacterial associations with CD [30]. Unlike RA and Type 1 Diabetes, CD shows more positive selection for alleles decreasing susceptibility to disease than for those increasing susceptibility. It may be the case that CD is in fact an ancient disease, the incidence of which was reduced due to natural selection against CD, only to see resurgence due to the advent of modern environments. However, many other possible scenarios could explain our findings, including shared genetic variants with a disease or trait that has undergone negative selection. CD is unique in the sense that while selection is detected as in RA and T1D, alleles decreasing susceptibility for CD are under positive selection, indicating a very different evolutionary history.

We acknowledge several limitations in our analysis. Controlling for LD by selecting only one SNP in each haplotype block after partitioning the genome may have complications in some regions of the genome. Haplotype blocks intuitively capture LD, but lack of complete haplotype block coverage (the fraction of the genome that is found neatly within haplotype blocks) complicates this approach [31]. More complex methods to control for LD will be considered for future works requiring a similar analysis. Another complicating issue is that both iHS and LRH belong to the same class of analytical methods for detecting selection, and it is not surprising that they indicate similar results. Yet, it has been shown that these two methods are in some ways complementary as they are better at detecting selected SNPs at different allele frequencies [16]. Overall, the results under iHS match the results produced with LRH with some changes in the magnitude of selection pressures on some diseases leading to more diseases appearing in the random neutral region in Fig 1 versus Figure S1 (more details on limitations in Materials and Methods S1). We acknowledge that it is unknown whether or not the most associated SNPs are causative; leading to confusion when we discuss selection for risk-associated alleles as the causal SNP may show the opposite selection pattern, that is, stronger selection of the protective allele. While this is certainly a possibility, it is unlikely to occur often. If a SNP has a very low p-value of association to a disease due to its proximity to the causative allele, it implies strong LD between the two SNPs. Due to strong LD, the risk-associated allele between the non-causative and the causative SNPs are more likely to be on the same haplotype block, making the risk-associated allele in a SNP in strong LD with the causative SNP an appropriate proxy. In addition, it should be noted that all discussion on the reasons for positive selection acting on these diseases necessarily remains speculation.

In summary, we observed stark heterogeneity in the overall patterns of positive selection across seven diseases. We find that the SNPs associated with T1D, RA, and CD show strong signs of positive selection. We also find that positive selection favors risk-associated alleles in T1D and protective alleles in CD, which is indicative of an evolutionary trajectory towards increasing and decreasing risk, respectively. In addition, we have demonstrated that selection analyses of GWAS results can complement and augment the basic p-value of association attributes (Fig. 2) as many regions appear to exclusively favor selection of risk or protective alleles.

Methods

In EHH (extended haplotype homozygosity) based positive selection methods, there are two selection scores for each SNP (one for each allele). Both iHS and LRH are based on the EHH calculation. These two methods, and variants thereof have been applied to uncover signals of positive selection within genes related to susceptibility and resistance to infectious disease [16], innate and adaptive immunity [32], LDL cholesterol levels [33], and autoimmune disorders [34]. This method exploits the principle that alleles in relatively larger and over-represented haplotype blocks imply positive selection. These two methods produce biased scores depending on the allele frequency and ancestral/derived allele state. These limitations were overcome by performing Z-score normalization and rank normalization of each iHS and LRH measurement, respectively. Each allele of each SNP was grouped with other alleles having the same allele frequency in addition to having the same ancestral/derived state prior to performing Z-

score (iHS) and inverse rank (LRH) normalization. All references to iHS and LRH score reference their normalized values.

The WTCCC study used the Affymetrix GeneChip 500K Array set to conduct a GWA study made up of two European cohorts for each disease. These include 2000 affected individuals for each of the seven diseases as well as a common control group of 3000 individuals. This study exploits the existence of hidden associations by including moderately associated SNPs. While this will undoubtedly capture hidden associations, diminishing returns of these "hidden associations" are expected as one increases the p-value (Fig. 1). The entire project pipeline is shown in Figure 3. We took all associated SNPs from the 7 diseases studied by the WTCCC using high-density assays [20] and used both iHS and LRH to probe for evidence of positive selection in these SNPs using haplotype information from the population having European ancestry in Phase 2 of the International HapMap project [35]. For every SNP showing association with disease (p-value <0.005) that has recently undergone positive selection (|iHS| >2.2), we determined whether the selected allele within the SNP is associated with susceptibility to disease versus protection from disease (Table 1 and Table S1). Figure 4 shows how risk versus protective SNPs are partitioned in this study.

In every case, the positive selection score assigned to a SNP is simply the score from the major and minor alleles showing the strongest signs of positive selection. As mentioned, there are two selection scores for each SNP, one for each allele. This makes it possible to investigate positive selection of a disease's risk-associated alleles separately from its protective alleles. In addition to controlling for allele frequency and for the ancestral/derived allele state, it is important to take into consideration whether or not a disease appears to be exhibiting positive selection due to a few high-scoring non-independently associated regions in Linkage Disequilibrium (LD). This analysis relies on the independence of each positive selection score measurement. In order to overcome

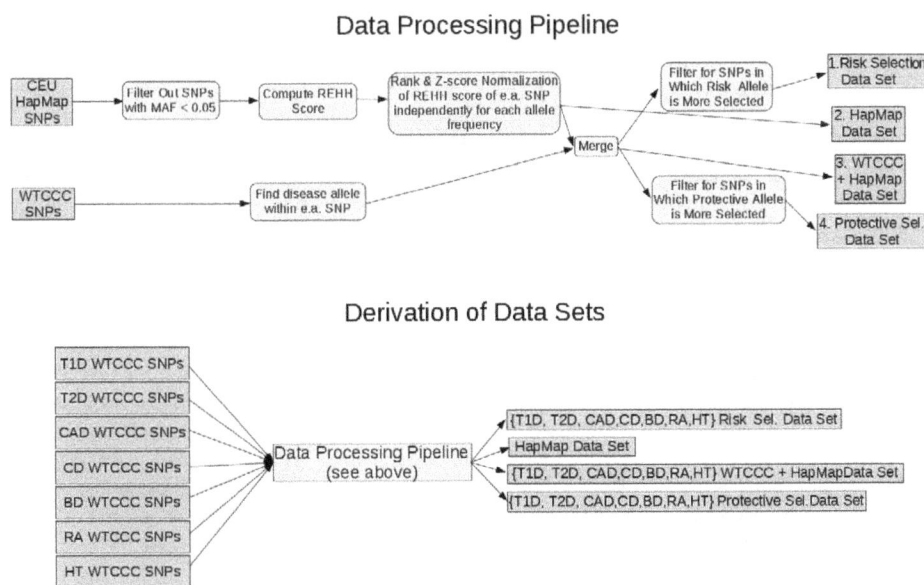

Figure 3. Project pipeline. The HapMap and WTCCC data sets are combined and partitioned to derive the data sets used for this study. First, the HapMap data set is filtered (SNPs with MAF <0.05 are excluded). iHS and LRH scores are then calculated for each SNP, which are Z-score and inverse rank normalized with respect to allele frequency and ancestral/derived allele state. The data is then merged with a WTCCC disease SNP data set after the "risk" allele has been extracted from the WTCCC SNP data set. This leads to 4 distinct SNP datasets; i) scored CEU HapMap SNPs, ii) the intersection of WTCCC SNPs and HapMap SNPs, iii) SNPs in which the susceptibility allele shows more selection iv) SNPs in which the protective allele show more selection. This data processing pipeline is used on all 7 WTCCC diseases, resulting in distinct data sets, which are then probed for disparities in positive selection.

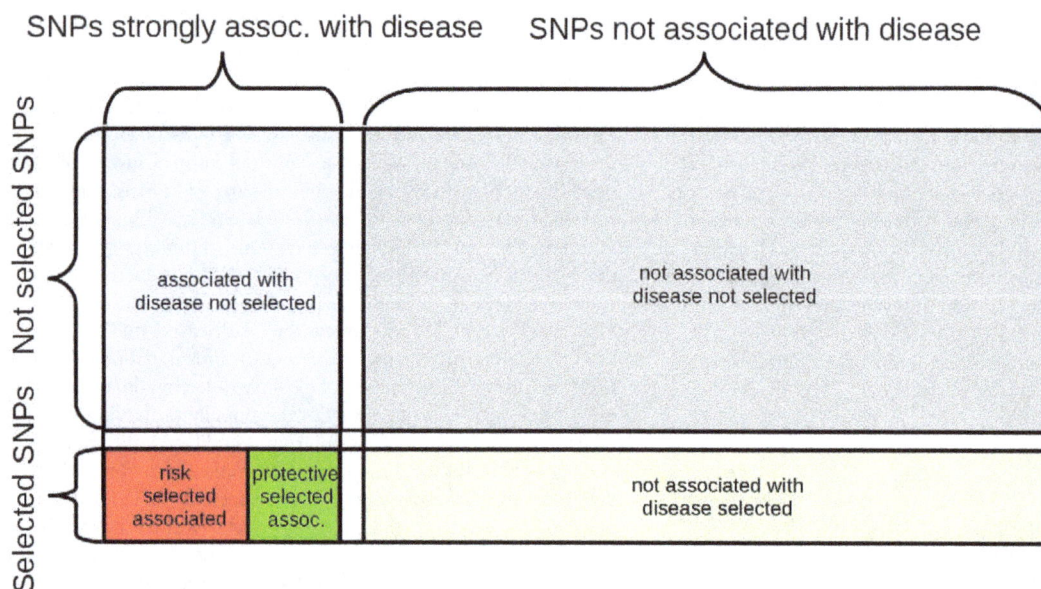

Figure 4. Partitioning the data set. The entire set of SNPs present in both the WTCCC and HapMap data sets was partitioned into five different categories. This study emphasizes associated SNPs partitioned into risk-associated selection and protective selected SNPs. The proportion of SNPs in these categories at cutoffs for selection and association (|iHS| >2.2 and rank normalized LRH score <0.01) is explored and used to test for differences in selection pressures among associated SNPs (p-value <0.005). Within associated SNPs, selection pressures between risk-associated selection (SNPs in which stronger selection is observed for the risk-associated allele), and protective selection are explored.

any potential issues with the non-independence of iHS and LRH calculations, the entire genome was partitioned into haplotype blocks using HapBlock software [36]. Haplotype blocks can be defined as regions of high |D'| or low haplotype diversity. The "Haplotype Diversity" method is used for partitioning the data into haplotype blocks [37] (more details provided in Materials and Methods S1). For each haplotype block, only the SNP most strongly associated with each of the 7 diseases (leading to a different data set for each disease) is chosen for this study, along with its corresponding iHS and LRH score (see Materials and Methods S1).

Randomized WTCCC and HapMap data was produced to detect deviations from neutral selection in Fig. 1 and Fig. S1. Each SNP comprising the 1000 neutral diseases (along with its positive selection score) are picked at random from each of the 7 diseases until the number of SNPs in each disease matched the number of SNPs in a WTCCC disease. The entire complement of the WTCCC disease panel resulting after the normalization and filtering procedures discussed was used to compute each random disease. Following this random selection of SNPs, the entire combined list of SNPs from the 7 diseases was randomly reassigned a positive selection score from this same combined list of SNPs, thereby creating 1000 "random neutral diseases" that have a random distribution of selection scores in associated SNPs. Figure 1 and Fig. 2 contain random neutral regions produced with this set of 1000 random diseases (see Materials and Methods S1 for more details).

Data for the seven diseases studied was obtained from the WTCCC1 data set [20]. WTCCC SNPs were intersected with CEU (Utah population) HapMap Phase II data (release 23a; only including autosomes). With the WTCCC data set, it is possible to deduce which allele within an associated SNP is increasing susceptibility to disease by looking at the genotype of the control group as well as those affected by the disease. Since LRH and iHS give scores for each allele of every SNP, we use the associated allele

for each disease (derived from the WTCCC data set) and each allele's LRH and iHS scores (computed from the HapMap data set) in order to assess whether the evolutionary trajectory is towards increased or decreased susceptibility to the diseases studied. The HapMap data adds frequency and haplotype data to each SNP included in the WTCCC study. Intersecting the HapMap and WTCCC data sets yielded 352,191 Type 1 Diabetes, 352,202 Type 2 Diabetes, 352,199 Rheumatoid Arthritis, 352,200 Hypertension, 352,198 Crohn's Disease, 352,198 Coronary Artery Disease, and 332,576 Bipolar Disorder SNPs. These SNPs were then normalized and filtered to control for LD effects. Finally, they are partitioned as shown in Fig. 4. Emphasis is placed on SNPs associated with each disease (defined as p-value <0.005 for this study). Among these, positively selected SNPs were identified (iHS >2.2 and normalized LRH score <0.01). Such positively selected SNPs were tested to see if the risk and/or protective alleles have recently undergone positive selection. Ancestral and derived alleles were determined by downloading DBSNP [38], which uses a method that derives the ancestral allele by comparing human DNA to chimpanzee DNA [39]. This study makes use of data generated by the Wellcome Trust Case Control Consortium. A full list of the investigators who contributed to the generation of the data is available from www.wtccc.org.uk. Funding for the Wellcome Trust Case Control Consortium was provided by the Wellcome Trust under award 076113. Version WTCCC1 of the dataset was used for this study [20].

Supporting Information

Materials and Methods S1 Materials and methods explaining limitations of this study, replication of the main results using LRH, and a list of SNPs associated with more than one disease showing some signs of selection.

Figure S1 Comparison of selection pressures reveals differences across the 7 diseases studied. The x-axis represents the p-value of association cutoff used for each disease when calculating the mean rank normalized LRH score (y-axis). Type 1 Diabetes shows extremely strong signs of positive selection. Crohn's Disease, Rheumatoid Arthritis, and Hypertension also exhibit evidence of positive selection. Figures S1b-S1c expose differences in the magnitude of selection strength. Crohn's Disease shows stronger positive selection of protective alleles versus susceptibility alleles. Hypertension shows positive selection almost exclusively for risk alleles. The gray regions represent a neutral random region used as a control which was made by randomizing the data (see Methods).

Table S1 Alleles of SNPs associated with disease (p-value <0.005) can either be SNPs in which the susceptibility allele shows more selection than the protective allele (risk SNPs) or SNPs in which the protective allele shows more selection (protective SNPs). When the intersection of Type 1 Diabetes associated SNPs (p-value 0.005) and strongly selected SNPs (LRH <0.01) are considered, 23 are SNPs in which the risk allele shows more selection than the protective allele, and only 8 are SNPs in which the protective allele shows more selection. This shows that risk alleles are more likely to have undergone positive selection (p-value = 0.01).

Table S2 In order to produce an inclusive list of all disease associated SNPs that have recently undergone positive selection,

all associated SNPs (p-value <0.005) having both a rank normalized LRH score below 0.05 and an iHS score greater than 1.645 (representing the 95th percentile in both LRH and iHS) are shown. SNPs in linkage disequilibrium with the SNPs appearing in these tables were not listed.

Table S3 Five of the SNPs listed in Table S2 appear in more than one disease. In particular, rs1525791 appears in four of the seven WTCCC diseases and the risk-associated allele in this SNP shows more selection than the protective allele. This is in contrast to rs204989, where the susceptibility allele for Type 1 Diabetes and the protective allele for Rheumatoid Arthritis are under selection.

Acknowledgments

We thank Marina Sirota from Stanford University for help in processing the SNP data, Alex Skrenchuk and Dr. Boris Oskotsky for computer support, and Sudhir Kumar from Arizona State University for helpful feedback regarding the initial draft of this manuscript.

Author Contributions

Conceived and designed the experiments: EC AJB. Performed the experiments: EC. Analyzed the data: EC AJB. Wrote the paper: EC JTD AJB.

References

1. Maddox J (1994) Migration out of Africa. Nature 372: 32.
2. Sabeti PC, Schaffner SF, Fry B, Lohmueller J, Varilly P, et al. (2006) Positive natural selection in the human lineage. Science 312: 1614–1620.
3. Currat M, Trabuchet G, Rees D, Perrin P, Harding RM, et al. (2002) Molecular analysis of the beta-globin gene cluster in the Niokholo Mandenka population reveals a recent origin of the beta(S) Senegal mutation. Am J Hum Genet 70: 207–223.
4. Chevin LM, Billiard S, Hospital F (2008) Hitchhiking both ways: effect of two interfering selective sweeps on linked neutral variation. Genetics 180: 301–316.
5. Plomin R, Haworth CM, Davis OS (2009) Common disorders are quantitative traits. Nat Rev Genet 10: 872–878.
6. Nejentsev S, Walker N, Riches D, Egholm M, Todd JA (2009) Rare variants of IFIH1, a gene implicated in antiviral responses, protect against type 1 diabetes. Science 324: 387–389.
7. Rothschild BM, Woods RJ, Rothschild C, Sebes JI (1992) Geographic distribution of rheumatoid arthritis in ancient North America: implications for pathogenesis. Semin Arthritis Rheum 22: 181–187.
8. Blekhman R, Man O, Herrmann L, Boyko AR, Indap A, et al. (2008) Natural selection on genes that underlie human disease susceptibility. Curr Biol 18: 883–889.
9. Mobley JL (2004) Is rheumatoid arthritis a consequence of natural selection for enhanced tuberculosis resistance? Med Hypotheses 62: 839–843.
10. Myles S, Davison D, Barrett J, Stoneking M, Timpson N (2008) Worldwide population differentiation at disease-associated SNPs. BMC Med Genomics 1: 22.
11. Thomas PD, Kejariwal A (2004) Coding single-nucleotide polymorphisms associated with complex vs. Mendelian disease: evolutionary evidence for differences in molecular effects. Proc Natl Acad Sci U S A 101: 15398–15403.
12. Di Rienzo A (2006) Population genetics models of common diseases. Curr Opin Genet Dev 16: 630–636.
13. Arbiza L, Duchi S, Montaner D, Burguet J, Pantoja-Uceda D, et al. (2006) Selective pressures at a codon-level predict deleterious mutations in human disease genes. J Mol Biol 358: 1390–1404.
14. Voight BF, Kudaravalli S, Wen X, Pritchard JK (2006) A map of recent positive selection in the human genome. PLoS Biol 4: e72.
15. Sirota M, Schaub MA, Batzoglou S, Robinson WH, Butte AJ (2009) Autoimmune disease classification by inverse association with SNP alleles. PLoS Genet 5: e1000792.
16. Sabeti PC, Varilly P, Fry B, Lohmueller J, Hostetter E, et al. (2007) Genome-wide detection and characterization of positive selection in human populations. Nature 449: 913–918.
17. Podder S, Ghosh TC (2009) Exploring the differences in evolutionary rates between monogenic and polygenic disease genes in human. Mol Biol Evol 27: 934–941.
18. Guinan KJ, Cunningham RT, Meenagh A, Gonzalez A, Dring MM, et al. (2010) Signatures of natural selection and coevolution between killer cell immunoglobulin-like receptors (KIR) and HLA class I genes. Genes Immun.
19. Babbitt CC, Fedrigo O, Pfefferle AD, Boyle AP, Horvath JE, et al. (2010) Both Noncoding and Protein-Coding RNAs Contribute to Gene Expression Evolution in the Primate Brain. Genome Biol Evol 2010. pp 67–79.
20. The Wellcome Trust Case Control Consortium (2007) Genome-wide association study of 14,000 cases of seven common diseases and 3,000 shared controls. Nature 447: 661–678.
21. Sabeti PC, Reich DE, Higgins JM, Levine HZ, Richter DJ, et al. (2002) Detecting recent positive selection in the human genome from haplotype structure. Nature 419: 832–837.
22. Richardson SJ, Willcox A, Bone AJ, Foulis AK, Morgan NG (2009) The prevalence of enteroviral capsid protein vp1 immunostaining in pancreatic islets in human type 1 diabetes. Diabetologia 52: 1143–1151.
23. Askling J, Fored CM, Brandt L, Baecklund E, Bertilsson L, et al. (2005) Risk and case characteristics of tuberculosis in rheumatoid arthritis associated with tumor necrosis factor antagonists in Sweden. Arthritis Rheum 52: 1986–1992.
24. Filler SG, Yeaman MR, Sheppard DC (2005) Tumor necrosis factor inhibition and invasive fungal infections. Clin Infect Dis 41 Suppl 3: S208–212.
25. Jimenez FG, Colmenero JD, Irigoyen MV (2005) Reactivation of brucellosis after treatment with infliximab in a patient with rheumatoid arthritis. J Infect 50: 370–371.
26. Center for Disease Control and Prevention (2004) Tuberculosis associated with blocking agents against tumor necrosis factor-alpha—California, 2002-2003. MMWR Morb Mortal Wkly Rep 53: 683–686.
27. Fabre S, Gibert C, Lechiche C, Jorgensen C, Sany J (2005) Primary cutaneous Nocardia otitidiscaviarum infection in a patient with rheumatoid arthritis treated with infliximab. J Rheumatol 32: 2432–2433.
28. Fung EY, Smyth DJ, Howson JM, Cooper JD, Walker NM, et al. (2009) Analysis of 17 autoimmune disease-associated variants in type 1 diabetes identifies 6q23/TNFAIP3 as a susceptibility locus. Genes Immun 10: 188–191.
29. Schaub MA, Kaplow IM, Sirota M, Do CB, Butte AJ, et al. (2009) A Classifier-based approach to identify genetic similarities between diseases. Bioinformatics 25: i21–29.
30. Kirsner JB (2001) Historical origins of current IBD concepts. World J Gastroenterol 7: 175–184.
31. Wall JD, Pritchard JK (2003) Haplotype blocks and linkage disequilibrium in the human genome. Nat Rev Genet 4: 587–597.

32. Walsh EC, Sabeti P, Hutcheson HB, Fry B, Schaffner SF, et al. (2006) Searching for signals of evolutionary selection in 168 genes related to immune function. Hum Genet 119: 92–102.

33. Ding K, Kullo IJ (2008) Molecular population genetics of PCSK9: a signature of recent positive selection. Pharmacogenet Genomics 18: 169–179.

34. Butty V, Roy M, Sabeti P, Besse W, Benoist C, et al. (2007) Signatures of strong population differentiation shape extended haplotypes across the human CD28, CTLA4, and ICOS costimulatory genes. Proc Natl Acad Sci U S A 104: 570–575.

35. The International HapMap Consortium (2003) The International HapMap Project. Nature 426: 789–796.

36. Zhang K, Qin Z, Chen T, Liu JS, Waterman MS, et al. (2005) HapBlock: haplotype block partitioning and tag SNP selection software using a set of dynamic programming algorithms. Bioinformatics 21: 131–134.

37. Patil N, Berno AJ, Hinds DA, Barrett WA, Doshi JM, et al. (2001) Blocks of limited haplotype diversity revealed by high-resolution scanning of human chromosome 21. Science 294: 1719–1723.

38. Sherry ST, Ward MH, Kholodov M, Baker J, Phan L, et al. (2001) dbSNP: the NCBI database of genetic variation. Nucleic Acids Res 29: 308–311.

39. Spencer CC, Deloukas P, Hunt S, Mullikin J, Myers S, et al. (2006) The influence of recombination on human genetic diversity. PLoS Genet 2: e148.

15

A Network-Based Approach to Prioritize Results from Genome-Wide Association Studies

Nirmala Akula[1]*, Ancha Baranova[2,3], Donald Seto[2], Jeffrey Solka[2], Michael A. Nalls[4], Andrew Singleton[4], Luigi Ferrucci[5], Toshiko Tanaka[5], Stefania Bandinelli[6], Yoon Shin Cho[7], Young Jin Kim[7], Jong-Young Lee[7], Bok-Ghee Han[7], Bipolar Disorder Genome Study (BiGS) Consortium[¶], The Wellcome Trust Case-Control Consortium, Francis J. McMahon[1]

1 Mood and Anxiety Section, Human Genetics Branch, National Institute of Mental Health, National Institutes of Health, Department of Health and Human Services, Bethesda, Maryland, United States of America, **2** School of Systems Biology, College of Science, George Mason University, Fairfax, Virginia, United States of America, **3** Research Center for Medical Genetics, RAMS, Moscow, Russian Federation, **4** Molecular Genetics Section, Laboratory of Neurogenetics, Intramural Research Program, National Institute on Aging, Bethesda, Maryland, United States of America, **5** Longitudinal Studies Section, Clinical Research Branch, Intramural Research Program, National Institute on Aging, National Institutes of Health, Baltimore, Maryland, United States of America, **6** Geriatric Unit, Azienda Sanitaria di Firenze, Florence, Italy, **7** Center for Genome Science, National Institute of Health, Seoul, Korea

Abstract

Genome-wide association studies (GWAS) are a valuable approach to understanding the genetic basis of complex traits. One of the challenges of GWAS is the translation of genetic association results into biological hypotheses suitable for further investigation in the laboratory. To address this challenge, we introduce Network Interface Miner for Multigenic Interactions (NIMMI), a network-based method that combines GWAS data with human protein-protein interaction data (PPI). NIMMI builds biological networks weighted by connectivity, which is estimated by use of a modification of the Google PageRank algorithm. These weights are then combined with genetic association p-values derived from GWAS, producing what we call 'trait prioritized sub-networks.' As a proof of principle, NIMMI was tested on three GWAS datasets previously analyzed for height, a classical polygenic trait. Despite differences in sample size and ancestry, NIMMI captured 95% of the known height associated genes within the top 20% of ranked sub-networks, far better than what could be achieved by a single-locus approach. The top 2% of NIMMI height-prioritized sub-networks were significantly enriched for genes involved in transcription, signal transduction, transport, and gene expression, as well as nucleic acid, phosphate, protein, and zinc metabolism. All of these sub-networks were ranked near the top across all three height GWAS datasets we tested. We also tested NIMMI on a categorical phenotype, Crohn's disease. NIMMI prioritized sub-networks involved in B- and T-cell receptor, chemokine, interleukin, and other pathways consistent with the known autoimmune nature of Crohn's disease. NIMMI is a simple, user-friendly, open-source software tool that efficiently combines genetic association data with biological networks, translating GWAS findings into biological hypotheses.

Editor: Thomas Mailund, Aarhus University, Denmark

Funding: This work was supported by the National Institute of Mental Health (NIMH) Intramural Research Program. The InCHIANTI study was supported as a "targeted project" (ICS 110.1RS97.71) by the Italian Ministry of Health, by the U.S. National Institute on Aging (Contracts N01-AG-916413, N01-AG-821336, 263 MD 9164 13, and 263 MD 821336) and in part by the Intramural Research Program, National Institute on Aging, National Institutes of Health, USA. Funding support for the Whole Genome Association Study of Bipolar Disorder was provided by NIMH, and the genotyping of samples was provided through the Genetic Association Information Network (GAIN). The funders had no role in study design, data collection and analysis, decision to publish, or preparation of the manuscript.

Competing Interests: The authors have declared that no competing interests exist.

* E-mail: akulan@mail.nih.gov

¶The member institutions of the Bipolar Disorder Genome Study (BiGS) Consortium are listed in the Acknowledgments.

Introduction

Genome-wide association studies (GWAS) have greatly facilitated the identification of genes involved in complex phenotypes [1,2]. However, replication of association findings has often been difficult, probably reflecting the relatively small effects of individual markers, and the genetic heterogeneity of complex traits [3]. The critical challenge now is to understand how multiple, modestly-associated genes interact to influence a phenotype [4–6]. Many studies have shown that there is a strong relationship between gene function and phenotype, and that functionally-related genes are more likely to interact [7–18]. Inspired by this insight, we undertook a systems-biology approach

to identify and prioritize groups of functionally-related genes that are enriched for genetic variants associated with a trait, what we call 'trait prioritized sub-networks.'

Previously described network and pathway-based methods of GWAS data are useful, but have limitations. Most 1) use licensed software, which is often costly and lacks transparency [19–22]; 2) depend on publicly available pathway databases that rely on a limited number of available pathways (<500) and that often ignore protein-protein interactions (PPIs) for recently studied genes [23–30]; 3) rely on simulated or model organism data only [11,31]; 4) require knowledge of programming [32]; or 5) limit the number of input genes [33]. Since signals with small effects not detectable at conventional levels of significance may account for substantial heritability [34], methods that can include all signals without arbitrary thresholds of statistical significance are needed. Such methods should extract more information from GWAS data by identifying susceptibility genes that have functional similarity. We hypothesized that such an approach might lead to a higher rate of replication in independent datasets, compared to studies that rely only on single markers. Replicated findings are more likely to generate sound biological hypotheses for subsequent laboratory studies.

To this end, we developed a novel software tool called Network Interface Miner for Multigenic Interactions (NIMMI). This tool generates biological networks using human PPI data, where proteins are considered as nodes and the interactions between proteins as edges. NIMMI assumes that proteins that show more interactions with other proteins in the same network (i.e., have higher connectivity) are more important than proteins with fewer interactions, and weights each protein by use of a modification of the Google PageRank algorithm [35]. This algorithm ranks proteins in much the same way as the popular search engine ranks websites on the internet, giving greater weight to proteins with more connections to other proteins, especially those that are themselves highly linked to additional proteins. Unlike the original Google PageRank algorithm, this modified algorithm uses the PPI data to calculate a "damping factor" dynamically for every gene in a network, accounting for differences in the topology of biological networks compared to computerized networks. To our knowledge, this approach has never been tested on biological networks. NIMMI combines these weights with the association signals from a GWAS to identify trait prioritized sub-networks. In this study we tested NIMMI in three GWAS datasets analyzed to assess genetic contributions to height, a classical polygenic trait. We further validate the method in a categorical phenotype, Crohn's disease. The results demonstrate that NIMMI can effectively identify genes involved in quantitative and categorical traits and group them into biologically-plausible networks that are highly replicable across independent studies.

Results

Summary of the statistical approach

NIMMI is a network-based approach that relies on three basic assumptions: 1) Genes, rather than SNPs are the functional units in biology; 2) Genes do not work in isolation, thus genes whose protein products show more interactions with other proteins in the same network (i.e., higher connectivity) are more important than proteins with fewer interactions; and 3) genetic association results for a trait and protein interactions within a network are complementary forms of information, reflecting a role for that network in that trait [36–38].

NIMMI prioritizes biological networks in three key steps. First networks are identified by use of human interactome data. Proteins are represented as nodes and interactions are represented as edges. Here we assumed that each gene corresponds to a single protein and used human protein-protein interaction (PPI) data to build the networks, but in principle any data that relates one gene to another could be used. Each gene in the same network is assigned a weight (w_i) based on connectivity to other genes in the same network, using a modification of the Google PageRank algorithm. Second, gene-based association p-values are calculated. Here we applied the Versatile Gene-based association study tool (VEGAS) (http://gump.qimr.edu.au/VEGAS/) [39] to GWAS data, but any method for mapping a SNP to a gene could be used. The gene-based p-value was converted to a z-score (z_i) and combined with w_i to generate the network-weighted score for that

gene. We used the Liptak-Stouffer method, which allowed us to weight the association p-value by the square-root of the sample size. Third, high-scoring genes are combined into what we call 'trait prioritized sub-networks', which were further tested by DAVID (http://david.abcc.ncifcrf.gov/) [40,41], a publicly available bioinformatics tool that identifies functionally related groups of genes. A flowchart of NIMMI's analysis steps is shown in Figure 1.

Comparison of single-locus method with NIMMI systems approach

In order to compare ranking by single-locus analysis with NIMMI, three independent height GWAS datasets were analyzed using both single-locus ranking and NIMMI network ranking methods. Percentile ranks of 34 candidate genes for height that were deemed confirmed candidates in recent review of GWAS for height were used as a standard of comparison [42–44].

The relative ranking of genes based on gene-wise association p-values alone was highly sample dependent, and ranks varied substantially in each GWAS dataset (Figure 2a). For the three height GWAS datasets we present the association p-values of susceptibility genes, gene-wise ranking, gene-wise percentile ranks (gene-wise PR), NIMMI-network ranking and NIMMI percentile ranks (Network PR) in Table S1. In contrast, the NIMMI-network ranking was very stable for 95% of the genes, despite differences in sample size and ancestry among the three height datasets (Figure 2b). Most of the confirmed height-associated candidate

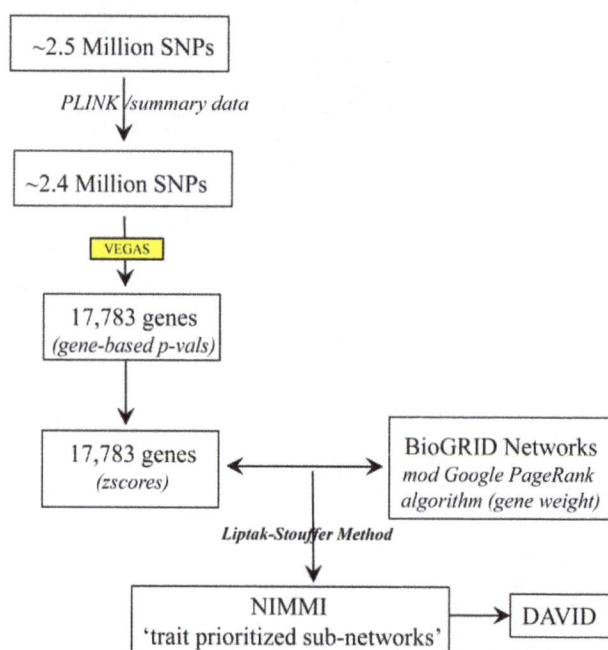

Figure 1. NIMMI flowchart. An overview of the dataflow in NIMMI is shown in Figure 1. The data shown here is drawn from the InCHIANTI height GWAS dataset. Approximately 2.5 million SNPs were analyzed using PLINK setting the parameters as specified under GWAS data module (see Design and Implementation). This resulted in ~2.4 million SNPs with association p-values, which were then assigned to 17,783 genes. Gene assignment and gene-based p-values were calculated using VEGAS. These gene-based p-values were converted to z-scores and combined with gene weights (calculated by the modified Google PageRank algorithm) in the network using the Liptak-Stouffer method to identify the 'trait prioritized sub-networks' that were evaluated in DAVID.

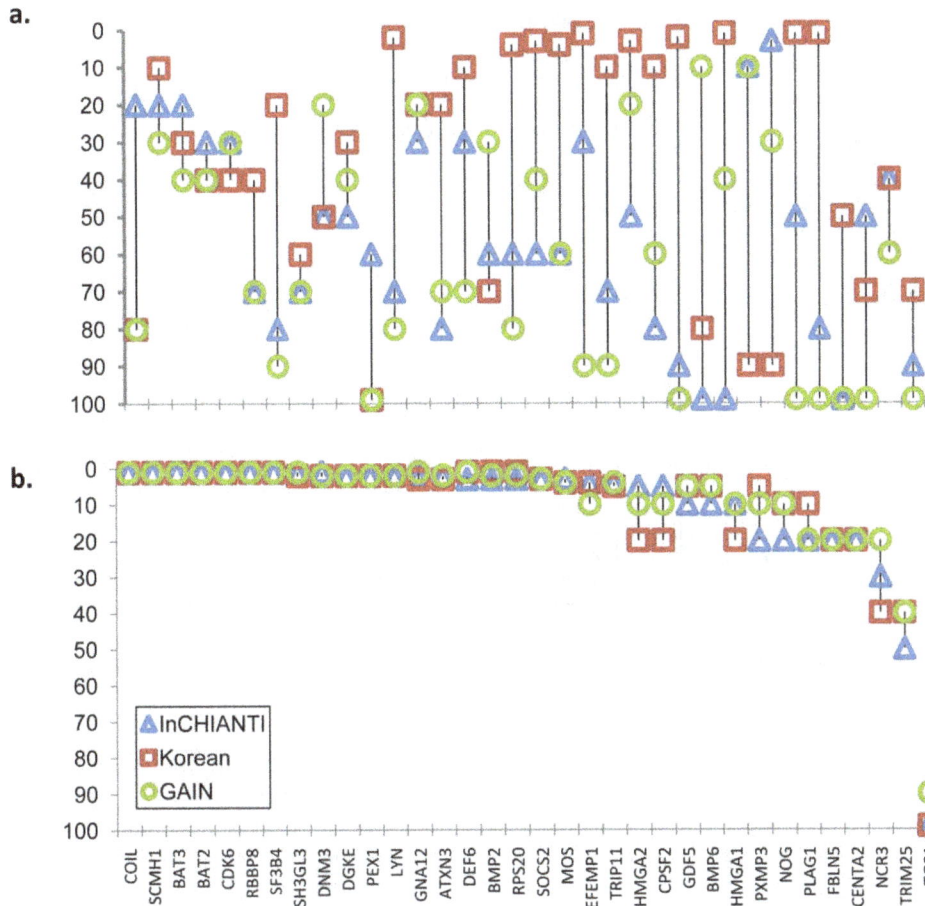

Figures 2. Comparison of gene-based percentile ranks with NIMMI's network percentile ranks. The x-axis shows the candidate genes for height and the y-axis shows the percentile rank. Blue triangles represent the InCHIANTI GWAS dataset, red squares represent the Korean height GWAS dataset and green circles represent the GAIN Controls height GWAS dataset. Figure 2a shows the single-locus ranking and Figure 2b shows NIMMI network-based ranking for 34 height candidate genes.

genes consistently fell in the top 2nd–5th percentile of the NIMMI ranking, and 95% of the genes fell in the top 20th percentile of all three datasets. For example, SCMH1 and CDK6, which belong to the same PPI network, were consistently ranked in the 1st percentile in all three datasets. This demonstrates that NIMMI's gene ranks are highly replicable and more stable across populations than those based on gene-based association p-values alone.

Identification and prioritization of 'trait prioritized sub-networks' for height GWAS datasets

Since 50% of the confirmed height-associated candidate genes (shown in Figure 2b) consistently fall in the top 2% of the NIMMI-ranked networks, these networks were compared in the three height datasets. A total of 38 'height prioritized sub-networks' were generated, which consistently replicated across the three datasets (Figure 3). There were 7 to 10 sub-networks that appeared to be specific to each dataset and 4 to 7 sub-networks that were common to any two datasets. The 38 height prioritized sub-networks common to all three datasets were further evaluated for gene-set enrichment using DAVID.

For each NIMMI prioritized sub-network, the p-values (corrected for the total number of genes in a GWAS and for the total number of networks in each of the datasets) are presented in

Table S2. A maximum of two significant Gene Ontology (GO) terms generated by DAVID are shown, along with the specific GO term, the number of genes associated with that GO term, and the corrected gene-set enrichment p-value (see Methods for GO term selection criteria). For example, one sub-network includes a total of 129 genes, of which 76 genes are involved in gene expression and 56 are involved in nucleic acid metabolism. Nineteen of the 38 sub-networks prioritized by NIMMI were significantly enriched for genes involved in nucleic acid metabolism. Eight sub-networks were enriched for genes that regulate gene expression and 12 sub-networks were enriched for zinc metabolism. Other associated GO terms implicated by NIMMI were transcription, signal transduction, transport, and phosphate and protein metabolism. Four sub-networks were excluded because they were not associated with any GO terms (not shown in Table S2).

NIMMI analysis of randomized data

Some networks identified by NIMMI may represent general relationships among well-studied genes that arise frequently due to "small-world" effects. To estimate the impact of this phenomenon in our data, we re-analyzed the height GWAS datasets after randomization by two methods: 1. Randomization of the network nodes; and 2. Permutation of gene labels in the GWAS data. Two sub-networks appeared consistently in the random networks

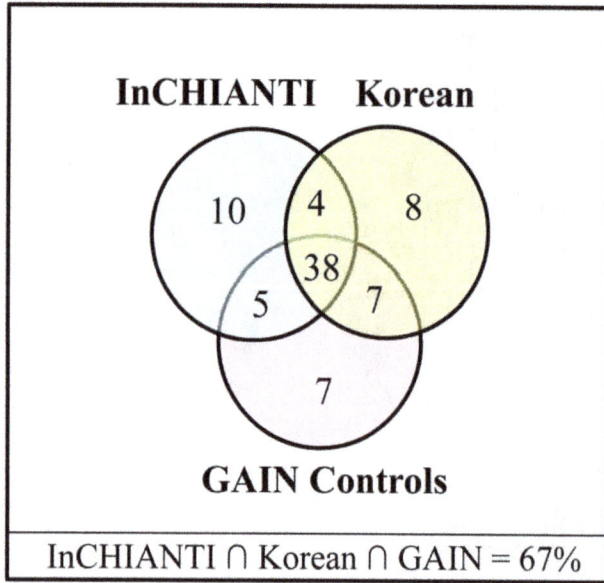

Figure 3. Network overlap. Top 2% overlap of NIMMI prioritized networks in InCHIANTI, Korean and GAIN controls datasets shows 38 networks that are common to all three datasets. Five networks are common to InCHIANTI and GAIN controls datasets only. Korean and GAIN controls datasets have seven networks in common and four networks are common between InCHIANTI and Korean datasets. Ten networks are specific to InCHIANTI dataset, whereas Korean and GAIN controls datasets have 8 and 7 networks, respectively.

Table 1. NIMMI 'height prioritized sub-networks' vs. Cytoscape.

GO-terms*	NIMMI sub-networks	Cytoscape sub-networks
E	x	x
H		x
M	x	x
N	x	x
P	x	x
R	x	x
S	x	x
T	x	x
Z	x	

*E-Gene Expression; H - Steroid Hormone receptor signaling; M-Protein metabolic process/protein modification process; N-Nucleic acid metabolism/ Nucliec acid binding/DNA-Replication; P-Phosphate/phosphorus metabolic process; R-RNA processing/RNA binding/RNA metabolic process/RNA splicing/ Transcription/Transcription Regulation; S-Signal transduction/Intracellular signaling/Cell communication; T-Transport/localization; Z-metal ion binding/ zinc ion binding.

analysis. Eight additional sub-networks appeared in >50% of NIMMI runs performed on the randomized GWAS results (Table S3). NIMMI analysis of randomized data is thus an important step in the identification of sub-networks that are most deserving of further study.

Comparison of NIMMI prioritized height sub-networks with Cytoscape

The three height GWAS datasets were also analyzed in Cytoscape using jActive modules and BiNGO plugins (as described in Baranzini et al [33]). Table 1 shows the 9 GO terms that were prioritized by either NIMMI or Cytoscape. There was substantial agreement between the two methods, with 7 out of 9 GO terms identified by both methods.

Identification and prioritization of Crohn's disease sub-networks by NIMMI

To test the performance of NIMMI with a categorical trait, we analyzed a published GWAS based on a case-control sample studied for Crohn's disease, an autoimmune disorder that has yielded about 20 risk loci by GWAS. NIMMI prioritized nine sub-networks that were significantly enriched for the GO terms "apoptosis", "response to organic substance", "intracellular signaling", "gene expression", "nucleic acid metabolism", "RNA metabolism", and "protein metabolism" (Table 2). KEGG and BioCarta pathway analysis of these nine prioritized sub-networks showed significant enrichment of apoptosis, B-cell receptor, T-cell receptor, chemokine, IL-2, IL-6, Jak-STAT, Wnt and TPO signaling pathways. These results are consistent with the known autoimmune nature of Crohn's disease. A complete list of significantly enriched pathways is presented in Table 3.

Discussion

NIMMI is a simple and efficient software tool that allows researchers to prioritize their GWAS results based on the functional relationships of the associated genes. To our knowledge, NIMMI is the first software tool that maps all the genes in a GWAS dataset to human interactome data using a modified Google PageRank algorithm. With NIMMI it is possible to identify 'trait prioritized sub-networks' in complex, multigenic traits and thus provide biological hypotheses for further study.

We hypothesized that NIMMI would produce more robust findings than single-locus analyses. To test this hypothesis, NIMMI was run on three independent samples rated for the classic polygenic trait of height. NIMMI produced a list of genes with very consistent ranking across all 3 datasets. This level of reproducibility was not achieved with gene-based analysis, probably reflecting small effect sizes of individual loci and differing sample sizes, reducing power to detect true signals. Despite population and sample size differences, NIMMI also identified networks that were enriched with confirmed height associated candidate genes. Furthermore, when height associated candidate genes were analyzed in DAVID, there were no significantly enriched GO terms suggesting that the functional relationships between genes that NIMMI networks represent could not be identified with single-locus analyses alone.

NIMMI's approach is unique. Previous studies that have used the Google PageRank algorithm to rank genes in a network relied on fixed damping factor values ($0.5 \leq d \leq 0.95$) (see Methods) [45,46,47]. Research by Fu et al has shown that a fixed damping factor can result in inconsistent ranking of the nodes in a network. Given that a flexible damping factor is needed, one of the natural approaches is to calculate it dynamically by using the ratio of interactions between neighboring genes [35]. Hence, NIMMI calculates the damping factor dynamically for every gene in a network which may be more appropriate for biological networks than the fixed damping factor typically used for ranking pages on the internet.

Most of the literature published on network and pathway-based approaches has focused on statistically significant findings from

Table 2. NIMMI prioritized sub-networks for Crohn's Disease.

Crohn's Disease Bonf. corrPval	David GO Set 1*	Genes in Set1	Enrichment Pval	David GO Set 2*	Genes in Set2	Enrichment Pval	David GO Set 3*	Genes in Set3	Enrichment Pval
9.51E-14	A	29/96	3.50E-08	N	31/96	7.30E-05	M	26/96	1.90E-10
2.12E-13		27/107	1.90E-03		33/107	1.70E-03	R	27/107	4.40E-11
3.30E-13		28/110	2.60E-03	O	27/110	1.00E-06	S	38/110	1.50E-07
3.53E-13		30/91	7.30E-07		23/91	4.90E-04			
3.23E-16	R	65/115	1.90E-20	O	28/115	4.90E-04	E	35/115	3.80E-15
4.10E-13		74/152	2.50E-18	N	41/152	9.00E-15	S	38/152	1.50E-04
2.89E-13	N	31/89	9.40E-05						
2.08E-14		31/123	1.80E-02						

A-Apoptosis; E-Gene Expression; M-Protein metabolic process/protein modification process; N-Nucleic acid metabolism/Nucliec acid binding/DNA-Replication; O-response to organic substance; R-RNA processing/RNA binding/RNA metabolic process/RNA splicing/Transcription/Transcription Regulation; S-Signal transduction/Intracellular signaling/Cell communication.

GWAS studies for replication or for downstream analysis [20,21,25,27,28,33], [48]. These studies are limited by the problem of finding an optimal p-value threshold. If the p-value threshold is set too low, then the number of genes might be too few to create a biological network and to find associated pathways [49]. Sets of findings with higher p-value thresholds, on the other hand, will contain more false positives. The magnitude of this problem was illustrated by the results of the International Schizophrenia GWAS Consortium, where optimal discrimination between cases and controls was achieved only after the inclusion of over 70,000 markers with p-values as high as 0.2 [34]. A major advantage of NIMMI's approach is that it includes all the findings in a GWAS dataset, weighting the findings by p-value and other factors that users may specify (such as effect size). This reduces the "top hits" selection bias. An example may illustrate this point. The gene BMP2, which encodes bone morphogenetic protein 2, has been implicated in several height GWAS studies [42], but it is not significant in any of the GWAS datasets used in the current study (gene-wise p-values of 0.57, 0.61 and 0.27). Although BMP2 plays a major role in bone development, this gene would not have been selected for downstream analysis with the classical p-value approach. However, NIMMI's network ranking correctly places this gene in the top 1st–3rd percentile. This is because NIMMI takes advantage of signals in genes whose protein products interact with BMP2, making NIMMI sensitive to statistical significance in any individual dataset.

The goal of NIMMI is to prioritize networks for further study. To aid decisions as to which networks to pursue, NIMMI can be applied to randomized networks and GWAS data. Of the 38 'height prioritized sub-networks' that successfully replicated in the three GWAS datasets, 2 appeared consistently in the random networks analysis, suggested that the Type I error rate was about 5% at the network level. When NIMMI was used to analyze 10,000 randomized GWAS datasets, a number of sub-networks appeared in >50% of the results sets (Table S3). We suggest that the users assess their own results in this way and ignore sub-networks that occur frequently in the results derived from randomized data. It is likely that such sub-networks represent general relationships among well-studied genes that arise frequently due to "small-world" effects. Sub-networks that occur rarely in the results derived from randomized data appear to have

good trait specificity. For example, 16 height-prioritized sub-networks that were observed in <5% of the randomized results included 7 sub-networks that were significantly enriched for zinc metabolism. This GO term was enriched only for height and not Crohn's disease. Zinc plays an important role in human growth. Studies in rats and tissue culture confirm that zinc stimulates DNA synthesis and protein synthesis in bone development [50,51]. Furthermore, zinc is a co-factor for zinc finger proteins that bind to methylated DNA to suppress transcription, thus regulating gene expression and protein synthesis [52].

Other GO terms significantly enriched among the height-prioritized sub-networks include nucleic acid metabolism, transcription, gene expression, signal transduction and transport, proteosome and protein metabolism. The effects of growth hormone on protein metabolism are well-documented in the literature, in both human and animal models. These studies suggest that growth hormone stimulates protein synthesis and decreases protein catabolism, a process that mainly occurs in the proteosome [53–56]. Additionally, keywords such as gene expression, signaling and proteases have recently been associated with height markers by GRAIL [57], a statistical text mining approach. Although most of the NIMMI detected 'height prioritized sub-networks' are well-supported by the literature, further functional studies are required to confirm these results.

NIMMI is reasonably sensitive in detecting true trait-related genes. For example, Table S1 includes 34 height associated genes, 16 of which were among the 1,232 genes identified within the top 2% of height prioritized sub-networks by NIMMI. This is a highly significant overlap, given that the total number of genes in all sub-networks created by NIMMI is 6035 (p-value = 1.11×10^{-4}, hypergeometric test). Although 38 sub-networks were prioritized for height, there is substantial overlap among these sub-networks (75%-90%). Each functional category consists of $\leq$100 genes. There is also overlap of genes between functional categories. For example, the category "gene expression" (E) includes ~100 genes, and "transcription" (R) includes ~75 genes, but at least 50% of the genes in set E overlap with those in set R.

Some of the functional categories (nucleic acid metabolism, gene expression) overlap between height and Crohn's disease prioritized sub-networks. These are broad categories and may reflect a true pathway overlap for these two otherwise disparate

Table 3. NIMMI prioritized Crohn's Disease enriched KEGG/ BioCarta pathways.

enriched KEGG/BioCarta pathways	enrichment p-value
Adherens junction	8.70E-07
Apoptosis	3.50E-05
B-cell receptor signaling	1.10E-02
Cell cycle	1.70E-07
Chemokine signaling	9.90E-03
Control of gene expression by vitamin D receptor	1.30E-07
EGF signaling	7.60E-04
ErbB signaling	8.10E-06
Erk1/Erk2 Mapk signaling	9.20E-05
Fc gamma R-mediated phagocytosis	5.80E-14
Focal adhesion	3.20E-06
IL-2 Receptor Beta Chain in T cell Activation	1.60E-02
IL6 signaling	2.80E-03
Insulin signaling	2.90E-04
Jak-STAT signaling	2.70E-03
Neurotrophin signaling	1.20E-02
p53 signaling	1.20E-03
Pathways in cancer	6.30E-11
Pelp1 Modulation of Estrogen Receptor Activity	1.20E-04
Role of PPAR-gamma Coactivators in Obesity and Thermogenesis	2.40E-04
T Cytotoxic Cell Surface Molecules	8.00E-03
T-cell receptor signaling	1.50E-04
TPO signaling	7.30E-03
Wnt signaling	1.70E-03

phenotypes [58]. A few functional categores, such as zinc metabolism and transport, were specific to height. Several functional categories were specific to Crohn's disease, including apoptosis, response to organic substance, Jak-Stat signalling and autoimmune pathways (B-cell receptor, T-cell receptor signaling,etc), consistent with the auto-immune nature of this disease. Although these pathways were detected by other studies [59], additional research is necessary to confirm the NIMMI results in additional samples.

Comparison of NIMMI prioritized height sub-networks to those from Cytoscape jActive modules illustrate that NIMMI gave similar results to the greedy algorithm implemented in Cytoscape. A major limitation of Cytoscape jActive modules is that it requires the input gene set be limited to those with p-value ≤0.05. NIMMI considers all genes implicated in a GWAS dataset, with no p-value threshold required. Consideration of all genes in the network analysis is important because GWAS p-values are inconsistent, especially when sample sizes are small. Including all genes in the Cytoscape analysis resulted in more than 1500 significantly associated GO terms, some of which could be false positives. Furthermore, NIMMI prioritizes trait networks within 3 seconds, which is 10 times faster than what we could achieve with Cytoscape. Cytoscape jActive modules and BiNGO also need more user intervention and formatting than is ordinarily necessary for NIMMI.

The goal of GWAS is to help illuminate the underlying molecular mechanism of a particular phenotype. To maximize the information provided by a GWAS, it is important to integrate functional data with GWAS results. NIMMI is a user-friendly software tool that will help researchers in their post-GWAS decisions by prioritizing genes and networks that are of the highest biological relevance.

Limitations

Some important limitations of network and pathway-based approaches should be mentioned. SNPs do not always bear a clear relationship to a particular gene, and may occur in non-genic regions. Some widely studied genes appear to have relatively greater connectivity, while less studied genes have less, due largely to publication bias. PPIs are sometimes inconsistent, or tissue dependent. Functional annotation systems, such as GO, have not yet been experimentally confirmed for most genes. In spite of these limitations, network and pathway-based approaches provide a unique insight into biology that is often not immediately evident in the GWAS results. As additional genome-wide functional studies are completed in the field, the quality of network and pathway information is likely to improve [29,60–63].

Conclusions

NIMMI is an open-source tool that takes into account information on biological relationships to help interpret GWAS data and to prioritize trait networks for further study. NIMMI offers several advantages over other network and pathway-based approaches. The results of this study demonstrate that NIMMI can identify important genes involved in a multi-genic trait with a high degree of consistency and reproducibility, even across datasets of differing size and ancestry.

The main aim of NIMMI is to help investigators prioritize genes and networks related to a particular phenotype after a GWAS. Although there are limitations to this approach, protein-protein networks and pathways are an excellent source of biological information that, when combined with genomics, could lead to a better understanding of molecular mechanisms. NIMMI efficiently combines genetic association data with protein networks, thus helping to effectively translate GWAS findings into biological hypotheses.

Materials and Methods

Height GWAS datasets

A total of three independent GWAS height samples were analyzed by NIMMI.

The Invechhiare in Chianti (InCHIANTI) GWAS dataset. The InCHIANTI Study is a population-based epidemiological cohort study in the Chianti region of Tuscany, Italy. The study employs two clinical sites, in the towns of Greve and Bagno a Ripoli, with participants recruited from the population registries of these immediate areas. Further details on this cohort have been previously published elsewhere [64]. DNA extracted from InCHIANTI participants was genotyped at the Laboratory of Neurogenetics, National Institute on Aging, using Illumina 550K beadchips. After standard QC measures, missing genotypes were imputed using MACH 1.0 software (http://www.sph.umich.edu/csg/abecasis/mach/) [65]. Maximum likelihood genotype dosages were filtered for quality of imputation prior to analysis (R^2 from MACH>0.30). Analyses were conducted on 975 unrelated members of the InCHIANTI cohort who had height data within +/-3SD from the mean of the sample. After outliers were removed height was log transformed. PLINK (http://pngu.mgh.harvard.

edu/~purcell/plink/), a whole genome association analysis toolset [66], was used for association analysis using study site and sex as covariates, resulting in a ~2.4 million SNPs after pruning. Genomic control inflation factor (λ) was 1.008. A λ close to 1 indicates that association of markers to the phenotype is real rather than due to population stratification. A total of 17,783 genes with gene-wise p-values were used in the downstream analysis (Table 4).

Korean GWAS dataset. Height GWAS data published by Cho et al. were obtained from the researchers [67]. Unimputed summary data for 8,842 Korean individuals was provided as well. Age, sex and study site were used as co-variates in the PLINK association analysis. λ was 1.061 and ~350K SNPs were left after pruning, resulting in 17,408 genes being analyzed by NIMMI (Table 4).

Genetic Association Information Network (GAIN) Controls GWAS height dataset. GWAS data for GAIN controls was obtained from GAIN (http://www.genome.gov/19518664) under a data access agreement. Self-reported height was available for 768 individuals. Only sex was used as a co-variate and ~720 K SNPs were left after pruning by PLINK. λ was 1.059 and a total of 17,720 genes were used in the final analysis by NIMMI (Table 4).

Crohn's disease (CD) GWAS dataset

Summary SNP association results for the CD GWAS dataset (~2000 cases and ~3000 controls) was obtained from the Wellcome Trust Case Control Consortium (WTCCC). Association analysis results are detailed elsewhere [68]. Approximately 409 K SNPs with their association p-values were assigned to 17,114 genes that were included in NIMMI network analysis (Table 4).

Algorithm

Modified Google PageRank Algorithm. Each protein in a network was considered a node, and the interactions between proteins were considered edges, resulting in an undirected graph. Some of the centrality measures available to rank networks are: 1) Degree centrality, which simply counts the number of interactions to a node; 2) Betweenness centrality, where nodes which fall in the shortest path of other nodes have high betweenness; 3) Closeness centrality, which is related to the topology of the nodes in a network; and 4) Eigenvector centrality which ranks the nodes in a network based on the its interacting neighbors, i.e., it takes into account the quantity and quality of connections to a particular node [69,70]. For example, when ranking a webpage (w_p), Google's PageRank algorithm not only considers the number of connections a w_p has, but also the connectivity of the pages linked to w_p. Therefore, w_p will receive a higher rank if it is connected to other highly ranked webpages. Since proteins in a biological

network should also be ranked based on the importance of their interacting partners, scoring them by eigenvector centrality seems to be a reasonable approach.

The PageRank algorithm, which is a based on eigenvector centrality, starts by creating an adjacency matrix (A) for all the proteins (nodes) in a network based on their interactions. $A_{i,j} = A_{j,i} = 1$ if protein 'i' interacts with protein 'j and vice versa, else $A_{i,j} = A_{j,i} = 0$. According to the Perron-Frobenius theorem in linear algebra, for a real square matrix with positive values there exists a largest positive eigenvalue and a corresponding positive dominant eigenvector [69]. The algorithm finds the dominant eigenvector for this adjacency matrix via power iteration (Figure S1) [45,71–73]. Thus, the resulting dominant eigenvector values are considered weights of proteins in a network.

The original Google PageRank algorithm suggested by Lawrance Page and Sergey Brin had a damping factor of 0.85 and excluded dangling links (nodes that have only incoming links but no outgoing links), before ranking the web networks. A damping factor is essential because it improves the speed of the algorithm and keeps it from hitting dead ends [74–77] (http://www.miislita.com/information-retrieval-tutorial/matrix-tutorial-3-eigenvalues-eigenvectors.html; http://www.webworkshop.net/PageRank.html). Investigators who previously applied the Google PageRank algorithm to rank SNPs or genes used a damping factor between $0.5 \leq d \leq 0.95$ [45,46]. The damping factor of 0.85 has been well evaluated for web networks and not for biological networks. Additionally, Fu et al have shown that a fixed damping factor value will lead to inconsistent ranking of nodes in a network [35]. Since all biological networks are not the same, having a fixed damping factor value for all networks might not be ideal. Furthermore, dangling links should be included while ranking a biological network. Given these limitations of the original Google PageRank algorithm, we used the modified Google PageRank algorithm suggested by Fu et al in 2006 [35] to rank the proteins in each of our 2,849 networks (see Design and Implementation).

Equation (1) depicts the modified Google PageRank algorithm

$$w_a = \left(1 - \frac{\sum g_i}{\sum l_i}\right) \times \frac{1}{2N} + \frac{\sum g_i}{\sum l_i} \times \left(\frac{w(g_1)}{l_1} + \frac{w(g_2)}{l_2} + \dots \frac{w(g_n)}{l_n}\right) (1)$$

where,

w_a = weight/PageRank of protein (gene) A in a network

g = all proteins that interact with protein A

Table 4. Summary of GWAS datasets.

Height Datasets	n	Observed [O] Imputed [I]	SNPs after QC	Total Genes
InCHIANTI	975	I	2,453,309	17,783
Korean	8,842	O	352,228	17,408
GAIN Controls	768	O	722,742	17,720
Crohn's Disease	**Cases**	**Controls**	**Observed [O] Imputed [I] SNPs after QC**	**Total Genes**
WTCCC Crohn's	1,748	2,953	O 409,541	17,114

$\sum l_i$ = sum of all proteins that interact with 'g' proteins

$\sum \dfrac{g_i}{l_i}$ = damping factor, which is the ratio of total proteins 'g' that interact with protein A to the sum of all proteins that interact with 'g' proteins

$w(g_1), w(g_2), \ldots w(g_n)$ = weight/PageRank of proteins H_1 to H_n that interact with protein A

$l_1, l_2, \ldots l_n$ = proteins that interact with proteins $g_1, g_2, \ldots\ldots g_n$ respectively

N = Total number of proteins in the network

The advantage of using the modified formula is that it considers all nodes in the network without any exclusion, and that the damping factor is calculated dynamically for every node in a network based on its interactions with neighboring nodes, making it more optimal to rank biological networks. Such an approach results in a damping factor value that is better reflective of the network. To scale the total probability of a given network between 0 and 1, the N in the above formula was doubled. Each protein in a network has a weight ranging between 0 and 1. The protein with weight closer to 1 plays an important role in the network than a protein with weight closer to 0, indicating that the higher the weight the higher the importance of a node in a network.

The Liptak-Stouffer method. The gene-wise association p-value, which is calculated by VEGAS, was integrated with gene weight (obtained from the modified Google PageRank algorithm) in a network. While several approaches are possible, for simplicity we chose the Liptak-Stouffer method. This method of combining p-values from independent experiments has previously been used in the analysis of genome-wide gene expression data [78-80] among others. At first, the association p-value of each gene was converted to its corresponding z-score as calculated in equation (2):

$$z_i = \frac{p_i - \mu}{\sigma} \qquad (2)$$

where,

z_i = z-score of a particular gene

p_i = empirical gene-wise p-value of a particular gene in a given GWAS dataset

μ = mean of all the p-values in a given GWAS dataset

σ = standard deviation of the p-values in a given GWAS dataset

Then, a combined z-score for a network was calculated using the Liptak-Stouffer formula shown in equation (3):

$$Z_{comb} = \frac{\sum_{i=1}^{n} w_i z_i}{\sqrt{\sum_{i=1}^{n} w_i^2}} \qquad (3)$$

where,

Z_{comb} = combined Z-score of a given network

w_i = weight of the protein (gene) obtained from modified Google PageRank in a given network

z_i = association z-score of the gene obtained from GWA data

n = number of proteins (genes) in a given network

Usually, the "w_i" in the Liptak-Stouffer formula refers to sample-size. However, we assigned gene weights based on the modified Google PageRank algorithm. A justification is provided in Methods S1 and Figure S2. The Z_{comb} is then transformed into its corresponding p-value and corrected for the number of genes in a network and total number of networks (by Bonferroni correction).

Architecture of Network Interface Miner for Multigenic Interactions (NIMMI)

NIMMI consists of three levels: SNPs, Genes and Networks. Each level in turn has sub-modules (Figure 4). At the SNPs level (or Level 1), the SNPs were analyzed in the GWAS data module, which were then assigned to genes at GENES level (Level 2) using VEGAS, a software tool. VEGAS also calculates a gene-based p-value for each gene. The Database Miner and Network generator module in Networks level (or Level 3) mined the BioGRID database for human PPIs and created two-step networks that were then ranked using the modified Google PageRank algorithm using Gene/Network ranker module. An association gene-wise p-value of a gene from VEGAS and gene weight from Gene/Network ranker module were then combined using Liptak-Stouffer method. The resulting 'trait prioritized sub-networks' were then evaluated in DAVID.

Level 1: SNPs: GWAS data module. Individual population-based samples from the "Invecchiare in the Chianti" (InCHIANTI) study and Genetic Association Information Network (GAIN) were genotyped on Illumina 550 K and Affymetrix 6.0 microarrays respectively. Genotype information from these SNPs and phased haplotype information on a reference dataset from the HapMap Phase 2 CEU samples (http://hapmap.ncbi.nlm.nih.gov/) were used to impute the allele frequencies of SNPs that are absent on these microarrays. Imputation was performed using MACH 1.0 software. The resulting data were analyzed using PLINK. The following criteria were applied while executing PLINK:

1. SNPs with minor allele frequency (MAF)$<$1% were excluded.
2. SNPs that deviate from Hardy-Weinberg equilibrium (HWE) may indicate genotyping errors [81–83]. Hence, SNPs with HWE p-value$<10^{-5}$ were excluded.
3. SNPs with failure rate$>$2% were excluded.
4. Any individuals with$>$2% missing genotypes were excluded.

A summary statistics file (SNP name along with its association p-value) of analyzed height GWA data was obtained from our collaborators in Korea and a similar file for Crohn's disease GWAS dataset was obtained from WTCCC.

At the end of Level 1, GWA data consisted of a SNP name and an association p-value which are annotated to their respective genes in Level 2.

Level 2: GENES: Versatile Gene-based Association Study (VEGAS). VEGAS is an open source software tool that assigns SNPs from Level 1 to their respective genes based on their position and calculates an empirical gene-based p-value using Monte Carlo simulations ($\leq$ 1 million) (http://gump.qimr.edu.au/VEGAS/) [39]. Any SNP that falls within a 50 kb flanking region of a gene will be assigned to that particular gene. Such an assignment will capture the regulatory regions and SNPs in LD. Although this value is arbitrary, it could be modified according to user specification. When a SNP belongs to more than one gene, that particular SNP was assigned to multiple genes in that location. Given that the PPI data is incomplete, such an assignment allows us to include all the possible genes with interaction data to be included in our downstream analysis. The linkage disequilibrium for each gene is estimated using HapMap populations. For InCHIANTI and GAIN controls height GWAS dataset, and CD GWAS dataset CEU population was used as a reference dataset, whereas CHB_JPT was used as a reference for Korean height GWAS dataset.

Level 3: NETWORKS. This level is made up of a Database Miner and Network generator module and a Gene/Network Ranker and prioritizer module. **(1) Database Miner:** The entire

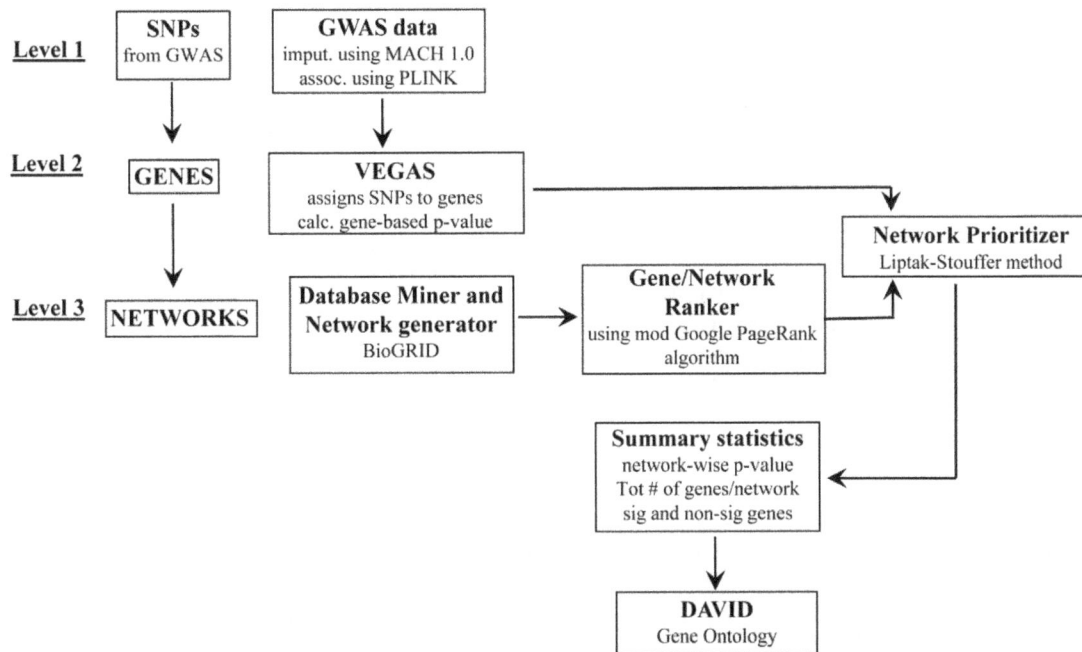

Figure 4. Architecture of Network Interface Miner for Multigenic Interactions (NIMMI). Network Interface Miner for Multigenic Interactions (NIMMI) consists of three levels: SNPs, Genes and Networks, and each level in turn has different modules necessary to prioritize 'trait prioritized sub-networks'. At the SNPs level (or Level 1), the SNPs are analyzed in the GWAS data module using PLINK. The SNPs are then assigned to genes and a gene-wise p-value is calculated using VEGAS (Level 2). The Database Miner and Network generator module in Networks level (or Level 3) mine the BioGRID database for human PPIs and created two-step networks that are then ranked using the modified Google PageRank algorithm in the Gene/Network ranker and prioritizer module. The association p-value of a gene from Level 2 and gene weight from Level 3 are then combined using the Liptak-Stouffer method. The resulting 'trait prioritized sub-networks' are then evaluated in DAVID.

human interactome consisting of 40,206 human PPIs was downloaded from the Biological General Repository for Interaction Datasets (BioGRID) database (http://www.thebiogrid.org/). After excluding human-nonhuman PPIs, a total of 38,509 human-human PPIs were left. Any PPIs detected by different experimental methods were integrated and self interacting proteins were deleted resulting in 24,101 unique human-human PPIs involving 7,646 unique proteins. These unique interactions were used to build biological networks. **(2) Network generator:** In the human PPI network, proteins are represented as nodes and the interaction between proteins are represented as edges. In order to find the optimal number of proteins per network, networks were created using single-step, two-step and three-step methods (data not shown). The median number of proteins per network with a single-step is three (too few) and with three-step was found to be 815 (too large). However, the median number of proteins per network created by two-step process was 58; this is an optimal number for computational efficiency as well as for the search space. A total of 7,646 networks were created by the network generator using the two-step method (Figure S3), of which 2,912 networks were complete subsets of other networks. Hence, these were excluded in the downstream analysis leaving 4,734 networks. These were then ranked using the modified Google PageRank algorithm (see Algorithm). Each of the 4,734 networks had between two and 1000 proteins. To reduce the search space, multiple-testing correction factor associated with the number of proteins and number of networks, and to avoid any false positive networks that could arise due to large size of the networks, we included networks that have only 20–200 proteins [29,48,84]. The algorithm was tested on various protein ranges in InCHIANTI dataset; this also led to the conclusion that the

optimal range of proteins in a network is 20–200 (data not shown) resulting in a total of 2,849 networks. **(3) Gene/Network Ranker module:** The resulting 2,849 networks from above Network generator module were ranked using the modified Google PageRank algorithm (see Algorithm). **(4) Network Prioritizer module:** In this module the association signals were combined with gene weights using the Liptak-Stouffer method (see The Liptak-Stouffer method).

Summary statistics module. In this module summary statistics for each network were generated. These consisted of names of significant genes and non-significant genes, number of significant and non-significant genes; total number of genes in a network; network number; combined Z-score (Z_{comb}); network p-value and corrected p-value.

DAVID, a functional annotation tool. To evaluate results obtained from NIMMI, genes in the top replicated networks were submitted to DAVID, a functional annotation tool [40,41]. There were a total of 7,646 unique proteins (genes) in BioGRID. The official names of these genes were converted to Genbank accession numbers and submitted as background to DAVID. Of the 7,646 genes, DAVID found 6,327 genes and set them as background. DAVID corrects the enrichment p-values for the number of background genes submitted. Then genes belonging to a particular network were submitted and results from the functional annotation tool were selected based on the following criteria:

- Each GO category should have at least 25% gene overlap with the input list.

- Enrichment p-value for each GO term had to be significant ($p \leq 0.05$).

- Benjamini-Hochberg p-value (False discovery rate (FDR)) should be ≤0.05.
- Medium to high stringency level was selected.
- General GO terms like plasmamembrane, membrane, cytoplasm, intracellular, etc were excluded.

To keep the tables concise, the top two GO categories that fit the abovementioned criteria were presented in the results.

Replication

Since NIMMI considers genes and networks as the functional units rather than individual SNPs, replication is expected at the gene/network level rather than at SNP level in the new sample. To test this, the networks NIMMI identified for height in the InCHIANTI GWAS dataset were tested in two independent GWAS datasets (Korean and GAIN Controls) for height.

Randomization of networks

Networks were randomized by permutation of the node labels. Although the number of nodes and edges per network remain the same as the original network, the identities of the nodes were changed resulting in randomization of the network. By this randomization procedure hubs will not remain as hubs. We performed 100 randomizations of the original networks.

Permuting GWAS data

In a given GWAS dataset the gene labels and the association p-values were permuted and NIMMI analysis was performed on each of the 10,000 permuted files.

Implementation of NIMMI

The user input file can either be in PLINK format (*.ped and *.map files) or a summary file with marker names along with association p-values. VEGAS then assigns these markers to their respective genes and calculates a gene-wise association p-value. The output file from VEGAS is then input to a perl script, weightedZscore_forVegasFiles.pl, which converts the association p-values to z-scores and integrates them with gene weights in networks to obtain a combined Z-score for a network (Z_{comb}), which is then converted to a p-value and corrected for the number of tests. The implementation of the modified Google PageRank algorithm in NIMMI has allowed it to identify 'trait prioritized sub-networks' in a given dataset within three seconds.

Availability and Future Directions

NIMMI software along with user manual can be downloaded from http://mapgenetics.nimh.nih.gov/datashare.html.

The current version of NIMMI includes only human PPIs, but this could easily be extended to PPIs from other model organisms. Future versions will incorporate gene expression data and micro RNA studies, whenever available, which could help in further pruning of the prioritized list of networks.

Supporting Information

Figure S1 Power iteration. An adjacency matrix was created based on the links of all the proteins in a network. The power iteration starts by initializing an eigenvector which is multiplied with the adjacency matrix resulting in a new eigenvector. This new eigenvector is normalized and multiplied with the original adjacency matrix until the algorithm finds a dominant eigenvector for this adjacency matrix. (PDF)

Figure S2 Standard error of the mean versus network size. The x-axis shows the number of genes in a network and y-axis shows the standard error of the mean (SEM).

Figure S3 Constructing Two-step networks. Building a two-step network starts with one protein-protein interaction (protein1-protein2). In STEP1 all the proteins interacting with protein1 and protein 2 are added to the network i.e., protein 3 interacts with protein 1 and protein 4 interacts with protein 1 and protein 2, so it is linked to both these proteins. In STEP2 all proteins interacting with proteins in STEP1 are added to the network, for e.g., proteins 6, 7 and 8 interact with protein 4 and protein 5 interacts with protein 3.

Methods S1 Rationale for using gene weight "w_i" in Liptak-Stouffer method.

Table S1 Comparison of single-locus ranking with NIMMI network ranking.

Table S2 'Trait prioritized sub-networks' for height.

Table S3 Empirical p-values of height-prioritized sub-networks.

Acknowledgments

This study makes use of data generated by the Wellcome Trust Case-Control Consortium. A full list of the investigators who contributed to the generation of the data is available from www.wtccc.org.uk. Special thanks to all the participants whose DNA was used in this analysis. We would like to thank the staff at the Center for Information Technology at National Institutes of Health for help with the computational analysis on Helix and Biowulf servers.

Bipolar Disorder Genome Study (BiGS) Consortium institutions:

Scripps Genomic Medicine and Scripps Translational Science Institute and Dept of Molecular and Experimental Medicine, The Scripps Research Institute, La Jolla, CA, USA; Dept of Psychiatry, Univ of Chicago, Chicago, IL, USA; Dept of Psychiatry, Portland VA Medical Center, Portland, OR, USA; Dept of Psychiatry, Johns Hopkins School of Medicine, Baltimore, MD, USA; Dept of Psychiatry, Univ of Pennsylvania, Philadelphia, PA, USA; Dept of Psychiatry, Univ of California, San Francisco, CA, USA; Dept of Psychiatry, Univ of Iowa, Iowa City, IA, USA; Neurogenomics Division, The Translational Genomics Research Institute, Phoenix, AZ, USA; Dept of Biochemistry and Molecular Biology, Indiana Univ School of Medicine, Indianapolis, IN, USA; Dept of Medical and Molecular Genetics, Indiana Univ School of Medicine, Indianapolis, IN, USA; Dept of Computer Science, Univ of California, Los Angeles, CA, USA; Dept of Psychiatry, Univ of California, San Diego, La Jolla, CA, USA; Dept of Psychiatry, Howard Univ, Washington, D.C., USA; Dept of Psychiatry, Indiana Univ School of Medicine, Indianapolis, IN, USA; Dept of Psychiatry, Univ of Michigan, Ann Arbor, MI, USA; Genetic Basis of Mood and Anxiety Disorders Unit, National Institute of Mental Health Intramural Research Program, National Institutes of Health, US Dept of Health and Human Services, Bethesda, MD, USA; Division of Biostatistics, Washington Univ, St. Louis, MO, USA; Dept of Psychiatry, Rush Univ, Chicago, IL, USA; Dept of Psychiatry, VA San Diego Healthcare System, La Jolla, CA, USA

Author Contributions

Conceived and designed the experiments: NA FJM. Analyzed the data: NA FJM. Contributed reagents/materials/analysis tools: MAN AS LF TT SB YSC YJK JYL BGH BiGS Consortium. Edited the manuscript: AB DS JS FJM. Wrote the manuscript: NA.

References

1. Risch N, Merikangas K (1996) The future of genetic studies of complex human diseases. Science 273: 1516–1517.
2. Altshuler D, Daly MJ, Lander ES (2008) Genetic mapping in human disease. Science 322: 881–888.
3. Kraft P, Zeggini E, Ioannidis JP (2009) Replication in genome-wide association studies. Stat Sci 24: 561–573.
4. Carlborg O, Haley CS (2004) Epistasis: too often neglected in complex trait studies? Nat Rev Genet 5: 618–625.
5. Marchini J, Donnelly P, Cardon LR (2005) Genome-wide strategies for detecting multiple loci that influence complex diseases. Nat Genet 37: 413–417.
6. Evans DM, Marchini J, Morris AP, Cardon LR (2006) Two-stage two-locus models in genome-wide association. PLoS Genet 2: e157.
7. Peri S, Navarro JD, Amanchy R, Kristiansen TZ, Jonnalagadda CK, et al. (2003) Development of human protein reference database as an initial platform for approaching systems biology in humans. Genome Res 13: 2363–2371.
8. Krauthammer M, Kaufmann CA, Gilliam TC, Rzhetsky A (2004) Molecular triangulation: bridging linkage and molecular-network information for identifying candidate genes in Alzheimer's disease. Proc Natl Acad Sci U S A 101: 15148–15153.
9. Gandhi TK, Zhong J, Mathivanan S, Karthick L, Chandrika KN, et al. (2006) Analysis of the human protein interactome and comparison with yeast, worm and fly interaction datasets. Nat Genet 38: 285–293.
10. Huang R, Wallqvist A, Covell DG (2006) Comprehensive analysis of pathway or functionally related gene expression in the National Cancer Institute's anticancer screen. Genomics 87: 315–328.
11. Lage K, Karlberg EO, Storling ZM, Olason PI, Pedersen AG, et al. (2007) A human phenome-interactome network of protein complexes implicated in genetic disorders. Nat Biotechnol 25: 309–316.
12. Feldman I, Rzhetsky A, Vitkup D (2008) Network properties of genes harboring inherited disease mutations. Proc Natl Acad Sci U S A 105: 4323–4328.
13. Ideker T, Sharan R (2008) Protein networks in disease. Genome Res 18: 644–652.
14. Iossifov I, Zheng T, Baron M, Gilliam TC, Rzhetsky A (2008) Genetic-linkage mapping of complex hereditary disorders to a whole-genome molecular-interaction network. Genome Res 18: 1150–1162.
15. Kohler S, Bauer S, Horn D, Robinson PN (2008) Walking the interactome for prioritization of candidate disease genes. Am J Hum Genet 82: 949–958.
16. Cordell HJ (2009) Detecting gene-gene interactions that underlie human diseases. Nat Rev Genet 10: 392–404.
17. Emily M, Mailund T, Hein J, Schauser L, Schierup MH (2009) Using biological networks to search for interacting loci in genome-wide association studies. Eur J Hum Genet 17: 1231–1240.
18. Pattin KA, Moore JH (2008) Exploiting the proteome to improve the genome-wide genetic analysis of epistasis in common human diseases. Hum Genet 124: 19–29.
19. Inada T, Koga M, Ishiguro H, Horiuchi Y, Syu A, et al. (2008) Pathway-based association analysis of genome-wide association screening data suggest that genes associated with the gamma-aminobutyric acid receptor signaling pathway are involved in neuroleptic-induced, treatment-resistant tardive dyskinesia. Pharmacogenet Genomics 18: 317–323.
20. Torkamani A, Topol EJ, Schork NJ (2008) Pathway analysis of seven common diseases assessed by genome-wide association. Genomics 92: 265–272.
21. Vink JM, Smit AB, de Geus EJ, Sullivan P, Willemsen G, et al. (2009) Genome-wide association study of smoking initiation and current smoking. Am J Hum Genet 84: 367–379.
22. Sun J, Jia P, Fanous AH, van den Oord E, Chen X, et al. (2010) Schizophrenia gene networks and pathways and their applications for novel candidate gene selection. PLoS One 5: e11351.
23. Askland K, Read C, Moore J (2009) Pathways-based analyses of whole-genome association study data in bipolar disorder reveal genes mediating ion channel activity and synaptic neurotransmission. Hum Genet 125: 63–79.
24. Chen L, Zhang L, Zhao Y, Xu L, Shang Y, et al. (2009) Prioritizing risk pathways: a novel association approach to searching for disease pathways fusing SNPs and pathways. Bioinformatics 25: 237–242.
25. Holmans P, Green EK, Pahwa JS, Ferreira MA, Purcell SM, et al. (2009) Gene ontology analysis of GWA study data sets provides insights into the biology of bipolar disorder. Am J Hum Genet 85: 13–24.
26. Hong MG, Pawitan Y, Magnusson PK, Prince JA (2009) Strategies and issues in the detection of pathway enrichment in genome-wide association studies. Hum Genet 126: 289–301.
27. O'Dushlaine C, Kenny E, Heron EA, Segurado R, Gill M, et al. (2009) The SNP ratio test: pathway analysis of genome-wide association datasets. Bioinformatics 25: 2762–2763.
28. Peng G, Luo L, Siu H, Zhu Y, Hu P, et al. (2010) Gene and pathway-based second-wave analysis of genome-wide association studies. Eur J Hum Genet 18: 111–117.
29. Wang K, Li M, Bucan M (2007) Pathway-Based Approaches for Analysis of Genomewide Association Studies. Am J Hum Genet 81.
30. Eleftherohorinou H, Wright V, Hoggart C, Hartikainen AL, Jarvelin MR, et al. (2009) Pathway analysis of GWAS provides new insights into genetic susceptibility to 3 inflammatory diseases. PLoS One 4: e8068.
31. Suthram S, Beyer A, Karp RM, Eldar Y, Ideker T (2008) eQED: an efficient method for interpreting eQTL associations using protein networks. Mol Syst Biol 4: 162.
32. Jia P, Zheng S, Long J, Zheng W, Zhao Z (2011) dmGWAS: dense module searching for genome-wide association studies in protein-protein interaction networks. Bioinformatics 27: 95–102.
33. Baranzini SE, Galwey NW, Wang J, Khankhanian P, Lindberg R, et al. (2009) Pathway and network-based analysis of genome-wide association studies in multiple sclerosis. Hum Mol Genet 18: 2078–2090.
34. International Schizophrenia Consortium, Purcell SM, Wray NR, Stone JL, Visscher PM, et al. (2009) Common polygenic variation contributes to risk of schizophrenia and bipolar disorder. Nature 460: 748–752.
35. Fu H, Lin DKJ, Tsai H (2006) Damping factor in Google page ranking. Applied Stochastic Models in Business and Industry 22: 431–444.
36. Lesnick TG, Papapetropoulos S, Mash DC, Ffrench-Mullen J, Shehadeh L, et al. (2007) A genomic pathway approach to a complex disease: axon guidance and Parkinson disease. PLoS Genet 3: e98.
37. Neale BM, Sham PC (2004) The future of association studies: gene-based analysis and replication. Am J Hum Genet 75: 353–362.
38. Tu Z, Wang L, Arbeitman MN, Chen T, Sun F (2006) An integrative approach for causal gene identification and gene regulatory pathway inference. Bioinformatics 22: e489–496.
39. Liu JZ, McRae AF, Nyholt DR, Medland SE, Wray NR, et al. (2010) A versatile gene-based test for genome-wide association studies. Am J Hum Genet 87: 139–145.
40. Dennis G, Jr., Sherman BT, Hosack DA, Yang J, Gao W, et al. (2003) DAVID: Database for Annotation, Visualization, and Integrated Discovery. Genome Biol 4: P3.
41. Huang da W, Sherman BT, Lempicki RA (2009) Systematic and integrative analysis of large gene lists using DAVID bioinformatics resources. Nat Protoc 4: 44–57.
42. Gudbjartsson DF, Walters GB, Thorleifsson G, Stefansson H, Halldorsson BV, et al. (2008) Many sequence variants affecting diversity of adult human height. Nat Genet 40: 609–615.
43. Lettre G, Jackson AU, Gieger C, Schumacher FR, Berndt SI, et al. (2008) Identification of ten loci associated with height highlights new biological pathways in human growth. Nat Genet 40: 584–591.
44. Weedon MN, Lango H, Lindgren CM, Wallace C, Evans DM, et al. (2008) Genome-wide association analysis identifies 20 loci that influence adult height. Nat Genet 40: 575–583.
45. Morrison JL, Breitling R, Higham DJ, Gilbert DR (2005) GeneRank: using search engine technology for the analysis of microarray experiments. BMC Bioinformatics 6: 233.
46. Davis NA, Crowe JE, Jr., Pajewski NM, McKinney BA (2010) Surfing a genetic association interaction network to identify modulators of antibody response to smallpox vaccine. Genes Immun 11: 630–636.
47. Draghici S, Khatri P, Tarca AL, Amin K, Done A, et al. (2007) A systems biology approach for pathway level analysis. Genome Res 17: 1537–1545.
48. Saccone SF, Saccone NL, Swan GE, Madden PA, Goate AM, et al. (2008) Systematic biological prioritization after a genome-wide association study: an application to nicotine dependence. Bioinformatics 24: 1805–1811.
49. Elbers CC, van Eijk KR, Franke L, Mulder F, van der Schouw YT, et al. (2009) Using genome-wide pathway analysis to unravel the etiology of complex diseases. Genet Epidemiol 33: 419–431.
50. Ma ZJ, Yamaguchi M (2001) Stimulatory effect of zinc on deoxyribonucleic acid synthesis in bone growth of newborn rats: enhancement with zinc and insulin-like growth factor-I. Calcif Tissue Int 69: 158–163.
51. Yamaguchi M, Oishi H, Suketa Y (1987) Stimulatory effect of zinc on bone formation in tissue culture. Biochem Pharmacol 36: 4007–4012.
52. Filion GJ, Zhenilo S, Salozhin S, Yamada D, Prokhortchouk E, et al. (2006) A family of human zinc finger proteins that bind methylated DNA and repress transcription. Mol Cell Biol 26: 169–181.
53. Biolo G, Bosutti A, Iscra F, Toigo G, Gullo A, et al. (2000) Contribution of the ubiquitin-proteasome pathway to overall muscle proteolysis in hypercatabolic patients. Metabolism 49: 689–691.
54. Biolo G, Iscra F, Bosutti A, Toigo G, Ciocchi B, et al. (2000) Growth hormone decreases muscle glutamine production and stimulates protein synthesis in hypercatabolic patients. Am J Physiol Endocrinol Metab 279: E323–332.
55. Hardin DS, Ellis KJ, Dyson M, Rice J, McConnell R, et al. (2001) Growth hormone decreases protein catabolism in children with cystic fibrosis. J Clin Endocrinol Metab 86: 4424–4428.
56. Schirra HJ, Anderson CG, Wilson WJ, Kerr L, Craik DJ, et al. (2008) Altered metabolism of growth hormone receptor mutant mice: a combined NMR metabonomics and microarray study. PLoS One 3: e2764.
57. Raychaudhuri S, Plenge RM, Rossin EJ, Ng AC, Purcell SM, et al. (2009) Identifying relationships among genomic disease regions: predicting genes at pathogenic SNP associations and rare deletions. PLoS Genet 5: e1000534.
58. Barabási AL, Gulbahce N, Loscalzo J (2011) Network medicine: a network-based approach to human disease. Nat Rev Genet. 12(1): 56–68.
59. Ballard D, Abraham C, Cho J, Zhao H (2010) Pathway analysis comparison using Crohn's disease genome wide association studies. BMC Med Genomics 3: 25.

60. Han JD (2008) Understanding biological functions through molecular networks. Cell Res 18: 224–237.

61. Kraft P, Raychaudhuri S (2009) Complex diseases, complex genes: keeping pathways on the right track. Epidemiology 20: 508–511.

62. Rhee SY, Wood V, Dolinski K, Draghici S (2008) Use and misuse of the gene ontology annotations. Nat Rev Genet 9: 509–515.

63. Schadt EE (2009) Molecular networks as sensors and drivers of common human diseases. Nature 461: 218–223.

64. Ferrucci L, Bandinelli S, Benvenuti E, Di Iorio A, Macchi C, et al. (2000) Subsystems contributing to the decline in ability to walk: bridging the gap between epidemiology and geriatric practice in the InCHIANTI study. J Am Geriatr Soc 48: 1618–1625.

65. Li Y, Abecasis GR (2006) Mach 1.0: Rapid Haplotype Reconstruction and Missing Genotype Inference. Am J Hum Genet S79: 2290.

66. Purcell S, Neale B, Todd-Brown K, Thomas L, Ferreira MA, et al. (2007) PLINK: a tool set for whole-genome association and population-based linkage analyses. Am J Hum Genet 81: 559–575.

67. Cho YS, Go MJ, Kim YJ, Heo JY, Oh JH, et al. (2009) A large-scale genome-wide association study of Asian populations uncovers genetic factors influencing eight quantitative traits. Nat Genet 41: 527–534.

68. Wellcome Trust Case Control Consortium (2007) Genome-wide association study of 14,000 cases of seven common diseases and 3,000 shared controls. Nature 447: 661–678.

69. Newman MEJ (2003) The mathematics of networks. Available: http://www-personal. umich.edu/~mejn/papers/palgrave.pdf. Accessed 2011 August 9.

70. Langville A, Meyer C (2006) Google's PageRank and Beyond: The Science of Search Engine Rankings. Princeton University Press, ISBN 0-691-12202-4.

71. Golub G, van Loan C (1996) Matrix computations. BaltimoreMD: Johns Hopkins Univ Press, 3rd edition.

72. Lohmann G, Margulies DS, Horstmann A, Pleger B, Lepsien J, et al. (2010) Eigenvector centrality mapping for analyzing connectivity patterns in FMRI data of the human brain. PLoS One 5: e10232.

73. Strang G (1988) Linear Algebra and Its Applications. New York: Saunders College Publishing.

74. Avrachenkov K, Litvak N, Pham KS (2006) A singular perturbation approach for choosing PageRank damping factor. arXiv:math/0612079v.

75. Brin S, Page L (1998) The Anatomy of a Large-Scale Hypertextual Web Search Engine, In: Seventh International World-Wide Web Conference.

76. Bryan K, Leise T (2006) The $25,000,000,000 Eigenvector, the linear algebra behind Google. Available: http://www.rose-hulman.edu/~bryan/googleFinalVersionFixed.pdf. Accessed 2011 August 9.

77. Vise D, Malseed M (2005) The Google Story. New York: Bantam Dell.

78. Hwang D, Rust AG, Ramsey S, Smith JJ, Leslie DM, et al. (2005) A data integration methodology for systems biology. Proc Natl Acad Sci U S A 102: 17296–17301.

79. Majeti R, Becker MW, Tian Q, Lee TL, Yan X, et al. (2009) Dysregulated gene expression networks in human acute myelogenous leukemia stem cells. Proc Natl Acad Sci U S A 106: 3396–3401.

80. Setlur SR, Royce TE, Sboner A, Mosquera JM, Demichelis F, et al. (2007) Integrative microarray analysis of pathways dysregulated in metastatic prostate cancer. Cancer Res 67: 10296–10303.

81. Clayton DG, Walker NM, Smyth DJ, Pask R, Cooper JD, et al. (2005) Population structure, differential bias and genomic control in a large-scale, case-control association study. Nat Genet 37: 1243–1246.

82. Hosking L, Lumsden S, Lewis K, Yeo A, McCarthy L, et al. (2004) Detection of genotyping errors by Hardy-Weinberg equilibrium testing. Eur J Hum Genet 12: 395–399.

83. Wittke-Thompson JK, Pluzhnikov A, Cox NJ (2005) Rational inferences about departures from Hardy-Weinberg equilibrium. Am J Hum Genet 76: 967–986.

84. Zhong H, Prentice RL (2008) Bias-reduced estimators and confidence intervals for odds ratios in genome-wide association studies. Biostatistics 9: 621–634.

16

Molecular Reclassification of Crohn's Disease by Cluster Analysis of Genetic Variants

Isabelle Cleynen[1]*, **Jestinah M. Mahachie John**[2,3], **Liesbet Henckaerts**[4], **Wouter Van Moerkercke**[1], **Paul Rutgeerts**[1], **Kristel Van Steen**[2,3], **Severine Vermeire**[1]

1 Department of Gastroenterology, KU Leuven, Leuven, Belgium, **2** Systems and Modeling Unit, Department of Electrical Engineering and Computer Science, University of Liège, Liège, Belgium, **3** Bioinformatics and Modeling, GIGA-R, University of Liège, Liège, Belgium, **4** Department of Medicine, UZ Leuven, Leuven, Belgium

Abstract

Background: Crohn's Disease (CD) has a heterogeneous presentation, and is typically classified according to extent and location of disease. The genetic susceptibility to CD is well known and genome-wide association scans (GWAS) and meta-analysis thereof have identified over 30 susceptibility loci. Except for the association between ileal CD and *NOD2* mutations, efforts in trying to link CD genetics to clinical subphenotypes have not been very successful. We hypothesized that the large number of confirmed genetic variants enables (better) classification of CD patients.

Methodology/Principal Findings: To look for genetic-based subgroups, genotyping results of 46 SNPs identified from CD GWAS were analyzed by Latent Class Analysis (LCA) in CD patients and in healthy controls. Six genetic-based subgroups were identified in CD patients, which were significantly different from the five subgroups found in healthy controls. The identified CD-specific clusters are therefore likely to contribute to disease behavior. We then looked at whether we could relate the genetic-based subgroups to the currently used clinical parameters. Although modest differences in prevalence of disease location and behavior could be observed among the CD clusters, Random Forest analysis showed that patients could not be allocated to one of the 6 genetic-based subgroups based on the typically used clinical parameters alone. This points to a poor relationship between the genetic-based subgroups and the used clinical subphenotypes.

Conclusions/Significance: This approach serves as a first step to reclassify Crohn's disease. The used technique can be applied to other common complex diseases as well, and will help to complete patient characterization, in order to evolve towards personalized medicine.

Editor: Antje Timmer, HelmholtzZentrum München, Germany

Funding: This work was supported by the Fund for Scientific Research (FWO) Flanders, Belgium, to I.C. and S.V.; the Geconcerteerde Onderzoekacties (GOA) of the KU Leuven [grant number GOA/11/015]; the Belgian Network BioMAGNet (Bioinformatics and Modelling: from Genomes to Networks), funded by the Interuniversity Attraction Poles Programme (Phase VI/4) and initiated by the Belgian State, Science Policy Office to J.M.M.J. and K.V.S.; the IST Programme of the European Community, under the PASCAL2 Network of Excellence (Pattern Analysis, Statistical Modelling and Computational Learning) [IST-2007-216886 to J.M.M.J. and K.V.S.]. The funders had no role in study design, data collection and analysis, decision to publish, or preparation of the manuscript.

Competing Interests: The authors have declared that no competing interests exist.

* E-mail: isabelle.cleynen@med.kuleuven.be

Introduction

Crohn's disease (CD) is a heterogeneous disorder with differences in severity, location, behavior and age at onset of inflammation. The heterogeneity of the disease has important implications towards clinical management: patients with a more severe disease course might benefit from early introduction of immunomodulators and/or biologicals, while patients with favorable disease prognosis could be spared from intense treatment and possible side-effects.

The genetic background of CD has been extensively evaluated. This has led to significant insights into the mechanism of the disease, such as a disturbed surveillance of bacteria of the microflora by the intestinal mucosa (*NOD2*), dysregulation of adaptive immunity (*IL23R*), or deficient autophagy (*ATG16L1*, *IRGM*). Meta-analysis of three CD GWAS have identified more than 30 loci associated to CD, with odds ratios (OR) ranging from 1.08 to 3.99 [1]. As a general principle of complex traits, particular

disease associated variants are found with increased frequency in patients when compared to controls. However, these variants appear neither unique nor necessary for the disease to express itself. Furthermore, attempts have been made to link the associated genetic variants with the classic clinical CD subphenotypes. A clear association has been found for *NOD2/CARD15* variants and ileal disease location [2–5]. However, for none of the other susceptibility genes, a robust association with any of these clinical subphenotypes could be shown. Our group recently examined whether the associated genes or a combination thereof could predict clinical outcome of CD. We showed that presence of risk alleles at some of the CD-associated genetic loci influenced disease progression, but overall the predictive power of these risk alleles was fairly poor [6].

The genetic contribution to Crohn's disease is without a doubt, as is the fact that not all CD patients have the same disease course. Although there are little robust genotype-phenotype associations described for CD, we hypothesize that subgroups of CD patients do exist on a molecular level. Here we report on our efforts to reclassify Crohn's disease into subgroups based on currently confirmed genetic markers. We then analyzed whether these subgroups are associated with the classically used clinical subphenotypes.

Methods

Study samples

875 CD patients previously described in [6] were included in this study. In brief, patients were recruited in the framework of the inflammatory Bowel Disease (IBD) genetics study that started in 1997 at the IBD unit of the University Hospital in Leuven (Belgium). Patients were unrelated and of Western European origin. Diagnosis of CD was based on the most recent international classification (Montreal classification) [7,8]. Median time of follow-up since diagnosis is 14 years (IQR 7–22 years). The control group consisted of 367 unrelated healthy volunteers (healthy control HC) of Western European origin, without a family history of IBD or other immune related disorders. Ethical approval was given by the Ethics Board of the University Hospital Leuven, and written informed consent was obtained from all participants. Samples and data were stored in a coded, anonymized database. Patient files were reviewed for phenotypic information as described in [6] (also see Table 1, 'Overall').

DNA extraction and genotyping

DNA extraction and genotyping was performed as described earlier [6]. A total of 46 markers identified from different GWAS performed on CD, and/or meta-analysis of these GWAS [1], were included in this study. Table S1 includes a list of all SNPs, with the reference where the SNP was selected from, as well as the odds ratio found in that study. In Table S2, allele and genotype counts in the CD patients and HCs studied here are listed. The minor

allele was defined as the less frequent allele in the control group. For the analysis performed in this study, coding for the additive genetic model was used with wild-type individuals (homozygous for the major allele) coded as 0, heterozygous individuals as 1, and individuals homozygous for the minor allele as 2.

Statistical analyses

Detailed information on the used statistical analyses can be found in the supporting information (Methods S1) online.

Cluster identification. To identify clusters, latent class analysis (LCA) was applied to the set of 46 genetic markers genotyped in CD patients and healthy controls. Analyses were performed in the patient and control group separately. LCA assumes that the population is composed of sub-populations (latent classes), each having its distinctive distribution of the included variables [9].

LCA was performed with Multimix, which can handle both continuous and categorical variables [10], as well as missing data [11]. Hence, for this study all individuals - including those with missing genotypes - were included. Class assignment was based on posterior probabilities. In particular, individuals were allocated to classes or clusters on the basis of highest membership probability. The number of latent classes (N) was derived from bootstrap p-values for the likelihood ratio (LR) test with the null hypothesis that the population is 'best' explained by N classes. The alpha level used for determining the number of latent classes is 0.05. Per model, 20 bootstrap samples were generated, making sure that the same percentages of missingness as in the original sample were attained.

Construction of classification trees. Once subjects were grouped into classes or clusters, on the basis of their available genetic information, we determined the genetic markers that contributed most to the formation of the clusters. To perform this step, i.e. to gain insight into the meaning of the formed clusters,

Table 1. Characteristics of all included CD patients (Overall), and of the six genetic-based subgroups (Cluster A–F).

Genetic-based subgroup	Overall	Cluster A	Cluster B	Cluster C	Cluster D	Cluster E	Cluster F
Subjects n	875	302	96	62	117	59	239
Gender n(%)							
Male	360 (41%)	120 (40%)	44 (46%)	30 (48%)	52 (44%)	25 (42%)	89 (37%)
Female	515 (59%)	182 (60%)	52 (54%)	32 (52%)	62 (56%)	34 (58%)	150 (63%)
Median age at diagnosis (Q25–Q75)	24 (18–31)	23 (18–31)	25 (18–32)	25 (19–32)	23 (17–30)	24 (20–32)	25 (18–33)
Location n(%)							
Colon§	113 (13%)	34 (11%)	15 (16%)	3 (5%)	17 (15%)	9 (15%)	35 (15%)
Ileum§	326 (37%)	107 (35%)	36 (38%)	32 (52%)	46 (39%)	19 (32%)	86 (36%)
Ileocolonic§	433 (50%)	161 (53%)	44 (46%)	27 (44%)	54 (46%)	31 (53%)	116 (49%)
Anal	331 (38%)	118 (39%)	33 (34%)	26 (42%)	51 (44%)	15 (25%)	88 (37%)
Behavior n(%)							
Inflammatory*	430 (49%)	144 (48%)	57 (59%)	23 (37%)	60 (51%)	30 (51%)	116 (49%)
Stenosing*	329 (38%)	115 (38%)	33 (34%)	31 (50%)	36 (31%)	18 (31%)	96 (40%)
Non-perianal fistulae	227 (26%)	82 (27%)	16 (17%)	18 (29%)	33 (28%)	16 (27%)	62 (26%)
Perianal fistulae*	267 (31%)	73 (29%)	31 (32%)	26 (42%)	34 (29%)	17 (29%)	73 (31%)
Surgery# n(%)	493 (57%)	171 (57%)	54 (56%)	45 (73%)	62 (53%)	31 (53%)	130 (54%)

§three missing values. Colonic, ileal, and ileocolonic location add up to 100% (are mutually exclusive). Anal disease can occur together with any of the other locations, and thus represents the % of patients in the respective cluster that also has anal involvement.
*one missing.
#four missing.

classification trees were generated with the R rpart package (R 2.9.1). Hence, trees were grown using the cluster variable obtained from Multimix as the (categorical) response and SNPs as potential explanatory variates. Goodness-of-fit of the obtained classification tree was compared to the cluster assignment of Multimix, by dropping individuals down the classification tree, and by comparing the R tree-based classification of subjects to the Multimix-based one.

Testing of the hypothesis of no overall status effect (case vs. control). To check for the effect of status (case vs. control), canonical discriminant analysis (CDA) was applied to LCA data of both CD patients and healthy controls (SAS 9.1.3). Two analyses were performed: (analysis 1) To globally look at the differences between CD patients and healthy controls, canonical variables were calculated for CD patients only (say Y1, Y2), and for healthy controls only (say X1, X2). In CDA, Y1,Y2 and X1,X2 are chosen so as to maximize separation between the clusters. (analysis 2) To test whether there is a difference in terms of clustering spread/separation rule between CD patients and healthy controls, canonical variables were computed for CD patients only (say Y1, Y2). The values of Y1 and Y2 were subsequently computed for the healthy controls using the "linear combination" rule derived for the CD patients. Mean values of Y1 and Y2 between CD patients and healthy controls were then compared using MANOVA.

Association of genetic-based subgroups and clinical characteristics. Univariate Chi-squares (or Fisher Exact tests when necessary) were performed using SPSS 15.0 to test for associations between each of the cluster memberships and the clinical subphenotypes gender; colonic, ileal, ileocolonic disease location at last follow-up; anal disease at last follow-up; inflammatory, stricturing, non-perianal fistulizing, or perianal fistulizing disease behavior at last follow-up; and need for surgery. Multiple logistic regression (using automated backward variable selection) was performed including those clinical parameters that showed at least a trend towards significance in univariate analysis (cut-off p-value = 0.1) using SPSS 15.0. These tests were complemented with Random Forest (RF) analysis in R (2.9.1; http://www.stat.berkeley.edu/~breiman/RandomForests/cc_home. htm). RF analysis estimates the importance of variables in determining classification and is able to highlight possible variable interactions.

Results

Cluster identification in CD patients

Latent class analysis (LCA) identified 6 genetic-based subgroups (clusters) in CD. For each patient, membership probabilities for each cluster were computed. As mentioned above, an individual was assigned to the cluster for which they had the highest probability. 90% of CD patients (n = 788) had a highest membership probability of >0.9, indicating clear membership. For 4% of CD patients (n = 37) the highest membership probability was <0.6, indicative of more uncertain membership (see Table S3 for all membership probabilities).

To investigate the relationship between subgroups identified in the different steps of the model building, the number of CD patients "flowing" from a cluster identified in one step ('Model i' (i≥1), e.g. a model with one cluster) to a cluster identified in the next step ('Model i+1', e.g. a model with two clusters) was determined (Figure 1A). Notably, the majority of patients who belong to a particular cluster in 'Model i', tend to be redistributed to a single cluster in 'Model i+1', as can be observed by inspecting connected clusters in Figure 1A: the white parallelograms connecting two clusters, one from 'Model i' and one from 'Model i+1', the area of which is proportional to the number of individuals that are common to the clusters.

The grouping into the 6 CD clusters was *best* explained by 3 SNPs (rpart analysis; Figure 1B): rs7869487 in *TNFSF15*, rs13361189 in *IRGM*, and rs946227 located on 6q23.3.

When dropping the CD patients down the SNP tree, only 39 CD patients (4.5%) were misclassified compared to the multimix cluster allocation. A total of 58 CD patients (6.6%) could not be allocated to any of the CD subgroups because of missing genotypes for at least one of the determining SNPs.

Cluster identification in control samples

If patient genotypes would cluster purely at random, then the same clusters are to be expected in the control samples. We therefore ran the Multimix program (LCA) also on 367 healthy controls (HC). A model with 5 clusters best explained the heterogeneity in healthy controls. A total of 83% of HC (n = 305) had a highest membership probability of >0.9, indicating clear membership. For 4.6% of HC (n = 17) the highest membership probability was <0.6, which is indicative of highly uncertain cluster membership assignments (data not shown).

The "flow" of control individuals through the clusters and formation of the clusters in the stepwise models is shown in Figure 1C. As we observed for the CD patients LCA analysis, identified clusters appeared to be stable across the different models.

Tree building with rpart showed that the following SNP combinations *best* explained the control clusters (Figure 1D): rs7869487 in *TNFSF15*, rs6927210 on chromosome 6, rs10883365 and rs7081330 in *NKX2-3*, and rs4958847 in *IRGM*. Cluster B could not be explained by specific SNPs, and may be interpreted as a waste bin: with the available genetic markers, no SNP appeared to be more important than others to explain cluster B.

We observed that 79 healthy controls (21.5%) were misclassified. Moreover, 39 HC (10.6%) were not allocated to a control cluster because of missing genotypes in at least one of the *best* determining SNPs, when dropped down the control SNP tree. This high prediction error rate is partly explained by the lack of any SNP-based rule for cluster B.

Comparing formed clusters between CD patients and healthy controls

Canonical discriminant analysis (CDA) was performed in CD patients and healthy controls, separately. The means derived for canonical variable 1 (X1, Y1) and canonical variable 2 (X2,Y2), with (X1, X2) for healthy controls and (Y1, Y2) for CD patients, were: mean value X1: 7.93E-17, SD 2.06; mean value Y1: 7.72E-17, SD 2.61; mean value X2: −2.68E-16, SD 2.36; mean value Y2: 1.96E-16, SD 1.55. When we constructed a plot based on the two main canonical variables for CD patients (Y1, Y2; Figure 2A) and on the two main canonical variables for healthy controls (X1,X2; Figure 2B), a clear difference between both groups in terms of spatial spread of the clusters could be observed (compare Figures 2A and 2B). This supports the existence of differential separation rules for CD patients and healthy controls. Indeed, when canonical variables for healthy controls were computed using the discriminant rule derived for CD patients (analysis 2; see Methods for details), the obtained mean values for the two first canonical variables for CD patients and healthy controls were significantly different ($p_{manova} < 0.0001$). Whereas the first two canonical variables nicely separated the CD clusters, the corresponding discriminant function did not clearly separate the clusters in healthy controls (compare Figures 2A and 2C).

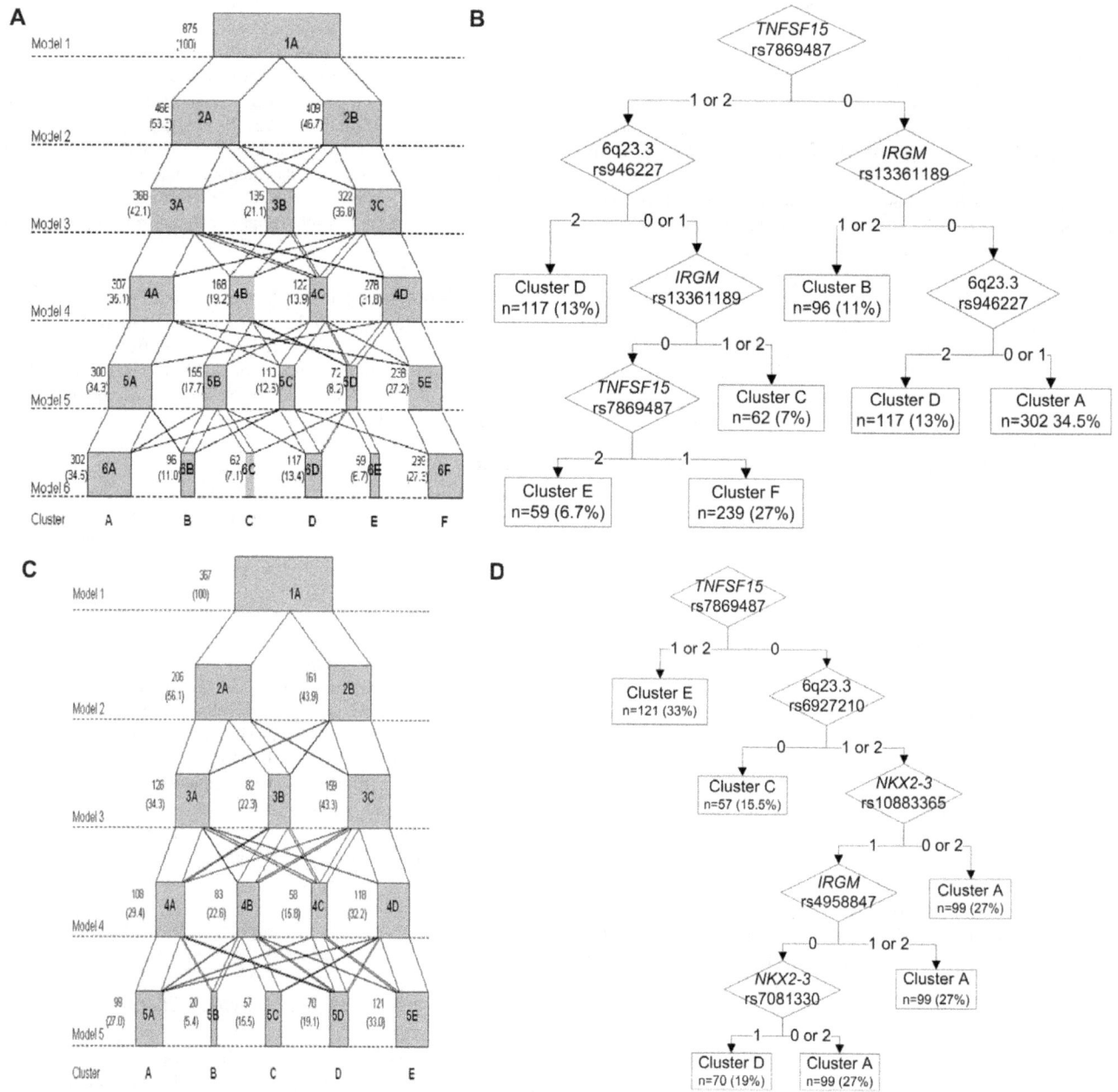

Figure 1. Modelbuilding process and classification trees for the final model. Formation of genetic-based subgroups when the number of clusters was increased stepwise for CD patients (**panel A**) or healthy controls (**panel C**) is shown. Data are presented as n (%). Box widths are proportional to the number of individuals in the respective cluster. The area of the white parallelograms connecting two clusters, one from Model i and one from Model i+1, is proportional to the number of individuals that are common between these clusters. Tree plot showing how SNPs determine the grouping of individuals into the different clusters for CD patients (**panel B**) and healthy controls (**panel D**). The diamond indicates where a decision is made (genotype 0 (wild-type), 1 (heterozygous) and/or 2 (homozygous mutant)). A rectangle indicates the decision (which cluster the patient belongs to when following the tree). The number and percentage of individuals in each cluster is presented as well.

Note that one cluster (cluster D in Figure 2A), was less confined to a particular spatial area than the other clusters derived for CD patients. This was to be expected since this cluster was determined by two different branches from the tree plot (see Figure 1B). Healthy controls were also nicely separated on the basis of the two first canonical variables for HC, although to a lesser extent than the CD clusters. This was also reflected in the higher prediction error rate in HC compared to CD patients. Here, cluster B seemed to smear out over the plotted area, which was in agreement with the SNP tree (see Figure 1D), where cluster B does not appear. As

stated above, for this cluster, no preference was given to any SNP to determine the cluster.

Comparing clinical subphenotypes across the identified clusters

The phenotypic characteristics of CD patients in the different genetic-based subgroups are summarized in Table 1. No obvious differences were observed for gender distribution and median age at diagnosis between the different clusters. However, a difference in distribution of disease location (colonic, ileal, or ileocolonic)

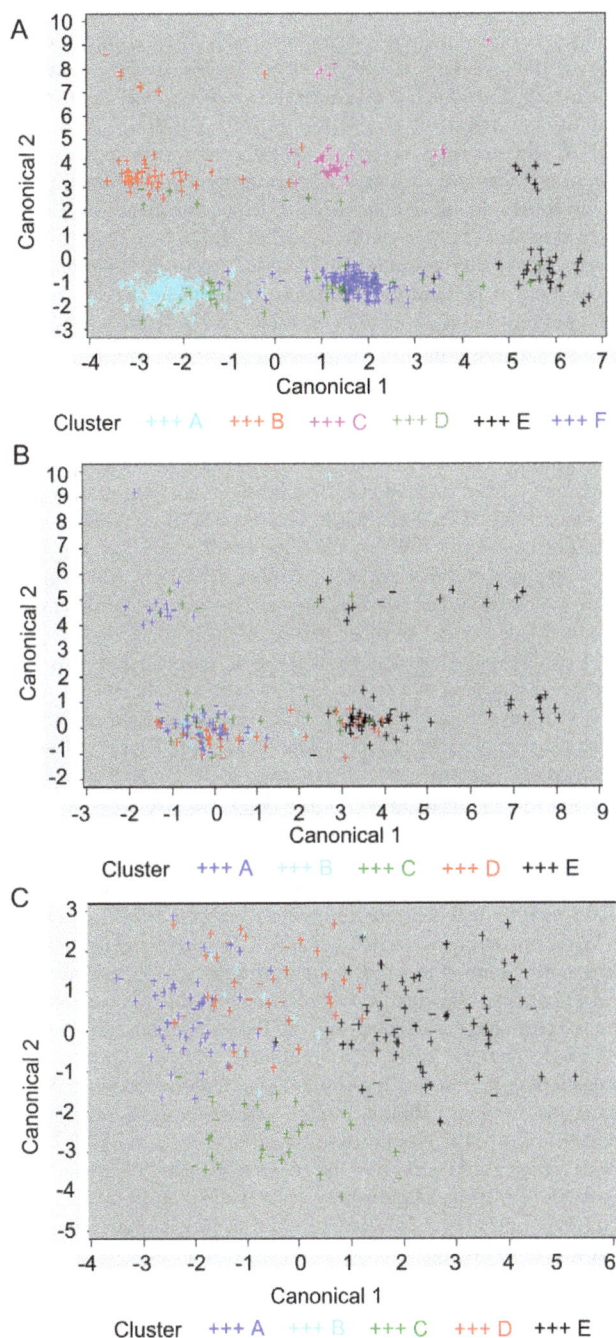

Figure 2. Cluster plots. Cluster plot based on canonical variables for CD patients (**panel A**) and for healthy controls (**panel B**). Cluster plot for healthy controls, when discriminant functions derived from CD patients were applied to the healthy control population (**panel C**).

37%). This difference (cluster B versus all other clusters) was, although borderline, statistically significant ($p_{Chi^2} = 0.04$, OR = 1.59[1.03–2.44]). In addition, cluster B contained the lowest prevalence of non-perianal fistulae (16/96, 17%), compared to 26%–29% in the other clusters ($p_{Chi^2} = 0.03$, OR = 0.54[0.31–0.94]). Stenosing disease behavior, and perianal fistulizing disease behavior, tended to be more prevalent in cluster C: 31/62 (50%) CD patients in cluster C had stenosing disease behavior versus 31%–40% in the other clusters ($p_{Chi^2} = 0.04$, OR = 1.73 [1.03–2.90]), and 26/62 (42%) CD patients had perianal fistulizing disease behavior versus 29%–31% in other clusters ($p_{Chi^2} = 0.04$, OR = 1.71 [1.01–2.90]). Also interesting was the high prevalence of surgery in cluster C: 45 out of 62 CD patients (73%) underwent surgery for their disease, compared to 53%–57% of CD patients in the other clusters. This difference (cluster C versus other clusters) was statistically significant ($p_{Chi^2} = 0.008$, OR = 2.13[1.2–3.79]). Multiple logistic regression analysis including all clinical parameters with $p < 0.1$, indicated that cluster B remained independently associated with non-perianal fistulizing disease behavior ($p = 0.03$, OR = 0.54 [0.31–0.95]; cluster C with perianal fistulizing disease behavior ($p = 0.03$, OR = 1.82 [1.07–3.14] and need for surgery ($p = 0.03$, OR = 1.92 [1.07–3.45]; and cluster E with anal disease ($p = 0.04$, OR = 0.54 [0.29–0.98]. It should be noted however, that all differences seen between the different clusters are modest in magnitude, and would not withstand correction for multiple testing.

On the other hand, random forest (RF) analysis applied to our data gave rise to large inconsistencies between the permutation-based mean decrease in accuracy criterion and the mean decrease Gini impurity criterion, indicating which variable would be the most and least important. From the observation that RF also showed a considerable classification error rate (71,31%) it could be presumed that the given clinical subphenotypes are inadequate or not sufficient to serve as sole class predictors.

Discussion

Crohn's disease (CD) is a heterogeneous disorder which is classically being classified according to extent and location of disease and its behavior (inflammatory, stenosing or fistulizing) [7,8]. Except for the association between *NOD2* and ileal disease location, no robust genotype-phenotype associations have been reported for CD. Because of the well-established role for genetics in the etiology of Crohn's disease, we looked whether subgroups of CD patients could also be identified based only on genetic marker information, and treating the clinical subphenotypes as unknown.

The applied technique distinguished six genetic-based subgroups in CD patients. Several genetic-based subgroups were also identified in healthy controls, but these clearly had a different pattern than in CD patients (Figure 2, panels A and B). The discriminant function for separation of clusters in CD patients indeed could not clearly separate the clusters in healthy controls (Figure 2, panel C; and CDA analysis 2). The genetic variants thus clustered in different ways within CD patients and healthy controls. Note that these clusters were derived directly from genetic marker data, completely independent from any *a priori* knowledge about clinical (sub)phenotypes.

Many of the genes/loci found to be associated with Crohn's disease segregate into particular pathways. Two of the key pathways are the autophagy and the Il23/Th17 pathway [12–15]. Among the most widely studied and replicated disease loci associated with CD are indeed the autophagy genes *ATG16L1* (rs2241880) [14] and *IRGM* (rs4958847, rs13361189) [15], *NOD2* (rs2066844, rs2066845, and rs2066847) [16,17], and *IL23R*

could be observed between cluster C, and the other clusters ($p_{Chi^2} = 0.02$). Prevalence of anal disease, which could occur irrespective of the other disease locations, was lowest in cluster E (15/59 CD patients, 25%), followed by cluster B (33/96, 34%), cluster F (88/239, 37%), cluster A (118/302, 39%), cluster C (26/62, 42%), and cluster D (51/117, 44%). With regards to disease behavior, the prevalence of inflammatory disease behavior was highest in cluster B (57/96 CD patients, 59%), less in cluster E (30/59, 51%) and D (60/117, 51%), followed by cluster F (116/239, 49%) and A (144/302, 48%), and lowest in cluster C (23/62, (rs11209026) [18]. Although these markers were included in this study, except for *IRGM*, they did not clearly pop up in the SNP classification tree as best predicting the identified clusters. In this study, we are actually searching for (a combination of) genetic factors that distinguish CD patients from one another, as opposed to factors that are common to all CD patients (versus healthy controls). These particular SNPs are *strong* susceptibility markers for CD when compared to healthy controls, and could thus be more generally applicable to all CD patients, which could explain why they do not appear in the classification trees. It is indeed believed that genetics of Crohn's disease consists of disease susceptibility genes/loci on the one side, and disease modifying genes/loci on the other. Recent work from the international IBD genetics consortium underscores this idea: re-analysis of GWAS data in function of disease behavior (mild versus aggressive disease) identified a number of SNPs that specifically predispose to a more aggressive disease course in CD. Interestingly, these SNPs were not associated with the disease in the original GWAS (Lee et al., ECCO 2010). Additionally, an important observation in our study was that the SNPs/genes that determine cluster formation in CD do not appear to group in specific pathways: eg *TNFSF15* and *IRGM*, which explain cluster B (Figure 1B) are – to the best of our knowledge – not part of one and the same pathway. It could thus be postulated that there are (more general) disease susceptibility pathways that lead to CD overall as compared to healthy controls: autophagy, Th17 pathway, innate immunity, … . But that the specific disease subphenotype (whether a patient will develop a severe disease phenotype with need for surgery for example) is dependent on single disease modifying genes that are not necessarily playing on different levels of the same pathway. Weersma et al. showed that an increase in the number of risk alleles is associated with an increased risk for Crohn's disease and with a more severe disease course [19]. Still, the absolute difference in the number of risk alleles between patients with Crohn's disease and controls was modest. Also, even in the extensive CD group studied by Weersma et al., the majority of patients carried up until 6 risk alleles, and only 5 CD patients carried 8 risk alleles [19]. It is expected that a plateau phase is reached with respect to the number of risk alleles patients carry. It could therefore be speculated that individuals carrying a specific set of risk alleles clustering in specific pathways (for example in *IRGM*, *ATG16L1* and *NOD2* – all implicated in autophagy), and maybe having been/being exposed to a same environmental factor(s), end up developing CD. When in these patients, a combination of genotypes at different risk loci – all of which part of different pathways – is present (cfr as in the SNP classification tree), the patient will end up developing a specific disease subphenotype, independent from the development of CD overall.

Among the clusters, modest differences in prevalence of disease location and/or behavior could be observed (Table 1). For example, cluster B contained less patients with non-perianal fistulizing disease behavior at last follow-up, and cluster C had a higher prevalence of patients with perianal fistulae and patients with need for surgery. Still, random forest analysis, which estimates the importance of variables in determining classification, showed that CD subgroups found based on genetic data could not be explained adequately by the known clinical (sub)phenotypes. This points to a poor relationship between the genetic-based subgroups and the used clinical subphenotypes. Different explanations could be put forward: (1) A relatively low number of SNPs was included in this exploratory study. It will be important to – in the future – include many more variants in this type of analysis, to look for subgroups within patients. At that time, it will also be important to re-assess the above-mentioned concept of disease

susceptibility *pathways* leading to disease *overall*, and *single disease modifying genes* defining the *specific disease course*. (2) As also mentioned above, the genetic variants included in this study are known *susceptibility* SNPs for CD versus healthy controls. The observation that the strongest associated loci to date (*CARD15*, *ATG16L1*, *IL23R*) did not pop up in the classification tree supports the hypothesis that they are indeed more general genes for CD, and might be less usefull to differentiate CD patients. More studies are needed to also discover markers for clinical subphenotypes. (3) CD has a heritability estimate of 50–60% (with λs~20–35). The proportion of heritability accounted for by the currently known susceptibility loci is about 20% [1]. The currently known variants might explain too little of the genetic part of disease risk to be of much clinical relevance. It is believed that part of the missing heritability is explained by gene-gene interactions, that might be even more important than the independent effects of the single susceptibility genes. A clustering analysis like performed in this study gives a first indication of potentially interacting markers: cfr on one branch of the tree (Figure 1B), one SNP is a potential effect modifier of another SNP on the same branch. Another aspect of the missing heritability are copy number variations, which in the future should be taken up as parameters in this type of analysis. (4) Although speculative, another reason might be that the currently used clinical parameters are not the best way to subclassify CD patients, or at least not in the genetic context. The classification based on extent and location of disease indeed is of limited practical use for clinical application, and for prediction of disease progression. Attempts have been made to better subclassify CD patients using clinical, as well as serological and genetic markers, but diagnostic and prognostic specificity and sensitivity of these methods are generally too low to be useful in clinical practice [7,20,21]. Still, from the clinical point of view, the clinical characteristics will continue to be most relevant.

With this study we could identify CD specific genetic-based subgroups, pointing to a non-random clustering of genetic markers in CD patients. The formed CD clusters are likely to contribute to disease pathogenesis. The specific SNP combinations determining the CD clusters could be promising disease (progression) predictors, and deserve future study once internationally ongoing efforts to develop a disability score will be finished. In order to further improve the classification based on genetic markers, in the future, more markers need to be included, even on a genome-wide level. Since this is an exploratory study, validation in independent data sets is necessary. Nevertheless, this technique may serve as a first step to reclassify Crohn's disease. Similar approaches could be interesting also for other complex diseases, and in for example pharmacogenetics where the goal is to find subgroups of patients benefiting most, or being most at risk for side-effects of certain therapies.

Supporting Information

Methods S1 Supporting methods

Table S1 Summary of included polymorphisms: reference and odds ratio as given in the discovery study.

Table S2 Allele and genotype counts in Crohn's disease (CD) patients and healthy controls.

Table S3 Membership probabilities for Crohn's disease patients.

Acknowledgments

The authors thank Ben Spycher for all professional advice with regards to the applied LCA clustering technique (Multimix), Vera Ballet for excellent database management, and Karolien Claes, Tamara Coopmans, Sophie Organe, and Nele Van Schuerbeek for the excellent technical and scientific support for sample selection, DNA extraction, and genotyping.

Author Contributions

Conceived and designed the experiments: IC PR KVS SV. Performed the experiments: IC JMMJ. Analyzed the data: IC. Contributed reagents/materials/analysis tools: LH WVM. Wrote the paper: IC JMMJ LH WVM PR KVS SV.

References

1. Barrett JC, Hansoul S, Nicolae DL, Cho JH, Duerr RH, et al. (2008) Genome-wide association defines more than 30 distinct susceptibility loci for Crohn's disease. Nat Genet 40: 955–962.
2. Vermeire S, Wild G, Kocher K, Cousineau J, Dufresne L, et al. (2002) CARD15 genetic variation in a Quebec population: prevalence, genotype-phenotype relationship, and haplotype structure. Am J Hum Genet 71: 74–83.
3. Hampe J, Grebe J, Nikolaus S, Solberg C, Croucher PJ, et al. (2002) Association of NOD2 (CARD 15) genotype with clinical course of Crohn's disease: a cohort study. Lancet 359: 1661–1665.
4. Cuthbert AP, Fisher SA, Mirza MM, King K, Hampe J, et al. (2002) The contribution of NOD2 gene mutations to the risk and site of disease in inflammatory bowel disease. Gastroenterology 122: 867–874.
5. Ahmad T, Armuzzi A, Bunce M, Mulcahy-Hawes K, Marshall SE, et al. (2002) The molecular classification of the clinical manifestations of Crohn's disease. Gastroenterology 122: 854–866.
6. Henckaerts L, Van Steen K, Verstreken I, Cleynen I, Franke A, et al. (2009) Genetic Risk Profiling And Prediction Of Disease Course In Crohn'S Disease Patients. Clin Gastroenterol Hepatol.
7. Silverberg MS, Satsangi J, Ahmad T, Arnott ID, Bernstein CN, et al. (2005) Toward an integrated clinical, molecular and serological classification of inflammatory bowel disease: Report of a Working Party of the 2005 Montreal World Congress of Gastroenterology. Can J Gastroenterol 19 Suppl A: 5–36.
8. Satsangi J, Silverberg MS, Vermeire S, Colombel JF (2006) The Montreal classification of inflammatory bowel disease: controversies, consensus, and implications. Gut 55: 749–753.
9. McLachlan G, Peel D (2000) Finite Mixture Models; Series W, editor. New York: John Wiley & Sons. 456 p.
10. Hunt L, Jorgensen M (1999) Mixture Model clustering using the MULTIMIX program. Aust N Z J Stat 41: 154–171.
11. Hunt L, Jorgensen M (2003) Mixture model clustering for mixed data with missing information. Computational Statistics & Data Analysis 41: 429–440.
12. Wang K, Zhang H, Kugathasan S, Annese V, Bradfield JP, et al. (2009) Diverse genome-wide association studies associate the IL12/IL23 pathway with Crohn Disease. Am J Hum Genet 84: 399–405.
13. McGovern DP, Rotter JI, Mei L, Haritunians T, Landers C, et al. (2009) Genetic epistasis of IL23/IL17 pathway genes in Crohn's disease. Inflamm Bowel Dis 15: 883–889.
14. Rioux JD, Xavier RJ, Taylor KD, Silverberg MS, Goyette P, et al. (2007) Genome-wide association study identifies new susceptibility loci for Crohn disease and implicates autophagy in disease pathogenesis. Nat Genet 39: 596–604.
15. Parkes M, Barrett JC, Prescott NJ, Tremelling M, Anderson CA, et al. (2007) Sequence variants in the autophagy gene IRGM and multiple other replicating loci contribute to Crohn's disease susceptibility. Nat Genet 39: 830–832.
16. Hugot JP, Chamaillard M, Zouali H, Lesage S, Cezard JP, et al. (2001) Association of NOD2 leucine-rich repeat variants with susceptibility to Crohn's disease. Nature 411: 599–603.
17. Ogura Y, Bonen DK, Inohara N, Nicolae DL, Chen FF, et al. (2001) A frameshift mutation in NOD2 associated with susceptibility to Crohn's disease. Nature 411: 603–606.
18. Duerr RH, Taylor KD, Brant SR, Rioux JD, Silverberg MS, et al. (2006) A genome-wide association study identifies IL23R as an inflammatory bowel disease gene. Science 314: 1461–1463.
19. Weersma RK, Stokkers PC, van Bodegraven AA, van Hogezand RA, Verspaget HW, et al. (2009) Molecular prediction of disease risk and severity in a large Dutch Crohn's disease cohort. Gut 58: 388–395.
20. Vasiliauskas EA, Kam LY, Karp LC, Gaiennie J, Yang H, et al. (2000) Marker antibody expression stratifies Crohn's disease into immunologically homogeneous subgroups with distinct clinical characteristics. Gut 47: 487–496.
21. Mow WS, Vasiliauskas EA, Lin YC, Fleshner PR, Papadakis KA, et al. (2004) Association of antibody responses to microbial antigens and complications of small bowel Crohn's disease. Gastroenterology 126: 414–424.

17

Genotype/Phenotype Analyses for 53 Crohn's Disease Associated Genetic Polymorphisms

Camille Jung[1,2,3], **Jean-Frédéric Colombel**[4], **Marc Lemann**[5], **Laurent Beaugerie**[6], **Matthieu Allez**[5], **Jacques Cosnes**[6], **Gwenola Vernier-Massouille**[4], **Jean-Marc Gornet**[5], **Jean-Pierre Gendre**[6], **Jean-Pierre Cezard**[3], **Frank M. Ruemmele**[7], **Dominique Turck**[8], **Françoise Merlin**[1,2], **Habib Zouali**[9], **Christian Libersa**[10], **Philippe Dieudé**[11], **Nadem Soufir**[12], **Gilles Thomas**[9], **Jean-Pierre Hugot**[1,2,3]*

1 Université Paris Diderot, UMR843, Paris, France, 2 UMR843, INSERM, Paris, France, 3 Service de Gastroentérologie Pédiatrique, Hôpital Robert Debré, APHP, Paris, France, 4 Service de Gastroentérologie, Hôpital Claude Huriez, Université de Lille, Lille, France, 5 Service de Gastroentérologie, Hôpital Saint-Louis, AP-HP, Université Paris- Diderot, Paris, France, 6 Department of Gastroenterology, Hôpital Saint-Antoine, AP-HP, and UPMC Univ Paris 06, Paris, France, 7 Université Paris Descartes and Service de Gastroentérologie Pédiatrique, Hôpital Necker Enfants-Malades, APHP, Paris, France, 8 Service de Gastroentérologie Pédiatrique, Hôpital Jeanne de Flandre, Université de Lille 2, Lille, France, 9 CEPH/Fondation Jean Dausset, Paris, France, 10 Centre D'Investigation Clinique 9301, Hôpital Cardiologique, INSERM, Lille, France, 11 Université Paris Diderot and Service de Rhumatologie, Hôpital Bichat, Paris, France, 12 Université Paris Diderot and Service de Biochimie Génétique, Hôpital Bichat, Paris, France

Abstract

Background & Aims: Recent studies reported a role for more than 70 genes or loci in the susceptibility to Crohn's disease (CD). However, the impact of these associations in clinical practice remains to be defined. The aim of the study was to analyse the relationship between genotypes and phenotypes for the main 53 CD-associated polymorphisms.

Method: A cohort of 798 CD patients with a median follow up of 7 years was recruited by tertiary adult and paediatric gastroenterological centres. A detailed phenotypic description of the disease was recorded, including clinical presentation, response to treatments and complications. The participants were genotyped for 53 CD-associated variants previously reported in the literature and correlations with clinical sub-phenotypes were searched for. A replication cohort consisting of 722 CD patients was used to further explore the putative associations.

Results: The *NOD2* rare variants were associated with an earlier age at diagnosis (p = 0.0001) and an ileal involvement (OR = 2.25[1.49–3.41] and 2.77 [1.71–4.50] for rs2066844 and rs2066847, respectively). Colonic lesions were positively associated with the risk alleles of *IL23R* rs11209026 (OR = 2.25 [1.13–4.51]) and 6q21 rs7746082 (OR = 1.60 [1.10–2.34] and negatively associated with the risk alleles of *IRGM* rs13361189 (OR = 0.29 [0.11–0.74]) and *DEFB1* rs11362 (OR = 0.50 [0.30–0.80]). The *ATG16L1* and *IRGM* variants were associated with a non-inflammatory behaviour (OR = 1.75 [1.22–2.53] and OR = 1.50 [1.04–2.16] respectively). However, these associations lost significance after multiple testing corrections. The protective effect of the *IRGM* risk allele on colonic lesions was the only association replicated in the second cohort (p = 0.03).

Conclusions: It is not recommended to genotype the studied polymorphisms in routine practice.

Editor: Nathan A. Ellis, University of Illinois at Chicago, United States of America

Funding: This work was financially supported by the Ministère de la Santé (PHRC n°P010904), Assistance-Publique Hôpitaux de Paris APHP, Institut National de la Recherche Scientifique (INSERM), Universités Paris Denis-Diderot, Paris Pierre et Marie-Curie, Paris René-Descartes and Lille 2 droit et santé, Agence Nationale de la Recherche (ANR), fondation Jean Dausset/CEPH, the Centre National de Génotypage (CNG), Société Nationale Française de Gastroentérologie, Fondation pour la Recherche Médicale and the Association François Aupetit. The funders had no role in study design, data collection and analysis, decision to publish, or preparation of the manuscript.

Competing Interests: The authors have declared that no competing interests exist.

* E-mail: jean-pierre.hugot@rdb.aphp.fr

Introduction

Crohn's disease (CD) is a complex genetic disorder resulting from the interplay between environmental and genetic risk factors. To date, more than 70 genes or loci have been associated with the susceptibility to CD, each with a small individual effect on disease risk [1–20]. A strong overlap with genes predisposing to ulcerative colitis was found among them [21]. The identified genes belong to several biological pathways including bacterial recognition/innate immunity/autophagy (*NOD2*, *ATG16L1*, *IRGM*), adaptative immunity (*IL23R*, *CCR6*, *IL12B*, *JAK2*, *STAT3*) and inflammatory response (*TNFSF15*, *PTPN2*). For some associated genes, there is no clear established role (*ZNF365*, *CCNY*), and even some CD-associated polymorphisms are located in gene desert regions.

CD is a heterogeneous disorder with different clinical presentations. The disease may occur at any point from childhood to old age, and some CD cases require surgery and/or immunosuppressive therapy while others are characterized by rare relapses that are easily treated with anti-inflammatory drugs. Complications such as severe colitis, strictures and fistulas are common but not constant. Finally, the responses to treatments vary between patients. Unfortunately, to date, only limited parameters are available to define the early clinical course of CD [22]. As a result, some patients can be undertreated while others can be exposed to the side effects of drugs without clear benefit.

Genetic factors can be regarded as good candidates for classifying patients in terms of disease location, severity, complications, extra-intestinal manifestations and drug response/toxicity. The impact of *NOD2* mutations has been extensively studied and its associations with a young age of onset, an ileal location and complicated behaviours are well established. However, *NOD2* status is not sufficient by itself to influence clinical practice [23,24]. Less consistent associations have been reported for other CD susceptibility genes, but again no recommendations have been formulated (for a review see [24]). In contrast, a few studies have investigated a large number of CD susceptibility alleles with special attention being paid to clinical items able to impact upon clinical practice. Henckaerts et al. identified positive associations between rs1363670 (close to *IL12B*), rs12704036 (in a gene desert region) and rs 6908425 (*CDKAL1*) polymorphisms and disease behaviour [25]. However, these results remain to be confirmed. The aim of this study was to further investigate 53 CD-associated variants in a large cohort of CD patients with detailed medical records in order to determine the genotype/phenotype relationships.

Subjects and Methods

Ethic Statements

The study received approval from the French national ethic committee (Hôpital Saint Louis, Paris, France) and all participants signed an informed consent form.

Patients

Six paediatric and adult gastroenterology tertiary centres recruited 798 CD cases as defined by the Lennard-Jones criteria [26]. The patients were included if the diagnosis of CD was made at least one year before inclusion and if they had attended continuous follow-up visits in the reference centres. More than 94% of the patients included had European origins while the others mainly originated from North Africa. The replication cohort consisted of 722 familial CD cases recruited through a European consortium [3]. A panel of 960 healthy blood donors without personal or familial history of inflammatory disorders [27] was also genotyped to evaluate the association of the studied SNPs with CD in the French population.

Phenotypic Data Recorded

Clinical, endoscopic, radiological and histological data were retrospectively collected on a standardized questionnaire by clinical research assistants, validated by the referring expert gastroenterologists of the patients and reviewed by the data managers of the study. The load factor of each item was up to 95%. In order to validate the quality of the data, the outlier values were searched for and verified and a sample of 200 questionnaires was checked twice. The items recorded included sex, date of birth, smoking habits (patients were classed as smokers in the case of any smoking habit) and presence of granulomas. Familial history of Inflammatory Bowel Diseases (IBD) was defined by a reported diagnosis of IBD in one or more first or second degree relatives.

The involvement of the digestive tract was registered at diagnosis and at the end of follow-up (cumulative locations) for the esophagus, stomach, duodenum, jejunum, proximal ileum, distal ileum, colon and rectum. Involvement was defined by macroscopic lesions. Disease behaviour' was classified according to the Montreal classification at last follow-up (B1: non-stricturing,

non penetrating disease; B2: stenosing behavior, B3 penetrating disease excluding perianal disease).

The use, response and side effects were recorded for corticosteroids, azathioprine/6-mercapopurine, methotrexate, infliximab and enteral feeding. Steroid exposure was classified as being mild (less than 2 months per year), moderate or frequent (more than 6 months per year). Patients who relapsed when the steroid dosage was tapered or within 3 months after treatment ended were defined as steroid dependent. There is no consensus definition of steroid resistance [28] and patients who showed no response after 2 weeks of full steroid doses (at least 1 mg/kg/d in children and 60 mg/d in adults) were defined as corticosteroid resistant. For the other drugs, treatment failure was determined by the IBD gastroenterologist. Indications of surgery were classed as follows: penetrating complications, stenosing disease, failure of medical treatment and anal surgery. Total gut resection was classified as major resection (total colectomy or small bowel resection >50 cm), limited resection or no resection. Proctologic surgery included all surgical procedures for perianal CD performed under general anaesthesia and with therapeutic actions.

Malnutrition (defined by a loss of two standard deviations on the weight curve in children or by the need of artificial nutrition in adults), bleeding requiring blood transfusion, severe colonic attacks and extra-intestinal manifestations were noted. Patients were classified as never hospitalized (excluding the initial diagnosis procedure and single day hospitalizations), frequently hospitalized (more than once a year) or intermediate. The evolution types were defined as frank relapses and remissions; chronic continuous evolution and other.

Genotyping

All patients and controls were genotyped for 53 reported CD susceptibility Single Nucleotide Polymorphisms (SNPs, Table 1) using an AB17900HT Sequence detection system Illumina GoldenGate assay (Illumina, San Diego, CA) by the Centre National de Génotypage (CNG, Evry, France) or by the Integragen company (Evry, France). This set of SNPs was retained on the basis of the available literature and corresponded to the 50 SNPs with the highest published OR and the three main *NOD2* associated variants. The genotyping rate of each SNP was higher than 90% (Table 1). All genotyped SNPs were in Hardy-Weinberg equilibrium in patients and in controls. No major discrepancies were observed between our calculated allele frequencies and those published in the SNP database. For rs916977, we observed a minor allele frequency of 0.25, whereas the published estimates varied between 0.13 and 0.42. The at-risk alleles were defined as the alleles previously associated with CD in the literature. For clarity, the nucleotides defining the risk alleles are indicated in table 1 and between brackets in the text.

Statistical Analyses

Qualitative variables were described in percentages and quantitative variables were described by their median with interquartile ranges (Q1–Q3). Comparisons of qualitative variables were performed using the Chi-square or Fisher's exact tests (when n<5 in the χ^2 contingency table). Comparisons of medians were performed using the Kruskal-Wallis or Mann-Whitney tests. The Odds-Ratio (OR) values were calculated using the logistic regression method in the univariate and multivariate analyses. Multivariate analyses took into account all of the risk factors associated (P<0.05) with the item studied in the univariate analyses, including the *NOD2* alleles. The cumulative incidences of first drug prescriptions and first surgery were drawn on Kaplan-Meier curves and compared using the log-rank test. The tests were

Table 1. Genetic polymorphisms studied.

SNP	chromosome	candidate genes	Major/Minor allele	risk allele	MAF (Controls)	MAF (CD)	p-value	OR	[CI 95%]	genotyping succes rate (%)
rs11209026 [4]	1p31	IL23R	G/A	G	0.08	0.02	1.94E-11	0.30	[0.20-0.43]	100
rs2476601 [2]	1p13	PTPN22	G/A	G	0.08	0.05	1.2E-03	0.62	[0.46-0.83]	99
rs2274910 [2]	1q23	ITLN1/CD244	C/T	C	0.34	0.31	1.9E-01	0.90	[0.77-1.05]	97
rs9286879 [2]	1q24	FASLG/TNFSF18/FNFSF4	A/G	G	0.26	0.3	2.1E-02	1.20	[1.02-1.41]	96
rs12035082 [7]	1q24	FASLG/TNFSF18/FNFSF4	C/T	T	0.45	0.46	2.7E-01	1.08	[0.94-1.24]	98
rs10801047 [6]	1q31	?	T/A	A	0.1	0.08	1.6E-01	0.83	[0.65-1.07]	98
rs11584383 [2]	1q32	C1orf106/KIF21B	T/C	T	0.24	0.23	5.5E-01	0.95	[0.80-1.12]	98
rs10733113 [14]	1q44	NLRP3	G/A	G	0.14	0.15	4.3E-01	1.08	[0.88-1.32]	98
rs2241880 [1]	2q37	ATG16L1	A/G	G	0.45	0.4	3.1E-03	0.80	[0.70-0.93]	98
rs3197999 [7]	3p21	MST1/GPX1/BSN	C/T	T	0.26	0.29	8.0E-02	1.15	[0.98-1.35]	94
rs16853571 [5]	4p12	PHOX2B	C/G	C	0.07	0.06	6.1E-01	0.93	[0.70-1.22]	98
rs17234657 [11]	5p13	PTGER4	T/G	G	0.12	0.15	1.4E-02	1.28	[1.05-1.56]	98
rs2631367 [9]	5q31	SCL22A4	G/C	C	0.49	0.55	1.0E-03	1.27	[1.10-1.47]	90
rs1050152 [9]	5q31	SCL22A5	C/T	T	0.43	0.48	3.6E-03	1.23	[1.07-1.42]	98
rs2188962 [2]	5q31	SLC22A4/A5. IRF1. IL3	C/T	T	0.43	0.48	3.0E-03	1.23	[1.07-1.42]	98
rs13361189 [6]	5q33	IRGM	T/C	C	0.13	0.18	6.6E-05	1.46	[1.21-1.77]	100
rs10045431 [2]	5q33	IL12B	C/A	C	0.28	0.25	3.6E-02	0.84	[0.71-0.99]	98
rs6908425 [2]	6p22	CDKAL1	C/T	C	0.21	0.19	0.15	0.89	[0.76-1.04]	97
rs7746082 [2]	6q21	PRDM1	G/C	C	0.25	0.28	9.3E-02	1.15	[0.97-1.35]	97
rs2301436 [2]	6q27	CCR6	G/C	C	0.47	0.48	0.32	1.07	[0.94-1.21]	98
rs1456893 [2]	7p12	IKZF1/ZPBP/FIGNL1	A/G	G	0.3	0.29	5.2E-01	0.95	[0.81-1.11]	98
rs2160322 [20]	7q21	MAGI2	C/G	C	0.39	0.36	8.4E-02	0.88	[0.76-1.01]	97
rs4728142 [17]	7q32	IRF5	G/A	A	0.43	0.43	8.5E-01	1.01	[0.87-1.17]	98
rs11362 [16]	8p23	DEFB1	G/A	G	0.42	0.42				98
rs1551398 [2]	8q24	?	A/G	A	0.42	0.39	4.7E-02	0.86	[0.74-0.99]	98
rs10758669 [2]	9p24	JAK2	A/C	C	0.35	0.38	9.6E-02	1.13	[0.97-1.31]	98
rs4263839 [2]	9q32	TNFSF15	G/A	G	0.31	0.27	1.7E-02	0.82	[0.70-0.96]	96
rs3936503 [7]	10p11	CCNY	G/A	A	0.35	0.28				98
rs17582416 [2]	10p11	CREM	T/G	G	0.33	0.4	7.6E-05	1.35	[1.16-1.57]	98
rs224136 [5]	10q21	ZNF365	A/G	A	0.49	0.54	3.8E-01	0.92	[0.77-1.10]	98
rs107161659 [7,8]	10q21	?	C/T	C	0.18	0.17	1.1E-02	1.20	[1.04-1.39]	99
rs1248696 [10]	10q23	DLG5	C/T	T	0.08	0.09	2.7E-01	1.14	[0.89-1.45]	98
rs10883365 [6]	10q24	NKX2-3	A/G	G	0.49	0.46	0.08	0.88	[0.77-1.01]	98
rs3814570 [15]	10q25	TCF7L2	C/T	T	0.28	0.24	1.5E-02	0.81	[0.69-0.96]	98

Table 1. Cont.

SNP	chromosome	candidate genes	Major/Minor allele	risk allele	MAF (Controls)	MAF (CD)	p-value	OR	[CI 95%]	genotyping succes rate (%)
rs1793004 [13]	11p15	NELL1	G/C	G	0.26	0.26	7.7E–01	1.02	[0.87–1.19]	98
rs7927894 [2]	11q13	C11orf30	C/T	T	0.36	0.42	**1.3E–03**	**1.27**	**[1.10–1.48]**	91
rs11175593 [2]	12q12	LRRK2/MUC19	C/T	T	0.02	0.03	1.3E–01	1.36	[0.91–2.03]	99
rs3764147 [2]	13q14	C13orf31	A/G	G	0.24	0.27	1.1E–01	1.14	[0.97–1.34]	98
rs916977 [7]	15q13	HERC2	G/A	A	0.3	0.25	**2.6E–03**	**0.78**	**[0.66–0.91]**	98
rs2066844 [3]	16q12	NOD2	C/T	T	0.07	0.14	**2.14E–11**	**2.17**	**[1.72–2.72]**	98
rs2066845 [3]	16q12	NOD2	G/C	C	0.01	0.05	**2.6E–07**	**2.71**	**[1.82–4.02]**	97
rs2066847 [3]	16q12	NOD2	0/insC	C	0.02	0.11	**1.3E–26**	**5.30**	**[3.78–7.42]**	97
rs8050910 [2]	16q24	FAM92B	T/G	G	0.41	0.4	4.2E–01	0.94	[0.81–1.09]	96
rs2872507 [2]	17q21	ORMDL3/GSMDL/ZPBP2/IKZF3	G/A	A	0.41	0.45	**4.0E–02**	**1.16**	**[1.00–1.34]**	95
rs744166 [2]	17q21	STAT3/MLX	A/G	A	0.42	0.41	3.8E–01	0.93	[0.81–1.08]	96
rs2542151 [2]	18p11	PTPN2	T/G	G	0.15	0.15	8.8E–01	1.01	[0.83–1.22]	98
rs2305767 [19]	19p13	MYO9B	T/C	T	0.42	0.41	4.0E–01	0.94	[0.81–1.08]	98
rs2315008 [12]	20q13	TNFRSF6B	C/A	C	0.28	0.26	1.6E–01	0.89	[0.75–1.04]	98
rs1736135 [2]	21q21	?	T/C	T	0.45	0.41	**2.1E–02**	**0.84**	**[0.73–0.97]**	97
rs762421 [2]	21q22	ICOSLG	A/G	G	0.35	0.4	**1.7E–02**	**1.19**	**[1.03–1.38]**	96
rs2836878 [12]	21q22	PSMG1	C/T	C	0.25	0.25	0.90	0.99	[0.85–1.14]	98
rs35873774 [18]	22q12	XBP1	A/C	T	0.04	0.04	6.8E–01	1.07	[0.77–1.49]	98
rs4821544 [5]	22q13	NCF4	T/C	C	0.33	0.38	**4.8E–03**	**1.23**	**[1.06–1.42]**	98

The minor and major alleles are derived from public databases. Significant associations (p<0.05) are in bold. SNP: Single Nucleotide Polymorphism. MAF: minor allele frequency. CD: Crohn's Disease. OR: Odds Ratio; CI: Confidence interval.

done for each (at-risk or protective) allele of each tested marker corresponding to a recessive/dominant model of inheritance. For *NOD2*, the three rare alleles (corresponding to independent mutations) were also analyzed jointly. Statistical analyses were performed using STATA 10 statistical software (Stata Corporation, College Station, Texas, USA).

The power of the cohort to detect an association depends on the respective frequencies of the sub-phenotypes tested and of the risk alleles in the subgroups compared. As an example, the cohort was powerful enough to detect an association with an OR of 1.5 between complicated and inflammatory behaviours for risk allele frequencies ranging from 0.3 to 0.7 in the reference group ($\alpha = 0.05$; $\beta = 0.8$). We report here a comprehensive overview of the most relevant positive tests with a nominal p-value lower than 0.05, with special attention paid to items exploring the Montreal classification, the responses to treatments and severity of the disease. For this study, we explored many phenotypic items for 53 markers and we thus performed several hundred statistical tests. These tests were not always independent but the coefficient for applying the Bonferroni correction needed to be higher than 500.

Under these conditions, only strong associations could remain significant. For this reason, associations with nominal p-values lower than 0.05 were further tested in the replication cohort no matter what their corrected P-values.

Results

Case-control Analyses

The allele frequencies of the 53 SNPs tested were compared between cases and controls. We confirmed an association between CD and 26 independent SNPs (Table 1). As expected, the most significant associations were observed for the CD susceptibility alleles with the highest reported OR, i.e. the *NOD2* mutations and the rare *IL23R* protective allele.

Sex, Family History, Tobacco Use and Age of Onset

The description of the exploratory cohort is shown in Table 2 and Table S1. The median duration of follow-up was 7 years (Q1–Q3: 4–12.5). The significant results are summarized in Table 3. The sex ratio was not altered by the SNPs tested. The *IL23R*

Table 2. Main characteristics of the cohorts of Crohn's Disease patients.

	Exploratory cohort (n = 798)		Replication cohort (n = 722)	
	Gender and age at diagnosis			
Gender	**Female: 56.7%**		**Female: 53.7%**	
Median age at diagnosis (1st and 3rd quartiles)	22 years (17–29)		22 years (16–30)	
	Location of the disease			
	At diagnosis	At follow-up	At diagnosis	At follow up
Upper digestive tract	14.5%	22%	16.2%	17.3%
Terminal ileum (TI)	70.7%	80.9%	73.3%	78%
Colon (including rectum)	73.7%	82.5%	71.2%	77%
Small bowel (excluding TI)	5.4%	10.4%	6.9%	11.6%
Rectum	31.5%	48.2%	25.2%	32.2%
Penetrating perianal disease	33.1%		32.9%	
	Behavior of the disease			
	At follow-up		At follow-up	
Inflammatory behavior (B1)	43.8%		29.7%	
Stricturing behavior (B2)	31.3%		22.7%	
Penetrating behaviour (B3)	24.8%		47.6%	
	Extra-digestive manifestations (at diagnosis)			
	22%		28.7%	
	Treatments			
Surgery	51.4%		55.7%	
Corticosteroids	90%		76.2%	
Immunosupressants (AZA+ MTX)	74.1%		37.4%	
Infliximab	24.9%		6.3%	
Nutritional therapy	14.2%		28.4%	
	Smoking habits (at the time of recruitment)			
Never	45.3%		52.8%	
Ex-smoker	29%		15.2%	
Current smoker	25.7%		32%	
	Familial history of IBD			
	16.9%		100%	

Table 3. Most significant results of the genotype/phenotype analyses obtained with the exploratory cohort.

best candidate susceptibility gene	polymorphism	associated allele	associated sub-phenotype	Nominal P-Value	Odds Ratio
NOD2	rs2066845	at risk allele	family history of IBD	0.034	OR = 1.80 [1.04–3.12]
NOD2	rs2066844	at risk allele	early age of onset	0.0001	NA
NOD2	rs2066845	at risk allele	early age of onset	0.0026	NA
NOD2	rs2066844	at risk allele	ileal disease	0.0001	OR = 2.25 [1.49–3.41]
NOD2	rs2066847	at risk allele	ileal disease	0.0001	OR = 2.77 [1.71–4.50]
NOD2	two SNPs versus none	at risk allele	non inflammatory disease	0.031	OR = 1.68 [1.04–2.69]
NOD2	rs2066847	protective allele	steroid dependance	0.04	OR = 0.36 [0.15–0.84]
NOD2	rs2066847	protective allele	earlier treatment with AZA	0.039	NA
NOD2	rs2066845	protective allele	earlier treatment with MTX	0.03	NA
NOD2	two SNPs versus none	at risk allele	surgery for penetrating disease	0.007	OR = 1.94 [1.19–3.15]
NOD2	two SNPs versus none	at risk allele	surgery for stenosing disease	0.005	OR = 1.90 [1.21–3.00]
NOD2	two SNPs versus none	protective	penetrating perianal disease	0.001	OR = 0.41 [0.24–0.67]
NOD2	two SNPs versus none	at risk allele	malnutrition	0.0001	OR = 3.21 [1.69–6.07]
IL23R	rs11209026	protective allele	family history of IBD	0.002	OR = 0.32 [0.15–0.64]
IL23R	rs11209026	at risk allele	colonic disease	0.021	OR = 2.25 [1.13–4.51]
IL23R	rs11209026	at risk allele	earlier surgery	0.031	NA
IL23R	rs11209026	protective allele	severe colonic attacks	0.009	OR = 0.16 [0.04–0.63]
DEFB1	rs11362	protective	colonic disease	0.004	OR = 0.50 [0.30–0.80]
DEFB1	rs11362	at risk allele	non inflammatory disease	0.007	OR = 1.73 [1.16–2.67]
DEFB1	rs11362	protective allele	severe colonic attacks	0.007	OR = 0.32 [0.14–0.74]
IRGM	rs13361189	protective	colonic disease	0.01	OR = 0.29 [0.11–0.74]
IRGM	rs13361189	at risk allele	non inflammatory disease	0.028	OR = 1.50 [1.04–2.16]
ATG16L1	rs2241880	at risk allele	non inflammatory disease	0.002	OR = 1.75 [1.22–2.53]
CDKAL1	rs6908425	at risk allele	better response rate to AZA/IFX	0.001	OR = 0.45 [0.29–0.71]
PTPN22	rs2476601	at risk allele	ileal disease	0.006	OR = 2.65 [1.32–5.30]
CCNY	rs3936503	at risk allele	better response rate to AZA/IFX	0.046	OR = 3.14 [1.02–9.71]
6q21	rs7746082	at risk allele	colonic disease	0.014	OR = 1.60 [1.10–2.34]
10q21	rs224136	at risk allele	better response rate to AZA/IFX	0.006	OR = 2.12 [1.24–3.65]

AZA = azathioprine. IFX = infliximab. NA: not applicable.

protective (A) allele and the *NOD2* (C) risk allele rs2066845 were associated with a positive family history of inflammatory bowel disease (Table 3). No differences were observed between smoking groups, arguing against a gene-environment interaction. As previously reported, patients with at least one *NOD2* variant had an earlier onset of disease (Table 3). No relationships were found between age at onset (or at diagnosis) and any other SNP.

Disease Location

For *NOD2*, the risk alleles rs2066844 (T) and rs2066847 (C) were associated with the involvement of the distal ileum. Patients carrying at least two *NOD2* mutations and with pure colonic disease were extremely rare (n = 3). The risk allele (G) of *PTPN22* (rs2476601) was associated with ileal lesions. Colonic disease (including rectum) was associated with the risk alleles of *IL23R* (G) and the chromosome 6q21 locus (T) and with the protective alleles of *IRGM* (T) and *DEFB1* (A). Analyzes performed on the bases of the Montreal classification system for disease location confirmed the associations obtained for each anatomical site but with lower P-values. After multivariate analysis, only *IL23R* and *DEFB1* remained associated with colonic disease. None of the at-risk alleles were associated with the presence of granulomas.

Behaviour

As previously reported, patients with two *NOD2* mutations more frequently had non-inflammatory disease behaviour at diagnosis compared to patients with wild-type *NOD2*. The risk alleles of *ATG16L1* (G), *IRGM* (C) *and DEFB1* (G) were also associated with a non-inflammatory behaviour (B2+B3). These associations remained significant after multivariate analysis, suggesting that these genes acted independently to modulate disease behaviour.

Medications

It was found that 52% of the patients were steroid-dependant and 12.5% were cortico-resistant. No associations were found with time of first steroid therapy, response to treatment or steroid exposure. The patients received an immunomodulatory treatment in 74% of cases. Patients who carried the *NOD2* protective allele rs2066847 (no insertion) (respectively rs2066845, (G)) received azathioprine treatment (respectively methotrexate) earlier (p: 0.04 respectively p: 0.03). Nevertheless, these associations disappeared when the three *NOD2* mutations were taken into account. The CD risk alleles of the *CCNY* (A), *CDKAL1* (C) and 10q21 (C) loci were weakly associated with a better response to immunosupressors

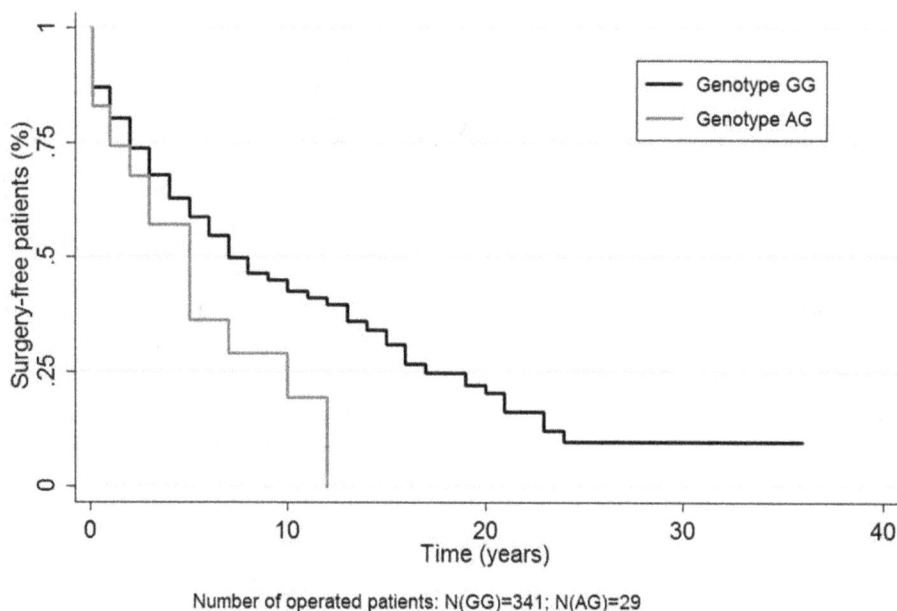

Number of operated patients: N(GG)=341; N(AG)=29

Figure 1. Time of the first non proctologic surgery according to IL23R rs11209026 genotype. Log Rank: P = 0.03.

and/or infliximab (Table 3). Multivariate logistic regression confirmed an association with *CDKAL1* and the 10q21 risk allele (OR = 2,70[4,54–1,61] and OR = 2,39[1,36–4,18], respectively). No association was found in multivariate analysis for the response to infliximab therapy.

Surgery

The time of first non proctologic surgery did not depend on any of the SNPs tested except for the *IL23R* risk allele (G) (log-rank, p = 0.031; Fig. 1). When the analyses were performed on the subgroup of patients with pure colonic disease, the *IL23R* protective allele (A) was also predictive of an earlier surgery (log-rank, p = 0.007). Patients who carried two *NOD2* mutations had a less frequent incidence of perforating perianal disease (p = 0.001) but they were more frequently operated on for penetrating or occlusive disease. However, after adjustment for ileal location, these latter associations did not remain significant.

Complications

Malnutrition was observed in 8.8% (n = 69) of patients at the time of diagnosis and in 10.7% (n = 84) at the end of follow-up. Patients who carried two *NOD2* mutations were more frequently exposed to this complication at diagnosis. This association was restricted to patients with ileal disease (9% for wild-type homozygotes vs. 28.3% for mutated patients, p = 0.0001) and remained significant in the subgroup of adult-CD onset. Severe colonic attacks were less frequent in patients who were homozygous for the at-risk alleles of *IL23R* (1.5% for genotype AA vs. 8.3% for genotype AG, p = 0.025) or *DEFB1* (6.3% for genotype GG vs. 0% for genotype AA, p = 0.005). No consistent associations were found with arthritis, arthralgias, mouth ulcers, cutaneous or ocular manifestations, ankylosing spondylitis, psoriasis or primary sclerosing cholangitis. No association was found with evolution type or frequency of hospitalization.

Replication Study

As anticipated, none of the above reported associations remained statistically significant after multiple testing corrections.

Therefore, we tested their relevance in the replication cohort. Because the impact of *NOD2* mutations on disease presentation was extensively studied previously (including patients from the replication cohort [28]), we only focused on the other 50 genetic markers. The exploratory and replication cohorts were not completely the same (Table 2). The main differences can be explained by the fact that the replication cohort included older patients (date of birth Q1–Q2–Q3: 1954–1967–1975 versus 1963–1972–1980, p<0.0001) with, on average, a longer follow-up (11 years). For these patients, the clinical use of immunosuppressants and biotherapies was less generalized. When comparing the patients within this cohort, we only confirmed that the risk allele (C) at rs13361189 of *IRGM* was less frequently encountered in cases of colonic disease at onset (p = 0.03).

Discussion

Genetic studies have recently identified a large number of susceptibility genes that play a role in the predisposition to CD. The aim of this work was to assess the clinical utility of these genetic associations in routine practice. This is an important issue for the development of personalized medicine in which the genetic profile of an individual patient would help to choose optimal treatment strategies.

We analysed the clinical course of 798 CD patients from referring paediatric and adult gastroenterology centres in detail. These centres treat patients with the most severe form of the disease, as shown by the comparison between the description of the current cohort and population-based studies [29]. For example, whereas approximately only half of the patients with CD received steroid therapy at some point in the disease course and a third had steroid dependency in the population-based studies, 90% of the patients in our cohort were treated by steroids and more than 50% were steroid dependant [29]. The participant centres were used to follow the international guidelines for CD management. However, differences between therapeutic practices were likely present considering that we saw differences in the proportion of patients having received steroids, immunosuppressors or surgery. However, if this heterogeneity between centres may affect disease behaviour, its impact on the here tested genotype/phenotype relationships is difficult to measure.

We studied the CD susceptibility alleles available at the time of genotyping and corresponding to the 50 alleles with the highest OR (in addition to the most common *NOD2* alleles). As shown by the case-control study, a large number of the alleles tested were positively associated with CD in our French cohort of patients, reinforcing their role in CD susceptibility. However, some alleles were not found to be associated with CD. This likely reflects the limited power of our case-control study when compared to the large meta-analyses required for identifying associations with the studied SNPs. However, some previously published CD-susceptibility alleles were not replicated, even in large cohorts of patients [19], suggesting that, in some cases, these SNPs do not indicate susceptibility to CD in all patient samples. In contrast, new SNPs have recently been added to the long list of CD susceptibility alleles [19] and additional SNPs will certainly follow. This work is thus limited by the knowledge available at the time of designing the study. However, it explored a panel of markers large enough to be representative of CD susceptibility genes. This panel contains the alleles that exhibit the strongest associations with CD. Another limitation of the study is that, except for *NOD2*, *IL23R*, *IRGM* and *ATG16L1*, CD-causing mutations have not yet been firmly established and thus the "genetic markers" tested might indirectly reflect the true causative alleles of the biological effects. However, recent in-depth sequencing of the best candidate genes does not argue for additional mutations with a larger effect in the studied candidate genes [30,31].

The first cohort was exploratory in nature. It was used to search for putative associations that could be relevant for clinical practice, and many items of disease presentation were explored. Under these conditions, the power of the cohort to detect relevant associations should be questioned. The cohort was comparable to the cohorts followed in medium-sized adult and paediatric IBD centres. It was thus supposed to be a good tool for exploring what is relevant for "real-life". In terms of power calculations, the cohort was large enough to detect an OR as low as 1.5 for the most common sub-phenotypes. This is in the range of what is expected to have a clinical impact. However, it is noteworthy that for less frequent sub-phenotypes (e.g. cancer or some extra-intestinal manifestations) and/or the less frequent polymorphisms, larger cohorts are required to efficiently explore this matter. In those situations, specific works focusing on specific genotype/phenotype relationships will be required, likely through large international consortia.

The exploratory cohort contained mainly Caucasian people from Europe (94%) or North Africa. Genetic heterogeneity may affect case-control studies. It is less clear that it may also affect genotype/phenotype correlation studies looking for phenotype modulating alleles. However, we performed the main analyzes again, excluding the patients with non-European ancestry. These analyzes did not significant change our conclusions (data not shown).

As previously published, the three *NOD2* SNPs were associated with ileal location and young age at onset [23,32–35]. However, we did not significantly extend the spectrum of *NOD2* associated-items, confirming the conclusion that *NOD2* genotyping only has a limited impact in routine practice [25]. Among the other 50 CD susceptibility alleles studied, only a few of them were associated with some of the clinical items in the first cohort. Considering that *NOD2* is the CD susceptibility gene with the strongest effect on the phenotype, this observation suggests that genetic markers with a

more limited role in CD risk may also have a limited impact on clinical presentation.

Even if some nominally significant associations were found with the first cohort, their number, nature and strength did not argue for their usefulness in clinical practice. In addition, after multiple testing corrections, none of these associations remained significant. Consequently, they would be seen by chance only. However, to better understand the significance of tests with a nominal P-value <0.05, we used a replication cohort. The replication cohort had a power comparable to the exploratory cohort but it contained familial cases only while the exploratory cohort mainly contained sporadic cases. Noteworthy, the genetic predisposition to familial and sporadic CD is the same with only limited differences observed for *NOD2* and *IL23R* (see above). In addition, there is no reason to suppose that genes involved in the modulation of CD phenotype are different in sporadic and familial CD. Thus the impact of the differences between cohorts, if any, should be limited. As a final result, we concluded that, individually, the newly identified risk alleles associated with CD do not notably contribute to the definition of clinical subgroups of patients.

In the literature, the *ATG16L1* risk allele has been inconsistently associated with ileal location, penetrating diseases and early onset [36–42]. We found a non-replicated association between *ATG16L1* and complicated disease behaviours. A modest association between rs4958847 of *IRGM* – which is partially correlated with rs13361189– and fistulizing behaviour/perianal fistulas has been reported [43]. The current study reports an association between the at-risk allele of rs13361189 with disease behaviour (in the first cohort) and an association between its protective allele and colonic disease at onset (in both cohorts). The last finding is in accordance with recent publications [44] but not with other ones [45,46]. It is thus difficult to definitively retain it. Finally, even if true, this association would have only a limited impact in practice.

Most studies failed to show an association between *IL23R* and CD subphenotypes [24,41,47–51]. We found here positive associations in the first cohort but failed to reproduce them in the replication cohort. An association between the risk allele of rs11362 located in the 5′-UTR of *DEFB1* and colonic location has been published [14]. In the first cohort the *DEFB1* protective allele was inversely associated with colonic location and severe colonic relapse, whereas it was positively associated with complicated behaviours. Finally, in a previous comparable exploratory study performed on 875 CD patients, Henckaerts et al. reported associations between rs1363670 at the *IL12B* locus and a stricturing behaviour; between rs12704036 on chromosome 5q and an early penetrating behaviour and between rs6908425 in *CDKAL1* and perianal fistulas [25]. The associations obtained here were not seen in this former study while we failed to replicate Henckaerts' results. As a whole, the comparison of our data and the literature further confirms the fact that associations between CD risk alleles and clinical sub-phenotypes are inconsistent (except for *NOD2*).

The prediction of responses to treatment is an important issue for the clinician. Unfortunately, no associations between the SNPs tested and responses to treatment and/or side effects could be obtained. The prediction of disease severity (at its best at the time of diagnosis) would also be welcome in order to propose personalized therapeutic options and to avoid rapid disease progression. As an example, a top-down strategy could be proposed to patients who are genetically at risk of developing a disabling disease while other patients with a lower risk of developing a severe course could be treated with the classic step-up strategy [52]. The definition of a severe or disabling disease is not consensual and there is a lack of validated parameters for exploring this issue [52,53]. We thus explored a large number of clinical parameters including disease behaviour, the presence of severe colonic attacks, malnutrition, extra-intestinal manifestations, time and indications of surgery, cumulative bowel resection, and the time and use of different medications, amongst others. We also looked at the type of evolution and the frequency of hospitalization. Finally, we approached this question using a visual analogue score of severity provided by the referring clinicians of the patients (data not shown). No matter what parameter was tested, we failed to identify a relevant association between severe outcome and any of the CD susceptibility genes.

If a single allele does not predict the phenotype, it is possible that a combination of genetic variants could impact disease clinical presentation. With the exception of *NOD2* variants, no allele dosage effects were observed for any of the allele tested. The exact mechanisms by which the CD susceptibility genes contribute to this disease is not known, but many of these genes are involved in two main biological functions: i) innate immunity, including bacterial recognition and killing and ii) the Th17 pathway and inflammation. It is thus tempting to imagine an epistatic interaction between the genes involved in the same (respectively complementary) biological functions. We tested this hypothesis using the logistic regression method but we failed to identify an epistatic interaction between the genetic variants involved in innate and/or adaptive immunity in the main disease subphenotypes (data not shown). This negative result may reflect a lack of statistical power but it is in accordance with other studies that also failed to find gene-gene interactions in the susceptibility to CD [33,36,37,40,47].

It is worth noting that if CD-causing genes do not seem to play a key role in the clinical presentation of CD, the possibility that other genetic factors may contribute towards modulating the clinical presentation of the disease cannot be excluded. Indeed, disease-modifier genes might be different from disease-causing genes. A re-analysis of the large genome-wide association studies taking into account sub-phenotype classifications of the patients will help to resolve this important issue in the development of personalized medicine.

Acknowledgments

This work was done in collaboration with D. Zelenica, Centre National de Génotypage, A. Zaouche, E. Jacz-Aigrain, C. Alberti from Centre d'Investigation Clinique, hôpital Robert Debré. We thank J.Demolin and L.Chedouba for their technical assistance.

Author Contributions

Conceived and designed the experiments: CJ JFC ML LB MA JC JPC GT JPH. Performed the experiments: CJ JFC ML LB MA JC GVM JMG JPG JPC FMR DT FM HZ CL PD NS GT JPH. Analyzed the data: CJ JPH. Contributed reagents/materials/analysis tools: CJ JFC ML LB MA JC GVM JMG JPC FMR DT PD NS JPH. Wrote the paper: CJ JFC LB MA FMR JPH.

References

1. Hampe J, Franke A, Rosenstiel P, Till A, Teuber M, et al. (2007) A genome-wide association scan of nonsynonymous SNPs identifies a susceptibility variant for Crohn disease in ATG16L1. Nat Genet 39: 207–11.
2. Barrett JC, Hansoul S, Nicolae DL, Cho JH, Duerr RH, et al. (2008) Genome-wide association defines more than 30 distinct susceptibility loci for Crohn's disease. Nat Genet 40: 955–62.
3. Hugot JP, Chamaillard M, Zouali H, Lesage S, Cézard JP, et al. (2001) Association of NOD2 leucine-rich repeat variants with susceptibility to Crohn's disease. Nature 411: 599–603.
4. Duerr RH, Taylor KD, Brant SR, Rioux JD, Silverberg MS, et al. (2006) A genome-wide association study identifies IL23R as an inflammatory bowel disease gene. Science 314: 1461–3.
5. Rioux JD, Xavier RJ, Taylor KD, Silverberg MS, Goyette P, et al. (2007) Genome-wide association study identifies new susceptibility loci for Crohn disease and implicates autophagy in disease pathogenesis. Nat Genet 39: 596–604.
6. Parkes M, Barrett JC, Prescott NJ, Tremelling M, Anderson CA, et al. (2007) Sequence variants in the autophagy gene IRGM and multiple other replicating loci contribute to Crohn's disease susceptibility. Nat Genet 39: 830–2.
7. Peltekova VD, Wintle RF, Rubin LA, Amos CI, Huang Q, et al. (2004) Functional variants of OCTN cation transporter genes are associated with Crohn disease. Nat Genet 36: 471–5.
8. Stoll M, Corneliussen B, Costello CM, Waetzig GH, Mellgard B, et al. (2004) Genetic variation in DLG5 is associated with inflammatory bowel disease. Nat Genet 36: 476–80.
9. Libioulle C, Louis E, Hansoul S, Sandor C, Farnr F, et al. (2007) Novel Crohn disease locus identified by genome-wide association maps to a gene desert on 5p13.1 and modulates expression of PTGER4. PLoS Genet 3:e58.
10. Kugathasan S, Baldassano RN, Bradfield JP, Sleiman PM, Imielinski M, et al. (2008) Loci on 20q13 and 21q22 are associated with pediatric-onset inflammatory bowel disease. Nat Genet 40: 1211–5.
11. Franke A, Hampe J, Rosenstiel P, Becker C, Wagner F, et al. (2007) Systematic association mapping identifies NELL1 as a novel IBD disease gene. PLoS ONE 2:e691.
12. Villani AC, Lemire M, Fortin G, Louis E, Silverberg MS, et al. (2009) Common variants in the NLRP3 region contribute to Crohn's disease susceptibility. Nat Genet 41: 71–6.
13. Koslowski MJ, Kubler I, Chamaillard M, Schaeffeler E, Reinisch W, et al. (2009) Genetic variants of Wnt transcription factor TCF-4 (TCF7L2) putative promoter region are associated with small intestinal Crohn's disease. PLoS One 4: e4496.
14. Kocsis AK, Lakatos PL, Somogyvari, Fuszek P, Papp J, et al. (2008) Association of beta-defensin 1 single nucleotide polymorphisms with Crohn's disease. Scand J Gastroenterol 43: 299–307.
15. Dideberg V, Kristjansdottir G, Milani L, Libioulle C, Sigurdsson S, et al. (2007) An insertion-deletion polymorphism in the interferon regulatory Factor 5 (IRF5) gene confers risk of inflammatory bowel diseases. Hum Mol Genet 16: 3008–16.
16. Kaser A, Lee AH, Franke A, Glickman JN, Zeissig S, et al. (2008) XBP1 links ER stress to intestinal inflammation and confers genetic risk for human inflammatory bowel disease. Cell 134: 743–56.
17. Cooney R, Cummings JR, Pathan S, Beckly J, Geremia A, et al. (2009) Association between genetic variants in myosin IXB and Crohn's disease. Inflamm Bowel Dis 15: 1014–21.
18. McGovern DP, Taylor KD, Landers C, Derkowski C, Dutridge D, et al. (2009) MAGI2 genetic variation and inflammatory bowel disease. Inflamm Bowel Dis 15: 75–83.
19. Franke A, McGovern DP, Barrett JC, Wang K, Radford-Smith GL, et al. (2010) Genome-wide meta-analysis increases to 71 the number of confirmed Crohn's disease susceptibility loci. Nat Genet. 42: 1118–25.
20. McCarroll SA, Huett A, Kuballa P, Chilewski SD, Landry A, et al. (2008) Deletion polymorphism upstream of IRGM associated with altered IRGM expression and Crohn's disease. Nat Genet 40: 1107–12.
21. Franke A, Balschun T, Karlsen TH, Sventoraityte J, Nikolaus S, et al. (2008) Replication of signals from recent studies of Crohn's disease identifies previously unknown disease loci for ulcerative colitis. Nat Genet 40: 713–5.
22. Beaugerie L, Seksik P, Nion-Larmurier I, Gendre JP, Cosnes J (2006) Predictors of Crohn's disease. Gastroenterology 130: 650–6.
23. Lesage S, Zouali H, Cézard JP, Colombel JF, Belaiche J, et al. (2002) CARD15/NOD2 mutational analysis and genotype-phenotype correlation in 612 patients with Inflammatory Bowel Disease. Am J Hum Genet 70: 845–57.
24. Mascheretti S, Schreiber S (2005) Genetic testing in Crohn disease: utility in individualizing patient management. Am J Pharmacogenomics 5: 213–22.
25. Henckaerts L, Van Steen K, Verstreken I, Cleyden I, Franke A, et al. (2009) Genetic risk profiling and prediction of disease course in Crohn's disease patients. Clin Gastroenterol Hepatol. 7: 972–980.
26. Lennard-Jones JE (1989) Classification of inflammatory bowel disease. Scand J Gastroenterol Suppl 170: 2–6.
27. Guedj M, Bourillon A, Combadières C, Rodero M, Dieudé P, et al. (2008) Variants of the MATP/SLAC gene are oprotective for melanoma in the French population. Human Mutat 29: 1154–60.
28. Faubion WA Jr, Loftus EV Jr, Harmsen WS, Zinsmeister AR, Sandborn WJ (2001) The natural history of corticosteroid therapy for inflammatory bowel disease: a population-based study. Gastroenterology 121: 255–60.

29. Peyrin-Biroulet L, Loftus EV, Jr., Colombel JF, Sandborn W (2010) The natural history of adult Crohn's disease in population-based cohorts. Am J Gastroenterol 105: 289–97.

30. Momozawa Y, Mni M, Nakamura K, Coppieters W, Almer S, et al. (2011) Resequencing of positional candidates identifies low frequency IL23R coding variants protecting against inflammatory bowel disease. Nat Genet 43: 43–7.

31. Rivas MA, Beaudoin M, Gardet A, Stevens C, Sharma Y, et al. (2011) Deep resequencing of GWAS loci identifies independent rare variants associated with inflammatory bowel disease. Nat Genet 43: 1066–73.

32. Radford-Smith G, Pandeya N (2006) Associations between NOD2/CARD15 genotype and phenotype in Crohn's disease–Are we there yet? World J Gastroenterol 12: 7097–103.

33. Prescott NJ, Fisher SA, Franke A, Hampe J, Onnie CM, et al. (2007) A nonsynonymous SNP in ATG16L1 predisposes to ileal Crohn's disease and is independent of CARD15 and IBD5. Gastroenterology 132: 1665–71.

34. Seiderer J, Schnitzler F, Brand S, Staudinger T, Pfennig S, et al. (2006) Homozygosity for the CARD15 frameshift mutation 1007fs is predictive of early onset of Crohn's disease with ileal stenosis, entero-enteral fistulas, and frequent need for surgical intervention with high risk of re-stenosis. Scand J Gastroenterol 41: 1421–32.

35. Adler J, Rangwalla SC, Dwamena BA, Higgins PD (2011) The prognostic power of the NOD2 genotype for complicated Crohn's disease: a meta-analysis. Am J Gastroenterol 106: 699–712.

36. Fowler EV, Doecke J, Simms LA, Zhao ZZ, Webb PM et al. (2008) ATG16L1 T300A shows strong associations with disease subgroups in a large Australian IBD population: further support for significant disease heterogeneity. Am J Gastroenterol 103: 2519–26.

37. Cummings JR, Cooney R, Pathan S, Anderson CA, Barrett JC, et al. (2007) Confirmation of the role of ATG16L1 as a Crohn's disease susceptibility gene. Inflamm Bowel Dis 13: 941–6.

38. Baldassano RN, Bradfield JP, Monos DS, Kim CE, Glessner JT, et al. (2007) Association of the T300A non-synonymous variant of the ATG16L1 gene with susceptibility to paediatric Crohn's disease. Gut 56: 1171–3.

39. Van Limbergen J, Russell RK, Nimmo ER, Drummond HE, Smith L, et al. (2008) Autophagy gene ATG16L1 influences susceptibility and disease location but not childhood-onset in Crohn's disease in Northern Europe. Inflamm Bowel Dis 14: 338–46.

40. Latiano A, Palmieri O, Valvano MR, D'Inca R, Cucchiara S, et al. (2008) Replication of interleukin 23 receptor and autophagy-related 16-like 1 association in adult- and pediatric-onset inflammatory bowel disease in Italy. World J Gastroenterol 14: 4643–51.

41. Roberts RL, Gearry RB, Hollis-Moffatt JE, Miller AL, Reid J, et al. (2007) IL23R R381Q and ATG16L1 T300A are strongly associated with Crohn's disease in a study of New Zealand Caucasians with inflammatory bowel disease. Am J Gastroenterol 102: 2754–61.

42. Hancock L, Beckly J, Geremia A, Cooney R, Cummings F, et al. (2008) Clinical and molecular characteristics of isolated colonic Crohn's disease. Inflamm Bowel Dis 14: 1667–77.

43. Latiano A, Palmieri O, Cucchiara S, Castro M, D'Inca R, et al. (2009) Polymorphism of the IRGM gene might predispose to fistulizing behavior in Crohn's disease. Am J Gastroenterol 104: 110–6.

44. Duraes C, Machado JC, Portela F, Rodrigues S, Lago P, et al. (2012) Phenotype-genotype profiles in Crohn's Disease predicted by genetic markers in autophagy related genes (GOIA study II). Inflamm Bowel Dis may 9 (epub ahead of print).

45. Waterman M, Xu W, Stempak JM, Milgrom R, Bernstein CN, et al. (2011) Distinct and overlapping genetic loci in Crohn's Disease and Ulcerative colitis: correlations with pathogenesis. Inflamm Bowel Dis 17: 1936–42.

46. Palomino-Morales RJ; Oliver J, Gomez-Garcia M, Lopez-Nevot MA, Rodrigo L, et al. (2009) Association of the ATG16L1 and IRGM genes polymorphisms with inflammatory bowel disease: a meta-analysis approach. Genes Immun 10: 356–64.

47. Tremelling M, Cummings F, Fisher SA, Mansfiled SA, Gwilliam R, et al. (2007) IL23R variation determines susceptibility but not disease phenotype in inflammatory bowel disease. Gastroenterology 132: 1657–64.

48. Weersma RK, Zhernakova A, Nolte IM, Lefebvre C, Rioux JD, et al. (2008) ATG16L1 and IL23R are associated with inflammatory bowel diseases but not with celiac disease in the Netherlands. Am J Gastroenterol 103: 621–7.

49. Van Limbergen J, Russell RK, Nimmo ER, Drummond HE, Smith L, et al. (2007) IL23R Arg381Gln is associated with childhood onset inflammatory bowel disease in Scotland. Gut 56: 1173–4.

50. Lappalainen M, Halme L, Turunen U, Saavalainen P, Einarsdottir E, et al. (2008) Association of IL23R, TNFRSF1A, and HLA-DRB1*0103 allele variants with inflammatory bowel disease phenotypes in the Finnish population. Inflamm Bowel Dis 14: 1118–24.

51. Marquez A, Mendoza JL, Taxonera C, Diaz-Rubio M, De La Concha EG, et al. (2008) IL23R and IL12B polymorphisms in Spanish IBD patients: no evidence of interaction. Inflamm Bowel Dis 14: 1192–6.

52. Peyrin-Biroulet L, Bigard MA, Malesci A, Danese S (2008) Step-up and top-down approaches to the treatment of Crohn's disease: early may already be too late. Gastroenterology 135: 1420–2.

53. Van Assche G, Dignass A, Bokemeyer B, Danese S, Gionchetti P, et al 2010) The second European evidence-based consensus on the diagnosis and management of Crohn's disease: Definitions and diagnosis. J Crohn's and Colitis 4: 7–27.

18

Dental Caries, Prevalence and Risk Factors in Patients with Crohn's Disease

Sara Szymanska[1], Mikael Lördal[2,3], Nilminie Rathnayake[1], Anders Gustafsson[1], Annsofi Johannsen[1]*

1 Department of Dental Medicine, Division of Periodontology, Karolinska Institutet, Huddinge, Sweden, **2** Department of Medicine, Division of Gastroenterology and Hepathology at Karolinska Institutet, Huddinge, Sweden, **3** Stockholm Gastro Center, Sophiahemmet, Stockholm, Sweden

Abstract

Objective: The present study tested the hypothesis that patients with Crohn's disease (CD) have a higher prevalence and risk for caries compared to people without CD.

Material and Methods: Patients with CD were divided into groups; 71 patients (50.7±13.9 years) who had gone through resective intestinal surgery and 79 patients (42.0±14.4 years) who had not. The patients were compared to 75 controls (48.6±13.4 years) regarding DMF-T and DMF-S, *Lactobacilli* (LB), *Streptococcus mutans* (SM), salivary flow and dental plaque. Statistical methods including ANOVA or Chi-square test for calculation of demographic differences between groups, analysis of covariance (ANCOVA) to compare the clinical variable and Post hoc analyses were done with Fischers Least Significant Difference test or Chi-square. Non-parametric Spearman's correlation matrix coefficient was estimated between clinical variables and disease duration.

Results: CD patients who had been subjected to resective surgery had a higher DMF-S score (50.7 *versus* 36.5; $p = 0.01$) compared to the control group after adjusting for age, gender and smoking. These patients had higher counts of SM (1.5 *versus* 0.9; $p = 0.04$) and LB (10000.0 *versus* 1000.0; $p = 0.01$), and more dental plaque (53.7 *versus* 22.6; $p = 0.001$). CD patients reported a more frequent consumption of sweetened drinks between meals compared to controls ($p = 0.001$).

Conclusions: The present study shows that patients with CD who had undergone resective surgery had a higher DMFs score, and higher salivary counts of *Lactobacilli* and *Streptococcus mutans* compared to the control group.

Editor: Salomon Amar, Boston University, United States of America

Funding: This study was supported by the Swedish Association of People with Stomach and Bowel Diseases, Swedish Patent Revenue Research Found, Praktikertjänst AB, Sweden, Swedish Society of Gastroenterology and Sophiahemmet Research Funds. The funders had no role in study design, data collection and analysis, decision to publish, or preparation of the manuscript.

Competing Interests: The authors have declared that no competing interests exist.

* E-mail: annsofi.johannsen@ki.se

Introduction

Crohn's disease (CD) is a granulomatous chronic inflammatory disease that can affect any region of the gastrointestinal tract, although it is usually localized to the small intestine and colon [1]. First described by Crohn et al. [2], the diagnosis of CD is based on clinical signs, endoscopy, histology, radiographic and/or biochemical findings [3]. CD shows episodes of disease activity, so called flares and asymptomatic intervals, or remissions [4]. This often leads to recurrent episodes of illness during which treatment with drugs and sometimes surgery is required to achieve symptomatic remission [5]. The aetiology of CD is unknown, however, studies have linked a possible genetic association [6]. In addition, a link between the microbiota and the lining of the gut mucosa has also been proposed as possible aetiological environmental factors [1,7]. The incidences of CD differ depending on geographical region. North America and the northern part of Europe have the highest incidence [8,9]. The prevalence of CD in adults in the US is 201 per 10^5 people [8].

Established risk factors for dental caries are increased number of *Lactobacilli* (LB) and *Steptococcus mutans* (SM), decreased salivary flow, insufficient oral hygiene, poor dietary habits including increased sugar consumption, as well as socioeconomic factors [10,11].

Earlier studies have reported higher caries prevalence in CD patients compared to controls [12]. Indeed CD patients exhibited higher levels of LB and SM [13,14]. Brito et al. [15] reported an increased mean value in the decayed, missed, filled teeth (DMF-T) score amongst CD patients compared to controls. Furthermore, a study from the US reported that patients with CD had more caries, increased mouth dryness and visited the dentist more often [16]. A questionnaire study from our group showed that patients with CD perceived their oral health to be poor and reported significantly more mouth-related problems and a greater requirement for dental treatment compared to a control group [17]. Thus, the aim of present study was to test the hypothesis that patients with CD have a higher prevalence and risk for caries compared to people without CD.

Materials and Methods

Patients with an established diagnosis of CD, according to Lennard-Jones criteria [18], attending the outpatient clinic at the Department of Gastroenterology and Hepathology at Karolinska Hospital were invited to participate in the study. Out of 309 patients that were consecutively asked to participate, 150 patients with CD were enrolled (73 females and 77 males), aged 18–77 years, between September 2008 and June 2010.

The control group were selected from 181 individuals that were randomly recruited through National Statistics Organization (SCB) in Sweden. 75 individuals (45 females and 30 males) accepted to participate in the study, aged 18–74 years. The selection of the control group was structured to achieve the same age and gender distribution as the patient group. All participants were living in Huddinge community of Stockholm and had no history of CD.

Ethical approval was obtained from the Karolinska Institutet Ethical Research Board (ref. nr.2007/2:11, 2009/1953-32), as well as oral and written informed consent from each participant before commencing the investigations.

Questionnaire

All participants completed a questionnaire that covered demographic data including age, gender, income, education level, medical history, medications, and smoking habits. Most of the questions in the questionnaire were of the multiple-chose type. The questions were based on the questionnaire from our earlier study ([17]). Smoking habits were reported as current smokers, former-smokers and never smokers, the response alternatives were yes or no. Questions concerning oral hygiene practice included frequency of tooth brushing, interproximal cleaning, and visits to the dentist and/or dental hygienist. Dental health was also registered by enquiring if they had reported any toothache, problems with oral ulcerations, dry mouth and bad breath during the last 12 months. The response alternatives to these questions were yes or no. In addition, all participants were asked about eating habits including frequency of meals and consumption of sweetened drinks between meals. The patients with CD were also asked how long they have had their disease, and if they had undergone surgical procedure.

Clinical Examination

Two investigators (SS/193 subjects, NR/32subjects) examined the participants. Prior to the clinical examination, an inter and intra calibration between the two examiners was conducted. Three participants (from CD group) were examined by both investigators to reach an agreement. In addition, repeated measurements within two patients were done by the same examiners.

The clinical examinations were conducted after saliva sampling, registration of the number of teeth and assessment of dental plaque (Visible Plaque Index, VPI) at six sites on all present teeth, excluding third molars.

Caries Registration

Caries was assessed by World Health Organization methods [19] and expressed by decayed, missing, or filled tooth (DMF-T) and surface index (DMF-S) in each person. The diagnosis was based on a clinical inspection and on x-rays. The diagnosis was based on a clinical inspection, visually and tactically with an examination probe and on radiographs. Clinically, caries was recorded when a lesion had a cavity, undermined enamel or an obviously softened surface, and the probe became stuck by using light pressure. Filled surfaces with caries were registered as both decayed and filled.

The radiographic examination was done with 4 bitewing radiographs. All tooth surfaces that could not be evaluated clinically were evaluated on the radiographs. Dental caries on the radiographs was recorded if the lesion reached the dentine.

The examiner of the radiographic images was blinded. An intra-examiner measurement analysis was performed in 10% of the patients and controls (randomly selected), and the measurements reached identical results in 89% of the cases.

Saliva Sampling

To avoid contamination of the oral cavity as a result of food intake or smoking, the subjects were instructed not to eat, drink, smoke or brush their teeth one hour before sampling. Unstimulated whole saliva and saliva stimulated by chewing paraffin wax was collected during a five minute period. Salivary flow rates were measured in millilitres per minute immediately after collection.

Analyses of Lactobacilli and Streptococcus Mutans

Salivary LB and SM counts were measured using Dentocult-LB Orion Diagnostica and Dentocult-SM Orion Diagnostica, according to the manufacturer's instructions. The salivary level of Lactobacilli is expressed as bacteria per mL and level of S. mutans in an arbitrary unit, 0–3. The numbers 0–1 represents less than 100 000 colony forming units (CFU)/mL, 2 represents 100 000–1000 000 CFU/mL and 3 represents more than 1000 000 CFU/mL.

Statistical Analysis

Analyses of the data were performed using the software package PASW Statistics 18 (PASW Inc., Chicago, IL, USA). The significance of the demographic differences (Table 1) between patients and controls were calculated with ANOVA, variables with only two factors were calculated with Chi-square test. Post hoc analyses were done with Fischers Least Significant Difference test or Chi-square. Analysis of covariance (ANCOVA) to control for age, gender and smoking were performed to compare the clinical variables between the groups, post hoc analyses were done with Fischers Least Significant Difference test (Table 2). P-values of 0.05 or below were considered significant. Non-parametric data were normalised with a logarithmation. Non-parametric Spearman's correlation matrix coefficient was estimated between clinical variables and disease duration.

Study Population

The number of patients with CD (n = 150) and the number of controls (n = 75) was chosen to allow us to observe differences in oral health of 10% of the population with a power of over 90%. Smaller differences were not considered clinically relevant. The power calculation was based on the differences reported by Brito et al. [15]. The power calculation revealed that 150 CD patients and 75 controls would provide 80% power to detect a difference in means of DMFT of 2.8 between the groups (22%), assuming that the common standard deviation is 7.0, with a 0.05 two-sided significance level.

Results

An initial analysis of the data showed that there were two distinct subgroups in the patient's population, those who had undergone resective surgery (RS) and those who had not (NRS). For this reason, the two groups were compared separately to the control group. Demographic data for all CD patients and the control group are presented in Table 1. There was a significant

Table 1. Demographic data, mean (SD) and percentages (number) for the CD patients (who had not and had undergone resective surgery) and the controls.

Variable	Control group n = 75	p 1	CD Patients No resective surgery n = 79	p 2	CD Patients Resective surgery n = 71	p 3
Gender F/M (n)	46/29		39/40		38/33	NS
Age (mean ± SD)	48.6 (±13.4)	0.003	42.0 (±14.4)	NS	50.7 (±13.9)	0.001
Weight, kg	74.4 (±13.0)		70.5 (±16.6)		74.3 (±14.4)	NS
Length cm	170.8 (±15.8)		170.8 (±9.8)		170.0 (±8.6)	NS
Smokers % (n)	6 (5)	0.030	19 (15)	0.005	25 (17)	0.012
Former smokers % (n)	46 (33)		41 (30)		37 (25)	NS
High blood pressure % (n)	9 (5)		19 (15)		17 (12)	NS
Cardiovascular disease % (n)	7 (5)		3 (2)		3 (2)	NS
Rheumatoid arthritis % (n)	5 (4)		13 (10)		7 (5)	NS
Kidney disease % (n)	4 (3)		5 (4)		7 (5)	NS
Diabetes % (n)	0 (0)		4 (3)		6 (4)	NS
Cancer % (n)	1.3 (1)		4(3)		6 (4)	NS
Osteoporosis % (n)	3 (2)		4 (3)		6 (4)	NS
Lung disease % (n)	1 (1)		8 (6)		7 (5)	NS
Asthma % (n)	21 (16)		29 (22)		23 (16)	NS
Use medication regularly % (n)	32 (23)	0.001	87 (66)	0.001	81 (54)	0.001
Behavior characteristic						
No Fibrostenotic/Penetrating,% (n)			71 (56)		35 (25)	
Fibrostenotic % (n)			23 (18)		51 (36)	
Penetrating % (n)			6 (5)		14 (10)	
CD duration (mean ± SD)			8 (8)		22 (14)	
Meal frequency	4.06 (1.5)		4.01 (1.4)		3.97 (1.5)	
Sweetened drinks % (n)	26 (20)	0.043	43 (34)	0.001	61 (43)	0.001
Toothache % (n)	14 (11)		24 (18)		19 (13)	NS
Dry mouth % (n)	11 (8)	0.001	38 (30)	0.011	29 (20)	0.001
Bad breath % (n)	12 (9)	0.003	33 (26)	NS	21 (15)	0.008
Ulcers % (n)	23 (17)		27 (21)		23 (16)	NS

p 1 indicates significance of the difference between controls and CD patients who had not undergone rescective surgery.
p 2 indicates significance of the difference between controls and CD patients who had undergone rescective surgery.
p 3 indicates significance of the difference between the 3 groups.
Significances were calculated with ANOVA and Chi-square test. Post doc analyses were done with Fischers' least significant difference test. NS = Not significant.
The difference in CD duration calculated with unpaired Student's t-test.

difference in age ($p = 0.001$) and duration of CD ($p = 0.01$) between the RS and NRS group. There were no significant differences between the groups regarding marital status, income and education.

There was no difference between the groups regarding frequency of meals. However, patients with CD reported significantly more frequent intake of sweetened drinks between the meals, such as soft drinks, compared to the control group (Table 1). There were significant differences between the groups regarding dry mouth and bad breath during the last 12 months as determined by a self-administrated questionnaire (Table 1).

Table 2 shows the clinical variables amongst the three groups, using ANCOVA and adjusted for age, gender and smoking. The RS group had a significantly higher DMF-S score. The difference was most pronounced regarding the number of filled surfaces (FS), although the difference did not reach statistical significance. The RS group had also a higher DMF-T score but the difference did not reach statistical significance ($p = 0.06$).

Both CD groups had significantly higher levels of LB and amounts of dental plaque compared to the control group. In addition, the RS group had more of SM compared to the control group (Table 2).

The results showed a weak positive correlation between disease duration and DMF-S ($r = 0.374$, $p = 0.01$), missing surface (MS) ($r = 0.272$, $p = 0.05$), and filled surface (FS) ($r = 0.424$, $p = 0.01$) in the RS group. These correlations could not be found in the NRS group.

When comparing the frequency of visits to the dentist and dental hygienist amongst the patients and controls, there were no significant differences. Oral hygiene habits did not differ regarding frequency of tooth brushing, and the use of approximal aids between the two groups (no data shown).

Gender Differences

Men in the CD group had significantly more decayed teeth (DT) (2.5 ± 3.7 vs. 1.5 ± 2.1, $p = 0.05$), and decayed surface (DS)

Table 2. Mean (SD) for the DMF-T/DMF-S index, *Steptococcus mutans*, volume of stimulated - and unstimulated saliva, the amount of dental plaque, and median (interquartile range) for *Lactobacilli*, in CD patients (who had not and had undergone resective surgery) and controls.

Variable	Control group n = 75	p 1	CD Patients No resective surgery n = 79	p 2	CD Patients Resective surgery n = 71	p 3
DMF-T	13.1 (6.5)		11.2 (7.1)		15.5 (8.3)	NS
DT	1.1 (2)		1.8 (2.9)		2.2 (3.2)	NS
MT	1.8 (3.3)		1.8 (2.9)		2.7 (4.1)	NS
FT	10.12 (5.4)		8.0 (5.4)		10.6 (6.4)	NS
DMF-S	36.5 (26.9)	NS	33.1 (28.6)	0.004	50.7 (36.2)	0.014
DS	1.5 (2.2)		2.7 (5.9)		3.6 (7.6)	NS
MS	8.5 (15.4)		8.9 (13.7)		13.3 (19.9)	NS
FS	26.5 (19.4)		22.6 (19.1)		33.7 (24.5)	NS
Modifiers						
Lactobacilli Bacteria/mL	1000 (1000)	0.008	10000 (99000)	0.012	10000 (99000)	0.011
Steptococcus mutans Arbitrary unit	0.9 (0.9)	NS	1.5 (0.9)	0.04	1.5 (1.1)	0.016
Stimulated saliva ml/min	2.0 (0.8)		2.2 (0.9)		2.0 (0.9)	NS
Unstimulated saliva ml/min	0.65 (0)		0.62 (0.4)		0.56(0)	NS
VPI	22.6 (22.1)	0.001	45.3 (25.9)	0.001	53.7 (29.2)	0.001

DMF-T = decayed, missed, filled teeth, DT = decayed teeth, MT = missing teeth, FT = filled teeth, DMF-S = decayed, missing, filled surface, DS = decayed surface, MS = missing surface, FS = filled surface, VPI = Visible Plaque index.
p 1 indicates statistical significance of the difference between controls and CD patients who had not undergone rescective surgery.
p 2 indicates statistical significance of the difference between controls and CD patients who had undergone rescective surgery.
p 3 indicates significances difference between all three groups.
Significances calculated with ANCOVA (analysis of covariance), adjusted for age, gender and smoking. Post hoc analyses done with Fischer's least significant difference test. NS = Not significant.

(4.3±8.6 vs. 2.1±4.1, $p = 0.05$) compared to women. The mean percentages of dental plaque were higher in men compared to women in the CD group (56.4±27.1 vs. 42.4±26.1, $p = 0.005$). There were no gender differences regarding dental caries assessment and the percentages of dental plaque in the control group.

Non-responders

Of those invited to participate 159 patients in the CD group and 106 individuals in the control group declined, albeit the reason was not asked. A statistical comparison between responders and non-responders showed no significant differences regarding age and gender.

Discussion

The present study revealed that CD patients who had undergone resective surgery had higher DMFs scores compared to patients without CD after adjusting for age, gender and smoking. More caries in CD patients have been shown by some previous studies [13,15,20]. Conversely, Grössner - Schreiber et al. [21] did not report any differences in the DMF-S index between patients with inflammatory bowel disease (IBD), but described a significantly higher prevalence of dentine caries amongst patients with IBD compared to the control group. An explanation for this discrepancy might be the different study groups, since patients with IBD include both CD and ulcerative colitis. The present study found more dental plaque in both CD patient groups, as compared to the controls, which could influence the prevalence of caries and is in agreement with a recent study by Habashneh et al. [22].

In this study both patient groups consumed more sweetened drinks between meals compared to the controls. This is in agreement with earlier epidemiological studies showing that patients with CD consumed larger amounts of highly refined carbohydrates, such as candy and/or soft drinks that are associated with increased dental caries risk [20,23]. Furthermore, several studies have shown that CD patients have a higher sugar intake compared to healthy controls even before the onset of disease [23,24]. Schütz et al. [20] demonstrated higher caries prevalence, higher sugar intake as well as lower zinc plasma levels in CD patients, but they were unable to relate these changes to each other. Zinc deficiency can influence sweet taste perception in patients with CD [25]. The mechanism of zinc deficiency remains unclear, and there are contradictory results as to whether in fact there are decreased plasma levels of zinc in CD patients compared to controls [25,26]. Our study did not show any differences in meal frequency between patients and controls.

The levels of LB and SM were higher in CD patients compared to the control group, which is in line with Sundh et al. [14]. Furthermore, several studies have found that these bacteria are involved in caries activity although it must be taken into consideration that species variations exist for these bacteria, for review see Takahashi and Nyvad [27]. The involvement of bacteria in the caries process is complex and remains unclear.

The biological agent, tumor necrosis factor alpha (TNFα) inhibitor, has an anti-inflammatory effect and is used when other medical treatment for Crohn's disease have failed [28]. TNFα-inhibitor is currently regarded as part of the treatment of choice for CD when other therapies have shown to be ineffective, but it has only been available during the last decade. This approach has reduced the need for resective surgery. In our study population very few patients had received the anti-TNF treatment. Thus, this treatment had no influence on the comparison between patient's undergone surgery or not. In the current study, patients that had undergone surgery had a higher DMFs score compared to the control group, while there were no difference between the patients who had not undergone surgery and the controls. This difference remains also after consideration for age and gender. Disease duration showed a weak but significant correlation with DMFs in resective group but not in the non-surgery group. The reason for this difference between the patient groups could be that the surgery group have had a more severe disease leading to a need for surgery. We found no differences in eating habits between the two patient groups. Another explanation could be that over the years of suffering with the disease prior to the resective surgery they experienced problems with their oral health status and many caries restorations were performed. It is well established that one of the risk factors for caries are old restorations and in turn might increase the risk for more cavities and oral health problems in this group.

Interestingly, in the present study, the men in the patient group had a significantly higher prevalence of dental plaque compared to the women in the same group, even if there are individual variations, whereas there were no gender differences in the control group. To date, no study exists considering gender perspective and oral health in patients with CD. The clinical significance of the present study is that patients with CD who had undergone RS, particularly men, seem to be in a need for individual caries prophylaxis.

The high numbers of drop-outs from the current study need consideration. All patients were contacted by phone and some of those who didn't want to participate in the study mentioned they were sick, or they had visited the dentistry recently and, some person gave no reason.

Living with CD, means coping with a lifelong condition sometimes requiring significant lifestyles adjustments that might influence oral hygiene behaviours and dietary habits. Keefer et al. [29] showed that patients with IBD who received behavioural interventions seemed to alter the disease course and improve their quality of life. Therefore it is important that patients with CD are instructed about the relationship between their disease and the increased risk for caries. In the clinical practice these patients must be informed about the consequences of altered dietary habits and the importance of prevention. Further research should focus on developing individual preventive programmes tailored to their needs.

The present study shows that patients with CD who had undergone resective surgery had a higher DMFs score, and higher salivary counts of *Lactobacilli and Streptococcus mutans* compared to the control group.

Author Contributions

Conceived and designed the experiments: SS ML AG AJ. Performed the experiments: SS NR. Analyzed the data: SS ML AG AJ. Contributed reagents/materials/analysis tools: SS ML NR AG AJ. Wrote the paper: SS ML AG AJ.

References

1. Head K, Jurenka JS (2004) Inflammatory bowel disease, Part ii: Crohn's disease-pathophysiology and conventional and alternative treatment options. Altern med Rev 9: 360–401.
2. Crohn Bb GLOG (1932) Regional ileitis: A pathologic and clinical entity. JAMA: The Journal of the American Medical Association 99: 1323–1329.
3. Stange EF, Travis SP, Vermeire S, Beglinger C, Kupcinkas L, et al. (2006) Organisation ECsaC: European evidence based consensus on the diagnosis and management of crohn's disease: Definitions and diagnosis. Gut 55: Suppl 1: i1–15.
4. Fatahzadeh M (2009) Inflammatory bowel disease. Oral Surg Oral Med Oral Pathol Oral Radiol Endod 108: e1–10.
5. Katz JA (2007) Management of inflammatory bowel disease in adults. J Dig Dis 8: 65–71.
6. Cho JH, Brant SR (2011) Recent insights into the genetics of inflammatory bowel disease. Gastroenterology 140: 1704–1712.
7. Gibson PR, Shepherd SJ (2005) Personal view: Food for thought–western lifestyle and susceptibility to crohn's disease. The fodmap hypothesis. Aliment Pharmacol Ther 21: 1399–1409.
8. Kappelman MD, Rifas-Shiman SL, Kleinman K, Ollendorf D, Bousvaros A, et al. (2007) The prevalence and geographic distribution of crohn's disease and ulcerative colitis in the united states. Clin Gastroenterol Hepatol 5: 1424–1429.
9. Vind I, Riis L, Jess T, Knudsen E, Pedersen N, et al. (2006) Increasing incidences of inflammatory bowel disease and decreasing surgery rates in copenhagen city and county, 2003–2005: A population-based study from the danish crohn colitis database. Am J Gastroenterol 101: 1274–1282.
10. Selwitz RH, Ismail AI, Pitts NB (2007) Dental caries. Lancet 369: 51–59.
11. Touger-Decker R, van Loveren C (2003) Sugars and dental caries. Am J Clin Nutr 78: 881S-892S.
12. Rooney TP (1984) Dental caries prevalence in patients with crohn's disease. Oral Surg Oral Med Oral Pathol 57: 623–624.
13. Bevenius J (1988) Caries risk in patients with crohn's disease: A pilot study. Oral Surg Oral Med Oral Pathol 65: 304–307.
14. Sundh B, Johansson I, Emilson CG, Nordgren S, Birkhed D (1993) Salivary antimicrobial proteins in patients with crohn's disease. Oral Surg Oral Med Oral Pathol 76: 564–569.

15. Brito F, de Barros FC, Zaltman C, Carvalho AT, Carneiro AJ, et al. (2008) Prevalence of periodontitis and dmft index in patients with crohn's disease and ulcerative colitis. J Clin Periodontol 35: 555–560.
16. Singhal S, Dian D, Keshavarzian A, Fogg L, Fields JZ, et al. (2011) The role of oral hygiene in inflammatory bowel disease. Dig Dis Sci 56: 170–175.
17. Rikardsson S, Jönsson J, Hultin M, Gustafsson A, Johannsen A (2009) Perceived oral health in patients with crohn's disease. Oral Health Prev Dent 7: 277–282.
18. Lennard-Jones JE (1984) Medical treatment of ulcerative colitis. Postgrad Med J 60: 797–802.
19. World Health Organization (1997) Oral Health Surveys: Basic Methods, 4th edition. Geneva: WHO.
20. Schütz T, Drude C, Paulisch E, Lange KP, Lochs H (2003) Sugar intake, taste changes and dental health in crohn's disease. Dig Dis 21: 252–257.
21. Grössner-Schreiber B, Fetter T, Hedderich J, Kocher T, Schreiber S, et al. (2006) Prevalence of dental caries and periodontal disease in patients with inflammatory bowel disease: A case-control study. J Clin Periodontol 33: 478–484.
22. Habashneh RA, Khader YS, Alhumouz MK, Jadallah K, Ajlouni Y (2011) The association between inflammatory bowel disease and periodontitis among jordanians: A case-control study. J Periodontal Res 3: 293–298.
23. Tragnone A, Valpiani D, Miglio F, Elmi G, Bazzocchi G, et al. (1995) Dietary habits as risk factors for inflammatory bowel disease. Eur J Gastroenterol Hepatol 7: 47–51.
24. Reif S, Klein I, Lubin F, Farbstein M, Hallak A, et al. (1997) Pre-illness dietary factors in inflammatory bowel disease. Gut 40: 754–760.
25. Solomons NW, Rosenberg IH, Sandstead HH, Vo-Khactu KP (1977) Zinc deficiency in crohn's disease. Digestion 16: 87–95.
26. Penny WJ, Mayberry JF, Aggett PJ, Gilbert JO, Newcombe RG, et al. (1983) Relationship between trace elements, sugar consumption, and taste in crohn's disease. Gut 24: 288–292.
27. Takahashi N, Nyvad B (2011) The role of bacteria in the caries process: Ecological perspectives. J Dent Res 90: 294–303.
28. Ferrante M, Van Assche G (2012) Medical therapy and mucosal healing. Curr Drug Targets 13: 1294–1299.
29. Keefer L, Kiebles JL, Martinovich Z, Cohen E, Van Denburg A, et al. (2011) Behavioral interventions may prolong remission in patients with inflammatory bowel disease. Behav Res Ther 49: 145–150.

19

PTGER4 Expression-Modulating Polymorphisms in the 5p13.1 Region Predispose to Crohn's Disease and Affect NF-κB and XBP1 Binding Sites

Jürgen Glas[1,2,3❀], Julia Seiderer[1❀], Darina Czamara[4], Giulia Pasciuto[1], Julia Diegelmann[1,2], Martin Wetzke[5], Torsten Olszak[1,6], Christiane Wolf[4], Bertram Müller-Myhsok[4], Tobias Balschun[7], Jean-Paul Achkar[8,9], M. Ilyas Kamboh[10], Andre Franke[7], Richard H. Duerr[10,11], Stephan Brand[1]*

1 Department of Medicine II - Grosshadern, University of Munich, Munich, Germany, 2 Department of Preventive Dentistry and Periodontology, University of Munich, Munich, Germany, 3 Department of Human Genetics, Rheinisch-Westfälische Technische Hochschule (RWTH) Aachen, Aachen, Germany, 4 Max-Planck-Institute of Psychiatry, Munich, Germany, 5 Center for Pediatrics, Hannover Medical School, Hannover, Germany, 6 Division of Gastroenterology, Brigham & Women's Hospital, Harvard Medical School, Boston, United States of America, 7 Institute of Clinical Molecular Biology, Christian-Albrechts-University, Kiel, Germany, 8 Department of Pathobiology, Lerner Research Institute, Cleveland Clinic, Cleveland, Ohio, United States of America, 9 Department of Gastroenterology and Hepatology, Digestive Disease Institute, Cleveland Clinic, Cleveland, Ohio, United States of America, 10 Department of Human Genetics, Graduate School of Public Health, University of Pittsburgh, Pittsburgh, Pennsylvania, United States of America, 11 Division of Gastroenterology, Hepatology and Nutrition, School of Medicine, University of Pittsburgh, Pittsburgh, Pennsylvania, United States of America

Abstract

Background: Genome-wide association studies identified a PTGER4 expression-modulating region on chromosome *5p13.1* as Crohn's disease (CD) susceptibility region. The study aim was to test this association in a large cohort of patients with inflammatory bowel disease (IBD) and to elucidate genotypic and phenotypic interactions with other IBD genes.

Methodology/Principal Findings: A total of 7073 patients and controls were genotyped: 844 CD and 471 patients with ulcerative colitis and 1488 controls were analyzed for the single nucleotide polymorphisms (SNPs) rs4495224 and rs7720838 on chromosome *5p13.1*. The study included two replication cohorts of North American (CD: n = 684; controls: n = 1440) and of German origin (CD: n = 1098; controls: n = 1048). Genotype-phenotype, epistasis and transcription factor binding analyses were performed. In the discovery cohort, an association of rs4495224 (p = 4.10×10^{-5}; 0.76 [0.67–0.87]) and of rs7720838 (p = 6.91×10^{-4}; 0.81 [0.71–0.91]) with susceptibility to CD was demonstrated. These associations were confirmed in both replication cohorts. *In silico* analysis predicted rs4495224 and rs7720838 as essential parts of binding sites for the transcription factors NF-κB and XBP1 with higher binding scores for carriers of the CD risk alleles, providing an explanation of how these SNPs might contribute to increased PTGER4 expression. There was no association of the *PTGER4* SNPs with IBD phenotypes. Epistasis detected between *5p13.1* and *ATG16L1* for CD susceptibility in the discovery cohort (p = 5.99×10^{-7} for rs7720838 and rs2241880) could not be replicated in both replication cohorts arguing against a major role of this gene-gene interaction in the susceptibility to CD.

Conclusions/Significance: We confirmed *5p13.1* as a major CD susceptibility locus and demonstrate by *in silico* analysis rs4495224 and rs7720838 as part of binding sites for NF-κB and XBP1. Further functional studies are necessary to confirm the results of our *in silico* analysis and to analyze if changes in PTGER4 expression modulate CD susceptibility.

Editor: Yong-Gang Yao, Kunming Institute of Zoology, Chinese Academy of Sciences, China

Funding: SB was supported by grants from Deutsche Forschungsgemeinschaft (BR 1912/6-1), the Else Kröner-Fresenius-Stiftung (Else Kröner Exzellenzstipendium 2010; 2010_EKES.32), by the Ludwig-Demling Grant 2007 from DCCV e.V. and by a grant from the Excellence Initiative of the Ludwig-Maximilians-University Munich (Investment Funds 2008). JS and JD were supported by grants from the University of Munich (FöFoLe Nr. 422; Habilitationsstipendium to JS and Promotionsstipendium to JD); JS also was supported by the Robert-Bosch-Foundation and the Else-Kröner-Fresenius-Stiftung. JG was supported by a grant from the Broad Medical Foundation (IBD-0126R2). TB and AF were supported by the German Ministry of Education and Research through the National Genome Research Network and infrastructure support through the Deutsche Forschungsgemeinschaft cluster of excellence 'Inflammation at Interfaces'. RHD is supported by National Institutes of Health (NIH)/NIDDK grant DK062420. MIK was supported by NIH grants AG030653, HL092397 and AG041718. JPA was supported by NIH grant DK068112. The funders had no role in study design, data collection and analysis, decision to publish, or preparation of the manuscript.

Competing Interests: The authors have declared that no competing interests exist.

* E-mail: Stephan.Brand@med.uni-muenchen.de

❀ These authors contributed equally to this work.

Introduction

Crohn's disease (CD) and ulcerative colitis (UC) are chronic inflammatory bowel diseases (IBD) characterized by a complex molecular pathogenesis resulting in an exaggerated immune response and mucosal destruction [1–3]. Recent insights in the interaction of various susceptibility genes with intestinal bacteria have substantially helped to unravel the pathogenesis of IBD [2,4]. Since the identification of *NOD2* as the first susceptibility gene for CD in 2001 [5,6], various studies including genome-wide association studies (GWAS) based on high-density SNP (single nucleotide polymorphism) arrays have identified CD-associated genetic variants of proteins involved in immune response, autophagy or bacterial recognition, such as *IL23R* [7,8], *ATG16L1* [9–11], and *IRGM* [12]. In addition, genotype-phenotype analysis by us and others also demonstrated significant associations for certain gene variants with particular CD phenotypes [13–20].

In 2007, a GWAS analyzing more than 318,000 SNPs identified a 250 kb region on chromosome *5p13.1* contributing to CD susceptibility [21]. The disease-associated alleles were found to correlate with expression levels of the prostaglandin receptor EP4, which binds prostaglandin E2 (PGE2) and is encoded by *PTGER4*, the gene located closest to the associated region [21]. Since *Ptger4*$^{-/-}$ mice develop severe dextran sodium sulphate (DSS)-induced colitis while treatment with EP4-selective agonists has protective effects against colitis through enhancement of epithelium survival and regeneration, *PTGER4* represents an attractive IBD candidate gene [22–24]. Prostaglandins are arachidonic acid metabolites produced by the action of the enzymes cyclooxygenase (COX)-1 and -2 and play a crucial role in the regulation of gastrointestinal homeostasis and IBD pathogenesis [25–27]. The novel *5p13.1* CD susceptibility locus in proximity of *PTGER4* was also replicated by a recent genome-wide association study [28].

Moreover, the data on the disease-modifying effect of this region on UC is very limited so far. In a recent GWAS of UC [29], a significant association between rs4613763 variant in the *5p13* region and UC has been reported. To analyze the effect of SNPs in the *5p13.1* region on IBD susceptibility in the German population, a large study was initiated and genomic DNA of 2803 individuals was genotyped for the two SNPs rs4495224 and rs7720838, identified in the initial study by Libioulle and co-workers as CD susceptibility locus [21]. Although other SNPs in the study by Libioulle et al. [21] showed moderately stronger association with CD, these two SNPs were selected for genotyping since they were both strongly associated with CD and showed the most significant effect on PTGER4 expression in that GWAS. In addition, the detailed phenotypic consequences of these gene variants in CD and UC were here analyzed for the first time. Moreover, we aimed to identify whether rs4495224 and rs7720838 are part of potential binding sites for transcription factors that might influence PTGER4 expression. As *5p13.1* may also interact with other IBD susceptibility genes, a detailed analysis for potential epistasis with the previously identified major CD susceptibility gene variants (in *NOD2*, *IL23R*, *ATG16L1* and in *SLC22A4/5* in the IBD5 region) was performed.

Methods

Ethics statement

This study was approved by the Ethics committee of the Medical Faculty of Ludwig-Maximilians-University Munich (discovery cohort), the University Hospital of the Christian-Albrechts-University Kiel (German replication cohort), the Cleveland Clinic and the University of Pittsburgh (North American replication

cohort). Written, informed consent was obtained from all patients prior to genotyping and inclusion into the study. In the case of minors, the consent was provided by the parents. The study protocol adhered to the ethical principles for medical research involving human subjects of the Helsinki Declaration (as described in detail under: http://www.wma.net/en/30publications/ 10policies/b3/index.html).

Study population and disease phenotype analysis

Overall, the German discovery study population (n = 2803) included 1315 IBD patients of Caucasian origin consisting of 844 patients with CD, 471 patients with UC, and 1488 healthy, unrelated controls. In order to replicate the association of chromosome *5p13.1* SNPs, a U.S. American Caucasian CD cohort (CD: n = 684; controls: n = 1440) from the University of Pittsburgh and the Cleveland Clinic and an additional German replication cohort from the University Hospital of Schleswig-Holstein at Kiel (CD: n = 1098; controls: n = 1048) were investigated. The diagnosis of CD or UC was based on established guidelines including endoscopic, radiological, and histopathological criteria [30]. Patients with CD were assessed according to the Montreal classification [31] analyzing age at diagnosis (A), location (L), and behavior (B) of disease. In patients with UC, anatomic location was also assessed in accordance to the Montreal classification, using the criteria ulcerative proctitis (E1), left-sided UC (distal UC; E2), and extensive UC (pancolitis; E3). Patients with indeterminate colitis were excluded from the study. Phenotypic characteristics were collected blind to the results of the genotypic data and included demographic and clinical parameters (behavior and anatomic location of IBD, disease-related complications, surgical or immunosuppressive therapy) which were recorded by analysis of patient charts and a detailed questionnaire including an interview at time of enrolment. The demographic

Table 1. Demographic characteristics of the German IBD discovery study population.

	Crohn's disease	Ulcerative colitis	Controls
	n = 844	n = 471	n = 1488
Gender			
Male (%)	51.4%	52.1%	62.9%
Age (yrs)			
Mean ± SD	39.5±13.1	41.8±14.5	45.9±10.7
Range	10–80	7–85	18–71
Body mass index			
Mean ± SD	23.1±4.2	23.9±4.2	
Range	13–40	15–41	
Age at diagnosis (yrs)			
Mean ± SD	27.7±11.7	32.0±13.4	
Range	1–78	9–81	
Disease duration (yrs)			
Mean ± SD	11.8±8.5	10.4±7.8	
Range	0–44	1–40	
Positive family history of IBD (%)	16.0%	16.1%	

characteristics of the IBD study population are summarized in Table 1.

DNA extraction and genotyping of SNPs in the 5p13.1 region

Genomic DNA was isolated from peripheral blood leukocytes by standard procedures using the DNA blood mini kit from Qiagen (Hilden, Germany). The SNPs rs4495224 and rs7720838 on chromosome $5p13.1$, for which significant associations with CD were found in a previous study [21], were genotyped by PCR and melting curve analysis using a pair of fluorescence resonance energy transfer (FRET) probes in a LightCycler 480 system (Roche Diagnostics, Mannheim, Germany), using a similar methodology as described previously [8,11]. The results of melting curve analysis were confirmed by analyzing samples representing all possible genotypes using sequence analysis. All sequences of primers and FRET probes and primer annealing temperatures used for genotyping and for sequence analysis are given in Tables S1 and S2.

In the U.S. American cohort, SNPs rs4532399, rs11955354, rs11957215, rs7720838, and rs10440635 in the $5p13.1$ region were genotyped using the Human Omni1-Quad chip (Illumina, Inc., San Diego, CA). In the German replication cohort, SNPs rs7720838 and rs10941508 (surrogate marker for rs4495224) in the $5p13.1$ region were genotyped using the SNPlex technology (Applied Biosystems) in an automated laboratory setup and all process data were written to and administered by a database-driven laboratory information management system.

Genotyping of variants in NOD2, IL23R, ATG16L1, and SLC22A4/5

From previous studies, the genotypes of CD-associated gene variants in $NOD2$ [16,17,19], $IL23R$ [8], $ATG16L1$ [11] and $SLC22A4/5$ [32] were available for the German discovery study cohort. Genotyping of the $NOD2$ variants p.Arg702Trp (rs2066844), p.Gly908Arg (rs2066845), and p.Leu1007fsX1008 (rs2066847) as well as analysis of the 1672 C→T SNP in $SLC22A4$ (rs1050152) encoding OCTN1 and the −207 G→C SNP (rs2631367) in $SLC22A5$ encoding OCTN2 were performed by PCR and restriction fragment length polymorphism analysis as described previously [32]. The primer sequences, the restriction enzymes used and the resulting fragment lengths are given in Table S3. The 10 CD-associated $IL23R$ SNPs (rs1004819, rs7517847, rs10489629, rs2201841, rs11465804, rs11209026 = p.Arg381Gln, rs1343151, rs10889677, rs11209032, rs1495965) described by Duerr and co-workers [7] and nine $ATG16L1$ SNPs (rs13412102, rs12471449, rs6431660, rs1441090, rs2289472, rs2241880 (= p.Thr300Ala), rs2241879, rs3792106, rs4663396) described by Hampe and co-workers [9] were genotyped by PCR and melting curve analysis as described previously [8,11]. All sequences of primers and FRET probes and primer annealing temperatures used for genotyping and for sequence analysis are given in Tables S4 and S5.

In the U.S. American cohort, $ATG16L1$ SNPs rs13412102, rs3828309, rs2289474, rs2241880 (= p.Thr300Ala), and rs2241879 were genotyped using the Human Omni1-Quad chip (Illumina, Inc.). In the German replication cohort, $ATG16L1$ SNPs rs13412102, rs12471449, rs6431660, rs1441090, rs2289472, rs2241880 (= p.Thr300Ala), rs2241879, rs3792106, rs4663396 were genotyped using the SNPlex technology (Applied Biosystems). Since genotyping was performed in the IBD centers in which the blood samples were centrally collected, each IBD center used its own "in house" genotyping protocol (Munich: PCR and melting curve analysis using a pair of FRET probes; Kiel: SNPlex technology (Applied Biosystems); Pittsburgh: Human Omni1-Quad chip (Illumina, Inc.)). Given the differences in the genotyping platforms, not all SNPs were identical; therefore, surrogate markers with high linkage disequilibrium were used where appropriate.

In silico analysis of transcription factor binding sites

SNPs rs4495224 and rs7720838 were analyzed for potential human transcription factor binding sites applying the online tool TFSEARCH which is based on the TRANSFAC database [33]. Transcription factors with predicted binding scores of ≥75 for each allele were included in the analysis (max. score = 100). For each SNP, major and minor alleles including the flanking 15 nucleotides upstream (5′) and downstream (3′) were analyzed.

Statistical analyses

Data were evaluated by using the SPSS 13.0 software (SPSS Inc., Chicago, IL, U.S.A.) and R-2.4.1. (http://cran.r-project.org). Each genetic marker was tested for Hardy-Weinberg equilibrium in the control population. Fisher's exact test was used for comparison between categorical variables, while Student's t test was applied for quantitative variables. Single-marker allelic tests were performed with Pearson's χ^2 test. All tests were two-tailed, considering p-values<0.05 as significant. Odds ratios were calculated for the minor allele at each SNP. For multiple comparisons, Bonferroni correction was applied where indicated. Interactions between different polymorphisms were tested using the −epistasis option provided in PLINK (http://pngu.mgh. harvard.edu/~purcell/plink/).

Results

The SNPs rs4495224 and rs7720838 in the 5p13.1 region are significantly associated with Crohn's disease

In all three subgroups (CD, UC, and controls) of the German discovery study cohort, the allele frequencies of the SNPs rs4495224 and rs7720838 were in accordance with the predicted Hardy-Weinberg equilibrium and are summarized in Table 2. Similar to the results of the study of Libioulle et al. (D′ = 0.84) [21], both $PTGER4$ expression-modulating SNPs were in linkage disequilibrium (controls: D′ = 0.843; CD: D′ = 0.795; UC: D′ = 0.871; all cohorts: D′ = 0.836).

Overall, significant differences in the frequencies of rs4495224 and rs7720838 were observed in CD patients compared to healthy controls (Table 2), identifying SNP rs4495224 and rs7720838 as significantly CD-associated genetic variants. In the CD group, the frequency of the rarer C allele of the rs4495224 polymorphism was 0.28, whereas in the controls it was 0.34 (p = 4.10×10^{-5}, OR 0.76 [0.67–0.87]). The frequencies of the minor G allele of the rs7720838 polymorphism were 0.375 in CD and 0.43 in the controls (p = 6.91×10^{-4}, OR 0.81 [0.71–0.91]), suggesting a protective effect of the minor allele in CD. In contrast, no associations were observed in UC patients. In UC, the frequencies of the rs4495224 C allele and of the rs7720838 G allele were 0.35 (p = 3.17×10^{-1}, OR 1.08 [0.93–1.26]) and 0.45 (p = 2.75×10^{-1}, OR 1.09 [0.94–1.26]), respectively. However, the lack of association with UC could be related to a lack of power. In a power analysis using the Genetics Power Calculator (http://pngu. mgh.harvard.edu/~purcell/gpc/), we used the settings unselected controls and, a minor allele frequency of 43%. Considering our sample size of 471 UC cases and 1488 controls, our study had 25% power for detecting differences in the minor allele frequencies between cases (UC) and controls corresponding to an OR of 1.10.

Table 2. Allele frequencies of the SNPs rs4495224 and rs7720838 in German discovery population of patients with Crohn's disease and ulcerative colitis and controls.

Gene marker	Minor allele	Crohn's disease n = 844			Ulcerative colitis n = 471			Controls n = 1488
		MAF	p value	OR [95% CI]	MAF	p value	OR [95% CI]	MAF
rs4495224	C	0.28	4.10×10^{-5}	0.76 [0.67–0.87]	0.35	3.17×10^{-1}	1.08 [0.93–1.26]	0.34
rs7720838	G	0.38	6.91×10^{-4}	0.81 [0.71–0.91]	0.45	2.75×10^{-1}	1.09 [0.94–1.26]	0.43

Note: Minor allele frequencies (MAF), allelic test p-values, and odds ratios (OR, shown for the minor allele) with 95% confidence intervals (CI) are shown.

In the North American CD cohort, all 5 SNPs investigated in the *PTGER4* region were strongly associated with CD susceptibility (Table 3). The SNPs rs4532399, rs11955354 and rs11957215, which were in nearly complete linkage disequilibrium according to the data of the Human HapMap project, were used as surrogate markers for SNP rs4495224. The minor allele frequencies of all these three SNPs were 0.28 in the North American CD cohort and 0.35 the in the North American control population (rs4532399: p = 3.07×10^{-6}; 0.72 [0.62–0.82], rs11955354: p = 5.45×10^{-6}; 0.72 [0.63–0.83], rs11957215: p = 7.08×10^{-6}; 0.72 [0.63–0.83]). The frequencies of the minor G allele of the SNP rs7720838 were 0.375 in CD and 0.45 in the controls (p = 2.19×10^{-7}; 0.71 [0.62–0.81]). For the SNP rs10440635, which is a surrogate marker for rs7720838, the minor allele frequencies were 0.36 in the CD cohort and 0.45 in the control population (p = 8.60×10^{-8}; 0.70 [0.61–0.80]).

In the German replication cohort, the SNP rs10941508, which was in nearly complete linkage disequilibrium within the data of the Human HapMap project and served as surrogate marker for rs4495224, was also strongly associated with CD susceptibility. The frequencies of the minor G allele of the SNP rs10941508 were 0.30 in the CD population and 0.34 in the controls (p = 8.60×10^{-8}; 0.70 [0.61–0.80]) (Table 4).

Genotype-phenotype analyses

So far, the phenotypic consequences of gene variants in the *5p13.1* region are unknown. We therefore performed a detailed genotype-phenotype correlation in the German IBD discovery cohort for which detailed phenotype data were available. In CD patients, the analysis revealed no significant associations of the SNPs rs4495224 and rs7720838 with phenotypic characteristics

such as age, male-to-female-ratio, body mass index (BMI), family history, incidence of stenoses and fistulas, use of immunosuppressive agents, or extraintestinal manifestations (Table S6 and S7). Weak associations with disease onset <16 years in CD patients heterozygous for SNP rs4495224 (p = 0.036) and with less colonic involvement according to the Montreal classification [31] in heterozygous carriers of the rs7720838 variant compared to the wildtype patients (p = 0.023) did not fulfill the significance criteria after Bonferroni correction (Table S6 and S7). Similarly, in UC, no significant associations between these SNPs and the main disease characteristics were found after Bonferroni correction (Table S8 and S9).

Analysis for epistasis between the 5p13.1 region and other CD susceptibility genes

Next, potential epistasis between the SNPs in the *5p13.1* region and other, replicated CD-associated gene variants was analyzed. This analysis included the three common *NOD2* variants p.Arg702Trp, p.Gly908Arg, and p.Leu1007fsX1008, 10 recently identified CD-associated *IL23R* variants [7,8] 9 variants in *ATG16L1* [9,11] and *SLC22A4/5* gene variants [32]. After Bonferroni correction, no evidence for epistasis between SNPs in the *5p13.1* region and gene variants in *NOD2*, *IL23R*, or *SLC22A4/5* was found (data not shown). In contrast, marked epistasis between the two SNPs of the *5p13.1* region (rs4495224 and rs7720838) and SNPs within the *ATG16L1* gene was demonstrated in the German CD discovery cohort (Table 5). The interactions were particularly strong between rs7720838 and *ATG16L1* polymorphisms, with p values ranging from 7.81×10^{-3} to 1.09×10^{-7} (Table 5). Strong interactions of rs7720838 occurred with rs13412102 in the 5'-flanking region (p = 1.09×10^{-7}), with

Table 3. Allele frequencies of the SNPs within the *5p13.1* region in North American replication cohort.

Gene marker	Gene/region	Minor allele	Crohn's disease n = 684			Controls n = 1440
			MAF	p value	OR [95% CI]	MAF
rs4532399*	*5p13.1*	A	0.28	3.07×10^{-6}	0.72 [0.62–0.82]	0.35
rs11955354*	*5p13.1*	A	0.28	5.45×10^{-6}	0.72 [0.63–0.83]	0.35
rs11957215*	*5p13.1*	G	0.28	7.08×10^{-6}	0.72 [0.63–0.83]	0.35
rs7720838	*5p13.1*	C	0.37	2.19×10^{-7}	0.71 [0.62–0.81]	0.45
rs10440635&	*5p13.1*	G	0.36	8.60×10^{-8}	0.70 [0.61–0.80]	0.45

Note: Minor allele frequencies (MAF), allelic test p-values, and odds ratios (OR, shown for the minor allele) with 95% confidence intervals (CI) are shown.
*surrogate markers for rs4495224;
&surrogate marker for, rs7720838.

Table 4. Allele frequencies of the SNPs within the *5p13.1* in German replication cohort with Crohn's disease patients and controls.

Gene marker	Gene/region	Minor allele	Crohn's disease			Controls
			n = 1098			n = 1048
			MAF	p value	OR [95% CI]	MAF
rs10941508§	*5p13.1*	G	0.30	1.96×10^{-3}	0.82 [0.72–0.93]	0.34

Note: Minor allele frequencies (MAF), allelic test p-values, and odds ratios (OR, shown for the minor allele) with 95% confidence intervals (CI) are shown.
§surrogate marker for rs4495224.

rs6431660 in the 5'-region of the gene ($p = 2.29 \times 10^{-7}$) and with rs2241880 (p.Thr300Ala) in the central region of *ATG16L1* ($p = 5.99 \times 10^{-7}$; Table 5). In the German CD discovery cohort, the epistasis between *ATG16L1* and rs4495224 was also strong, but less pronounced than that of rs7720838; the strongest interaction with rs4495224 involved rs6431660 ($p = 8.37 \times 10^{-5}$) and the coding SNP rs2241880 (p.Thr300Ala) ($p = 3.81 \times 10^{-4}$; Table 5). In addition, the *ATG16L1* SNP rs2241879, which was associated with CD in several studies [9–11], displayed strong interactions with both *5p13.1* SNPs (rs7720838: $p = 1.10 \times 10^{-6}$, rs4495224: $p = 3.07 \times 10^{-4}$).

Despite the pronounced epistasis between *ATG16L1* and the *5p13.1* region regarding CD susceptibility in the German discovery cohort, no significant epistatic effect of these genetic regions on the CD or UC phenotype could be detected after Bonferroni correction (Table S8 and S9) which was partly related to the great number of interactions tested for (n = 189 for CD; n = 144 for UC).

To analyze if the epistasis between the *5p13.1* region and *ATG16L1* could be replicated in other CD populations, we investigated a U.S. American and a German CD replication cohort. In the U.S. American cohort, both *5p13.1* (Table 3) and *ATG16L1* (Table S10) were strongly associated with CD susceptibility. Using different genotyping platforms (Human Omni1-

Quad chip from Illumina in the U.S. American and SNPlex technology from Applied Biosystems in the German replication cohort), a slightly different panel of SNPs in the *5p13.1* region and *ATG16L1* SNPs was available (Tables 3 and 4, Table S11). In the U.S. American study population, rs4532399 in the *5p13.1* region served as surrogate marker for rs4495224, and rs2289474 was used as surrogate marker for rs6431660. In the German replication cohort, rs10941508 in the *5p13.1* region served as surrogate marker for rs4495224. However, as shown in Tables S12 and S13, there was no significant epistasis detected between these gene markers, suggesting that the strong epistasis between *5p13.1* and *ATG16L1* found in the German CD discovery cohort is not a general phenomenon in Caucasian CD populations.

Analysis of potential transcription factor binding sites in the 5p13.1 region harboring SNPs rs4495224 and rs7720838

The study of Libioulle et al. analyzed the influence of 26 SNPs within the gene desert on chromosome *5p13.1* regarding *PTGER4* gene expression [21]. They found that, amongst all analyzed SNPs, the CD risk alleles in rs4495224 and rs7720838 were most strongly associated with increased PTGER4 expression [21]. However, the underlying mechanisms explaining of how these SNPs might influence PTGER expression, were not examined so far. We therefore analyzed *in silico* for potential transcription factor binding sites in the genomic sequences containing SNPs rs4495224 or rs7720838 and the respective surrounding nucleotides. As depicted in table 6, several predicted transcription factor binding sites with high binding scores could be identified for the CD risk alleles in rs4495224 and rs7720838, suggesting a stronger transcription factor binding and hence higher expression of the neighboring *PTGER4* gene as it has been described by Libioulle et al. [21] for the respective CD risk alleles.

Interestingly, rs4495224 is part of a nearly perfect NF-κB consensus sequence (with only one nucleotide not matching the consensus sequence; Table 6). Accordingly, the highest binding scores for the DNA sequence containing the CD risk allele were predicted for the transcription factor NF-κB (p50/p65 heterodimer) as well as for the NF-κB subunits NF-κB p65 (RelA), NF-κB2 (p52) and c-Rel (Table 6). Binding of these factors to DNA containing the protective allele was predicted to be considerably weaker suggesting lower transcriptional activation of neighboring genes.

For rs7720838, the IBD-associated transcription factor XBP1, that has recently been identified as important modulator of intestinal inflammation [34], was predicted to bind strongly to a DNA sequence with the CD risk allele while predicted binding to a sequence with the protective allele was substantially lower (Table 6).

Table 5. Epistasis analysis between SNPs rs4495224 and rs7720838 in the *5p13.1* region and SNPs within the *ATG16L1* gene regarding CD susceptibility in the German discovery study population.

ATG16L1 SNPs	5p13.1/PTGER4 SNPs	
	rs4495224	rs7720838
	P value	P value
rs13412102	4.84×10^{-4}	1.09×10^{-7}
rs12471449	1.09×10^{-2}*	1.39×10^{-2}*
rs6431660	8.37×10^{-5}	2.29×10^{-7}
rs1441090*	8.36×10^{-2}*	5.66×10^{-2}*
rs2289472	3.05×10^{-4}	1.34×10^{-6}
rs2241880 (Thr300Ala)	3.81×10^{-4}	5.99×10^{-7}
rs2241879	3.07×10^{-4}	1.10×10^{-6}
rs3792106	2.65×10^{-4}	1.40×10^{-5}
rs4663396*	9.86×10^{-3}*	7.81×10^{-3}*

Note:
*All p values given are uncorrected for multiple comparisons. After applying Bonferroni correction, all associations remained significant (p<0.05) with the exceptions of those marked with an asterisk.

Table 6. Analysis of transcription factor binding sites in the DNA sequences surrounding SNPs rs4495224 and rs7720838 applying the program TFsearch.

rs4495224 (approx. 200 kb upstream of *PTGER4*):

5'-CAGAGTTTAAATTGG*[A/C]*ACTTCCCCTGAGGAC-3' plus strand

3'-GTCTCAAATTTAACC*[T/G]*TGAAGGGGACTCCAG-5' minus strand

Transcription factor	Consensus sequence #(5'→3')	DNA strand	Position relative to SNP (5'→3')	Binding score risk allele‡	Binding score protective allele‡
NF-κB (p50/p65 heterodimer)	GGGAMTTYCC	minus	−7 to +2	**92.2**	**86.0**
c-Rel	SGGRNWTTCC	minus	−7 to +2	**89.3**	**82.6**
NF-κB p65 (RelA)	GGGRATTTCC	minus	−7 to +2	*88.7*	*78.8*
NF-κB2 (p52)	NGGGACTTTCCA	minus	−8 to +3	**86.3**	**79.1**
MZF1	NGNGGGGA	plus	+4 to +11	82.6	82.6
Elk-1	NNNACMGGAAGTNCNN	minus	−12 to +3	80.5	80.5
STATx	TTCCCRKAA	plus	+3 to +11	79.8	79.8
SRY	AAACWAM	minus	+8 to +14	77.3	77.3
Tst-1	NNKGAWTWANANTKN	minus	−7 to +7	**77.1**	**68.8**
HSF2	NGAANNWTCK	plus	−2 to +7	**76.3**	**67.3**
HSF1	RGAANTRRCN	plus	−2 to +7	*75.7*	*65.2*
p300	NNNRGGAGTNNNNS	minus	−9 to +4	73.3	77.2

rs7720838 (approx. 193 kb upstream of *PTGER4*):

5'-CAGGGCTTTGACATG*[T/G]*CATCACCAATGCATC-3' plus strand

3'-GTCCCGAAACTGTAC*[A/C]*GTAGTGGTTACGTAG-5' minus strand

Transcription factor	Consensus sequence # (5'→3')	DNA strand	Position relative to SNP (5'→3')	Binding score risk allele‡	Binding score protective allele‡
GATA-1	SNNGATNNNN	minus	−7 to +2	85.3	88.6
XBP-1	NNGNTGACGTGKNNNWT	minus	−6 to +10	*83.2*	*73.3*
GATA-2	NNNGATRNNN	minus	−7 to +2	80.6	83.0
Oct-1	CWNAWTKWSATRYN	minus	−7 to +6	**79.6**	**73.5**
CREB	NNGNTGACGYNN	minus	−9 to +2	79.5	82.8
C/EBPb	RNRTKNNGMAAKNN	minus	−8 to +5	78.6	79.2
C/EBP	NNTKTGGWNANNN	minus	−12 to 0	78.5	80.8
MZF1	NGNGGGGA	minus	−10 to −3	77.4	77.4
c-Myc/Max	NANCACGTGNNNW	minus	−4 to +7	*77.3*	*64.1*

Note:
#Nucleotides in the genomic sequences according with the consensus sequences are underlined and the polymorphic nucleotide is marked in **bold**.
‡Predicted binding scores differing more than 5 points between CD risk alleles and protective alleles are depicted in **bold**. Scores differing 10 points and more are depicted in ***bold italic***. Binding score threshold for each allele was set to 75.0. Nucleotide codes: K = G or T, M = A or C, R = A or G, S = C or G, W = A or T, Y = C or T, N = A, G, C or T.

Discussion

In summary, our study confirms the *5p13.1* region as susceptibility locus in CD. This finding is in agreement with the genome-wide association studies by Libioulle and co-workers [21] and Franke et al. [35]. In contrast, we could not replicate a contribution of the *5p13.1* region to UC susceptibility which was demonstrated by recent meta-analyses of GWAS [29,36] and may be related to the limited sample size of our cohort and the weaker effect of the *5p13.1* region on UC susceptibility compared to CD susceptibility. Very recently, the largest meta-analysis ever performed in IBD, including more than 75,000 cases and controls, demonstrated an association with UC, which convincingly

confirms that there is a very strong association of the *PTGER4* locus with CD (p = 1.81×10^{-82}), while there is only a weak association with UC (p = 1.68×10^{-5} for the immunochip UC cohort) which reached only in all UC cohorts combined genome-wide significance (p = 1.36×10^{-10} for all UC cohorts combined) [37]. This clearly illustrates that extremely large cohorts are required to show significant results for weak associations as for *PTGER4* and UC. Following Bonferroni correction, we could not identify a specific IBD subphenotype associated with the investigated SNPs in the *5p13.1* region.

In CD, the observed ORs for the minor alleles of the analyzed *PTGER4* SNPs are below a value of 1.0 and thus, are most likely protective while the major alleles represent the CD risk alleles for both SNPs. The rs4495224 A and rs7720838 T risk alleles (=major alleles) were associated with increased PTGER4 expression in the study of Libioulle et al. [21]. Although protective functions of EP4 against inflammation have been described, [22–24,38], other studies reported a proinflammatory role for EP4 in models of rheumatoid arthritis or experimental autoimmune encephalitis [39–41]. Interestingly, EP4 has been shown to drive the differentiation of Th1 cells and proliferation of Th17 [40–42]. Since these two proinflammatory T cell subsets play very important roles in the pathogenesis of CD [43], increased expression of PTGER4 and therefore increased EP4 signaling in carriers of the CD risk alleles of the two SNPs rs4495224 and rs7720838 is plausible. The transcription factors NF-κB and XBP1 were identified as very likely candidates for binding to the respective genomic regions and thereby increasing PTGER4 expression. NF-κB is a transcription factor involved in many inflammatory signaling pathways and has been implicated in the pathogenesis of IBD [44]. XBP1 has very recently been described as an important transcription factor that links endoplasmatic reticulum stress to the development of intestinal inflammation [34]. However, further functional studies are necessary to clarify the influence of these transcription factors on PTGER4 expression and to further elucidate the role of this chromosomal region in the CD pathogenesis.

Prostaglandins are arachidonic acid metabolites produced by the action of the enzymes cyclooxygenase-1 and -2 (COX-1 and COX-2) which have been identified to play a crucial role in the physiological regulation of inflammation and gastrointestinal homeostasis [45–47] as well as in the defense of the intestinal mucosa [48]. Moreover, a haplotype of prostaglandin synthase 2/cyclooxygenase 2 has been found to be involved in IBD susceptibility [25] and microsomal prostaglandin E synthase-1 is overexpressed in IBD [26]. Interestingly, prostaglandin 15-deoxy-delta(12,14)-PGJ2 attenuates the development of intestinal injury caused by dinitrobenzene sulphonic acid (DNBS) in rats [27].

Recently, PTGER4 polymorphisms have been found to be associated with asthma [49] including aspirin-intolerant asthma [50], suggesting a role also in inflammation of the respiratory tract. Prostaglandin E2-EP4 signaling was further found to play a key role in skin immune responses by promoting migration and maturation of Langerhans cells, specialized antigen-presenting cells (APCs) [51]. Since APCs such as dendritic cells (DCs) are critical for the defense against intestinal bacterial microbiota [52], prostaglandin E2-EP4 signaling might also contribute to IBD via the regulation of intestinal DCs. Interestingly, we and others demonstrated that the capacity of lamina propria DCs to form transepithelial dendrites for sampling of luminal antigens depends on the chemokine receptor CX3CR1 [52] which was identified by us as an important genetic modifier of the CD phenotype [13].

In addition, we report strong epistasis between PTGER4 expression-modulating SNPs in the 5p13.1 region and the ATG16L1 gene in the German discovery cohort. Based on the p-value of 1×10^{-7} for the strongest interaction (between rs7720838 and rs13412102), this is the strongest epistasis signal reported so far and nearly 3-log fold stronger than the most significant gene-gene interaction reported in the meta-analysis by Barrett et al. [53]. However, this gene-gene interaction was only observed in the German discovery population but not in the U.S. American and the German replication cohorts, suggesting that the epistasis between the two gene regions is not a general phenomenon contributing to CD susceptibility in all Caucasian populations. This is supported by the recent meta-analyses of GWAS [35,53] which did not find epistasis between SNPs in the PTGER4 and ATG16L1 regions.

The lack of replication of the gene-gene interaction between PTGER4 and ATG16L1 regions may be related to population differences, although this is unlikely given the close genetic similarity between the South and North German population representing the discovery and the replication cohort, respectively. However, some minor genetic differences were shown between the populations analyzed in this study (e.g., association of CD with DLG5 only in the North German population [54,32] and association with PHOX2B, NCF4 and FAM92B only in the North American population [10] but not the German population [55]). Furthermore, methodological issues could explain the lack of replication of the gene-gene interaction between PTGER4 and ATG16L1 since a different genotyping platform was used in the U.S. American and in the German CD replication cohorts requiring the use of surrogate markers instead of the original SNPs used in the German discovery population. However, given the high linkage disequilibrium between original SNPs and surrogate markers, this is very unlikely. The observed gene-gene interaction could also be coincidental which illustrates the need for extremely large sample sizes to find convincing association evidence and separate true signals from noise for complex trait loci that have small effect sizes.

The potential intergenic interaction between ATG16L1 and the 5p13.1 region would be of particular interest since the exact functional consequences of polymorphisms in the 5p13.1 chromosomal region are largely unknown. In the study of Libioulle and co-workers [21], the disease-associated alleles were found to correlate with expression levels of PTGER4 which was the gene located closest to the associated region. The finding of PTGER4 as an important CD target gene in the 5p13.1 region is also in line with reports of Ptger4 knock-out mice developing severe DSS-induced colitis [22,23].

In summary, our study confirms the chromosome 5p13.1 region as a susceptibility locus in CD. For the first time, we demonstrate the strongly CD-associated PTGER4 SNPs rs4495224 and rs7720838 as part of binding sites for NF-κB and XBP1, suggesting that these transcription factors may modulate PTGER4 expression. However, further functional assays are necessary to clarify if the SNPs analyzed in our study modulate binding of transcription factors and thereby regulating PTGER4 expression and IBD susceptibility. We could not identify a specific IBD phenotype associated with the SNPs rs4495224 and rs7720838, although the cohort used in this study convincingly demonstrated other strong association such as for the NOD2 variant p.Leu1007fsX1008 with ileal CD involvement, stenosis and need for surgery [16,17,56,57], suggesting that the sample size in CD was sufficient to detect clinically relevant associations. In addition, a strong epistasis signal between rs4495224 and rs7720838 with SNPs in the ATG16L1 gene region was observed in the German CD discovery cohort. However, this gene-gene interaction could not be replicated in the North American CD cohort and in the German CD replication cohort, arguing against a major role of this interaction in the CD pathogenesis. Further functional studies are required to clarify the exact role of the 5p13.1 region in the CD pathogenesis.

Supporting Information

Table S1   Primer sequences, FRET probe sequences, and primer annealing temperatures used for genotyping of rs4495224 and rs7720838.
(DOC)

Table S2   Primer sequences used for sequence analysis of rs4495224 and rs7720838.
(DOC)

Table S3 Primer sequences and restriction enzymes used for genotyping of *NOD2* and *SLC22A4/5* variants.
(DOC)

Table S4 Primer sequences, FRET probe sequences, and primer annealing temperatures used for genotyping *IL23R* variants.
(DOC)

Table S5 Primer sequences, FRET probe sequences, and primer annealing temperatures used for genotyping *ATG16L1* variants.
(DOC)

Table S6 Association between rs4495224 genotype and CD disease characteristics based on the Montreal classification [31].
(DOC)

Table S7 Association between rs7720838 genotype and CD disease characteristics based on the Montreal classification [31].
(DOC)

Table S8 Association between rs4495224 genotype and UC disease characteristics based on the Montreal classification [31].
(DOC)

Table S9 Association between rs7720838 genotype and UC disease characteristics based on the Montreal classification [31].
(DOC)

Table S10 Allele frequencies of the SNPs within the *ATG16L1* gene in the North American replication cohort with Crohn's disease and controls.
(DOC)

Table S11 Allele frequencies of the SNPs within the *ATG16L1* gene region in the German replication cohort with Crohn's disease patients and controls.
(DOC)

Table S12 Epistasis analysis between SNPs rs4495224 and rs7720838 in the *5p13.1* region and SNPs within the *ATG16L1* gene regarding CD susceptibility in the North American (NIDDK IBD Genetics Consortium) replication cohort.
(DOC)

Table S13 Epistasis analysis between SNPs rs10941508 and rs7720838 in the *5p13.1* region and SNPs within the *ATG16L1* gene regarding CD susceptibility in the German replication cohort.
(DOC)

Author Contributions

Conceived and designed the experiments: JG TB JPA MIK AF RHD SB. Performed the experiments: JG GP JD MW TB JPA MIK AF RHD. Analyzed the data: JD DC GP CW BMM TB JPA MIK AF RHD SB. Contributed reagents/materials/analysis tools: JG DC JD TO CW BMM TB JPA MIK AF RHD SB. Wrote the paper: JS JG SB. Organized the collaboration between the different centers: SB.

References

1. Podolsky DK (2002) Inflammatory bowel disease. N Engl J Med 347: 417–429.
2. Xavier RJ, Podolsky DK (2007) Unravelling the pathogenesis of inflammatory bowel disease. Nature 448: 427–434.
3. Sartor RB (2006) Mechanisms of disease pathogenesis of Crohn's disease and ulcerative colitis. Nat Clin Pract Gastroenterol Hepatol 3: 390–407.
4. Cho JH, Weaver CT (2007) The genetics of inflammatory bowel disease. Gastroenterology 133: 1327–1339.
5. Ogura Y, Bonen DK, Inohara N, Nicolae DL, Chen FF, et al. (2001) A frameshift mutation in NOD2 associated with susceptibility to Crohn's disease. Nature 411: 603–606.
6. Hugot JP, Chamaillard M, Zouali H, Lesage S, Cezard JP, et al. (2001) Association of NOD2 leucine-rich repeat variants with susceptibility to Crohn's disease. Nature 411: 599–603.
7. Duerr RH, Taylor KD, Brant SR, Rioux JD, Silverberg MS, et al. (2006) A genome-wide association study identifies IL23R as an inflammatory bowel disease gene. Science 314: 1461–1463.
8. Glas J, Seiderer J, Wetzke M, Konrad A, Török HP, et al. (2007) rs1004819 is the main disease-associated IL23R variant in German Crohn's disease patients: combined analysis of IL23R, CARD15, and OCTN1/2 variants. PLoS ONE 2: e819.
9. Hampe J, Franke A, Rosenstiel P, Till A, Teuber M, et al. (2007) A genome-wide association scan of nonsynonymous SNPs identifies a susceptibility variant for Crohn disease in ATG16L1. Nat Genet 39: 207–211.
10. Rioux JD, Xavier RJ, Taylor KD, Silverberg MS, Goyette P, et al. (2007) Genome-wide association study identifies new susceptibility loci for Crohn disease and implicates autophagy in disease pathogenesis. Nat Genet 39: 596–604.
11. Glas J, Konrad A, Schmechel S, Dambacher J, Seiderer J, et al. (2007) The ATG16L1 gene variants rs2241879 and rs2241880 (T300A) are strongly associated with susceptibility to Crohn's disease in the German population. Am J Gastroenterol 103: 682–691.
12. Parkes M, Barrett JC, Prescott NJ, Tremelling M, Anderson CA, et al. (2007) Sequence variants in the autophagy gene IRGM and multiple other replicating loci contribute to Crohn's disease susceptibility. Nat Genet 39: 830–832.
13. Brand S, Hofbauer K, Dambacher J, Schnitzler F, Staudinger T, et al. (2006) Increased expression of the chemokine fractalkine in Crohn's disease and association of the fractalkine receptor T280M polymorphism with a fibrostenosing disease phenotype. Am J Gastroenterol 101: 99–106.
14. Brand S, Staudinger T, Schnitzler F, Pfennig S, Hofbauer K, et al. (2005) The role of Toll-like receptor 4 Asp299Gly and Thr399Ile polymorphisms and CARD15/NOD2 mutations in the susceptibility and phenotype of Crohn's disease. Inflamm Bowel Dis 11: 645–652.
15. Schnyder-Candrian S, Togbe D, Couillin I, Mercier I, Brombacher F, et al. (2006) Interleukin-17 is a negative regulator of established allergic asthma. J Exp Med 203: 2715–2725.
16. Seiderer J, Schnitzler F, Brand S, Staudinger T, Pfennig S, et al. (2006) Homozygosity for the CARD15 frameshift mutation 1007fs is predictive of early onset of Crohn's disease with ileal stenosis, entero-enteral fistulas, and frequent need for surgical intervention with high risk of re-stenosis. Scand J Gastroenterol 41: 1421–1432.
17. Seiderer J, Brand S, Herrmann KA, Schnitzler F, Hatz R, et al. (2006) Predictive value of the CARD15 variant 1007fs for the diagnosis of intestinal stenoses and the need for surgery in Crohn's disease in clinical practice: results of a prospective study. Inflamm Bowel Dis 12: 1114–1121.
18. Thalmaier D, Dambacher J, Seiderer J, Konrad A, Schachinger V, et al. (2006) The +1059G/C polymorphism in the C-reactive protein (CRP) gene is associated with involvement of the terminal ileum and decreased serum CRP levels in patients with Crohn's disease. Aliment Pharmacol Ther 24: 1105–1115.
19. Schnitzler F, Brand S, Staudinger T, Pfennig S, Hofbauer K, et al. (2006) Eight novel CARD15 variants detected by DNA sequence analysis of the CARD15 gene in 111 patients with inflammatory bowel disease. Immunogenetics 58: 99–106.
20. Glas J, Seiderer J, Nagy M, Fries C, Beigel F, et al. (2010) Evidence for STAT4 as a common autoimmune gene: rs7574865 is associated with colonic Crohn's disease and early disease onset. PLoS One 5: e10373.
21. Libioulle C, Louis E, Hansoul S, Sandor C, Farnir F, et al. (2007) Novel Crohn disease locus identified by genome-wide association maps to a gene desert on 5p13.1 and modulates expression of PTGER4. PLoS Genet 3: e58.
22. Kabashima K, Saji T, Murata T, Nagamachi M, Matsuoka T, et al. (2002) The prostaglandin receptor EP4 suppresses colitis, mucosal damage and CD4 cell activation in the gut. J Clin Invest 109: 883–893.
23. Nitta M, Hirata I, Toshina K, Murano M, Maemura K, et al. (2002) Expression of the EP4 prostaglandin E2 receptor subtype with rat dextran sodium sulphate colitis: colitis suppression by a selective agonist, ONO-AE1-329. Scand J Immunol 56: 66–75.
24. Jiang GL, Nieves A, Im WB, Old DW, Dinh DT, et al. (2007) The prevention of colitis by E Prostanoid receptor 4 agonist through enhancement of epithelium survival and regeneration. J Pharmacol Exp Ther 320: 22–28.
25. Cox DG, Crusius JB, Peeters PH, Bueno-de-Mesquita HB, Pena AS, et al. (2005) Haplotype of prostaglandin synthase 2/cyclooxygenase 2 is involved in the susceptibility to inflammatory bowel disease. World J Gastroenterol 11: 6003–6008.
26. Subbaramaiah K, Yoshimatsu K, Scherl E, Das KM, Glazier KD, et al. (2004) Microsomal prostaglandin E synthase-1 is overexpressed in inflammatory bowel

disease. Evidence for involvement of the transcription factor Egr-1. J Biol Chem 279: 12647–12658.

27. Cuzzocrea S, Ianaro A, Wayman NS, Mazzon E, Pisano B, et al. (2003) The cyclopentenone prostaglandin 15-deoxy-delta(12,14)- PGJ2 attenuates the development of colon injury caused by dinitrobenzene sulphonic acid in the rat. Br J Pharmacol 138: 678–688.

28. Franke A, Hampe J, Rosenstiel P, Becker C, Wagner F, et al. (2007) Systematic association mapping identifies NELL1 as a novel IBD disease gene. PLoS ONE 2: e691.

29. McGovern DP, Gardet A, Törkvist L, Goyette P, Essers J, et al. (2010) Genome-wide association identifies multiple ulcerative colitis susceptibility loci. Nat Genet 42: 332–337.

30. Lennard-Jones JE (1989) Classification of inflammatory bowel disease. Scand J Gastroenterol Suppl 170: 2–6; discussion 16–19.

31. Silverberg MS, Satsangi J, Ahmad T, Arnott ID, Bernstein CN, et al. (2005) Toward an integrated clinical, molecular and serological classification of inflammatory bowel disease: Report of a Working Party of the 2005 Montreal World Congress of Gastroenterology. Can J Gastroenterol 19 Suppl A: 5–36.

32. Török HP, Glas J, Tonenchi L, Lohse P, Müller-Myhsok B, et al. (2005) Polymorphisms in the DLG5 and OCTN cation transporter genes in Crohn's disease. Gut 54: 1421–1427.

33. Heinemeyer T, Wingender E, Reuter I, Hermjakob H, Kel AE, et al. (1998) Databases on transcriptional regulation: TRANSFAC, TRRD and COMPEL. Nucleic Acids Res 26: 362–7.

34. Kaser A, Lee AH, Franke A, Glickman JN, Zeissig S, et al. (2008) XBP1 links ER stress to intestinal inflammation and confers genetic risk for human inflammatory bowel disease. Cell 134: 743–56.

35. Franke A, McGovern DP, Barrett JC, Wang K, Radford-Smith GL, et al. (2010) Genome-wide meta-analysis increases to 71 the number of confirmed Crohn's disease susceptibility loci. Nat Genet 42: 1118–1125.

36. Anderson CA, Boucher G, Lees CW, Franke A, D'Amato M, et al. (2011) Meta-analysis identifies 31 additional ulcerative colitis risk loci, increasing the number of confirmed associations to 49. Nat Genet 43: 246–252.

37. Jostins L, Ripke L, Weersma R, Duerr RH, McGovern DP, et al. (2012). Host-microbe interactions have shaped the genetic architecture of inflammatory bowel disease. Nature 491: 119–24.

38. Okamoto T, Uemoto S, Tabata Y (2012) Prevention of trinitrobenzene sulfonic acid-induced experimental colitis by oral administration of a poly(lactic-coglycolic acid microsphere containing prostaglandin E2 receptor subtype 4 agonist. J Pharmacol Exp Ther 341: 340–349.

39. Clark P, Rowland SE, Denis D, Mathieu MC, Stocco R, et al. (2008) MF498 [N-{[4-(5,9-Diethoxy-6-oxo-6,8-dihydro-7H-pyrrolo[3,4-g]quinolin-7-yl)-3-methylbenzyl]sulfonyl}-2-(2-methoxyphenyl)acetamide], a selective E prostanoid receptor 4 antagonist, relieves joint inflammation and pain in rodent models of rheumatoid and osteoarthritis. J Pharmacol Exp Ther 325: 425–434.

40. Chen Q, Muramoto K, Masaaki N, Ding Y, Yang H, et al. (2010) A novel antagonist of the prostaglandin E(2) EP(4) receptor inhibits Th1 differentiation and Th17 expansion and is orally active in arthritis models. Br J Pharmacol 160: 292–310.

41. Yao C, Sakata D, Esaki Y, Li Y, Matsuoka T, et al. (2009) Prostaglandin E2-EP4 signaling promotes immune inflammation through Th1 cell differentiation and Th17 cell expansion. Nat Med 15: 633–640.

42. Boniface K, Bak-Jensen KS, Li Y, Blumenschein WM, McGeachy MJ, et al. (2009) Prostaglandin E2 regulates Th17 cell differentiation and function through cyclic AMP and EP2/EP4 receptor signaling. J Exp Med 206: 535–548.

43. Brand S (2009) Crohn's disease: Th1, Th17 or both? The change of a paradigm: new immunological and genetic insights implicate Th17 cells in the pathogenesis of Crohn's disease. Gut 2009 58: 1152–1167.

44. Atreya I, Atreya R, Neurath MF (2008) NF-kappaB in inflammatory bowel disease. J Intern Med 263: 591–596.

45. Morteau O (2000) Prostaglandins and inflammation: the cyclooxygenase controversy. Arch Immunol Ther Exp (Warsz) 48: 473–480.

46. Dey I, Lejeune M, Chadee K (2006) Prostaglandin E2 receptor distribution and function in the gastrointestinal tract. Br J Pharmacol 149: 611–623.

47. Gookin JL, Galanko JA, Blikslager AT, Argenzio RA (2003) PG-mediated closure of paracellular pathway and not restitution is the primary determinant of barrier recovery in acutely injured porcine ileum. Am J Physiol Gastrointest Liver Physiol 285: G967–G979.

48. Morteau O, Morham SG, Sellon R, Dieleman LA, Langenbach R, et al. (2000) Impaired mucosal defense to acute colonic injury in mice lacking cyclooxygenase-1 or cyclooxygenase-2. J Clin Invest 105: 469–478.

49. Kurz T, Hoffjan S, Hayes MG, Schneider D, Nicolae R, et al. (2006) Fine mapping and positional candidate studies on chromosome 5p13 identify multiple asthma susceptibility loci. J Allergy Clin Immunol 118: 396–402.

50. Kim SH, Kim YK, Park HW, Jee YK, Bahn JW, et al. (2007) Association between polymorphisms in prostanoid receptor genes and aspirin-intolerant asthma. Pharmacogenet Genomics 17: 295–304.

51. Kabashima K, Sakata D, Nagamachi M, Miyachi Y, Inaba K (2003) Narumiya S. Prostaglandin E2-EP4 signaling initiates skin immune responses by promoting migration and maturation of Langerhans cells. Nat Med 9: 744–749.

52. Niess JH, Brand S, Gu X, Landsman L, Jung S, et al. (2005) CX3CR1-mediated dendritic cell access to the intestinal lumen and bacterial clearance. Science 307: 254–258.

53. Barrett JC, Hansoul S, Nicolae DL, Cho JH, Duerr RH, et al. (2008) Genome-wide association defines more than 30 distinct susceptibility loci for Crohn's disease. Nat Genet 40: 955–962.

54. Stoll M, Corneliussen B, Costello CM, Waetzig GH, Mellgard B, et al. (2004) Genetic variation in DLG5 is associated with inflammatory bowel disease. Nat Genet 36: 476–480.

55. Glas J, Pasciuto G, Tillack C, Diegelmann J, et al. (2009) rs224136 on chromosome 10q21.1 and variants in PHOX2B, NCF4, and FAM92B are not major genetic risk factors for susceptibility to Crohn's disease in the German population. Am J Gastroenterol 104: 665–672.

56. Glas J, Seiderer J, Tillack C, Pfennig S, Beigel F, et al. (2010) The NOD2 single nucleotide polymorphisms rs2066843 and rs2076756 are novel and common Crohn's disease susceptibility gene variants. PLoS One 5:e14466.

57. Jürgens M, Brand S, Laubender RP, Seiderer J, Glas J, et al. (2010) The presence of fistulas and NOD2 homozygosity strongly predict intestinal stenosis in Crohn's disease independent of the IL23R genotype. J Gastroenterol 45:721–31.

20

A Randomized Controlled Trial of the Efficacy and Safety of CCX282-B, an Orally-Administered Blocker of Chemokine Receptor CCR9, for Patients with Crohn's Disease

Satish Keshav[1], Tomáš Vaňásek[2], Yaron Niv[3], Robert Petryka[4], Stephanie Howaldt[5], Mauro Bafutto[6], István Rácz[7], David Hetzel[8], Ole Haagen Nielsen[9], Séverine Vermeire[10], Walter Reinisch[11], Per Karlén[12], Stefan Schreiber[13], Thomas J. Schall[14], Pirow Bekker[14]*, for the Prospective Randomized Oral-Therapy Evaluation in Crohn's Disease Trial-1 (PROTECT-1) Study Group¶

1 John Radcliffe Hospital, University of Oxford, Oxford, United Kingdom, 2 Hepato-Gastroenterologie HK, Hradec Králové, Czech Republic, 3 Rabin Medical Center, Petach Tikva, Israel, 4 NZOZ Vivamed, Zespół Lekarzy Specjalistów, Warszawa, Poland, 5 Praxis für Innere Medizin, Hamburg, Germany, 6 Instituto Goiano de Gastroenterologia e Endoscopia Digestiva Ltda., Goiânia, Brazil, 7 Petz Aladár County and Teaching Hospital, Győr, Hungary, 8 Royal Adelaide Hospital, Adelaide, Australia, 9 Department of Gastroenterology, Herlev Hospital, Herlev, Denmark, 10 UZ Gasthuisberg, Leuven, Belgium, 11 Allgemeines Krankenhaus Wien, Universitätsklinik für Innere Medizin III, Klinische Abteilung für Gastroenterologie und Hepatologie, Vienna, Austria, 12 Department of Clinical Science and Education, Karolinska Institutet, Södersjukhuset, Stockholm, Sweden, 13 Department of Medicine I, Christian Albrechts University, University Hospital Schleswig Holstein, Kiel, Germany, 14 ChemoCentryx, Inc., Mountain View, California, United States of America

Abstract

CCX282-B, also called vercirnon, is a specific, orally-administered chemokine receptor CCR9 antagonist that regulates migration and activation of inflammatory cells in the intestine. This randomized, placebo-controlled trial was conducted to evaluate the safety and efficacy of CCX282-B in 436 patients with Crohn's disease. Crohn's Disease Activity Index (CDAI) scores were 250–450 and C-reactive protein >7.5 mg/L at study entry. In addition to stable concomitant Crohn's medication (85% of subjects), subjects received placebo or CCX282-B (250 mg once daily, 250 mg twice daily, or 500 mg once daily) for 12 weeks. They then received 250 mg CCX282-B twice daily, open-label, through week 16. Subjects who had a clinical response (a ≥70 point drop in CDAI) at week 16 were randomly assigned to groups given placebo or CCX282-B (250 mg, twice daily) for 36 weeks. Primary endpoints were clinical response at Week 8 and sustained clinical response at Week 52. During the 12-week Induction period, the clinical response was highest in the group given 500 mg CCX282-B once daily. Response rates at week 8 were 49% in the placebo group, 52% in the group given CCX282-B 250 mg once daily (odds ratio [OR] = 1.12; p = .667 vs placebo), 48% in the group given CCX282-B 250 mg twice daily (OR = 0.95; p = .833), and 60% in the group given CCX282-B 500 mg once daily (OR = 1.53; p = .111). At week 12, response rates were 47%, 56% (OR = 1.44; p = .168), 49% (OR = 1.07; p = .792), and 61% (OR = 1.74; p = .039), respectively. At the end of the Maintenance period (week 52), 47% of subjects on CCX282-B were in remission, compared to 31% on placebo (OR = 2.01; p = .012); 46% showed sustained clinical responses, compared to 42% on placebo (OR = 1.14; p = .629). CCX282-B was well tolerated. Encouraging results from this clinical trial led to initiation of Phase 3 clinical trials in Crohn's disease.

Trial Registration: ClinicalTrials.gov NCT00306215.

Editor: Lise Lotte Gluud, Copenhagen University Hospital Gentofte, Denmark

Funding: The authors have no support or funding to report.

Competing Interests: The authors have the following interests. P. Bekker is an employee and shareholder of ChemoCentryx, and T. Schall is an employee, shareholder, and holder of patent number US2005-0137179 on bis-aryl sulfonamides., the funder of this clinical trial. Robert Petryka, is an employee of NZOZ Vivamed, which is a network of medical care specialists. NZOZ Vivamed does not have any commercial interest or stake in the drug candidate, CCX282-B, tested in the clinical trial which is the subject of this manuscript. There are no further patents, products in development or marketed products to declare.

* E-mail: pbekker@chemocentryx.com

¶ The investigators who contributed to the Prospective Randomized Oral-Therapy Evaluation in Crohn's Disease Trial-1 (PROTECT-1) are listed in Appendix S1.

Introduction

Crohn's disease is characterized by leukocyte infiltration of segments of the intestine, most commonly in the terminal ileum and colon, leading to mucosal erosion, ulceration, fistulization, and stenosis. [1] Chemokine receptors are G-protein coupled cell-surface proteins that interact with their chemokine ligands, which are low-molecular weight cytokine-like proteins, forming an elaborate system that regulates the migration and movement of inflammatory and immune cells within the body. [2] The C-C chemokine receptor CCR9 is expressed on a certain subset of circulating lymphocytes and is the principal chemokine receptor mediating homing to the intestinal mucosa, with enrichment of CCR9-positive cells in the intestine. [3] CCL25, or thymus-expressed chemokine (TECK), is the only identified CCR9 ligand [4], and is highly expressed in the intestine and thymus. CD8-positive T lymphocytes, plasmablasts, plasma cells, and plasma-cytoid dendritic cells expressing CCR9 are involved in cellular interactions contributing to the pathogenesis of Crohn's disease [5–8].

CCX282-B, also called Traficet-EN, GSK1605786A, or vercirnon, is a small molecule CCR9 antagonist that inhibits CCR9- and CCL25-dependent chemotaxis. Preclinical and early clinical studies suggested that orally-administered CCX282-B could reduce intestinal inflammation in inflammatory bowel disease (IBD). [9] This clinical trial, termed PROTECT-1 for Prospective Randomized Oral-Therapy Evaluation in Crohn's disease, is the first major study to evaluate the safety and efficacy of a chemokine receptor antagonist in IBD.

Methods

The protocol for this trial and supporting CONSORT checklist are available as supporting information; see Checklist S1 and Protocol S1.

Ethics Statement

All subjects provided written informed consent prior to any study procedures. The names of ethics committees that reviewed and approved the clinical trial are provided in the Appendix.

All study procedures were governed by International Conference on Harmonisation Good Clinical Practice standards and the Declaration of Helsinki.

Study Subjects

Ninety study centers in 17 countries in North America, Europe, Australia, Brazil, and South Africa enrolled and treated subjects from March 2006 to May 2009. The clinicaltrials.gov registration number is NCT00306215 (http://clinicaltrials.gov/ct2/show/NCT00306215?term = CCX282-B&rank = 2). This clinical trial was sponsored by ChemoCentryx. Adult subjects with moderate to severe small bowel and/or colonic Crohn's disease were enrolled. The Crohn's Disease Activity Index (CDAI) [10] at screening was required to be 250 to 450, with fasting serum C-reactive protein (CRP) above 7.5 mg/L. Subjects receiving immunosuppressants or glucocorticoids (up to 20 mg prednisone-equivalent) had to be on stable doses for at least 4 weeks prior to randomization, and concomitant stable use of these drugs during the study was allowed. Concomitant 5-ASA treatment was also allowed. Anti-TNF or anti-α4 integrin treatment within 12 weeks prior to randomization was prohibited, and concomitant use during the study was not allowed.

Study Design

This was a randomized, double-blind, placebo-controlled clinical trial to assess the efficacy and safety of CCX282-B in patients with moderate to severe Crohn's disease. During the initial 12-week Induction period, subjects were randomized to receive placebo or CCX282-B, either 250 mg once daily (q.d.), 250 mg twice daily (b.i.d.), or 500 mg q.d. in a 1.5:1:1:1 ratio. Randomization was performed centrally using an interactive voice response system. A blocked randomization schedule was generated by a biostatistician who was otherwise not involved in the study. Since efficacy in each CCX282-B group was compared to placebo, and for sample size efficiency, 1.5 times the number of subjects

were randomized to the placebo group compared to each CCX282-B group. To conceal the allocation sequence, placebo and CCX282-B capsules, containing 250 mg CCX282-B, and bottles were identical in appearance and subjects received one kit (box) with three bottles of study medication every 4 weeks. The placebo kits contained three bottles of placebo capsules, the 250 mg q.d. kits contained one bottle of CCX282-B capsules (bottle 1) and two bottles of placebo (bottles 2 and 3), the 250 mg b.i.d. kits contained two bottles of CCX282-B capsules (bottles 1 and 3) and one bottle of placebo (bottle 2), and the 500 mg q.d. kits contained two bottles of CCX282-B capsules (bottles 1 and 2) and one bottle of placebo (bottle 3). Subjects were asked to take one capsule from each of the first two bottles every morning and one capsule from the third bottle every evening, 12 hours after the morning dose. Study medication was taken with water and could be taken with or without a meal.

The placebo-controlled portion of the study was double-blind. Blinding of the study was achieved by the following measures: (1) Study medication bottle and capsule appearances were identical; (2) Limited access was provided to the randomization code: Study site personnel, study subjects, personnel responsible for study monitoring, and biostatisticians and data managers involved in data analysis of the study, remained blinded to treatment assignment for the duration of the study; (3) While laboratory personnel conducting the pharmacokinetic (PK) assays were not blinded to treatment assignment, unblinded CCX282 plasma concentration results were not shared with the study site personnel or the study staff with direct contact with study sites during the study; (4) Efficacy data that could potentially be unblinding, such as serum CRP and CDAI scores, were not made available to study site personnel, study subjects, personnel responsible for study monitoring, and biostatisticians and data managers during the study unless required for safety monitoring.

After trial initiation, the protocol was amended to extend the study period from 12 weeks to 52 weeks to add a 4-week Active period and a 36-week Maintenance period. The amendment was implemented prior to having knowledge of the Induction period results. Subjects who had completed the Induction period of the study by the time of implementation of the protocol amendment, were allowed to enter the 4-week Active treatment period if they were within 3 months after completing the Induction period. All consenting subjects who completed 12 weeks in the Induction period received 250 mg CCX282-B b.i.d. from week 12 to 16 in an open-label Active period. This Active period was inserted between the Induction and Maintenance periods to allow all subjects, including those receiving placebo during the Induction period, to receive CCX282-B treatment and potentially to be included in the CDAI ≥70-point responder population for the Maintenance period. All consenting subjects who showed a clinical response at week 16 (CDAI decrease of ≥70 points compared to study baseline value), were re-randomized to receive placebo or CCX282-B 250 mg b.i.d., in a ratio of 1:1.5 in the Maintenance period, from week 16 to 52. This change in the study allowed for evaluation of CCX282-B in both induction and maintenance settings. Corticosteroids, if used at week 16, were to be tapered to zero over a period not exceeding 6 weeks.

CDAI and CRP (high sensitivity assay with 3 mg/L as upper limit of normal) were recorded at baseline and weeks 4, 8, 12, 16, 20, 28, 36, 44, and 52. Consenting subjects, at study sites that agreed to participate, underwent colonoscopy at baseline and week 12. The Crohn's Disease Endoscopic Index of Severity (CDEIS) was calculated using a modification of the method described by Mary and Modigliani. [11] The length of disease involvement and ulceration was recorded as actual lengths, in cm, rather than

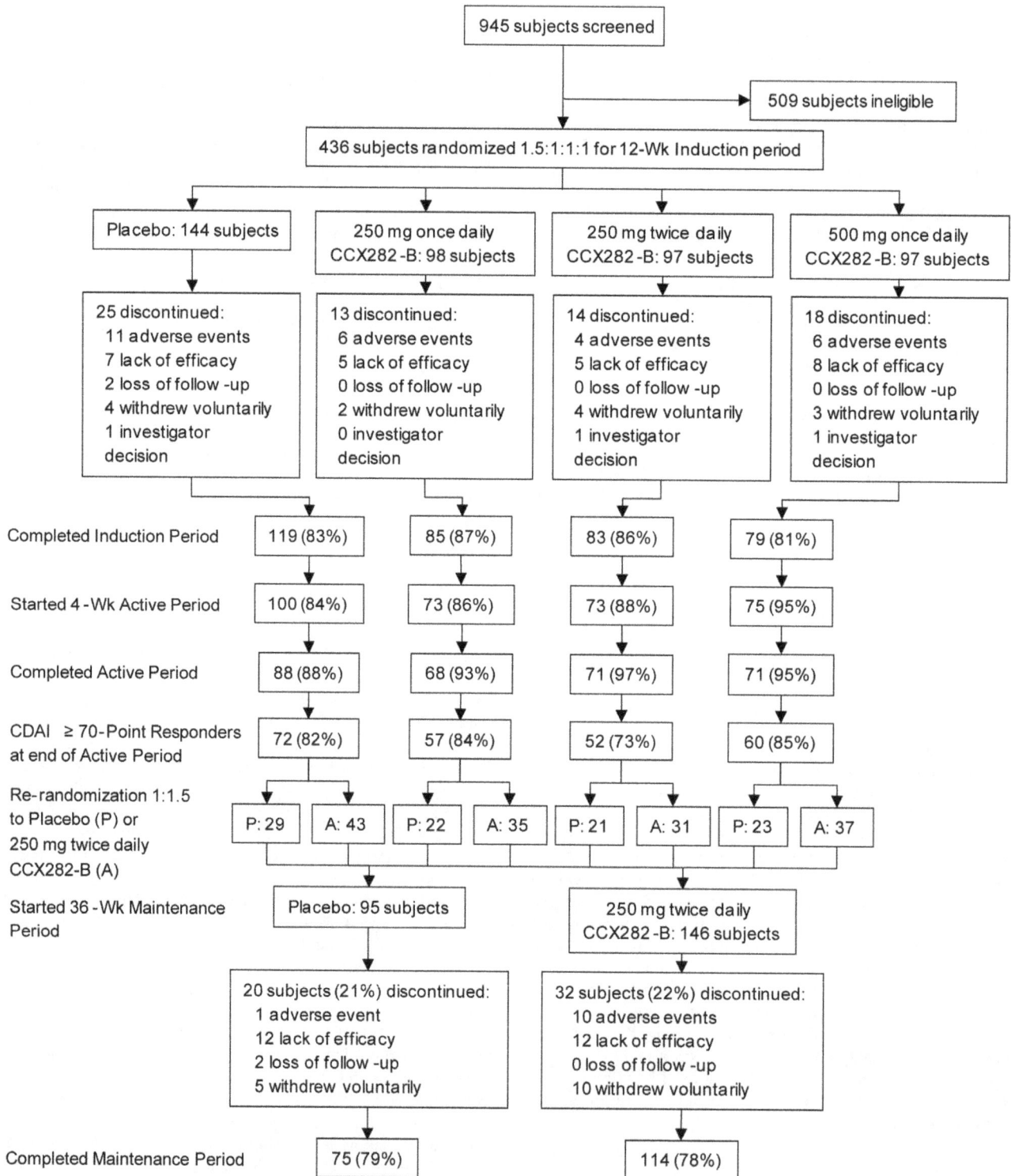

Figure 1. Subject Disposition. A total of 945 subjects were screened of whom 436 were randomized. Screen failure occurred most commonly for low CRP (57%) and low CDAI (24%). In the Induction period, 144 subjects were randomized to placebo, and 98, 97, and 97 to CCX282-B 250 mg q.d., 250 mg b.i.d., or 500 mg q.d., respectively. One subject, in the 250 mg b.i.d. group was excluded from the ITT population in the Induction period because the subject did not take any study medication. In the four groups, 83%, 87%, 86%, and 81% completed the Induction period. Most common primary reasons for withdrawal were adverse events and lack of efficacy with similar distributions across treatment groups. A total of 321 subjects started the 4-week open-label Active period, receiving CCX282-B 250 mg b.i.d.; 298 subjects completed this period, and of these, 241 clinical responders were enrolled in the Maintenance period. These subjects were re-randomized to placebo (95 subjects) or 250 mg b.i.d. CCX282-B (146 subjects). One subject, in the 250 mg b.i.d. group was excluded from the ITT population in the Maintenance period because the subject did not take any study medication. Of the two groups, 79% and 78%, respectively, completed the Maintenance period. The most common primary reason for withdrawal in the placebo group was lack of efficacy, 13% (12 of 95 subjects), compared to 8% (12 of 145 subjects) in the CCX282-B group, whereas the most common primary reason for withdrawal from the CCX282-B group was adverse events, 7% (10 of 145 subjects), compared to 1% (1 of 95

subjects) in the placebo group. Most of the adverse events leading to withdrawal in the CCX282-B group (9 of 10 cases) were related to Crohn's disease. Arguably, withdrawal for lack of efficacy is similar to withdrawals because of Crohn's disease-related adverse events. In both instances, the Crohn's worsen or fail to improve. Therefore, when the number of withdrawals due to Crohn's disease-related adverse events and lack of efficacy are added, the incidence is similar for the placebo and CCX282-B groups, i.e., 13/95 (14%) for placebo and 21/145 (14%) for CCX282-B.

normalized on a 10-cm scale. CCX282 plasma concentrations were measured in samples taken at single random time points from all subjects at each study visit using high performance liquid chromatography with tandem mass spectrometric detection (lower limit of detection 2 ng/mL).

Definition of Endpoints and Statistical Analysis

The primary efficacy endpoint for the Induction period was attainment of a clinical response, defined as a decrease in CDAI of at least 70 points from baseline, at week 8. Safety endpoints included the incidence of adverse events, serious adverse events, and withdrawals due to adverse events. Pre-defined secondary

Table 1. Demographics and Baseline Characteristics of the Induction Period and Maintenance Period Intention-to-Treat Populations.

| | Induction Period | | | | Maintenance Period | |
| | | CCX282-B Groups | | | | |
	Placebo (N = 144)	250 mg q.d. (N = 98)	250 mg b.i.d. (N = 96)	500 mg q.d. (N = 97)	Placebo (N = 95)	250 mg b.i.d. (N = 145)
Mean age–yr	36.6±12.24	37.2±11.69	37.3±13.24	34.9±12.14	34.6±12.63	37.2±11.77
Female–no. (%)	84 (58)	52 (53)	53 (55)	47 (49)	46 (48)	76 (52)
Mean body mass index–kg/m^2	23.6±5.68	23.7±5.04	22.8±4.59	23.7±4.92	24.1±5.35	23.7±4.58
Current smoker–no. (%)	48 (33)	24 (25)	35 (37)	29 (30)	28 (30)	44 (30)
Median (range) duration of Crohn's disease–yr	6 (0–31)	6 (0–33)	5 (0–25)	6 (0–44)	5 (0–35)	5 (0–26)
Median (range) of CDAI	321 (250–454)	334 (249–449)	327 (249–471)	335 (249–446)	136 (3–371)	128 (0–355)
Median (range) of CRP–mg per liter*	22 (4–200)	22 (3–124)	22 (4–166)	21 (7–182)	14 (1–78)	13 (0–97)
Location of Crohn's disease–no. (%)						
Small intestine	117 (81)	83 (85)	83 (87)	76 (78)	81 (85)	118 (81)
Colon	117 (81)	81 (83)	72 (75)	71 (73)	71 (75)	111 (77)
Small intestine and colon	90 (63)	66 (67)	60 (63)	50 (52)	57 (60)	85 (59)
Rectum	67 (47)	38 (39)	38 (40)	38 (39)	37 (39)	67 (46)
Perianal	43 (30)	31 (32)	25 (26)	29 (30)	35 (37)	39 (27)
Previous bowel resection–no. (%)	30 (21)	29 (30)	24 (25)	26 (27)	26 (27)	29 (20)
Crohn's medication use at start of study–no. (%)					–	–
none	24 (17)	14 (14)	10 (10)	16 (17)		
5-aminosalicylic acid	91 (63)	56 (57)	63 (66)	61 (63)		
azathioprine	41 (29)	32 (33)	27 (28)	22 (23)		
6-mercaptopurine	0	4 (4)	3 (3)	4 (4)		
methotrexate	7 (5)	4 (4)	4 (4)	2 (2)		
corticosteroids	55 (38)	38 (39)	40 (42)	33 (34)		
Previous biologic treatment–no. (%)					–	–
infliximab	32 (22)	28 (29)	25 (26)	23 (24)		
adalimumab	11 (8)	6 (6)	5 (5)	9 (9)		
natalizumab	10 (7)	3 (3)	5 (5)	5 (5)		
No. of subjects with baseline and week 12 colonoscopies	37	16	21	16	–	–
Median (range) of CDEIS, per protocol	16.8 (2–58)	25.5 (3–65)	14.0 (1–48)	23.0 (3–78)	–	–
Median (range) of CDEIS, as defined in ref. 11	9.7 (1–24)	12.4 (3–28)	7.8 (0–19)	11.3 (3–32)	–	–

*A total of 8 subjects (2, 3, 2, and 1 in the placebo, 250 mg q.d., 250 mg b.i.d., and 500 mg q.d. groups, respectively) had baseline CRP values ≤ 7.5 mg/L, a deviation from the study protocol inclusion criteria.

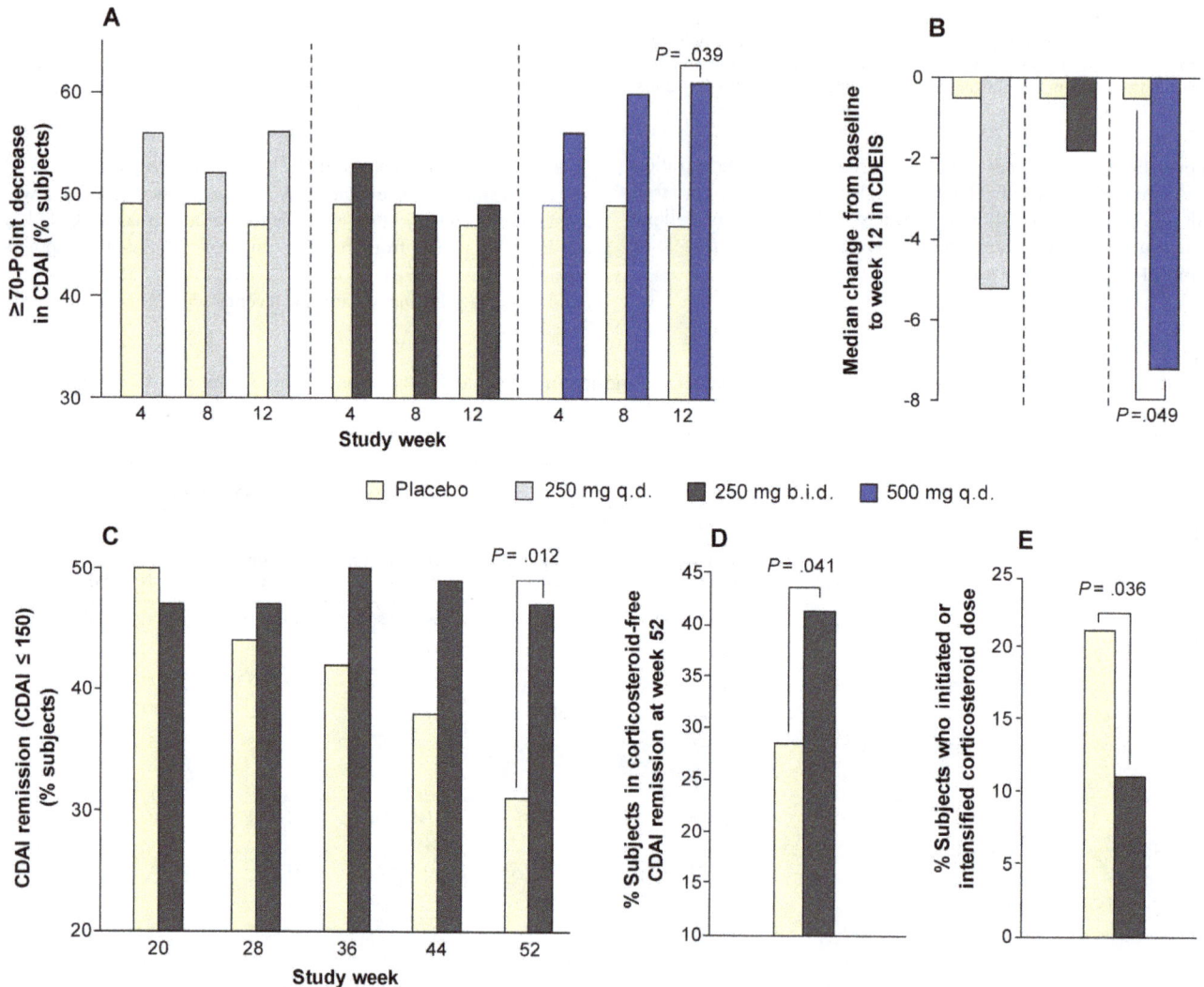

Figure 2. Clinical Efficacy Results. The percentage of subjects who had a CDAI decrease of at least 70 points is shown at each Induction period study visit after the baseline (A). Placebo n = 144, CCX282-B 250 mg q.d. n = 98, CCX282-B 250 mg b.i.d. n = 96, CCX282-B 500 mg q.d. n = 97; (B) The median change from baseline to week 12 in CDEIS, calculated per protocol (Placebo n = 37, CCX282-B 250 mg q.d. n = 16, CCX282-B 250 mg b.i.d. n = 21, CCX282-B 500 mg q.d. n = 16); (C) The percentage of subjects in each treatment group who were in remission (CDAI ≤150) at each visit over the course of the Maintenance period (Placebo n = 95 and CCX282-B 250 mg b.i.d. n = 145); (D) The percentage of subjects by treatment group who achieved corticosteroid-free remission, i.e., CDAI ≤150, at the end of the Maintenance period of the clinical trial, and (E) The percentage of subjects by treatment group who required an increase in corticosteroid dose or initiation of new corticosteroid use during the Maintenance period of the clinical trial.

efficacy endpoints included clinical response at week 12, as well as clinical remission (CDAI ≤150) [12] and ≥100-point decrease in CDAI from baseline at weeks 8 and 12. The primary endpoint for the Maintenance period was maintenance of response from week 16 to week 52. Loss of response was defined as an increase in CDAI of more than 70 points and an increase to above 250, or a missing CDAI measurement. The main secondary endpoint was maintenance of remission through week 52. Loss of remission was defined as a CDAI above 150.

The primary analysis was in the intention-to-treat population for both Induction and Maintenance periods, including all randomized subjects who received study medication. Subjects who discontinued treatment, who had missing CDAI scores, or who received rescue treatment or surgery, were considered treatment failures from that point forward. For the primary and main pre-specified secondary endpoints, the statistical analysis was

based on Mantel-Haenszel tests, stratified according to geographic region, comparing each CCX282-B group with the placebo group. Repeated measures mixed effect ANOVA models, including terms for treatment, time point, treatment by time point interaction, and geographic region were employed for continuous variables. All interactions were tested at an alpha level of 0.1 and statistical testing was two-sided.

Power calculations were based on a 25% placebo clinical response and a 50% clinical response in at least one CCX282-B group at week 8. A target number of 423 subjects would achieve 90% power at an overall alpha level of 0.05, 0.017 for each CCX282-B group compared to placebo, based on Bonferroni-adjusted Mantel-Haenszel testing. The protocol made allowance for an optional interim analysis when all subjects participating in the Maintenance period of the study had completed the Week 28 visit. A decision was made by the sponsor, upon review of the

Table 2. Clinical Response and Remission Results During the 12-Week Induction Period.

	Placebo (N = 144)	250 mg q.d. CCX282-B (N = 98)	250 mg b.i.d. CCX282-B (N = 96)	500 mg q.d. CCX282-B (N = 97)
Clinical response[a]				
Week 4, n (%)[b]	70 (48.6)	55 (56.1)	51 (53.1)	54 (55.7)
Week 8, n (%)	71 (49.3)	51 (52.0)	46 (47.9)	58 (59.8)
Week 12, n (%)	68 (47.2)	55 (56.1)	47 (49.0)	59 (60.8)*
Clinical remission[c]				
Week 4, n (%)	21 (14.6)	16 (16.3)	13 (13.5)	15 (15.5)
Week 8, n (%)	37 (25.7)	23 (23.5)	16 (16.7)	23 (23.7)
Week 12, n (%)	39 (27.1)	25 (25.5)	21 (21.9)	29 (29.9)
CDAI decrease from baseline ≥100				
Week 4, n (%)	58 (40.3)	40 (40.8)	40 (41.7)	40 (41.2)
Week 8, n (%)	61 (42.4)	40 (40.8)	42 (43.8)	47 (48.5)
Week 12, n (%)	58 (40.3)	47 (48.0)	40 (41.7)	53 (54.6)**

[a]Clinical response is defined as a decrease in CDAI score from baseline ≥70.
[b]n (%) = number and percentage of subjects in each group; % calculated as n/N x 100.
[c]Clinical remission is defined as a CDAI score ≤150.
*p = 0.039; p-value was obtained from Mantel-Haenszel test, stratified according to geographic region, comparing each CCX282-B group with the placebo group.
**p = 0.029; p-value was obtained from Mantel-Haenszel test, stratified according to geographic region, comparing each CCX282-B group with the placebo group.

Induction period results, not to conduct this interim analysis, but to allow the study to run uninterrupted to completion. This decision was made to preserve the integrity of the Maintenance period of the trial. Therefore, the alpha level for the final analysis was 0.05.

Results

Study Subjects

Subject disposition is shown in Figure 1. Demographics and baseline characteristics of the study population were similar across treatment groups for the Induction period and the Maintenance period (Table 1). Of 945 subjects screened, 436 were randomized. Low CDAI and CRP were the main reasons for exclusion. Over 80% of subjects completed the Induction period, and nearly 80% the Maintenance period.

Efficacy

Subjects underwent an aggregate treatment regimen of 52 weeks: a 12-week Induction period followed by a 4-week open-label Active period and a 36-week Maintenance period. Table 2 shows the CDAI response and remission results from the 12-week Induction period. The CCX282-B 500 mg q.d. group showed the highest CDAI response rates (≥70 point decrease in CDAI): 56%, 60%, and 61% at weeks 4, 8, and 12, respectively (Table 2 and Figure 2a). The placebo group response rates were 49%, 49%, and 47%, respectively, at these time points. The odds ratio (OR) between 500 mg q.d. CCX282-B and placebo was 1.53; 98.3% Confidence Interval [CI] 0.81, 2.89; p = 0.111 at Week 8, the predefined primary time point, and the OR was 1.74; 98.3% CI 0.92, 3.29; p = 0.039 at week 12, the predefined secondary time point. The 250 mg CCX282-B groups showed no significant differences in CDAI response compared to placebo at any time point. The 500 mg q.d. group showed higher clinical response rates compared with placebo and the 250 mg groups across all gender, Crohn's disease anatomic location strata, including colonic Crohn's disease, as well as other concomitant Crohn's medication use strata (Table 3). Age, race, gender, disease

location, and Crohn's medication did not show significant interaction (at p<0.1) with CDAI response. During the Induction period, the CDAI remission (≤150) rate was not significantly different across treatment groups (Table 2). The proportion of subjects with ≥100 point decrease in CDAI was 41%, 49%, and 55%, at weeks 4, 8, and 12, respectively, in the 500 mg q.d. group compared to 40%, 42%, and 40%, respectively, for the placebo group (Table 2); the OR between 500 mg CCX282-B q.d. and placebo at Week 12 was 1.79; 98.3% CI 0.95, 3.37; p = 0.029. The 250 mg groups did not show significant differences compared to placebo.

Approximately 26% of subjects (112 of 435) had previously received anti-TNF therapies, and 53 of these were non-responsive to one or more of these anti-TNF therapies based on data collected during screening. CDAI results from an exploratory analysis in the anti-TNF-experienced subjects are shown in Table S1. In the subset of subjects who were non-responsive to one or more anti-TNF drugs, CDAI ≥70 and ≥100 point responses at week 12 occurred in 8 of 14 (57%) subjects on CCX282-B 500 mg q.d., compared to 5 of 18 (28%) on placebo. Remission was observed in 3 of 14 (21%) on CCX282-B 500 mg q.d. and 1 of 18 (6%) on placebo.

The 321 subjects who entered the Active period, during which all subjects received CCX282-B 250 mg b.i.d., had a median CDAI of 184. At the end of the 4-week Active period, the median CDAI was 160. Of subjects completing the Active period, 241 (75.1%) showed a clinical response with a drop in CDAI of ≥70 (relative to their baseline value), and were re-randomized in a 1:1.5 ratio to receive placebo or CCX282-B 250 mg b.i.d. in the 36-week Maintenance period.

CDAI response and remission results for the Maintenance period are shown in Figure 2 and elaborated in Table 4. At week 52, 47% of subjects on CCX282-B were in remission compared with 31% on placebo (OR 2.01; 95% CI 1.16, 3.49; p = 0.012; Figure 2c). In a pre-specified last-observation-carried-forward sensitivity analysis, remission was achieved in 74 of 145 subjects (51%) in the CCX282-B group and 32 of 95 subjects (34%) in the placebo group (OR 2.05, 95% CI 1.20, 3.51; p = 0.009).

Table 3. CDAI Clinical Response at Week 12 by Gender, Crohn's Disease Location, and Other Concomitant Crohn's Medication Use.

	Placebo (N = 144)	250 mg q.d. CCX282-B (N = 98)	250 mg b.i.d. CCX282-B (N = 96)	500 mg q.d. CCX282-B (N = 97)
Gender				
Male				
N′	60	46	43	50
n (%)	27 (45.0%)	27 (58.7%)	20 (46.5%)	33 (66.0%)*
Female				
N′	84	52	53	47
n (%)	40 (47.6%)	28 (53.8%)	27 (50.9%)	26 (55.3%)
Crohn's Disease Location				
Small intestine				
N′	117	83	83	76
n (%)	56 (47.9%)	46 (55.4%)	41 (49.4%)	47 (61.8%)#
Colon				
N′	117	81	72	71
n (%)	58 (49.6%)	45 (55.6%)	33 (45.8%)	44 (62.0%)
Small intestine and colon				
N′	90	66	60	50
n (%)	46 (51.1%)	36 (54.5%)	28 (46.7%)	32 (64.0%)
Rectum and perianal				
N′	28	19	12	20
n (%)	13 (46.4%)	12 (63.2%)	6 (50.0%)	15 (75.0%)#
Other Concomitant Crohn's Medication Use[a]				
Users				
N′	111	86	81	75
n (%)	52 (46.8%)	50 (58.1%)	42 (51.9%)	45 (60.0%)#
Non-Users				
N′	33	12	15	22
n (%)	16 (48.5%)	5 (41.7%)	5 (33.3%)	14 (63.6%)

N′ = number of subjects in the ITT population for each subgroup; % = n/N′ x 100.

[a]Other concomitant Crohn's medications include 5-ASA, corticosteroids, 6-mercaptopurine, azathioprine, and methotrexate.

*p<0.05 for comparison with placebo based on Fisher's exact test.

#p<0.10 for comparison with placebo based on Fisher's exact test.

Furthermore, at week 52, 41% (60 of 145 subjects) on CCX282-B were in corticosteroid-free remission compared to 28% (27 of 95 subjects) on placebo (p = 0.041; see Figure 2d). A sustained response at every visit during the Maintenance period was seen in 46% of subjects in the CCX282-B 250 mg b.i.d. group compared to 42% in the placebo group (OR 1.14, 95% CI 0.67, 1.92; p = 0.629), and sustained remission (CDAI ≤150) was observed in 41% in the CCX282-B group and 30% in the placebo group (OR 1.60, 95% CI 0.77, 3.30; p = 0.205). In a pre-specified last-observation-carried-forward sensitivity analysis, sustained remission was achieved in 42 of 87 subjects (48%) in the CCX282-B group and 17 of 53 subjects (32%) in the placebo group (OR 1.94, 95% CI 0.95, 3.95; p = 0.066).

The changes from baseline to week 12 in CDAI, CRP, and CDEIS are shown in Table 5. The CCX282-B 500 mg q.d. group showed the largest mean decreases from baseline to week 12 in CDAI, CRP, and CDEIS. Mean change from baseline to week 12 in CDEIS was −3.0 in placebo, compared with −8.7, 2.0, and −10.8 (p = 0.049 vs. placebo; Figure 2b) in the CCX282-B groups, respectively. Mean change from baseline to week 12 in CDEIS,

calculated using normalized lengths of Crohn's involvement [11], was −1.1 in placebo, compared with −3.1, 0.9, and −4.4 (p = 0.049 vs. placebo) in the CCX282-B groups, respectively.

During the 36-week Maintenance period, median CDAI decreased from 128 to 95 in the CCX282-B group and increased from 136 to 146 in the placebo group. Median CRP levels decreased from 12.6 mg/L to 8.7 mg/L in the CCX282-B group, and from 14.1 mg/L to 12.3 mg/L in the placebo group from week 16 to 52. Systemic corticosteroid therapy was initiated or intensified in 21% (20/95 subjects) of the placebo group and 11% (16/145 subjects) of the CCX282-B group (p = 0.036; see Figure 2e). Conversely, corticosteroid therapy in CCX282-B subjects was stopped in 57% (32/56 subjects on corticosteroids at the start of the Maintenance period) compared to 43% (13/30 subjects) in the placebo group. Anti-TNF rescue treatment was given to 4% (4 of 95 subjects) in the placebo group and 1% (1 of 145 subjects) in the CCX282-B group. One subject, withdrawn from CCX282-B treatment, received natalizumab during the Maintenance period.

Table 4. Clinical Response and Remission Results for the 36-Week Maintenance Period.

	Placebo (N = 95)	250 mg b.i.d. CCX282-B (N = 145)	Placebo (N = 53)	250 mg b.i.d. CCX282-B (N = 87)	Placebo (N = 95)	250 mg b.i.d. CCX282-B (N = 145)
	Sustained response[a]		Sustained remission[b]		Remission at each time point	
Week 16, n (%)[c]	95 (100.0%)	145 (100.0%)	53 (100.0%)	87 (100.0%)	53 (55.8%)	88 (60.7%)
Week 20, n (%)	75 (78.9%)	118 (81.4%)	39 (73.6%)	59 (67.8%)	47 (49.5%)	68 (46.9%)
Week 28, n (%)	62 (65.3%)	93 (64.1%)	28 (52.8%)	47 (54.0%)	42 (44.2%)	68 (46.9%)
Week 36, n (%)	54 (56.8%)	82 (56.6%)	23 (43.4%)	47 (54.0%)	40 (42.1%)	73 (50.3%)
Week 44, n (%)	48 (50.5%)	75 (51.7%)	20 (37.7%)	43 (49.4%)	36 (37.9%)	71 (49.0%)
Week 52, n (%)	40 (42.1%)	66 (45.5%)	16 (30.2%)	36 (41.4%)	29 (30.5%)	68 (46.9%)*

[a]Sustained response was defined as a decrease in CDAI score from baseline (last non missing value before the first dose in the Induction period) ≥ 70 at Week 16 and no loss of the response during the 36-week Maintenance period. Loss of clinical response was defined as a CDAI score increase at any visit after the Week 16 visit of ≥ 70 from the Week 16 value and an absolute CDAI value of >250, or the need for intervention after Week 16. Missing values were also imputed as loss of response.
[b]Sustained remission was defined as a CDAI score ≤ 150 at Week 16 and Week 52 and all visits in between. If data from any time point between Week 16 and 62 were missing for a subject, sustained remission was not achieved.
[c]n (%) = number and percentage of subjects in each group; % calculated as n/N x 100.
*p = 0.012; p-value was obtained from Mantel-Haenszel test, stratified according to geographic region, comparing the CCX282-B group with the placebo group.

Population pharmacokinetic data from the Induction period indicated that the highest maximum plasma concentration (C_{max}) occurred with 500 mg q.d. CCX282-B. The modeled estimated mean ($\pm$SD) C_{max} was 736 ($\pm$141), 812 ($\pm$147), and 1032 ($\pm$163) ng/mL in the CCX282-B 250 mg q.d., 250 mg b.i.d., and 500 mg q.d. groups, respectively.

Safety

Safety results are summarized in Table 6. In the Induction period, 63% (90 subjects) on placebo reported at least one adverse event compared to 60% (174 subjects) on CCX282-B. The incidence of the most common adverse events was similar across treatment groups. Serious adverse events occurred in 10% placebo versus 9% in the CCX282-B group (15/144 subjects compared to 25/291, respectively). Study drug withdrawals due to adverse events in the CCX282-B group occurred in 7% (20 subjects) compared to 13% (19 subjects) in the placebo group. A lower incidence of withdrawals attributed to gastrointestinal adverse events and exacerbation of Crohn's disease was also observed in the CCX282-B group overall compared to placebo. One subject, in the placebo group, died during the study from septic complications following intestinal perforation. Another subject, in the 250 mg b.i.d. group, who had lack of response after the week 16 visit, died 39 days later due to complications of Crohn's disease that were deemed unrelated to study medication. Infections occurred in 16% of both placebo and CCX282-B groups during the Induction period (23/144 on placebo and 47/291 on CCX282-B). No opportunistic infections were reported. No clinically significant changes in laboratory parameters occurred in any of the treatment groups.

The incidence of the most common adverse events during the Maintenance period was similar across treatment groups, and 58 of 95 subjects (61%) in the placebo group reported at least one adverse event compared to 98 of 145 subjects (68%) in the CCX282-B 250 mg b.i.d. group. Serious adverse events occurred in 10% of placebo group versus 9% in the CCX282-B group (9/95 subjects versus 13/145, respectively). No serious infections or opportunistic infections were observed during the Maintenance period and no deaths occurred.

Discussion

CCX282-B, an orally-administered CCR9 antagonist, is the first chemokine receptor antagonist to be tested in IBD. In this clinical trial, the efficacy, safety and tolerability of CCX282-B were evaluated in a 12-week Induction period, followed by a 4-week Active period, and then a 36-week Maintenance period. Blocking CCR9 is a new approach to Crohn's disease therapy and a test of this mechanism has not been attempted previously in clinical trials. Accordingly, the trial design largely reflected that of other agents, predominantly the anti-TNF modalities. While primary endpoints of this trial were not achieved, pre-specified secondary endpoints were met.

Patients with both small and large bowel disease were eligible for the trial. The decision to include patients with large bowel disease was based on experimental evidence that CCR9 and TECK are expressed in both small and large bowel[13–15], and emerging experimental evidence that CCR9 inhibition is effective in the MDR1a$^{-/-}$ mouse model of colitis [15].

In the Induction period of the study, the CCX282-B 500 mg q.d. group showed the highest CDAI response. The difference in clinical response rate (drop in CDAI $\geq$70 points) between 500 mg q.d. CCX282-B and placebo (ΔCDAI) was 7%, 11%, and 14% at weeks 4, 8, and 12, respectively. This increasing ΔCDAI was also observed for CDAI $\geq$100-point response (1%, 6%, and 14%, respectively). This suggests that the full effect of CCX282-B may take longer than 8 weeks to manifest clinically, and week 12 might have been a more appropriate primary time point for the Induction period.

The ΔCDAI of 14% at week 12 for CDAI $\geq$70-point response between 500 mg q.d. CCX282-B and placebo is generally comparable to results from clinical trials of other therapies that have found a place in clinical practice. For example, at 12 weeks, the ΔCDAI was 10 to 16% with natalizumab [16,17] and 9% with certolizumab. [18] There are no 12-week time point data available for adalimumab [19].

CDAI clinical response differences between 500 mg q.d. CCX282-B and placebo were seen across all GI location strata (Table 3); the treatment difference was most pronounced in patients with rectal and perianal disease (ΔCDAI 29%). There are insufficient patient numbers in each GI location stratum to be

Table 5. Change from Baseline to Week 12 in CDAI, CRP, and CDEIS.

	Placebo (N = 144)	250 mg q.d. CCX282-B (N = 98)	250 mg b.i.d. CCX282-B (N = 96)	500 mg q.d. CCX282-B (N = 97)
Crohn's Disease Activity Index				
Baseline				
Mean (SD)	329.9 (49.47)	340.1 (54.29)	332.3 (52.36)	332.5 (55.68)
Median	321.0	333.5	326.5	335.0
Min, Max	250, 454	249, 449	249, 471	249, 446
n	144	98	96	97
Week 12–Change from baseline				
Mean (SD)	−115.9 (116.07)	−134.2 (99.87)	−121.7 (101.21)	−136.0 (102.05)
Median	−126.9	−147.1	−125.3	−146.2
Min, Max	−368, 251	−345, 88	−375, 105	−338, 109
n	120	85	85	87
C-reactive protein, mg/L				
Baseline				
Mean (SD)	30.8 (27.87)	28.0 (22.62)	27.6 (22.63)	30.3 (27.13)
Median	21.6	22.3	21.8	21.4
Min, Max	4.4, 200.0	2.7, 124.0	4.3, 165.5	6.6, 182.0
n	144	98	96	97
Week 12–Change from baseline				
Mean (SD)	−4.4 (34.08)	−4.1 (26.50)	−1.4 (31.06)	−6.6 (34.84)
Median	−2.9	−3.1	−4.5	−6.7
Min, Max	−199.6, 115.2	−123.7, 72.1	−82.6, 133.6	−175.4, 117.0
N	138	97	96	94
Crohn's Disease Endoscopic Index of Severity (CDEIS)[a]				
Baseline				
Mean (SD)	19.1 (15.02)	23.5 (20.56)	18.7 (14.14)	29.5 (23.28)
Median	14.0	16.2	16.5	23.0
Min, Max	2, 58	1, 65	1, 48	2, 78
n	48	24	26	22
Week 12–Change from baseline				
Mean (SD)	−3.0 (11.44)	−8.7 (11.60)	2.0 (10.75)	−10.8 (17.70)*
Median	−0.5	−5.2	−1.8	−7.2
Min, Max	−28, 30	−30, 6	−12, 35	−51, 17
n	37	16	21	16

[a]CDEIS calculated using a modification of the method described by Mary and Modigliani[13]. The length of disease involvement and ulceration was recorded as actual lengths, in cm, rather than normalized on a 10-cm scale.
*$p = 0.049$; p-value based on a repeated measures mixed effect ANOVA model, including terms for treatment, time point, treatment by time point interaction, and geographic region.

definitive, but this finding, if confirmed, would support a role for CCX282-B in treatment of patients with both small and large bowel disease.

Differences in the pharmacokinetic profiles between the 500 mg and 250 mg dosage regimens might explain the apparent differences in efficacy results. Chemotaxis studies of human lymphocytes in 100% human serum indicate that 800 ng/mL CCX282 is required to block 90% of CCR9 receptors (serum IC_{90}). Furthermore, full efficacy in pre-clinical studies required CCX282 plasma concentrations above the serum IC_{90}. [9] Based on modeled population pharmacokinetic profiles, plasma concentrations with 500 mg q.d. CCX282-B exceeded the serum IC_{90} for at least 8 hours following dosing. However, the mean maximum

CCX282 plasma concentrations at the 250 mg b.i.d dose were probably sub-therapeutic in the Induction setting. This difference in CCX282 plasma exposure between the 500 mg q.d. and 250 mg b.i.d. dosing regimens may explain the different clinical efficacy profiles in the Induction period. Since plasma samples were taken only at single time points at study visits, sparse data were available for each subject, and full pharmacokinetic profiles are not available for individual subjects. Therefore, correlations of individual pharmacokinetic parameters such as C_{max} or AUC with CDAI response could not be made reliably. CCX282-B 250 mg b.i.d. was selected as the dose for the Active and Maintenance periods before data from the Induction period, showing that 500 mg q.d. might be more effective, were available. Although the

Table 6. Adverse Events in the Safety Population.

Event	Induction Period					Active Period	Maintenance Period	
	CCX282-B							
	Placebo (N=144)	250 mg q.d. (N=98)	250 mg b.i.d. (N=96)	500 mg q.d. (N=97)	All (N=291)	250 mg b.i.d. CCX282-B (N=318)	Placebo (N=95)	250 mg b.i.d. CCX282-B (N=145)
	No. of subjects (%)							
Any event	90 (63)	62 (64)	56 (58)	56 (58)	174 (60)	88 (28)	58 (61)	98 (68)
Event in ≥5% of placebo or CCX282-B group overall								
Abdominal pain	19 (13)	16 (17)	18 (19)	12 (12)	46 (16)	14 (4)	19 (20)	19 (13)
Crohn's disease	10 (7)	9 (9)	14 (14)	6 (6)	29 (10)	12 (4)	7 (7)	17 (12)
Diarrhoea	11 (8)	10 (10)	7 (7)	7 (7)	24 (8)	12 (4)	14 (15)	15 (10)
Nausea	10 (7)	8 (8)	10 (10)	6 (6)	24 (8)	4 (1)	7 (7)	6 (4)
Dyspepsia	5 (4)	7 (7)	3 (3)	9 (9)	19 (7)	1 (0.3)	0	5 (3)
Headache	7 (5)	6 (6)	8 (8)	5 (5)	19 (7)	2 (1)	3 (3)	3 (2)
Arthralgia	8 (6)	10 (10)	3 (3)	3 (3)	16 (6)	3 (1)	7 (7)	14 (10)
Pyrexia	8 (6)	5 (5)	4 (4)	5 (5)	14 (5)	8 (3)	2 (2)	7 (5)
Abdominal tenderness	3 (2)	3 (3)	5 (5)	4 (4)	12 (4)	1 (0.3)	6 (6)	4 (3)
Vomiting	5 (4)	4 (4)	5 (5)	3 (3)	12 (4)	8 (3)	2 (2)	8 (6)
Serious adverse events	15 (10)	5 (5)	11 (11)	9 (9)	25 (9)	12 (4)	9 (10)	13 (9)
Events leading to study treatment withdrawal	19 (13)	8 (8)	5 (5)	7 (7)	20 (7)	9 (3)	6 (6)	10 (7)
Gastrointestinal events leading to study treatment withdrawal	14 (10)	6 (6)	3 (3)	5 (5)	14 (5)	9 (3)	4 (4)	9 (6)
Crohn's disease leading to study treatment withdrawal	6 (4)	3 (3)	0	1 (1)	4 (1)	5 (2)	1 (1)	4 (3)
Adverse events leading to death	1 (1)	0	0	0	0	1 (0.3)[a]	0	0
Infection or infestation	23 (16)	11 (11)	18 (19)	18 (19)	47 (16)	20 (6)	19 (20)	35 (24)
Transaminase increase >3× upper limit	1 (1)	0	1 (1)	0	1 (0.3)	0	1 (1)	1 (0.7)

[a]Event occurred 39 days after study discontinuation.

250 mg b.i.d. dose was apparently ineffective in the Induction period, this dose provided some evidence of efficacy in the Maintenance period. One potential explanation for these observations is that higher CCX282 plasma concentrations may be required to induce a clinical response in active disease, while lower plasma concentrations may effectively sustain remission subsequently when disease activity is lower. Such findings are not uncommon for maintenance dosing during remission with a variety of therapeutic modalities in chronic disease.

Changes in CRP and CDEIS support the efficacy of 500 mg q.d. CCX282-B in the Induction period. Of all four groups, 500 mg q.d. CCX282-B showed the largest decrease in serum CRP, of approximately 30%, at 12 weeks. The higher CRP level entry criterion of >7.5 mg/L in PROTECT-1 compared to other clinical trials, which resulted in a higher mean baseline CRP compared to these trials, [16,18,19] limits comparison across studies. Nonetheless, the absolute decrease in CRP with 500 mg CCX282-B is generally comparable to the changes observed with anti-TNF agents [18,19] and with natalizumab. [17] Subjects receiving 500 mg q.d. CCX282-B also showed a greater decrease in CDEIS compared to placebo, suggesting that CCX282-B treatment may improve intestinal mucosal lesions.

The percentage of subjects reaching clinical remission (CDAI of ≤150), was significantly higher in the CCX282-B group compared to placebo at the end of the Maintenance period, even though remission rates were not significantly different among groups in the Induction period. The baseline CDAI of the study population in PROTECT-1 was 333 (±53), or approximately 30 points higher than in other recent studies, [16,18,19] so that a larger absolute drop in CDAI was required to reach the CDAI score of 150, which was used to define remission. This high baseline CDAI could therefore have reduced the chance of achieving remission in a 12-week Induction trial, and of demonstrating a difference between CCX282-B and placebo groups. Some support for this contention was provided by an exploratory analysis indicating that with CDAI "near-remission" 5-point incremental thresholds of 155 up to 170, the near-remission rate in the CCX282-B 500 mg q.d. group was up to 10% higher than the placebo group (38.1% compared to 28.5% with 170 as threshold; Table S2).

In the Maintenance period, the incidence of relapse in the placebo group was 58% over 36 weeks, which was lower than anticipated. In a comparable natalizumab clinical trial, the incidence of relapse was 72% at the 36-week time point in the placebo group. [16] Therefore, the placebo response rate in our study was higher than expected. A possible reason is that the majority of subjects in this study (85%), including the subjects receiving placebo, were receiving background medications for Crohn's disease including corticosteroids. This difference may also reflect variations in clinical trial design. For example, in PROTECT-1, all subjects received 4 weeks of CCX282-B treatment at the end of the Induction period and before entering the Maintenance period. In the natalizumab clinical trial, [16] there was no active treatment period between the Induction period and the Maintenance period.

Although subjects who have previously received anti-TNF agents often have lower response rates to other treatments, in this study, exploratory analyses showed that CCX282-B might have utility in these subjects. This finding is a topic of further study in ongoing Phase 3 clinical trials.

The apparent safety and tolerability of CCX282-B observed in this study are encouraging as most other medications for Crohn's disease have limitations such as increased risk of infection. Thiopurines, widely used to maintain remission, are also associated with an increased risk of neoplasia, particularly of the lymphohemopoietic system. [20] Preclinical and early phase CCX282-B clinical studies have supported the favorable safety and tolerability profile, [9] and if confirmed in larger studies, would be beneficial.

Limitations of this study include the relatively small sample size, the strict inclusion criteria, defining patients with moderately to severely active Crohn's disease, so that results cannot yet be generalized to less or more severely affected patients. Furthermore, as this is the first major trial of a CCR9 antagonist, the design of the trial and selection of time points relied on evidence from mechanistically unrelated medical treatments. Lastly, the placebo response rates observed during both the Induction and Maintenance periods of this trial were relatively high.

In conclusion, this study suggests that CCX282-B, an orally-administered and specific CCR9 antagonist, provides a novel approach to modulating intestine-specific inflammatory responses, and if results are confirmed might be an effective therapy for IBD. Targeting the chemokine system offers the prospect of organ specific immunotherapy for a wide variety of immunologically-activated diseases. Phase 3 clinical trials are now being conducted to further evaluate the safety and efficacy of CCX282-B (also called GSK1605786A or vercirnon) in groups of patients with broader inclusion criteria.

Supporting Information

Table S1 CDAI Results in Anti-TNF Users. A total of 112 patients previously used anti-TNF drugs, adalimumab or infliximab, for treatment of their Crohn's disease. The number and percentage of patients who had a decrease of at least 70 points in CDAI, CDAI ≤150 (remission), and a decrease of at least 100 points in CDAI at week 12 in the clinical trial are shown by treatment group in this table.

Table S2 CDAI "Near Remission" Results. The number and percentage of patients who reached CDAI thresholds of ≤155, ≤160, ≤165, and ≤170 at week 12 in the clinical trial are shown in this table.

Checklist S1 CONSORT Checklist.

Protocol S1 Study Protocol.

Appendix S1 Study Centers and Ethics Committees.

Author Contributions

Critically reviewed and contributed to paper: TV YN RP SH MB IR DH ON SV WR PK SS. Conceived and designed the experiments: SK TS PB. Performed the experiments: SK TV YN RP SH MB IR DH ON SV WR PK SS. Analyzed the data: SK PB. Wrote the paper: SK PB.

References

1. Farmer RG, Hawk WA, Turnbull RB Jr (1975) Clinical patterns in Crohn's disease: a statistical study of 615 cases. Gastroenterology 68: 627–635.

2. Charo IF and Ransohoff RM. (2006) The many roles of chemokines and chemokine receptors in inflammation. N Engl J Med 354: 610–21.

3. Zabel BA, Agace WW, Campbell JJ, Heath HM, Parent D, et al. (1999) Human G protein-coupled receptor GPR-9-6/CC chemokine receptor 9 is selectively expressed on intestinal homing T lymphocytes, mucosal lymphocytes, and thymocytes and is required for thymus-expressed chemokine-mediated chemotaxis. J Exp Med 190: 1241–1256.

4. Zaballos A, Gutierrez J, Varona R, Ardavin C, and Márquez G. (1999) Cutting edge: identification of the orphan chemokine receptor GPR-9-6 as CCR9, the receptor for the chemokine TECK. J Immunol 162: 5671.

5. Marsal J, Svensson M, Ericsson A, Iranpour AH, Carramolino L, et al. (2002) Involvement of CCL25 (TECK) in the generation of the murine small-intestineal CD8αα+CD3+ intraepithelial lymphocyte compartment. Eur J Immunol 32: 3488–3497.

6. Svensson M, Marsal J, Ericsson A, Carramolino L, Brodén T, et al. (2002) CCL25 mediates the localization of recently activated CD8αβ+ lymphocytes to the small-intestinal mucosa. J Clin Invest 110: 1113–1121.

7. Pabst O, Ohl L, Wendland M, Wurbel MA, Kremmer E, et al. (2004) Chemokine receptor CCR9 contributes to the localization of plasma cells to the small intestine. J Exp Med 199: 411–416.

8. Wendland M, Czeloth N, Mach N, Malissen B, Kremmer E, et al. (2007) CCR9 is a homing receptor for plasmacytoid dendritic cells to the small intestine. Proc Natl Acad Sci USA 104: 6347–6352.

9. Walters MJ, Wang Y, Lai N, Baumgart T, Zhao BN, et al. (2010) Characterization of CCX282-B, an orally bioavailable antagonist of the CCR9 chemokine receptor, for treatment of inflammatory bowel disease. J Pharmacol Exp Ther 335: 65–69.

10. Best WR, Becktel JM, Singleton JW, and Kern F. (1976) Development of a Crohn's disease activity index. Gastroenterology 70: 439–444.

11. Mary JY and Modigliani R. (1989) Development and validation of an endoscopic index of the severity for Crohn's disease: a prospective multicenter study. Gut 30: 983–989.

12. Sandborn WJ, Feagan BG, Hanauer SB, Lochs H, Lofberg R, et al. (2002) A review of activity indices and efficacy endpoints for clinical trials of medical therapy in adults with Crohn's disease. Gastroenterology 122: 512–530.

13. Papadakis KA, Prehn J, Nelson V, Cheng L, Binder SW, et al. (2000) The role of thymus-expressed chemokine and its receptor CCR9 on lymphocytes in the regional specialization of the mucosal immune system. J Immunol 165: 5069–5076.

14. Papadakis KA, Prehn J, Moreno ST, Cheng L, Kouroumalis EA, et al. (2001) CCR9-positive lymphocytes and thymus-expressed chemokine distinguish small bowel from colonic Crohn's disease. Gastroenterology 21: 246–254.

15. Walters MJ, Berahovich R, Wang Y, Wei Z, Ungashe S, et al. (2008) Presence of CCR9 and its ligand CCL25/TECK in the colon: scientific rationale for the use of CCR9 small molecule antagonist CCX282-B in colonic disorders. Gut 57 (Suppl II): A39 (OP184).

16. Sandborn WJ, Colombel JF, Enns R, Feagan BG, Hanauer SB, et al. (2005) Natalizumab induction and maintenance therapy for Crohn's disease. N Engl J Med 353: 1912–1925.

17. Targan SR, Feagan BG, Fedorak RN, Lashner BA, Panaccione R, et al. (2007) Natalizumab for the treatment of active Crohn's disease: results of the ENCORE trial. Gastroenterology 132: 1672–1683.

18. Sandborn WJ, Feagan BG, Stoinov S, Honiball PJ, Rutgeerts P, et al. (2007) Certolizumab pegol for the treatment of Crohn's disease. N Engl J Med 357: 228–238.

19. Hanauer SB, Sandborn WJ, Rutgeers P, Fedorak RN, Lukas M, et al. (2006) Human anti-tumor necrosis factor monoclonal antibody (adalimumab) in Crohn's disease: the CLASSIC-I trial. Gastroenterology 130: 323–333.

20. Beaugerie L, Brousse N, Bouvier AM, Colombel JF, Lemann M, et al. (2009) Lymphoproliferative disorders in patients receiving thiopurines for inflammatory bowel disease: a prospective observational cohort study. Lancet 374; 1617–1625.

21

Peripheral Monocyte Functions and Activation in Patients with Quiescent Crohn's Disease

David Schwarzmaier[1], Dirk Foell[1,2], Toni Weinhage[1], Georg Varga[1], Jan Däbritz[1,2,3]*

1 Department of Pediatric Rheumatology and Immunology, University Children's Hospital Münster, Münster, NRW, Germany, **2** Interdisciplinary Center of Clinical Research, University of Münster, Münster, NRW, Germany, **3** The Royal Children's Hospital Melbourne, Murdoch Children's Research Institute, Parkville, VIC, Australia

Abstract

Recent developments suggest a causal link between inflammation and impaired bacterial clearance in Crohn's disease (CD) due to alterations of intestinal macrophages. Studies suggest that excessive inflammation is the consequence of an underlying immunodeficiency rather than the primary cause of CD pathogenesis. We characterized phenotypic and functional features of peripheral blood monocytes of patients with quiescent CD (n = 18) and healthy controls (n = 19) by analyses of cell surface molecule expression, cell adherence, migration, chemotaxis, phagocytosis, oxidative burst, and cytokine expression and secretion with or without lipopolysaccharide (LPS) priming. Peripheral blood monocytes of patients with inactive CD showed normal expression of cell surface molecules (CD14, CD16, CD116), adherence to plastic surfaces, spontaneous migration, chemotaxis towards LTB4, phagocytosis of *E. coli*, and production of reactive oxygen species. Interestingly, peripheral blood monocytes of CD patients secreted higher levels of IL1β (p<.05). Upon LPS priming we found a decreased release of IL10 (p<.05) and higher levels of CCL2 (p<.001) and CCL5 (p<.05). The expression and release of TNFα, IFNγ, IL4, IL6, IL8, IL13, IL17, CXCL9, and CXCL10 were not altered compared to healthy controls. Based on our phenotypic and functional studies, peripheral blood monocytes from CD patients in clinical remission were not impaired compared to healthy controls. Our results highlight that defective innate immune mechanisms in CD seems to play a role in the (inflamed) intestinal mucosa rather than in peripheral blood.

Editor: T. Mark Doherty, Glaxo Smith Kline, Denmark

Funding: The study was supported by grants of the Broad Medical Research Program (BMRP Reference No. IBD0201, to DF and JD), the German Research Foundation (DFG Reference No. DA1161/4-1, to JD and DF), and the Innovative Medical Research Program of the University of Münster (IMF Reference No. DÄ120904, to JD and DF). The funders had no role in study design, data collection and analysis, decision to publish, or preparation of the manuscript.

Competing Interests: The authors have declared that no competing interests exist.

* E-mail: Jan.Daebritz@uni-muenster.de

Introduction

Recent developments in immunology and genetics have consolidated the view of Crohn's disease (CD) as a form of immunodeficiency and studies continue to highlight defects of the initially involved innate immune system [1–4]. Segal *et al.* performed several *in vitro* studies using monocyte-derived macrophages of CD patients in clinical remission to identify a defective mechanism, which could explain the diminished acute inflammatory response in CD patients. They observed that diminished neutrophil recruitment and bacterial clearance result from insufficient macrophage cytokine secretion on bacterial challenge. As a result, secondary macrophage activation may lead to the formation of granulomas and chronic inflammation [5,6]. Furthermore, it has been suggested that blood monocytes are the exclusive source of macrophages in inflamed intestinal mucosa [7,8] and that both peripheral monocytes as well as their derivative cells play an important role in the pathophysiology of CD. We were thus interested in the characterization of peripheral blood monocytes in CD, specifically in the underlying constitutive intrinsic alterations of monocyte subpopulations. The aim of the study was to identify possible functional and phenotypic abnormalities of monocytes already at a stage before their recruitment into the intestinal mucosa. We investigated i) the expression of cell surface molecules; ii) functional characteristics including adherence, migration, chemotaxis, oxidative burst, and phagocytosis; and iii) the expression and secretion of chemokines and pro- and anti-inflammatory cytokines. In addition, priming studies were performed using lipopolysaccharide (LPS) in order to simulate the exposure and subsequent activation of monocytes to proinflammatory bacterial products in the intestinal mucosa.

Materials and Methods

Ethics Statement

Written informed consent was obtained from all patients. The study was approved by the ethics committee of the University of Münster, Germany (reference number 2009-434-f-S, J.D.).

Patients and Controls

Patients who met the inclusion criteria were recruited from January 2010 to December 2011 to participate in the study. All patients had definitive diagnoses of CD, which were confirmed by standard diagnostic criteria, with quiescent disease (Harvey Bradshaw Index [HBI] ≤5) [9]. Patients receiving either no medication, a stable maintenance dose of 5-aminosalicylates (2.5 g/d) or a tapering dose of budesonide for the previous 3 months were included. None of the patients had received conventional/systemic corticosteroids, immunosuppressants, anti-tumor necrosis factor, or metronidazole therapy within 3 months

Table 1. Characteristics of Crohn's disease patients and healthy controls.

	Crohn's disease	Controls
Number, n	18	19
Age, years (range)	45 (27–59)	30 (23–47)
Sex, n (%)		
- female	10 (55%)	9 (47%)
- male	8 (45%)	10 (53%)
BMI, kg/m² (range)	23.6 (18.0–38.2)	21.5 (19.4–32.8)
Duration of disease, years (range)	7 (0–45)	–
Location, n (%)		
- ileal	6 (33%)	–
- colonic	2 (11%)	–
- ileo-colonic	8 (45%)	–
- other	2 (11%)	–
Harvey-Bradshaw index, score (range)	1 (0–5)	–
Medication, n (%)		
- Budesonide	4 (22%)	0 (0%)
- Mesalazine	4 (22%)	0 (0%)
- None	10 (56%)	19 (100%)

of enrolment. Healthy volunteers approximately matched for age and sex were used as controls. No subject was studied more than once in each of the different experiments. Details of included patients and healthy control subjects are provided (Table 1).

Isolation of Peripheral Blood Monocytes and Flow Cytometry

Human peripheral blood mononuclear cells (PBMCs) were isolated from patients and healthy controls by Ficoll-Hypaque (Pharmacia, Freiburg, Germany) density gradient centrifugation. Monocytes were further enriched by using the CD16 monocyte isolation kit in combination with CD14 microbeads according to the manufacturer's instructions (Miltenyi Biotec, Bergisch Gladbach, Germany). In brief, 1×10^8 PBMCs were incubated with 100 µl FcR blocking reagent together with 100 µl non-monocyte depletion cocktail containing anti-CD15 and anti-CD56 microbeads to magnetically deplete CD16 expressing NK cells and granulocytes. Subsequently, the flow-through was incubated with 100 µl anti-CD16 and 200 µl anti-CD14 microbeads and CD14/CD16 expressing monocytes were positively selected by magnetic separation.

To determine purity of isolated monocytes and to investigate CD14, CD16 and CD116 expression on naïve PBMC monocytes, 5×10^5 cells of each PBMCs and isolated monocytes, were stained in 50 µl FACS-buffer (PBS +1% FSC) with anti-CD14-FITC (clone 61D3, eBioscience, San Diego, CA, USA), anti-CD116 Pe (clone 4H1, eBioscience, San Diego, CA, USA) and anti-CD16-APC (clone eBioCB16, eBioscience, San Diego, CA, USA) antibodies for 30 min at room temperature in the dark. After washing twice with FACS-buffer, cells were analyzed using a FACSCalibur and CellQuest software (both from Becton Dickinson, Heidelberg, Germany). Purity after isolation was routinely higher than 90% for CD14/CD16 expressing monocytes.

Monocytes were then cultured (1×10^6 cells/ml) in hydrophobic teflon bags (Heraeus, Hanau, Germany) in McCoy's 5a medium supplemented with 15% heat-inactivated FCS, 2 mM L-glutamine, 200 IU/ml penicillin, 100 µg/ml streptomycin and $1 \times$ non-essential amino acids (all from Biochrom, Berlin, Germany).

Priming of Monocytes

For priming of isolated monocytes, cells were harvested after resting for 40 hours at $37°C$ and 7% CO_2, washed once with complete McCoy's 5a medium and resuspended (1×10^6 cells/ml). The resting period was chosen to minimize potential effects of cell activation during isolation procedure. Cells were then stimulated with *E. coli* 055:B5 derived LPS for 2 hours (10 ng/ml, Sigma-Aldrich, Taufkirchen, Germany).

Adhesion, Migration and Chemotaxis

For determination of cell adhesion, 96-well flat-bottom plastic tissue-culture plates were treated with human fibronectin (50 µg/ml, BD Biosciences, Heidelberg, Germany) for 1 hour at $37°C$. Monocytes (2×10^5) were seeded in triplicates and incubated at $37°C$ and 7% CO_2 for 4 hours. Non-adhering cells were removed by washing twice; remaining adherent cells were fixed with 2% glutaraldehyde (Sigma-Aldrich, Taufkirchen, Germany) for 10 min. Wells were washed two times with H_2O and subsequently stained with 0.5% crystal violet (Merck, Darmstadt, Germany) in 2% EtOH (pH 6.0) for an additional 15 min at room temperature. Finally, wells were washed three times and lysed. 10% acetic acid was added and staining was quantified measuring the OD at 560 nm using an Asys Expert 96 Microplate ELISA reader (Anthos Mikrosysteme, Krefeld, Germany).

Monocyte migration and chemotaxis assays were performed in transwell plates (5 µm pore size) using Leukotriene B4 (LTB4, 100 nM, Cayman Chemical, Ann Arbor, MI, USA) as an additional chemoattractant. The modified Boyden chamber assay was used according to the manufacturer's instructions (Corning, Lowell, MA, USA). Monocytes (2.5×10^5) were seeded on top of the membrane and cell numbers in the lower chamber were quantified by counting after 4 hours of incubation at $37°C$ and 7% CO_2. All analyses were performed in triplicate.

Escherichia coli Phagocytosis

Cultured cells were harvested and resuspended (1×10^6 cells/ml) in complete McCoy's 5a medium together with 10 MOI fluorescein labeled *E. coli* supplemented with 15 µl human AB-serum and mixed thoroughly. The cells were incubated with *E. coli* at $37°C$ for 30 minutes. After incubation cells were washed two times with ice-cold McCoy's 5a medium and analyzed by flow cytometry as described above. Phagocytic internalization of *E. coli* was confirmed by fluorescence microscopy.

Oxidative Burst

Monocytes were stimulated for 2 hours at $37°C$ with *E. coli* 055:B5 derived LPS (10 ng/ml, Sigma-Aldrich, Taufkirchen, Germany) in the presence of 15 µM Dihydrorhodamine 123 (DHR, Merck, Darmstadt, Germany) for the final 15 min. Monocytes were placed on ice after incubation and analyzed by flow cytometry as described above.

Analysis of Cytokine and Chemokine Levels

Cytokine and chemokine secretion of monocytes before and after LPS treatment was measured in cell supernatants. Human TNFα, IL1β, IL6, IL10, CCL2, CCL5, CXCL9, and CXCL10 were measured by Cytometric Bead Array (CBA, human chemokine kit and human inflammatory cytokine kit, BD Bio-science, Heidelberg, Germany) according to the manufacturer's instructions and subsequently analyzed by flow cytometry. Human IL8 was measured using a commercial enzyme-linked immuno-sorbent assays (ELISA) according to the manufacturer's instructions (BD Biosciences, Heidelberg, Germany).

Quantitative Real-time PCR

Complementary DNA was synthesized from 1 µg of total RNA using SuperScript II RNase H-reverse transcriptase (Invitrogen, Carlsbad, CA, USA) with oligo$_{18}$ dT primers. Primers used for RT-PCR analysis are given in Table 2. Real-time RT-PCR was performed by using an ABI PRISM 7900 (Applied Biosystems, Foster City, CA, USA) with a KAPA SYBR® FAST qPCR Kit (Kapa Biosystems, Woburn, MA, USA) as described previously [10]. Gene expression was normalized to the endogenous housekeeping control gene ribosomal protein L13a (RPL) and relative expression of respective genes was calculated by the comparative threshold cycle method. All analyses were performed in duplicate.

Statistics

Data are expressed as mean ± standard error of the mean (SEM) except when stated otherwise and were assessed using the Student's t-test. P values less than 0.05 were considered to be statistically significant. All calculations were performed using SPSS version 14 (SPSS Inc, Chicago, IL, USA).

Results

Expression of Cell Surface Molecules

We investigated whether differences exist in the CD14/CD16 subsets of monocytes from patients with quiescent CD as described for patients with active disease [11]. However, we found that there is no difference among these subsets (Figure 1A and C). The CD14++/CD16− subset represented 69.1% ±2.3% of monocytes of healthy controls (HC) and 71.3% ±2.1% of monocytes of included patients with CD, respectively. In addition, we found no significant differences in the CD14++/CD16++ and the CD14+/CD16++ subsets of HC and CD patients. Furthermore, we analyzed the expression of the GM-CSF-receptor (CD116) as there are reports of defective leukocyte CD116 expression and function in IBD [12]. In our analyses CD116 expression did not differ between monocytes derived from HC (MFI 39.5±5.6) and CD (MFI 40.3±4.9).

Monocyte Functions

To determine whether CD monocytes are functionally impaired, we performed several functional assays. We found that CD monocytes have no impairment in adhesion (OD [560 nm] HC 0.057% ±0.012% vs. CD 0.076% ±0.015%), migration (HC 11.1% ±1.2% vs. CD 10.4% ±0.9%) and chemotaxis towards LTB4 (HC 15.3% ±2.1% vs. CD 14.6% ±1.8%) (Figure 2A and B).

Phagocytosis of bacteria is a fundamental capacity of monocytes. CD monocytes showed similar phagocytosis capabilities in the presence of FITC-labeled *Escherichia coli (E. coli)* (MFI 9.6±1.8) compared with monocytes of HC (MFI 12.2±1.9) (Figure 2C).

We found no differences in the production of reactive oxygen species (ROS) by monocytes from patients with quiescent CD compared to healthy controls, neither in the presence of LPS (MFI HC 41.7±2.3 vs. CD 40.8±2.3) nor without LPS (MFI HC 28.8±1.3 vs. CD 26.9±1.5).

Chemokine and Cytokine Expression

We analyzed cytokine and chemokine secretion of freshly isolated monocytes after resting for 40 hours. Monocytes of CD patients in remission showed significantly higher levels of IL1β (HC 18.2 pg/ml ±4.3 pg/ml vs. CD 34.7 pg/ml ±4.5 pg/ml; P<0.05). There was no significant difference in the levels of TNFα, IL6, IL8, IL10, CCL2, CCL5, CXCL9, and CXCL10 (Figure 3A).

In addition, peripheral blood monocytes from patients with CD in remission showed a significantly higher secretion of the chemokines CCL2 (HC 126.8 pg/ml ±17.4 pg/ml vs. CD 472.8 pg/ml ±89.3 pg/ml; P<0.001) and CCL5 (HC 28.4 pg/ml ±3.2 pg/ml vs. CD 51.0±7.6 pg/ml; P<0.05) after priming with LPS. In contrast, the levels of anti-inflammatory IL10 were significantly lower in monocytes of included CD patients (HC 8.8 pg/ml ±1.9 pg/ml vs. CD 4.5 pg/ml ±0.9 pg/ml; P<0.05). Production of TNFα, IL1β, IL6, IL8, CXCL9, and CXCL10 was not different between monocytes from healthy controls compared to CD patients (Figure 3B).

Quantitative real-time PCR analysis also showed that there were no differences in gene expression of IL1β, IL6, IL8, IL10, TNFα, CCL2, CCL5, CXCL9, and CXCL10 in naïve monocytes (Figure 3C).

Discussion

It was realized more than 30 years ago that the acute inflammatory response and neutrophil recruitment is impaired

Table 2. Primer sequences for RT-PCR.

Gene	Forward Primer Sequence (5'-3')	Reverse Primer Sequence (5'-3')
TNFα	CTT CTC GAA CCC CGA GTG AC	TGA GGT ACA GGC CCT CTG ATG
IL1β	GCG GCC AGG ATA TAA CTG ACT TC	TCC ACA TTC AGC ACA GGA CTC TC
IL6	AGA GGC ACT GGC AGA AAA CAA C	AGG CAA GTC TCC TCA TTG AAT CC
IL8	CTT GTT CCA CTG TGC CTT GGT T	GCT TCC ACA TGT CCT CAC AAC AT
IL10	GCT GAG AAC CAA GAC CCA GAC A	CGG CCT TGC TCT TGT TTT CA
CCL2	TCG CCT CCA GCA TGA AAG TC	TTG CAT CTG GCT GAG CGA G
CCL5	CAG TGG CAA GTG CTC CAA CC	CCA TCC TAG CTC ATC TCC AAA GAG T
CXCL9	GAC CTT AAA CAA TTT GCC CCA AG	TCC TTC ACA TCT GCT GAA TCT GG
CXCL10	GCA AGC CAA TTT TGT CCA CG	ACA TTT CCT TGC TAA CTG CTT TCA G

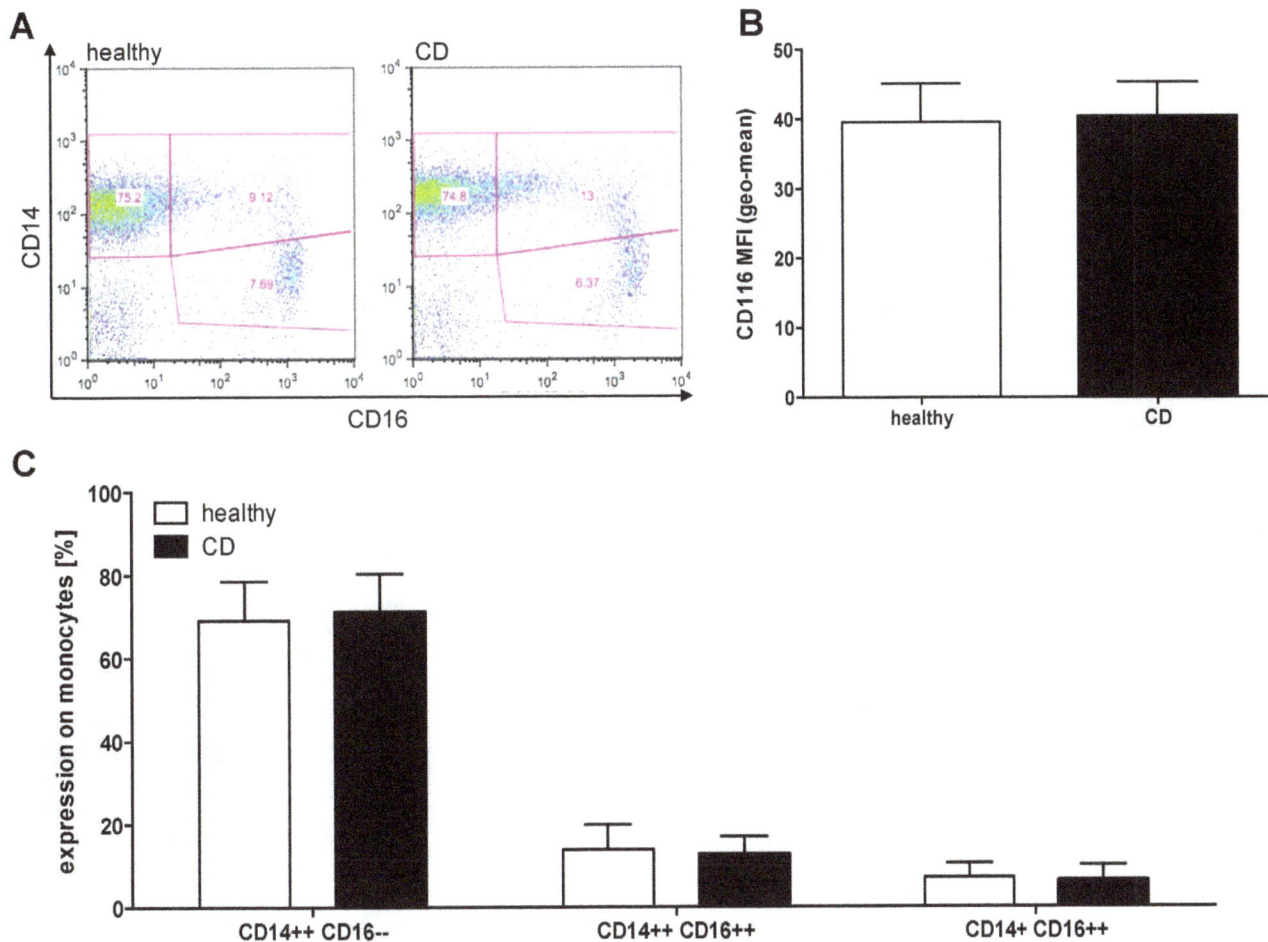

Figure 1. Cell surface molecule expression. (A) Example of CD14 and CD16 expression on naïve PBMCs after Ficoll isolation gated for viable monocytes. Upper left quadrant shows CD14++/CD16– monocytes, upper right quadrant shows CD14++/CD16++ monocytes, and CD14+/CD16++ monocytes are represented in the lower right quadrant. (B) Shown is the CD116 expression on naïve monocytes of healthy controls (n = 11) and patients with CD in remission (n = 12) as mean fluorescence intensity. (C) Cell surface expression of CD14 and CD16 on viable PBMC monocytes of healthy controls (n = 17) and patients with CD (n = 18) analyzed by flow cytometry as shown in (A). All bars represent means ± SEM.

in CD [13]. Recent studies on the pathogenesis of inflammatory bowel diseases (IBD) further support the immunodeficiency model of Crohn's disease. The focus has shifted from the primary defect in adaptive immunity to deficient acute inflammation in the intestinal mucosa with diminished macrophage cytokine production and neutrophil recruitment leading to a reduced bacterial clearance. Given that blood monocytes are the exclusive source of macrophages in the inflamed intestinal mucosa, here we have attempted to characterize peripheral blood monocyte populations in CD patients. The aim was to explore whether functional changes in resulting tissue macrophages are already detectable in blood monocytes. Our results suggest, that peripheral blood monocytes of CD patients in clinical remission are phenotypically and functionally indistinguishable from those of healthy controls.

Previous studies investigating functions of peripheral blood monocytes in CD have reported conflicting results. Mee *et al.* showed that peripheral blood monocyte counts, phagocytosis (*Staphylococcus aureus*), and intracellular killing are not impaired in CD. They concluded that peripheral blood monocytes in CD patients are rather activated and that granulomata in CD are unlikely to result from a defect in the microbicidal functions of monocytes [14,15]. A study on the expression of cell surface

molecules showed an increased MFI of surface molecules CD86/B7-2, CD18, and ICAM-1 on peripheral blood monocytes from patients with CD, which also indicates that monocytes from CD patients are activated and may have an increased antigen-presenting function by providing increased costimulatory signals (e.g. CD86/B7-2) [16]. Okabe *et al.* observed a reduced immunologic activity in CD monocytes [17], an increased superoxide production in peripheral blood monocytes of CD patients (determined by chemiluminescence) [18] as well as diminished phagocytic activity (determined by automated laser flow cytometry) [19]. On the other hand, Whorwell *et al.* reported that phagocytosis (*Candida albicans*) and undirected motility are significantly increased in blood monocytes of CD patients when compared with controls. In addition, they found no difference in the chemotaxis (towards zymosan-activated serum) between the disease and control group [20]. Baldessano *et al.* showed that freshly isolated monocytes from patients with inactive CD release equivalent amounts of superoxide anion (measured by superoxide dismutase inhibitable reduction of ferricytochrome c) when compared with monocytes from healthy controls. However, freshly isolated monocytes from patients with active CD showed a significantly enhanced respiratory burst and responded in a similar fashion to LPS-

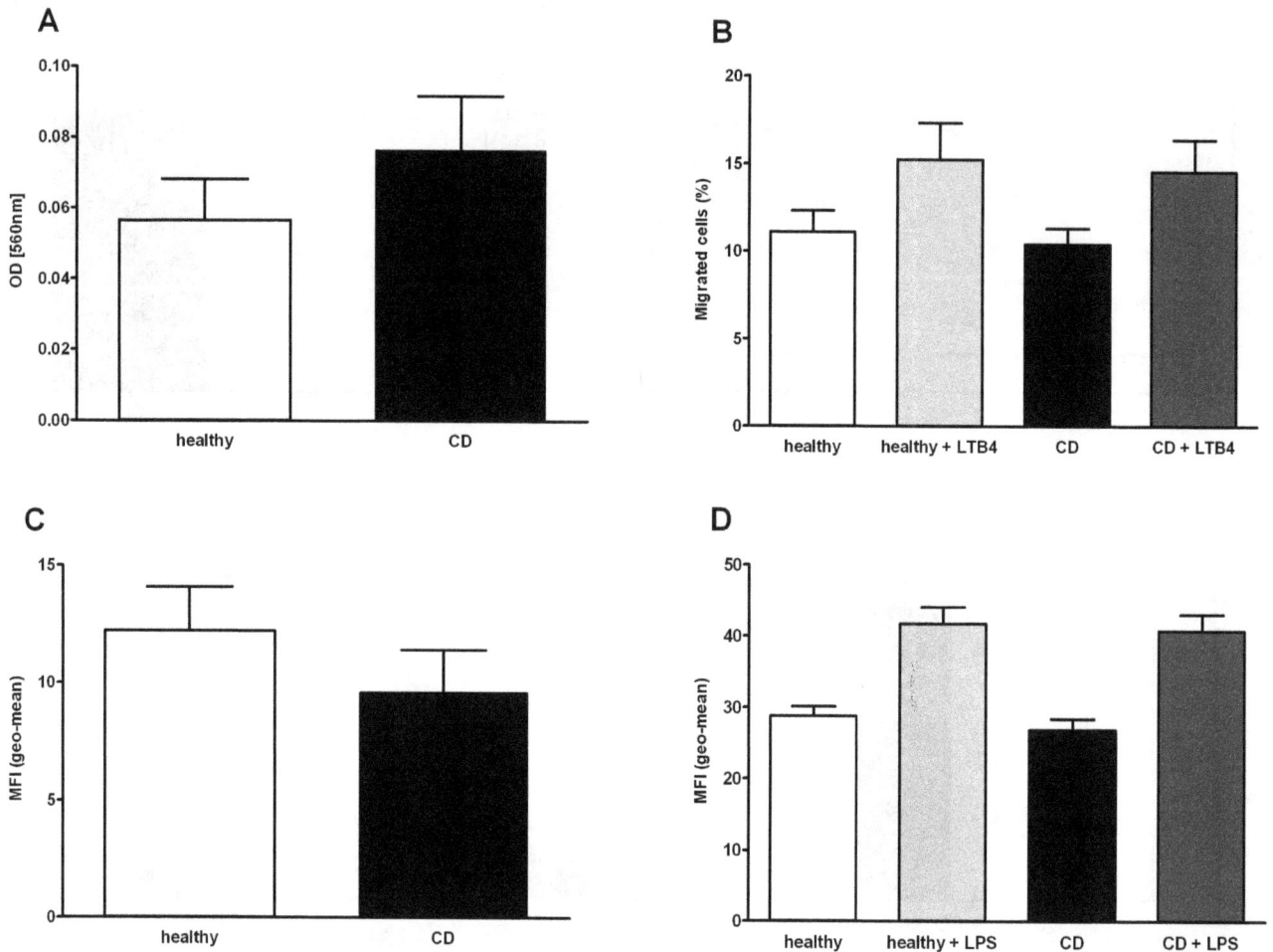

Figure 2. Functional cell assays. (A) Adhesion of monocytes of healthy controls (n = 15) and CD (n = 16) to fibronectin-coated plastic surface. (B) Migration and chemotaxis studies of monocytes of healthy controls (n = 5) and patients with CD (n = 5) using a modified Boyden chamber and LTB4 as a chemoattractant. (C) Phagocytosis of FITC-labeled *E. coli* by monocytes of healthy controls (n = 12) and patients with CD (n = 11). (D) Production of reactive oxygen species (ROS) by monocytes of healthy controls (n = 11) and patients with CD (n = 12) with and without further LPS stimulation for 2 hours. All bars represent means ± SEM.

primed monocytes [21]. Miura *et al.* investigated the phagocytosis (yeast particles), monocyte polykaryon formation and accessory cell function of monocyte/macrophages in CD patients. They postulated that peripheral blood monocytes from patients with CD have abnormal functions, which may be involved in the pathogenesis of the granuloma and giant cell formation in CD patients [22].

Differences in the methodology used and the heterogeneity of the included study patients in previous studies may have led to the divergent data. Thus, we systematically studied phenotypic and functional characteristics of peripheral blood monocytes of patients with definitive but inactive CD compared with healthy controls. In order to specifically characterize potential intrinsic alterations of monocyte subpopulations in CD patients and to exclude potential *in vivo* effects of immunosuppressive and immunomodulatory medications, we exclusively included CD patients in clinical remission. This approach allowed comparison of our results with findings from a recent study by Smith *et al.* that utilized monocyte-derived macrophages from quiescent CD patients to identify a defective mechanism [5]. In the present study we report that adherence to plastic surfaces, spontaneous migration, chemotaxis towards Leukotriene B4, phagocytosis of

E. coli, and production of reactive oxygen species is not impaired in peripheral blood monocytes of patients with inactive CD. LTB4 was chosen for our chemotaxis studies because of its ability to induce the adhesion and activation of leukocytes on the endothelium, allowing their extravasation into (intestinal) tissue. *E. coli* was chosen for the phagocytosis studies because of its abundance in intestinal flora. Our results show that cell functions of peripheral blood monocytes of CD patients are not intrinsically defective *per se*. However, the immunological activity of monocytes may potentially differ in the context of active disease, in the milieu of the inflamed intestinal mucosa, or after further cell differentiation/maturation. Hence, Smith *et al.* have revealed deficient secretion of the (pro-) inflammatory cytokines TNFα, IL4, IL6, IL5, IL13, IL15, IL12, IL17, IFNγ, and IL1β by macrophages from patients with inactive CD following exposure to *E. coli* [5]. In the present study we were able to demonstrate that the expression and release of TNFα, IFNγ, IL4, IL6, IL8, IL13, IL17, CXCL9, and CXCL10 from peripheral blood monocytes is not altered in patients with inactive CD compared to healthy controls. Furthermore, we observed that peripheral blood monocytes of CD patients secreted significant higher levels of pro-inflammatory IL1β and,

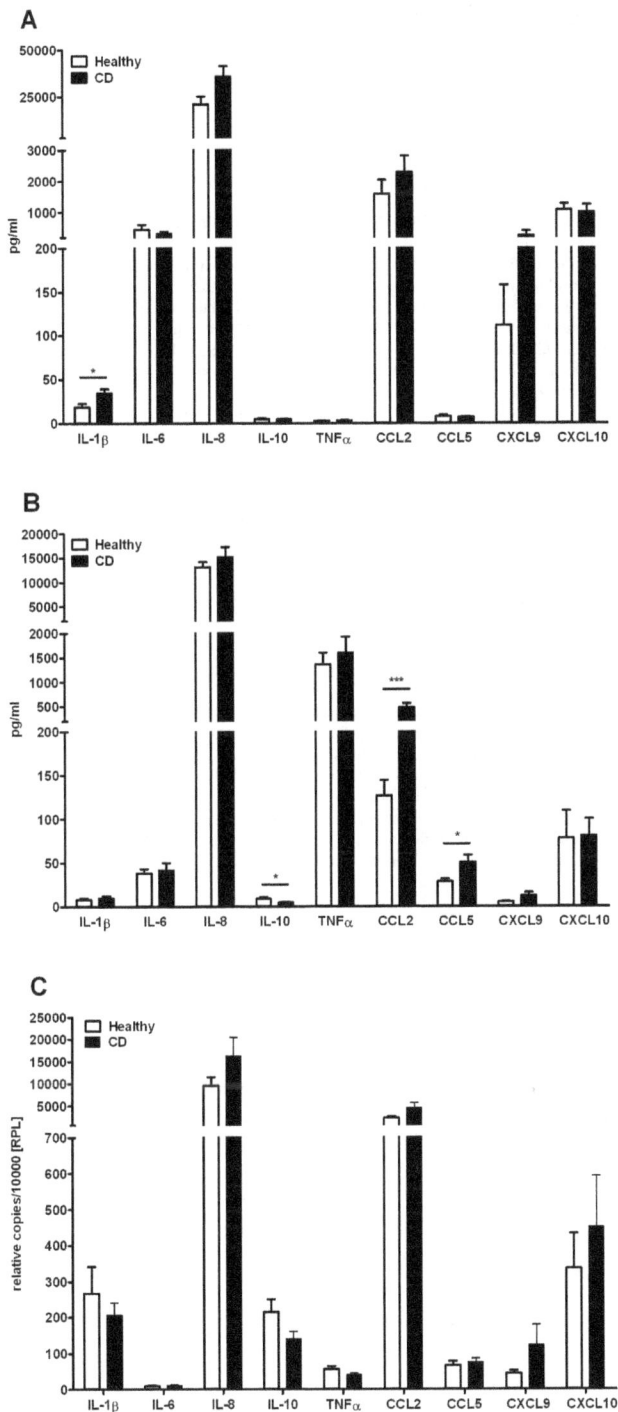

Figure 3. Cytokine expression and secretion. (A) Cytokine and chemokine secretion by resting monocytes of healthy controls (n = 19) and patients with CD in remission (n = 17). (B) Cytokine and chemokine secretion by monocytes of healthy controls (n = 13) and patients with CD (n = 13) stimulated with LPS for 2 hours. (C) mRNA expression levels of resting monocytes of healthy controls (n = 13) and patients with CD (n = 14). Error bars indicate SEM. *, P<0.05; ***, P<0.001.

[5]. However, we cannot exclude that some of the patients were not in complete remission, even though the majority of the included patients with CD had a HBI score <3, and were thus very likely in remission according to the Crohn's disease activity index (CDAI) [9]. However, clinical disease activity scores cannot sufficiently reflect subclinical intestinal inflammation and might be hindered by inaccuracy as a result of subjective components.

A subset of blood monocytes expressing LPS co-receptor CD14 and the low-affinity FCγ receptor CD16 (CD14+CD16+) has been identified previously as a major proinflammatory cell population characterized by low production of IL10 and high levels of IL1β, TNFα and IL12 [23]. CD14+CD16+ peripheral blood monocytes are increased in active CD and CD14+CD16+ cells are a major contributor to the inflammatory infiltrate in CD mucosa [24,25]. Thus, our findings further support the assumption that peripheral blood monocytes from CD patients with quiescent disease are immunological competent rather than functionally impaired. CD14+CD16+ peripheral blood monocytes showed normal levels and were not increased in our CD cohort compared to healthy controls, possibly due the fact that the patients were in clinical remission. Furthermore, it has been reported that the expression of circulating granulocyte-macrophage colony-stimulating factor receptor (CD116) on IBD monocytes from IBD patients is decreased compared to healthy controls (independent of disease activity) [12]. However, we did not observe lower CD116 expression levels on peripheral blood monocytes of patients with quiescent CD, which could be explained by the fact that the IBD-associated CD116 repression is more prominent in patients with ulcerative colitis compared to Crohn's disease [12].

In addition, we found a significantly enhanced release of the chemokines CCL2 (MCP-1) and CCL5 (RANTES) of LPS-primed peripheral blood monocytes of patients with quiescent CD. Both chemokines play an active role in the recruitment of leukocytes to the sites of inflammation. The elevated secretion of chemokines by peripheral blood monocytes of patients with inactive CD provides further evidence for our observation that the monocyte compartment is not functionally impaired in quiescent CD but instead represents immunocompetent cells having the potential to initiate an effective immune response.

Despite the relatively small number of included CD patients, our data were highly consistent within each group of subjects. Nevertheless, further studies may elucidate the impact of the disease activity on monocyte functions in CD patients. Furthermore, comparative studies in peripheral blood monocytes as well as tissue macrophages in patients with active CD patients may further illuminate the underlying immune mechanisms. In addition, other stimulants of Toll-like receptors (TLRs), as well as nucleotide oligomerization domains (NODs), should be investigated, and CD patients should be characterized for their genetic carriage of innate immune gene polymorphisms.

In conclusion, based on our phenotypic and functional studies, peripheral blood monocytes from CD patients in clinical remission were not impaired compared to healthy controls. Our results highlight that defective innate immune mechanisms in CD seems to play a role in the (inflamed) intestinal mucosa rather than in peripheral blood.

Acknowledgments

We thank Melanie Saers and Susanne Schleifenbaum for excellent technical work. Lastly, we thank our study nurse Nicole Voos (Network for Coordinating Centers for Clinical Trials, Münster, NRW, Germany)

upon LPS priming, significantly lower levels of anti-inflammatory IL10 compared to those of healthy controls. Interestingly, Smith *et al.* found no difference in the secretion of IL1β and IL10 by macrophages from CD patients in response to *E. coli*

for her outstanding support. The authors thank Dr Trevelyan Menheniott for carefully reading the manuscript.

Author Contributions

Conceived and designed the experiments: JD DF. Performed the experiments: DS. Analyzed the data: DS DF TW GV JD. Contributed reagents/materials/analysis tools: DS DF TW GV JD. Wrote the paper: DS JD.

References

1. Marks DJ (2011) Defective innate immunity in inflammatory bowel disease: a Crohn's disease exclusivity? Curr Opin Gastroenterol 27: 328–334.
2. Casanova JL, Abel L (2009) Revisiting Crohn's disease as a primary immunodeficiency of macrophages. J Exp Med 206: 1839–1843.
3. Korzenik JR (2007) Is Crohn's disease due to defective immunity? Gut 56: 2–5.
4. Folwaczny C, Glas J, Torok HP (2003) Crohn's disease: an immunodeficiency? Eur J Gastroenterol Hepatol 15: 621–626.
5. Smith AM, Rahman FZ, Hayee B, Graham SJ, Marks DJ, et al. (2009) Disordered macrophage cytokine secretion underlies impaired acute inflammation and bacterial clearance in Crohn's disease. J Exp Med 206: 1883–1897.
6. Marks DJ, Harbord MW, MacAllister R, Rahman FZ, Young J, et al. (2006) Defective acute inflammation in Crohn's disease: a clinical investigation. Lancet 367: 668–678.
7. Zhou L, Braat H, Faber KN, Dijkstra G, Peppelenbosch MP (2009) Monocytes and their pathophysiological role in Crohn's disease. Cell Mol Life Sci 66: 192–202.
8. Burgio VL, Fais S, Boirivant M, Perrone A, Pallone F (1995) Peripheral monocyte and naive T-cell recruitment and activation in Crohn's disease. Gastroenterology 109: 1029–1038.
9. Sandborn WJ, Feagan BG, Hanauer SB, Lochs H, Lofberg R, et al. (2002) A review of activity indices and efficacy endpoints for clinical trials of medical therapy in adults with Crohn's disease. Gastroenterology 122: 512–530.
10. Dabritz J, Friedrichs F, Weinhage T, Hampe J, Kucharzik T, et al. (2011) The functional -374T/A polymorphism of the receptor for advanced glycation end products may modulate Crohn's disease. Am J Physiol Gastrointest Liver Physiol 300: G823–832.
11. Grip O, Bredberg A, Lindgren S, Henriksson G (2007) Increased subpopulations of CD16(+) and CD56(+) blood monocytes in patients with active Crohn's disease. Inflamm Bowel Dis 13: 566–572.
12. Goldstein JI, Kominsky DJ, Jacobson N, Bowers B, Regalia K, et al. (2011) Defective leukocyte GM-CSF receptor (CD116) expression and function in inflammatory bowel disease. Gastroenterology 141: 208–216.
13. Segal AW, Loewi G (1976) Neutrophil dysfunction in Crohn's disease. Lancet 2: 219–221.
14. Mee AS, Berney J, Jewell DP (1980) Monocytes in inflammatory bowel disease: absolute monocyte counts. J Clin Pathol 33: 917–920.
15. Mee AS, Szawatakowski M, Jewell DP (1980) Monocytes in inflammatory bowel disease: phagocytosis and intracellular killing. J Clin Pathol 33: 921–925.
16. Liu ZX, Hiwatashi N, Noguchi M, Toyota T (1997) Increased expression of costimulatory molecules on peripheral blood monocytes in patients with Crohn's disease. Scand J Gastroenterol 32: 1241–1246.
17. Okabe N, Matsuoka Y, Ueda I, Fujita K, Mashiba H, et al. (1988) Immunological studies on Crohn's disease. VII. Reduced immunologic activity in monocytes. J Clin Lab Immunol 25: 69–72.
18. Okabe N, Kuroiwa A, Fujita K, Shibuya T, Yao T, et al. (1986) Immunological studies on Crohn's disease. VI. Increased chemiluminescent response of peripheral blood monocytes. J Clin Lab Immunol 21: 11–15.
19. Okabe N, Ikura S, Uchida Y, Fujita K, Yao T (1990) Immunological studies on Crohn's disease. VIII. Diminished phagocytic activity in peripheral blood monocytes. J Clin Lab Immunol 32: 29–31.
20. Whorwell PJ, Bennett P, Tanner AR, Wright R (1981) Monocyte function in Crohn's disease and ulcerative colitis. Digestion 22: 271–275.
21. Baldassano RN, Schreiber S, Johnston RB, Jr., Fu RD, Muraki T, et al. (1993) Crohn's disease monocytes are primed for accentuated release of toxic oxygen metabolites. Gastroenterology 105: 60–66.
22. Miura M, Hiwatashi N (1987) Impaired monocyte macrophages function in patients with Crohn's disease. J Clin Lab Immunol 24: 167–170.
23. Ziegler-Heitbrock L (2007) The CD14+ CD16+ blood monocytes: their role in infection and inflammation. J Leukoc Biol 81: 584–592.
24. Koch S, Kucharzik T, Heidemann J, Nusrat A, Luegering A (2010) Investigating the role of proinflammatory CD16+ monocytes in the pathogenesis of inflammatory bowel disease. Clin Exp Immunol 161: 332–341.
25. Grimm MC, Pavli P, Van de Pol E, Doe WF (1995) Evidence for a CD14+ population of monocytes in inflammatory bowel disease mucosa-implications for pathogenesis. Clin Exp Immunol 100: 291–297.

22

Gram-Negative Enterobacteria Induce Tolerogenic Maturation in Dexamethasone Conditioned Dendritic Cells

Raquel Cabezón[1], **Elena Ricart**[1,2], **Carolina España**[1], **Julián Panés**[1,2], **Daniel Benitez-Ribas**[2]*

1 Department of Gastroenterology, Hospital Clínic de Barcelona, IDIBAPS, Barcelona, Spain, **2** Centro de Investigación Biomédica en Red de Enfermedades Hepáticas y Digestivas (CIBERehd) and Centre Esther Koplowitz, Barcelona, Spain

Abstract

Dendritic cells have been investigated in clinical trials, predominantly with the aim of stimulating immune responses against tumours or infectious diseases. Thus far, however, no clinical studies have taken advantage of their specific immunosuppressive potential. Tolerogenic DCs may represent a new therapeutic strategy for human immune-based diseases, such as Crohn's disease, where the perturbations of the finely tuned balance between the immune system and the microflora result in disease. In the present report, we describe the generation of tolerogenic DCs from healthy donors and Crohn's disease patients using clinical-grade reagents in combination with dexamethasone as immunosuppressive agent and characterize their response to maturation stimuli. Interestingly, we found out that dexamethasone-conditioned DCs keep their tolerogenic properties to Gram-negative bacteria. Other findings included in this study demonstrate that the combination of dexamethasone with a specific cytokine cocktail yielded clinical-grade DCs with the following characteristics: a semi-mature phenotype, a pronounced shift towards anti-inflammatory versus inflammatory cytokine production and low T-cell stimulatory properties. Importantly, in regard to their clinical application, the tolerogenic phenotype of DCs remained stable after the elimination of dexamethasone and after a second stimulation with LPS or bacteria. All these properties make this cell product suitable to be tested in clinical trials of inflammatory conditions including Crohn's disease.

Editor: Phillip A. Stumbles, Murdoch University, Australia

Funding: This work was supported by grant SAF 2009-07272 from the Ministerio de Ciencia e Innovacion, grant TRA-097 from the Ministerio de Sanidad y Politica Social, and by Centro de Investigación Biomédica en Red de Enfermedades Hepáticas y Digestivas (CIBERehd). DB-R is supported by CIBERehd and by the Instituto de Salud Carlos III, RC is funded by a FI fellowship from the Generalitat de Catalunya. The funders had no role in study design, data collection and analysis, decision to publish, or preparation of the manuscript.

Competing Interests: The authors have declared that no competing interests exist.

* E-mail: daniel.benitez@ciberehd.org

Introduction

Dendritic cells (DCs) represent the most potent antigen-presenting cells linking innate and adaptive immune responses. DCs express a set of receptors involved in pathogen recognition. Known as pattern-recognition receptors (PRR), they include Toll-like receptors (TLR), C-type lectins and the cytoplasmic NOD family, as well as RIG-I and MDA-5 molecules [1]. Interaction of these receptors with their specific ligands leads to DC differentiation to an activated state. Their role in the immune system is crucial, either by initiating effective immune responses or by inducing tolerance, depending on the presence or absence of danger associated molecular patterns within endocytosed particles [2].

Due to their physiological properties [3] DCs have been safely and successfully used in clinical trials aimed at stimulating an efficient immune response against tumors in humans [4,5]. However, only one recent study has taken advantage of their specific tolerogenic properties by utilizing CD40, CD80 and CD86 antisense transfected DCs to treat diabetic patients [6]. The tolerogenic properties of immature autologous DCs have already been documented in healthy human volunteers, providing proof of

principle that systemic antigen-specific T-cell tolerance can be achieved using this approach in humans [7]. However, an important concern when designing DC-based immunotherapy protocols is whether immature DCs might inadvertently receive *in vivo* maturation signals in an inflammatory microenvironment, either from pro-inflammatory cytokines and/or pathogen-derived molecules or whole microorganisms [8]. An alternative to the use of immature DCs is to generate tolerogenic DCs (tol-DCs). The addition of immunosuppressive agents, pharmacological modulation, or inhibitory cytokines during the process of DC differentiation from monocytes influences the functional properties of the resulting cells [9,10]. Recently, a study between clinical-grade DCs compared the phenotypic characterization of human DCs using different tolerogenic agents [11]. These studies demonstrate that activation of tol-DCs might actually be a critical step in optimizing the re-stimulation and/or expansion of functional Tregs rather than in maintaining their immaturity [12,13]. Alternative activated DCs differentially regulated naïve and memory T cells; specifically, naïve T cells were sensitized and polarized towards a low IFN-γ/high IL-10 cytokine profile, whereas memory T cells were anergized in terms of proliferation and cytokine production [14]. The studies described above were carried out using animal models or DC lines [15,16]. However, the use of reagents that fail to fulfil GMP requirements, such as LPS, cytokines or fetal calf/bovine serum [17], makes this approach unfeasible for human trials [18]. An important obstacle to overcome in translating this method to a human setting is the need for reproducible, high-quality stable tol-DCs [19]. Furthermore, given the importance of genetic predisposition in the majority of immune mediated inflammatory disorders, it needs to be proven that tol-DCs produced from patients' monocytes have the same tolerogenic functions as those of healthy controls.

In this study, we characterized the tolerogenic properties of monocyte-derived DCs from healthy donors and Crohn's disease patients generated under clinical-grade conditions. In addition, we evaluated not only the stability of the tolerogenic phenotype after washing out all of the factors, but also the activation profile of those cells when exposed to different Gram-negative enterobacteria a physiologic stimuli that tol-DCs will likely encounter after administration to patients. This approach takes advantage of the complexity of the microbes that provide, at the same time, a variety of stimuli for innate receptors to elicit polarizing cytokines.

Materials and Methods

Generation of Human DCs and Cell Cultures

The present study was approved by the Ethics Committee at the Hospital Clinic of Barcelona. Buffy coats were obtained from Banc de Sang i Teixits and written informed consent was obtained from all blood donors. PBMC from Crohn's disease patients were obtained with written informed consent to participate in the study. DCs were generated from the peripheral blood samples as previously reported [4]. In summary, PBMCs were allowed to adhere for 2 h at 37°C. Non-adherent cells peripheral blood lymphocytes (PBLs) were gently removed, washed, and cryopreserved. The adherent monocytes were cultured in X-VIVO 15 medium (BioWhittaker, Lonza, Belgium) supplemented with 2% AB human serum (Sigma-Aldrich, Spain), IL-4 (300 U/ml), and GM-CSF (450 U/ml) (Both from Miltenyi Biotec, Madrid, Spain) for 6 days in order to obtain immature DCs (iDCs). The maturation cocktail consisted of IL-1β, IL-6 (both at 1000 IU/ml), TNF-α (500 IU/ml) (CellGenix, Freiburg, Germany) and Prostaglandin E2 (PGE2, 10 μg/ml; Dinoprostona, Pfizer) and was added on day 6 for 24 h. Mature DCs (mDCs) were harvested and analyzed on day 7. Dexamethasone (10^{-6} M; Fortecortin, MERCK, Spain) was added on day 3. For cell stability, DCs were washed and further stimulated for 24 h with 100 ng/ml LPS (Sigma Aldrich) or 1 μg/ml of recombinant soluble CD40 ligand (Bender Medsystems, Vienna, Austria). We did not observe differences in viability and yield between iDCs, mDCs and tol-DCs generation. The protocol and reagents for tol-DC generation are fully compatible with cGMP regulations and it has been approved by Agencia Española del Medicamento y Productos Sanitarios.

Heat-killed *Escherichia coli*, *Protheus mirabillis*, *Klebsiella pneumoniae* and *Salmonella thyphimurium* were incubated at 1:10 (DC:bacteria) ratio with DCs for 24 h. After co-incubation, supernatant was collected for cytokines determination and DCs phenotype was then analyzed.

Flow Cytometry

To characterize and compare the phenotype of the DC populations, flow cytometry was performed. The following mAbs or appropriate isotype controls were used: anti- CD14 (eBioscience, San Diego, CA), CD80, CD83, CD86 (BD-Pharmingen), CCR7, MHC class I (W6/32 a generous gift from

Dr. Ramon Vilella, Dept of Immunology Hospital Clinic de Barcelona) and FITC-labeled MHC class II (BD-Pharmingen). Primary antibodies were followed by staining with PE-labelled goat-anti-mouse (from BD Pharmingen™). Flow cytometry was performed using a FACSCalibur™ with CellQuest software (BD Biosciences) and data were analyzed using WinMDI software (version 2.9; http://facs.scripps.edu/software.html), FACSCanto II, and analyzed with BD FACSDiva 6.1™ software.

T-cell Stimulation

For co-culture experiments, PBLs and naïve CD4$^+$ T cells were isolated from healthy individuals using the CD4$^+$ and naïve CD4$^+$ T isolation kit (Miltenyi Biotec, Spain), according to the manufacturer's instructions. The allo-response was tested in a mixed lymphocyte reaction; allogeneic T cells were co-cultured with DCs differently generated in a 96-well microplate. For Ag-specific T-cell responses, 1 μg/ml of tetanus toxoid (TT) (Sigma-Aldrich, Spain) or 10 ng/ml of superantigen toxic shock syndrome toxin-1 (TSST-1) (Sigma-Aldrich, Spain) loaded DCs were co-cultured with autologous T lymphocytes in a 96-round well microplate. For the proliferation assay, a tritiated thymidine (1 μCi/well, Amersham, UK) was added to the cell cultures on day six and an incorporation assay was measured after 16 h. For some experiments T cells were labelled with CFSE and plated in fixed amounts of 10^5 cells/well. T-cell proliferation was determined by the sequential dilution of CFSE fluorescence in positive cells, as detected by flow cytometry. TT-specific cell lines were generated by adding 1 μg/ml of TT to PBMCs for one week and further cell expansion with 50 IU/ml of IL-2 for an extra week.

Anergy Induction

For anergy induction, $1*10^6$ of highly (>98%) purified naïve CD4$^+$ CD45RA$^+$ T cells were co-cultured with DCs (iDCs, mDCs and tol-DCs) in a 6-well plate for 1 week (ratio 1:10; DC:T). After extensive washing, T cells were expanded and rested in the presence of IL-2 and IL-7 for an additional week. T lymphocytes were washed and re-stimulated by co-culturing $1*10^5$ T cells with matured DCs from the original donor at 1:20 ratio in 96-well plates. After 6 days, plates were pulsed with ^{3}H-thymidine and measured as described above.

Cytokine Production

DC supernatants were collected and frozen after 24 h of activation. IL-10, IL-12p70, IL-23 and TNF-α from the DCs supernatants and IFN-γ and IL-10 from the T-cell cultures were analyzed by ELISA according to the manufacturer's guidelines.

mRNA Isolation, cDNA Synthesis, and Real-time PCR

Total RNA was isolated from DCs using an RNeasy Mini Kit (Qiagen, Germany). RNA was transcribed to cDNA using a High-Capacity cDNA Archive RT kit (Applied Biosystems, USA), and was then used to perform quantitative real-time PCR in triplicate wells with a TaqMan Universal PCR Master Mix (Applied Biosystems) containing IL-10 and IL-12p35 and ß-actin (TaqMan primers and probes; Applied Biosystems). PCRs were performed using an Applied Biosystems 7500 Fast Real-Time PCR System sequence detection system. mRNA content (x) was calculated using the formula $x = 2^{-\Delta Ct}$ (where $\Delta Ct = Ct$ target gene-Ct housekeeping gene) were calculated for each gene and setting using ß-actin as a housekeeping gene. Fold-increase expression of target genes in mDCs or in tol-DCs was determined relative to iDCs.

Statistical Analysis

Results are shown as the mean ± SD. To determine statistical differences between the means of two data sets, the paired or independent sample two-tailed Student t-tests were used. Statistically significant difference was set at $p < 0.05$.

Results

Tolerogenic DCs Display a Semi-mature Phenotype

The presence of dexamethasone during DC differentiation partially impaired the upregulation of co-stimulatory molecules such as CD80 (38% reduction, $p < 0.001$), the maturation marker CD83 (40% reduction, $p < 0.001$), and the HLA-DR (39% reduction, $p < 0.05$) compared with fully mDCs (**Figure 1A**). CD86 was highly expressed on iDCs and we did not observe any significant changes in the expression of CD86 upon activation in tol-DCs compared to mDCs. Consistently, similar phenotypic results were obtained by stimulation of dexamethasone-treated DCs with TLR ligands, such as LPS (data not shown), as elsewhere described [20,21,11]. The maturation of DCs resulted in a tightly regulated production of pro- and anti-inflammatory cytokines, depending on the type of stimuli. In accordance with the tolerogenic phenotype shown in **Figure 1A**, tol-DC cytokine secretion resulted in significantly higher production of the anti-inflammatory cytokine IL-10 (mean = 510±453 pg/ml) compared with either iDCs (68±69 pg/ml, $p < 0.001$) or mDCs (51±59 pg/ml, $p < 0.001$) (**Figure 1B**). The inflammatory cytokines IL-12p70 and IL-23 remained undetectable in the supernatants of either tol-DCs or mDCs, which is coherent with the absence to TLR-L on the maturation cocktail [22,23]. In order to confirm these results, we analyzed the transcripts of these cytokines by real-time PCR. mRNA levels for the pro-inflammatory cytokine IL-12p35 were significantly reduced in tol-DCs compared to mDCs (**Figure 1C**), whereas the RNA levels of IL-10 exhibited a significant six-fold increase in tol-DCs compared with mDCs, thus corroborating our results at the protein level.

Tolerogenic DCs Show Reduced T-cell Stimulatory Capacity

To determine the functional properties of clinical-grade tol-DCs, we analyzed their T-cell stimulatory capacity. Tol-DCs induced a lower proliferative allo-response (mean cpm = 40.879, $p < 0.05$) compared to mDCs (cpm = 74.651), whereas the response to iDCs was also low (mean cpm = 23.634, $p < 0.001$ vs mDCs) as expected, **Figure 2A**. We also investigated the capacity of tol-DCs to present exogenous antigen to autologous T cells. As depicted in **Figure 2B**, tol-DCs exhibited a reduced antigen-presenting capacity to autologous T cells compared with control DCs, when the latter were loaded with either the superantigen toxic shock syndrome toxin-1 (TSST-1) or tetanus toxoid (TT). Thus, tol-DCs were poorer stimulators of allo- or antigen-specific T-lymphocyte responses (in allogeneic and autologous settings) than mDCs.

Tolerogenic DCs Generate Antigen-specific Anergic T cells

To evaluate the ability of tol-DCs to induce CD4[+] T-cell hypo-responsiveness, allogeneic highly purified CD4[+] naïve T cells (purity 98% CD4[+]CD45RA[+]) were initially primed for 14 days during the first round with iDCs, mDCs or tol-DCs (initial challenge) and then were re-stimulated (re-challenged) with iDCs or fully competent mDCs from the original donor. T cells exposed to tol-DCs exhibited a reduced capacity to proliferate as well as reduced IFN-ÿ secretion when re-challenged with fully competent

mDCs. In contrast, T cells exposed to control DCs proliferated and secreted IFN-γ to a high degree (**Figure 3A**). To confirm the capacity of tol-DCs to mitigate effector T cells, tetanus toxoid (TT)-specific T cell lines were re-stimulated with TT loaded or control (non-loaded) mDCs. Whereas T cells primarily exposed to mDCs vigorously responded to TT, as measured by T-cell proliferation and IFN-γ production (**Figure 3B**), those exposed to tol-DCs showed a significantly reduced proliferation and an absolute inability to induce IFN-γ during a secondary response to TT-loaded DCs.

Tolerogenic DCs are Stable and Resistant to Further Stimulation

To address the stability of tol-DCs, dexamethasone and cytokines were carefully washed away and the DCs were re-stimulated with secondary maturation stimulus. Tol-DCs were refractory to further stimulation with LPS (**Figure 4A**, data from **n = 6** independent experiments) and CD40L (**n = 4**), maintaining a stable semi-mature phenotype. Interestingly, tol-DCs retained their ability to further produce high levels of IL-10, but failed to generate IL-12 or IL-23 following stimulation with LPS (**Figure 4B**) data not included for negative IL-12 and IL-23), we did not detect any cytokine after CD40L stimulation. Furthermore, tol-DCs re-challenged with LPS or CD40L were unable to induce a proliferative T-cell response (**Figure 4C**). In addition, the lower levels of IFN-γ cytokine secretion by T cells stimulated with LPS-treated tol-DCs compared with mDCs (mean 6332±1514 vs 1700±700 pg/ml $p = 0.07$) suggest inhibition of the Th1-type response (**Figure 4C**).

Tolerogenic Response of Dexamethasone-conditioned DCs to Gram-negative Bacteria

Whole microorganisms contain multiple PAMPs capable of stimulating DCs by different pathways. This capacity exemplifies a more physiological setting, versus the use of restricted TLR agonists or exogenous recombinant cytokines. DCs were incubated with Gram-negative heat-inactivated *Escherichia coli* (*E. coli*). Interestingly, the presence of dexamethasone during DCs differentiation profoundly influenced cell maturation, exhibiting strong inhibitory effect on their phenotype (**Figure 5A**) with significant reduction in CD83, CD86 and MHC class I and II expression, when compared with DCs without *E. coli*. Importantly, it caused a robust inhibition of pro-inflammatory cytokines (IL-12p70, IL-23 and TNF-α), increased IL-10 secretion (**Figure 5B**), and modified the immune response of T lymphocytes (**Figure 5C**) inhibiting T cell proliferation and Th1 induction. The production of IFN-γ by T cells was inhibited (mean 21550±11782 pg/ml vs 7869±6198 pg/ml; $p = 0.07$) when DCs were conditioned with dexamethasone previously to *E. coli* stimulation. We did not detect any IL-10 in the supernatant of activated T cells.

Tolerogenic DCs are Stable and Resistant to Further Gram-negative Bacteria

To address the stability of tol-DCs, dexamethasone and maturation cytokine cocktail were carefully washed away as described above and DCs were incubated with *E. coli* for further 24 h without dexamethasone or other factors present in the culture. Tol-DCs were refractory to further stimulation with Gram-negative bacteria. Interestingly, tol-DCs produced significantly higher levels of IL-10 in response to *E. coli* than mDCs (mean 1252±694 vs 249±306 pg/ml; $p = 0.01$) even after DC maturation with a cytokine cocktail, whereas the levels of pro-inflammatory cytokines were hardly detected (**Figure 6A**). Fur-

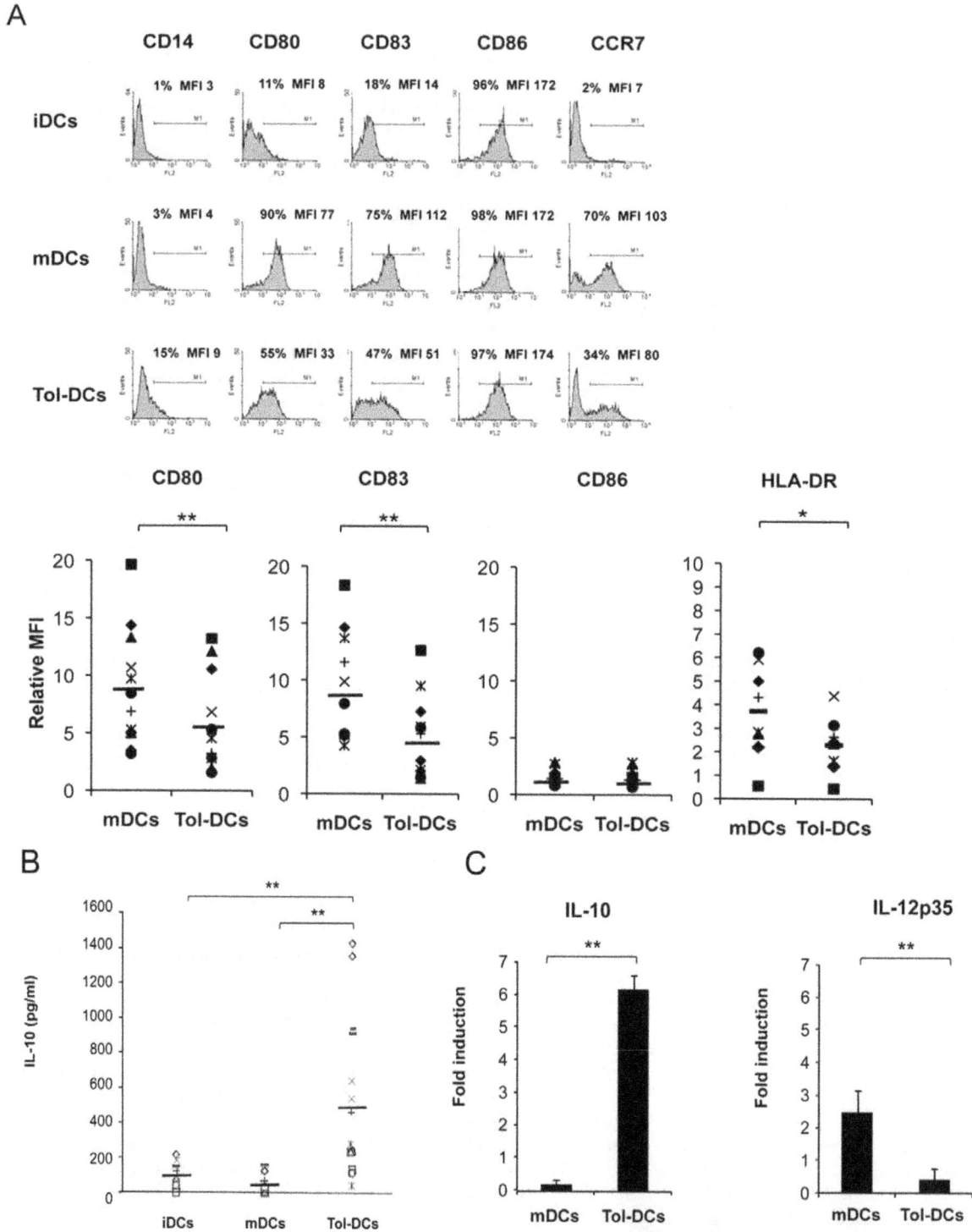

Figure 1. Dexamethasone modulates cytokine cocktail-induced DC maturation. (A) Phenotypic analysis of untreated (iDCs), cytokine-activated (mDCs) and 10^{-6} M dexamethasone cytokine-activated dendritic cells (Tol-DCs) was performed by flow cytometry. Representative histogram data set from 12 independent experiments is shown. Maturation associated molecules are depicted in the lower graph as mean fluorescent intensity of expression (MFI) of mDCs and Tol-DCs relative (fold-change expression) to iDCs. **(B)** IL-10 and IL-12p70 were measured in supernatants harvested from DCs. Concentration of IL-10 (in pg/ml) is shown (n = 15). In none of the conditions analyzed were IL-12p70 or IL-23 produced (lowest detection limit 7.6 pg/ml). **(C)** Transcripts levels of IL-10 and IL-12p35 were determined by real-time PCR using β-actin as the endogenous reference gene. Data represent fold-change induction relative to iDCs (n = 3). Student's t-test: *$p<0.05$, **$p<0.001$.

thermore, when we evaluated the capacity of DCs to generate Th1 response we observed that tol-DCs induced significant lower IFN-γ levels compared to mDCs (**Figure 6B**). The results obtained with *E. coli* were further confirmed and strengthened when

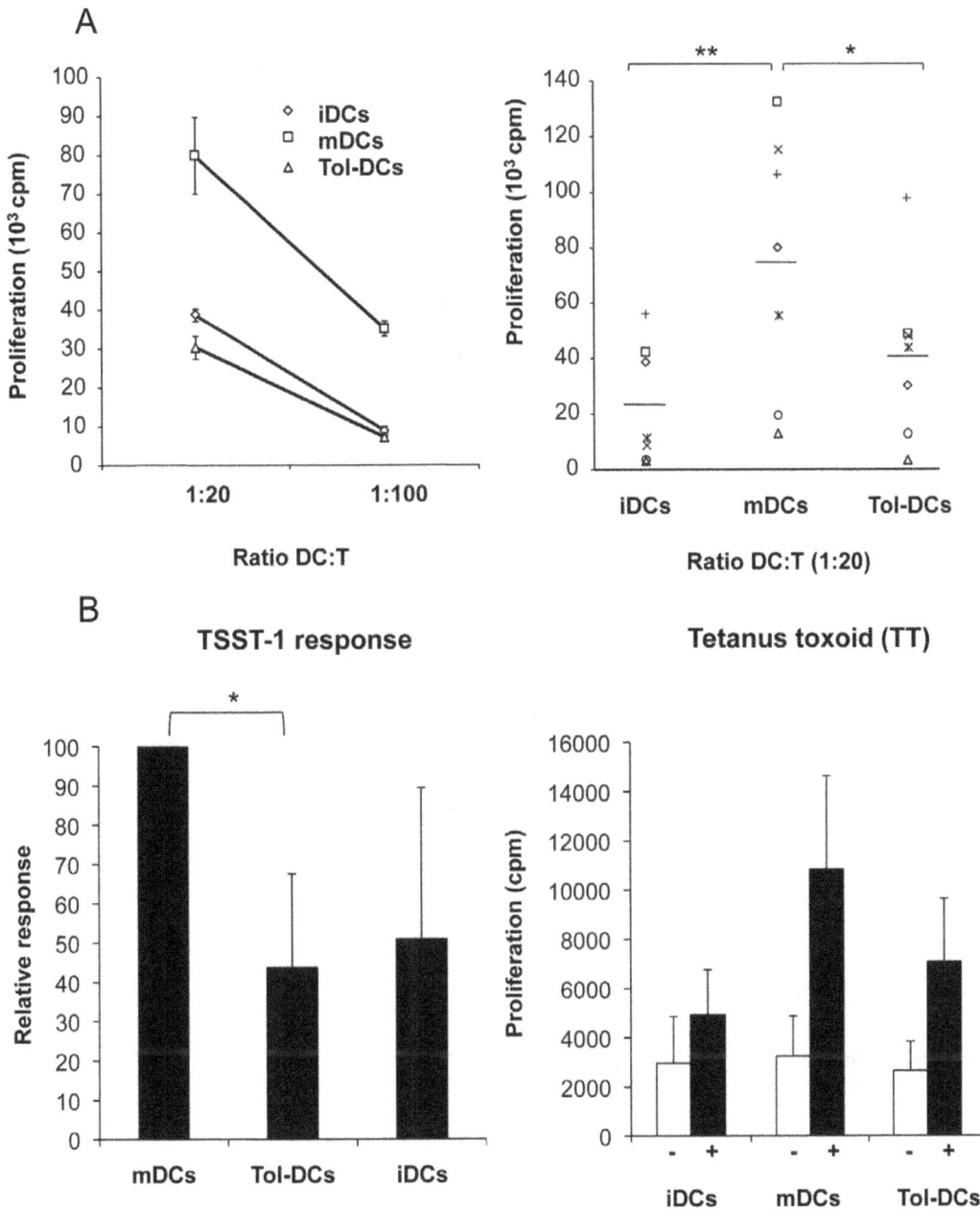

Figure 2. Tol-DCs have a reduced capacity to stimulate T lymphocytes. (A) DCs were cultured with allogeneic PBL at different ratio (1:20 or 1:100) for seven days. Upper-left panel data represent the mean ± SD of a representative experiment carried out in triplicate of the seven (upper-right graph) that were independently performed. **(B)** Antigen-specific T-cell responses. CD4[+] T cells we cultured with autologous DCs pre-loaded with the superantigen TSST-1 (left graph) or with tetanus toxoid (+ presence and – absence of TT) at a 1:20 ratio for seven days. T-cell proliferation was determined in triplicate by ^{3}H thymidine incorporation. Data represent the mean ± SD of n = 3 independently performed experiments. Student's t-test: *$p < 0.05$, **$p < 0.001$.

different Gram-negative enterobacteria. *P. mirabillis*, *K. pneumoniae* and *S. thyphimurium* were incubated with dexamethasone-conditioned DCs (**Figure 7A**) or with tol-DCs (dex-DCs plus maturation cocktail) (**Figure 7B**) after washing out the immunosuppressive agent and cytokines. Although, mDCs and tol-DCs stimulated with bacteria provoked a comparable T cell proliferative response, the IFN-γ secretion was significantly reduced in both culture conditions (no IL-10 was detected in any condition) (**Figure 7**). These results show the incapacity of dex-DCs or tol-DCs to generate Th1 response measured by IFN-γ production

revealing the stability of the tolerogenic properties, even after strong and activation induced by Gram-negative bacteria.

DCs from Crohn's Disease Patients can be also Educated towards a Tolerogenic Phenotype

In order to validate the tol-DCs generation in the context of an inflammatory disease, DCs from Crohn's disease patients were generated and analysed. As depicted in **figure 8A**, tol-DCs generated from Crohn's disease patients showed a statistically significant impairment in the upregulation of CD80, CD83 and

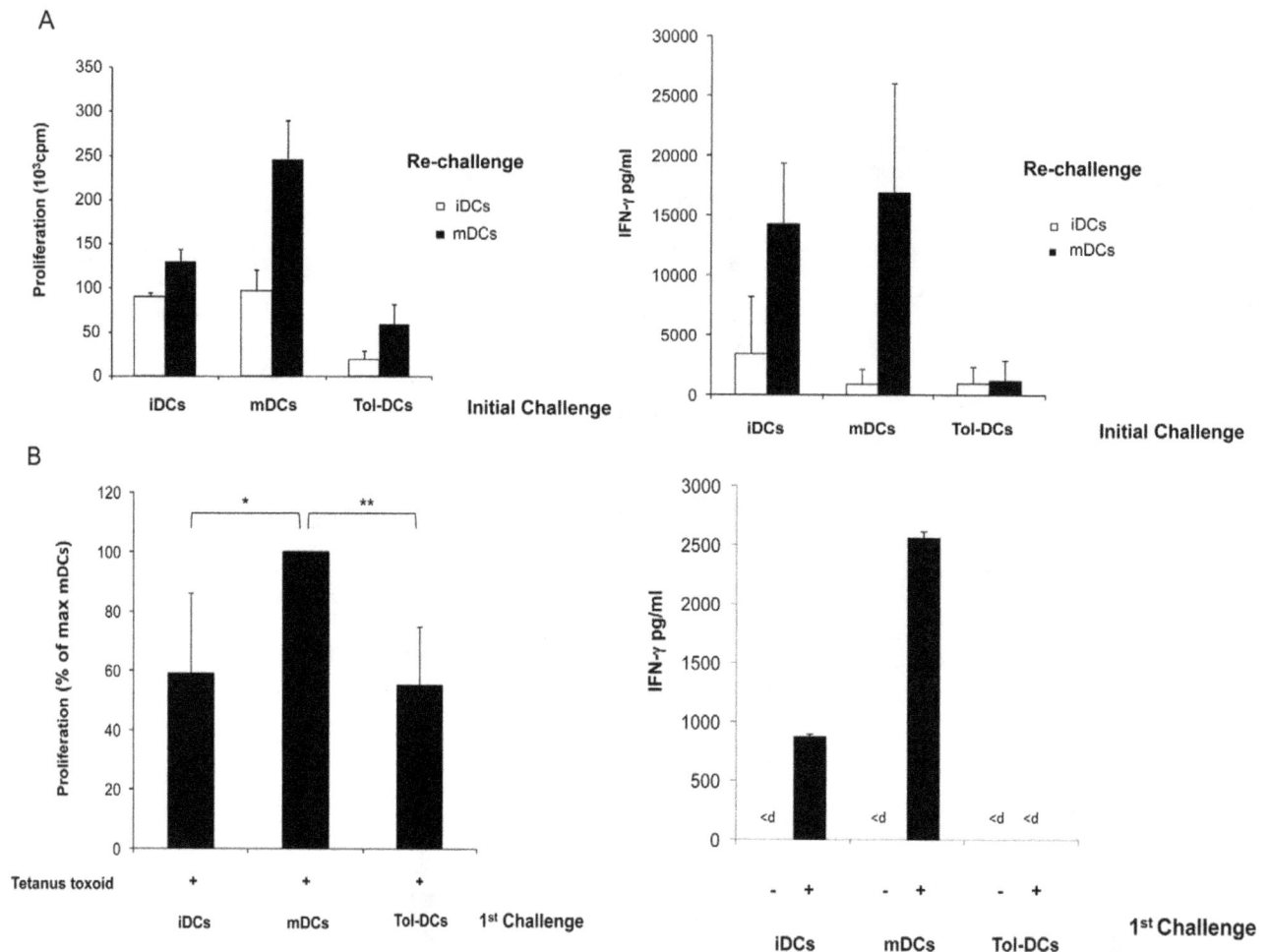

Figure 3. Tol-DCs induce anergic T cells. (A) Naïve CD4[+] CD45RA[++] T cells were primarily primed with allogeneic iDCs, mDCs or tol-DCs for 7 days. After 5 days, anergy induction was examined by re-stimulation of primed CD4[+] T cells with iDCs or mDCs from the original donor. **(B)** TT-specific CD4[+] T cells were primed with TT-loaded autologous iDCs, mDCs or tol-DCs for 6 days (initial challenge). After *in vitro* expansion with TT loaded-DCs anergy induction was examined by re-stimulation of TT-specific CD4[+] T cells with mDCs loaded (+) with TT at a 1:20 ratio. Data represent the mean ± SD of n = 5 experiments that were independently performed. Proliferation was normalized relative to mDCs loaded with TT (100%) for each independent experiment. Cytokines were determined in the supernatant of cell cultures by ELISA (<d; below detection limit; IFN-γ data represent mean ± SD of n = 3).

HLA-DR compared to iDCs, with no CD86 modification. Interestingly, the levels of IL-10 were significantly increased in the supernatants of tol-DCs of Crohn's disease patients compared to mDCs and iDCs (**figure 8B**) and did not produce pro-inflammatory cytokines like IL-12 or IL-23 (data not included). Furthermore, T cells exposed to tol-DCs from Crohn's disease patients exhibited a significantly reduced capacity to proliferate (mean cpm = 20561 ± 13058 vs 38181 ± 18177; p = 0.037) compared to mDCs, as well as reduced IFN-γ secretion when co-cultured with fully competent mDCs (**figure 8C**). These results show the ability to generate tol-DCs in patients with Crohn's disease.

Discussion

The generation of reproducible and stable clinical-grade tolerogenic DCs is a critical step towards developing therapeutic trials for the treatment of human disorders such as allergies, autoimmune diseases, chronic inflammation, and transplant rejection [19] [24]. The addition of immunosuppressive agents,

pharmacological modulation, or inhibitory cytokines when DCs are being generated from monocytes influences the functional properties of the resulting DCs [9,10]. Several agents, including glucocorticoids [25] such as dexamethasone [26,27], mycophenolic acid [28], vitamin D3 (1α,25-dyhydroxyvitamin D_3) [29], retinoic acid [30], the combination of dexamethasone and vitamin D3 [31], or IL-10 [32] have been used to render DCs resistant to maturation [33].

Tolerogenic DCs have been shown to induce T-cell anergy [34], suppress effector T cells, and promote the generation of regulatory T cells (Tregs) [14,35]. Interestingly, some studies [14] have reported that the maturation of dex-conditioned DCs with LPS potentiates the tolerogenic phenotype of DCs.

We performed a detailed phenotype analysis in order to compare iDCs and fully mature DCs with tol-DCs from healthy donors and patients with Crohn's disease and address the stability of tol-DCs. DCs conditioned with dexamethasone displayed a semi-mature phenotype, which is consistent with the tolerogenic DC phenotypes described elsewhere [36]. We also observed an alteration in the DC maturation process; characterized by low-

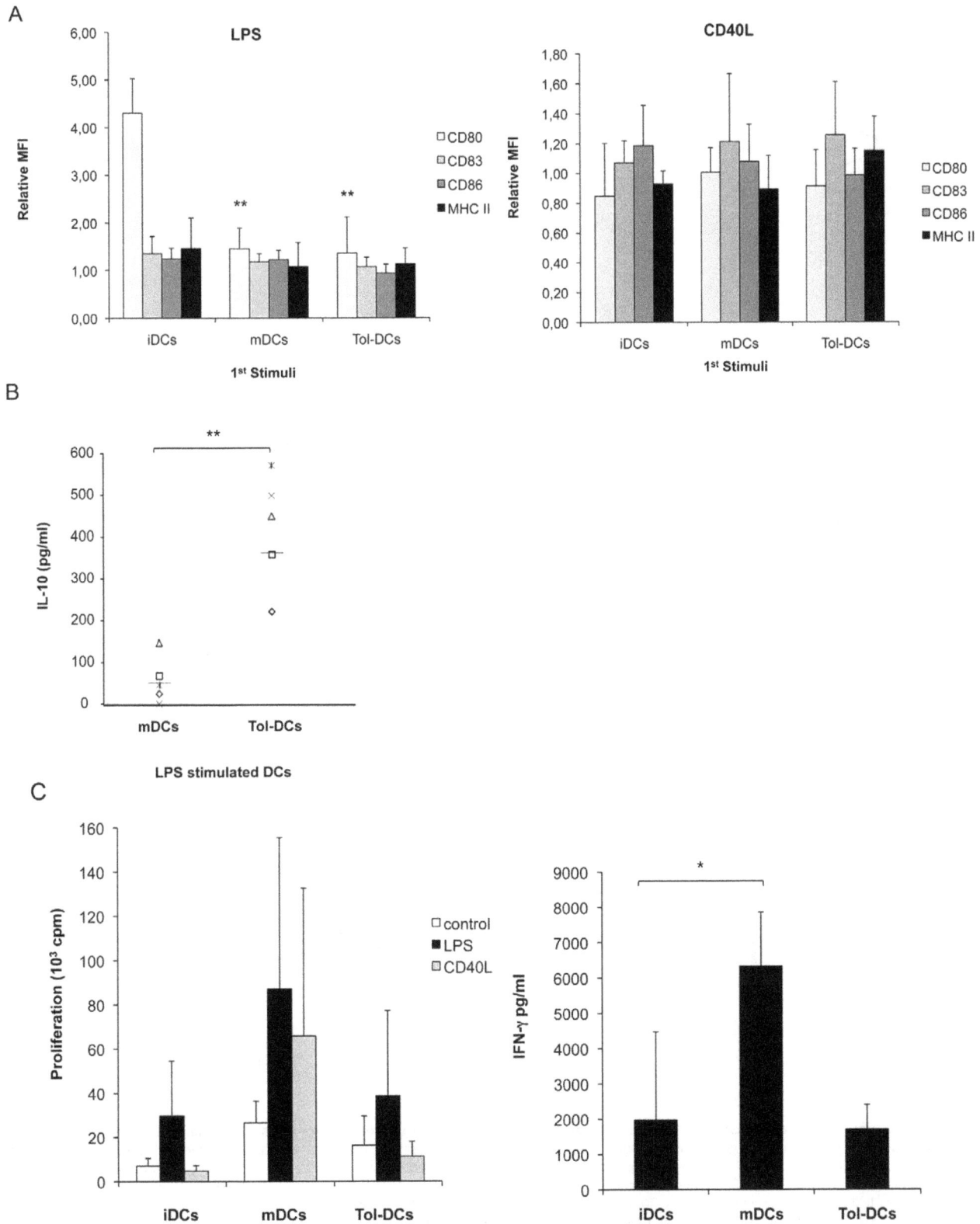

Figure 4. Tol-DCs possess a stable phenotype. DCs were carefully washed to eliminate cytokines and dexamethasone, and viable DCs were further re-challenged with 100 ng/ml of LPS or 1 μg/ml of soluble CD40L as second stimuli. After 24 h, the phenotype (**A**) was analyzed by flow cytometry. Data represent relative MFI increase induced by LPS (n = 6) or CD40L (n = 4) compared to unstimulated iDCs, mDCs or tol-DCs as control. (**B**) IL-10 concentration is shown in pg/ml. IL-12p70 and IL-23 were not detected (detection limit = 7.8 pg/ml). Student's t-test: *p<0.05, **p<0.001. (**C**) Tol-DCs do not recover the ability to stimulate T cells after re-challenge. T-cell proliferation was determined in triplicate by ^{3}H-thymidine incorporation. IFN-γ and IL-10 production in the supernatant was analyzed.

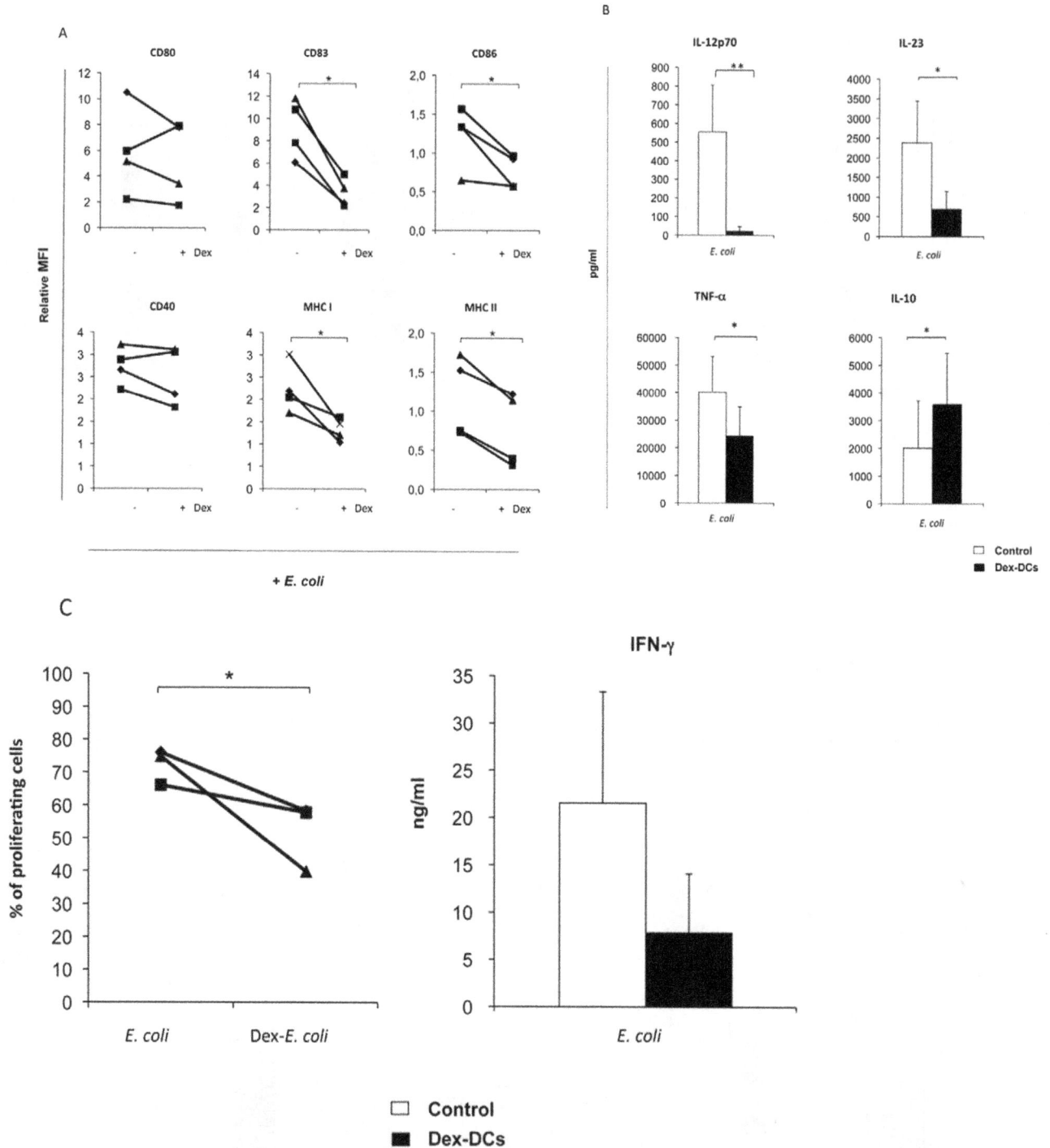

Figure 5. Gram-negative bacteria do not break the tolerogenic properties of dexamethasone-DCs. Heat-killed bacteria were added at ratio 1:10 for 48 h to mo-DCs treated with dexamethasone or untreated as a positive control. **A.** Phenotypic analysis revealed statistically significant reduction of CD83, CD86, and MHC I and class II expression. Maturation associated molecules are depicted as mean fluorescent intensity of expression (MFI) of *E. coli* stimulated-DCs relative (fold-change expression) to control DCs without *E. coli*. (**B**) Cytokines produced by *E. coli*-stimulated DCs. Reduction of IL-12p70 (95.9%; $p<0.05$), IL-23 (70.5%; $p<0.05$) and TNF-α (40%; $p<0.05$) and elevation of IL-10 (78% increase; $p<0.05$) in Gram-negative treated DCs. (**C**) Gram-negative stimulated DCs were cultured after being carefully washed with allogenic PBLs (ratio 1:20) for 7 days. The % of proliferating cells was measured by CFSE dilution using flow cytometry. Significant allo-response inhibition of *E. coli* dex-DC (inhibition 28%; $p<0.05$) compared to control DCs. IFN-γ secretion was analyzed in the supernatant by standard ELISA. Results represent the mean and standard deviation of three independent donors. Student's *t*-test: *$p<0.05$, **$p<0.001$.

intermediate CD80, CD83, CCR7, MHC class I and MHC class II expression. The high levels of CD86 on DCs can be explained by the presence either of human serum or steroids in the culture [37]. Indeed, dexamethasone has been shown to increase CD86

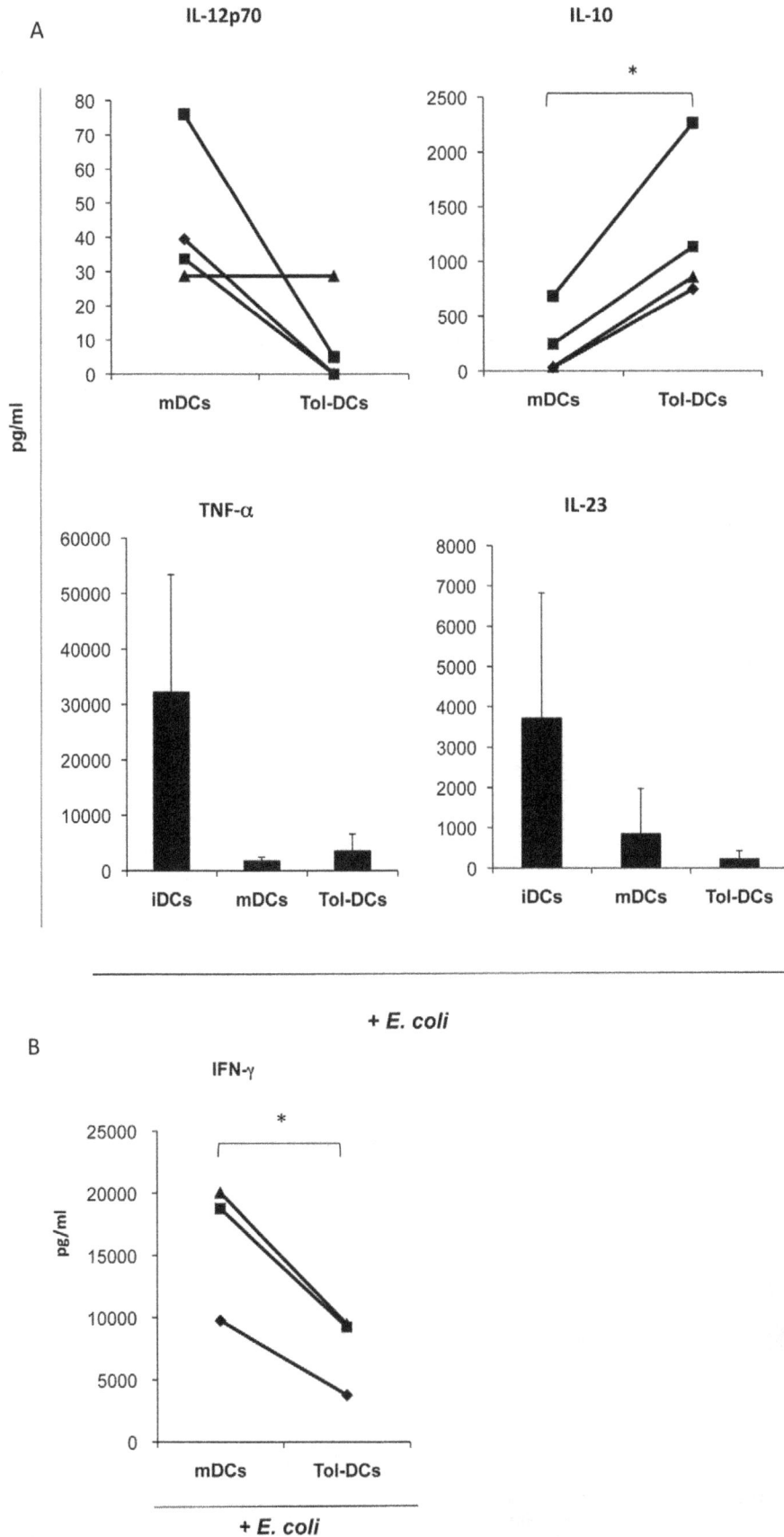

Figure 6. Gram negative *E. coli* induces tolerogenic activation on Tol-DCs. DCs were carefully washed to eliminate cytokines and dexamethasone at day 7, and viable DCs were further re-challenged with *E. coli* (ratio 1:10) without cytokines or dexamethasone. (**A**) Tol-DCs (dex

matured-DCs) produced significant higher levels of IL-10 whereas levels of pro-inflammatory cytokines were very low compared with mDCs or iDCs in response to *E. coli* (n = 4, from each donor, iDCs, mDCs and tol-DCs were generated in parallel). (**B**) The production of IFN-γ was evaluated in the supernatant of allogenic T cells cultured for 7 days with *E. coli* stimulated mDCs or tol-DCs. IFN-γ production was significantly (p = 0.024) reduced in T cells stimulated with tol-DCs plus *E. coli*. IL-10 was not detected in any condition (data not included). Student's *t*-test: *$p<0.05$, **$p<0.001$.

expression through GILZ (glucocorticoid-induced leucine zipper) induction [38]. Furthermore, interactions involving CD80/86 are needed in order to expand Tregs, as was revealed when Treg expansion was inhibited via the use of CD86-blocking antibodies [39]. CCR7 mediates the migration of peripheral DCs to lymph nodes [40]. Although CCR7 expression is induced on DCs by PGE2 [41], we were unable to detect CCR7 expression in tol-DCs by increasing PGE2 concentration (unpublished results). Our data clearly demonstrate that a phenotypic description alone without functional studies appears insufficient for ascertaining the nature of tol-DCs. Comparisons between different tolerogenic agents have revealed the differences among these so-called tol-DCs [11,33]. The cytokine balance determines the type of T-cell effector response when DC-T cell interaction occurs. Pro-inflammatory cytokines like IL-12p70 and IL-23 were absent in tol-DCs at both the protein and mRNA transcripts levels. Interestingly, levels of

IL-10 in response to maturation stimuli, which is one of the most important anti-inflammatory cytokines having powerful tolerogenic properties, were significantly higher in tol-DCs compared with mDCs. The balance between IL-12/IL-10 might be crucial both for the induction of tolerance and for Th1 inhibition.

Tol-DCs exhibited a low stimulatory capacity in an allogeneic-mixed leucocyte reaction, as well as skewed T-cell polarization toward an anti-inflammatory phenotype. Importantly, this immunosuppressive function was also observed in autologous settings when superantigen TSST-1 or TT antigens were used as recall antigens. DCs can be manipulated to induce T-cell anergy and regulatory T-cell activity depending on the maturation level and the interaction with naïve $CD4^+CD45RA^+$ or memory T cells. The induction of anergy on naïve T cells could represent another mechanism of tolerance induction. In our study, we demonstrate that naïve T cells expanded with tol-DCs were unable to

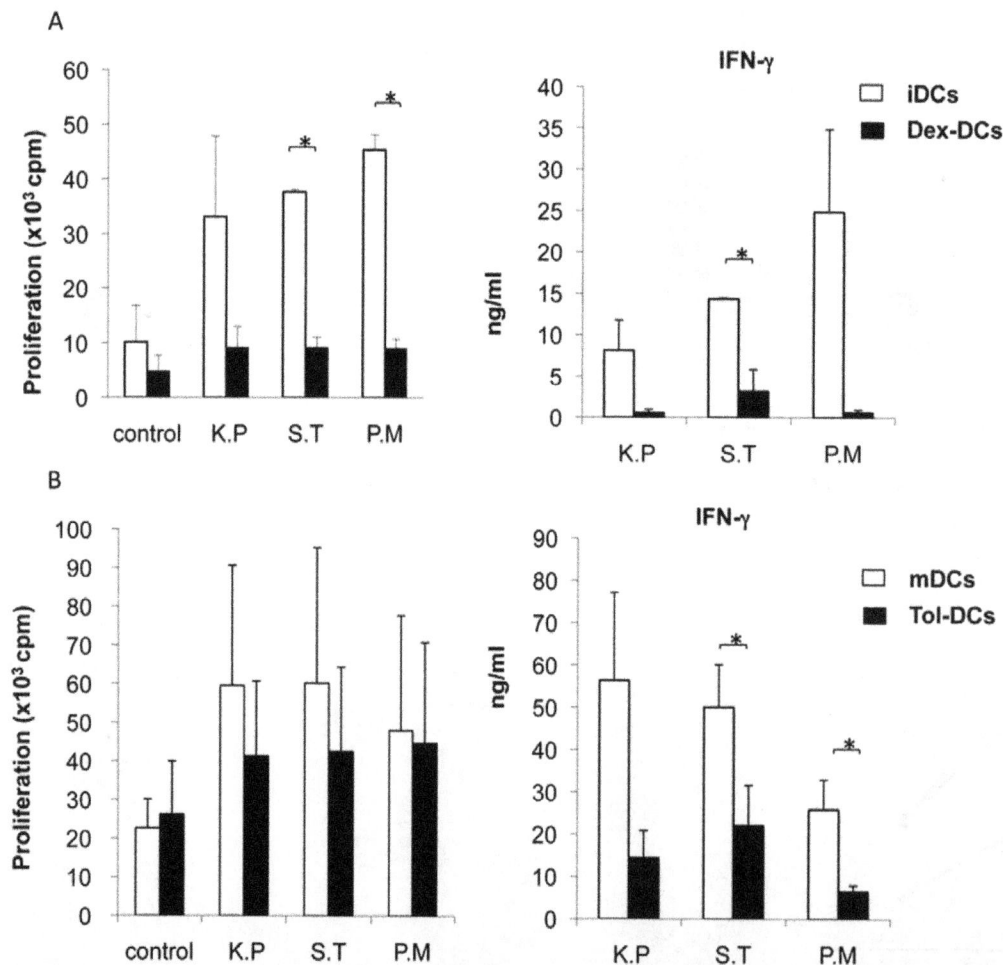

Figure 7. Tol-DCs interaction with Gram-negative enterobacteria inhibits Th1 response. Tol-DCs were treated as described in figure 5 and 6. Proliferative response and IFN-γ production induced by Gram-negative enterobacteria (*P. mirabillis, K. pneumoniae* and *S. thyphimurium*) stimulation of dex-DCs (**A**) and tol-DCs (dex matured-DCs) (**B**) were evaluated in allogeneic T cell culture. IFN-γ production was reduced in T cells stimulated with tol-DCs plus Gram-negative enterobacteria. IL-10 was not detected. Data represent mean ± SD of four independent experiments. Student's *t*-test: *$p<0.05$.

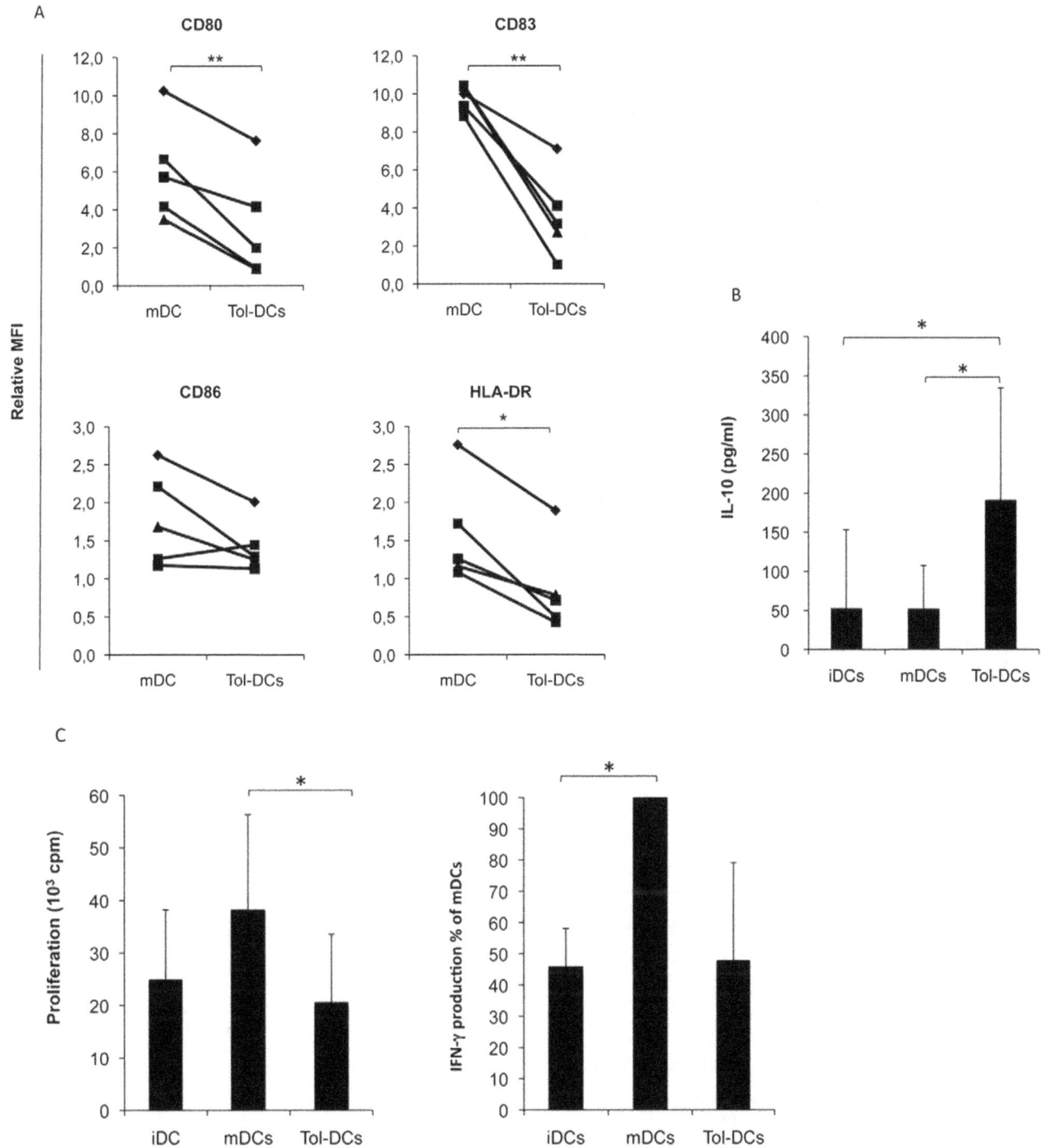

Figure 8. Crohn's disease patients' DCs are educated towards tolerogenic phenotype. (**A**) Maturation associated molecules upregulation in DCs from Crohn's disease patients are depicted as mean fluorescent intensity of expression (MFI) in mDCs and tol-DCs relative to iDCs (fold-change expression). (**B**) IL-10 was measured in supernatants harvested from DCs. Concentration of IL-10 (in pg/ml) is shown as mean $\pm$ SD (n = 6). (**C**) Proliferative response and IFN-γ production induced by tol-DCs from patients were evaluated in allogeneic T cell culture. Both, proliferation and IFN-γ production were reduced in T cells stimulated with tol-DCs compared to mDCs (data represent mean $\pm$ SD (n = 4)). IFN-γ production was normalized relative to mDCs (100%) for each independent experiment (n = 3). Student's t-test: *$p < 0.05$.

proliferate, even after further stimulation with fully mature DCs from the same donor. Interestingly, we observed the same pattern of inhibition when TT was used as specific antigen. While TT induces strong IFN-γ secretion following interaction with mDCs [42], in our study tol-DCs completely inhibited such Th1

polarization. Increasing evidence suggests that mature DCs that lack the ability to deliver signal 3 preferentially promote the differentiation of CD4$^+$ T cells into IL-10 producing T cells (reviewed by Joffre O et al. [22]). Interestingly, our results reveal that tol-DCs have the capacity to tolerize memory T cells, which are generally viewed as very difficult cell type to tolerize. However, we failed to generate *de novo* Treg (Foxp3 positive) from purified naïve $CD4^+$ T lymphocyte when cultured with tol-DCs.

An important concern to be considered when designing DC-based immunotherapy protocols is their stability. In this regard, it is important to point out that tol-DCs maintained their tolerogenic properties (particularly relevant for IL-10 production) once the immunosuppressive agent was removed from the culture and the DCs were further stimulated with LPS or CD40L.

It is important to stress that the tolerogenic effects of dexamethasone were evident after adding whole microorganisms (Gram-negative enterobacteria), taking into account the presence of multiple PAMPs capable of stimulating DCs by various pathways [43,44]. Interestingly, it has been recently described how glucocorticoids alter DC maturation in response to TLR7 or TLR8 through a mechanism involving GR transcriptional activity [45]. These results indicate that the response to commensal bacteria is directly related to any pre-conditioning DCs receive, underscoring the importance of the interaction between DCs and their surrounding environment [46]. Although pre-conditioning might entail some risk of infection in treated patients, it may also constitute a critical component in the treatment of immune-mediated inflammatory disorders, particularly of those in which an inappropriate response to commensal bacteria is believed to play a role, such as inflammatory bowel diseases. The clinical relevance of such interaction between enterobacteria with clinical-grade tol-DCs would take place in the inflamed lamina propria of IBD patients in the context of a cellular-based therapy. Importantly, we confirm for the first time that this protocol could be used for the production of tol-DCs from Crohn's disease patients, in line with studies in other immune-based diseases like rheumatoid arthritis [47] or multiple sclerosis [48]. This is a key aspect for considering this form of cell therapy in Crohn's disease, because it might have occurred that genetic variants conferring susceptibility for Crohn's disease might alter the biology of DCs.

In conclusion, we herein report that DCs generated by the addition of dexamethasone in combination with a cocktail of pro-inflammatory cytokines yield clinical-grade DCs with tolerogenic properties. Tol-DCs remain stable after Gram-negative bacteria interaction. These properties may serve as the basis for modulating abnormal immune responses and for developing effective strategies for the treatment of immune-mediated diseases.

Acknowledgments

We would like to thank Dr. Xavier Romero Ros and Dr. Elisabeth Calderón-Gómez for discussion and critical reading of the manuscript and the DC.CAT group (the Catalan group for DCs studies) for suggestions.

We would like to thank Dr. Jordi Vila and Elisabet Guiral for providing the microorganisms included in this study.

Author Contributions

Conceived and designed the experiments: RC JP DB-R. Performed the experiments: RC CE DB-R. Analyzed the data: RC ER JP DB-R. Wrote the paper: RC JP DB-R.

References

1. Medzhitov R (2007) Recognition of microorganisms and activation of the immune response. Nature 449: 819–826.
2. Mellman I, Steinman RM (2001) Dendritic cells: specialized and regulated antigen processing machines. Cell 106: 255–258.
3. Napoletano C, Pinto D, Bellati F, Taurino F, Rahimi H, et al. (2007) A comparative analysis of serum and serum-free media for generation of clinical grade DCs. J Immunother 30: 567–576.
4. de Vries IJ, Eggert AA, Scharenborg NM, Vissers JL, Lesterhuis WJ, et al. (2002) Phenotypical and functional characterization of clinical grade dendritic cells. J Immunother 25: 429–438.
5. Figdor CG, de Vries IJ, Lesterhuis WJ, Melief CJ (2004) Dendritic cell immunotherapy: mapping the way. Nat Med 10: 475–480.
6. Giannoukakis N, Phillips B, Finegold D, Harnaha J, Trucco M (2011) Phase I (Safety) Study of Autologous Tolerogenic Dendritic Cells in Type 1 Diabetic Patients. Diabetes Care. 34(9): 2026–32.
7. Dhodapkar MV, Steinman RM, Krasovsky J, Munz C, Bhardwaj N (2001) Antigen-specific inhibition of effector T cell function in humans after injection of immature dendritic cells. J Exp Med 193: 233–238.
8. Laffont S, Siddiqui KR, Powrie F (2010) Intestinal inflammation abrogates the tolerogenic properties of MLN CD103+ dendritic cells. Eur J Immunol 40: 1877–1883.
9. Hackstein H, Thomson AW (2004) Dendritic cells: emerging pharmacological targets of immunosuppressive drugs. Nat Rev Immunol 4: 24–34.
10. Pulendran B, Tang H, Manicassamy S (2010) Programming dendritic cells to induce T(H)2 and tolerogenic responses. Nat Immunol 11: 647–655.
11. Naranjo-Gomez M, Raich-Regue D, Onate C, Grau-Lopez L, Ramo-Tello C, et al. (2011) Comparative study of clinical grade human tolerogenic dendritic cells. Journal of Translational Medicine 9: 89.
12. Emmer PM, van der Vlag J, Adema GJ, Hilbrands LB (2006) Dendritic cells activated by lipopolysaccharide after dexamethasone treatment induce donor-specific allograft hyporesponsiveness. Transplantation 81: 1451–1459.
13. Watanabe N, Wang YH, Lee HK, Ito T, Cao W, et al. (2005) Hassall's corpuscles instruct dendritic cells to induce CD4+CD25+ regulatory T cells in human thymus. Nature 436: 1181–1185.
14. Anderson AE, Sayers BL, Haniffa MA, Swan DJ, Diboll J, et al. (2008) Differential regulation of naive and memory CD4+ T cells by alternatively activated dendritic cells. J Leukoc Biol 84: 124–133.
15. Fazekasova H, Golshayan D, Read J, Tsallios A, Tsang JY, et al. (2009) Regulation of rat and human T-cell immune response by pharmacologically modified dendritic cells. Transplantation 87: 1617–1628.
16. Bros M, Jahrling F, Renzing A, Wiechmann N, Dang N-A, et al. (2007) A newly established murine immature dendritic cell line can be differentiated into a mature state, but exerts tolerogenic function upon maturation in the presence of glucocorticoid. Blood 109: 3820–3829.

17. Peng JC, Thomas R, Nielsen LK (2005) Generation and maturation of dendritic cells for clinical application under serum-free conditions. J Immunother 28: 599–609.
18. Feldmann M, Steinman L (2005) Design of effective immunotherapy for human autoimmunity. Nature 435: 612–619.
19. Steinman RM, Banchereau J (2007) Taking dendritic cells into medicine. Nature 449: 419–426.
20. Chamorro S, Garcia-Vallejo JJ, Unger WW, Fernandes RJ, Bruijns SC, et al. (2009) TLR triggering on tolerogenic dendritic cells results in TLR2 up-regulation and a reduced proinflammatory immune program. J Immunol 183: 2984–2994.
21. Anderson AE, Swan DJ, Sayers BL, Harry RA, Patterson AM, et al. (2009) LPS activation is required for migratory activity and antigen presentation by tolerogenic dendritic cells. J Leukoc Biol 85: 243–250.
22. Joffre O, Nolte MA, Sporri R, Reis e Sousa C (2009) Inflammatory signals in dendritic cell activation and the induction of adaptive immunity. Immunol Rev 227: 234–247.
23. Boullart AC, Aarntzen EH, Verdijk P, Jacobs JF, Schuurhuis DH, et al. (2008) Maturation of monocyte-derived dendritic cells with Toll-like receptor 3 and 7/8 ligands combined with prostaglandin E(2) results in high interleukin-12 production and cell migration. Cancer Immunol Immunother 57: 1589–1597.
24. Moreau A, Varey E, Beriou G, Hill M, Bouchet-Delbos L, et al. (2012) Tolerogenic dendritic cells and negative vaccination in transplantation: from rodents to clinical trials. Front Immunol 3: 218.
25. Woltman AM, de Fijter JW, Kamerling SW, Paul LC, Daha MR, et al. (2000) The effect of calcineurin inhibitors and corticosteroids on the differentiation of human dendritic cells. Eur J Immunol 30: 1807–1812.
26. Piemonti L, Monti P, Allavena P, Sironi M, Soldini L, et al. (1999) Glucocorticoids affect human dendritic cell differentiation and maturation. J Immunol 162: 6473–6481.
27. Rozkova D, Horvath R, Bartunkova J, Spisek R (2006) Glucocorticoids severely impair differentiation and antigen presenting function of dendritic cells despite upregulation of Toll-like receptors. Clin Immunol 120: 260–271.
28. Lagaraine C, Lemoine Y, Baron C, Nivet H, Velge-Roussel F, et al. (2008) Induction of human CD4+ regulatory T cells by mycophenolic acid-treated dendritic cells. J Leukoc Biol 84: 1057–1064.
29. Penna G, Adorini L (2000) 1 Alpha,25-dihydroxyvitamin D3 inhibits differentiation, maturation, activation, and survival of dendritic cells leading to impaired alloreactive T cell activation. J Immunol 164: 2405–2411.
30. Jin CJ, Hong CY, Takei M, Chung SY, Park JS, et al. (2009) All-trans retinoic acid inhibits the differentiation, maturation, and function of human monocyte-derived dendritic cells. Leuk Res. 34(4): 513–20.

31. Pedersen AE, Schmidt EG, Gad M, Poulsen SS, Claesson MH (2009) Dexamethasone/1alpha-25-dihydroxyvitamin D3-treated dendritic cells suppress colitis in the SCID T-cell transfer model. Immunology 127: 354–364.

32. Steinbrink K, Wolfl M, Jonuleit H, Knop J, Enk AH (1997) Induction of tolerance by IL-10-treated dendritic cells. J Immunol 159: 4772–4780.

33. Boks MA, Kager-Groenland JR, Haasjes MS, Zwaginga JJ, van Ham SM, et al. (2012) IL-10-generated tolerogenic dendritic cells are optimal for functional regulatory T cell induction–a comparative study of human clinical-applicable DC. Clin Immunol 142: 332–342.

34. Berger TG, Schulze-Koops H, Schafer M, Muller E, Lutz MB (2009) Immature and maturation-resistant human dendritic cells generated from bone marrow require two stimulations to induce T cell anergy in vitro. PLoS One 14; 4(8): e6645.

35. Kuwana M, Kaburaki J, Wright TM, Kawakami Y, Ikeda Y (2001) Induction of antigen-specific human CD4(+) T cell anergy by peripheral blood DC2 precursors. Eur J Immunol 31: 2547–2557.

36. Verginis P, Li HS, Carayanniotis G (2005) Tolerogenic semimature dendritic cells suppress experimental autoimmune thyroiditis by activation of thyroglobulin-specific CD4+CD25+ T cells. J Immunol 174: 7433–7439.

37. Duperrier K, Eljaafari A, Dezutter-Dambuyant C, Bardin C, Jacquet C, et al. (2000) Distinct subsets of dendritic cells resembling dermal DCs can be generated in vitro from monocytes, in the presence of different serum supplements. J Immunol Methods 238: 119–131.

38. Cohen N, Mouly E, Hamdi H, Maillot MC, Pallardy M, et al. (2006) GILZ expression in human dendritic cells redirects their maturation and prevents antigen-specific T lymphocyte response. Blood 107: 2037–2044.

39. Chung DJ, Rossi M, Romano E, Ghith J, Yuan J, et al. (2009) Indoleamine 2,3-dioxygenase-expressing mature human monocyte-derived dendritic cells expand potent autologous regulatory T cells. Blood 114: 555–563.

40. Kim CH (2005) The greater chemotactic network for lymphocyte trafficking: chemokines and beyond. Curr Opin Hematol 12: 298–304.

41. Legler DF, Krause P, Scandella E, Singer E, Groettrup M (2006) Prostaglandin E2 is generally required for human dendritic cell migration and exerts its effect via EP2 and EP4 receptors. J Immunol 176: 966–973.

42. Sabin EA, Araujo MI, Carvalho EM, Pearce EJ (1996) Impairment of tetanus toxoid-specific Th1-like immune responses in humans infected with Schistosoma mansoni. J Infect Dis 173: 269–272.

43. Kassianos AJ, Hardy MY, Ju X, Vijayan D, Ding Y, et al. (2012) Human CD1c (BDCA-1)(+) myeloid dendritic cells secrete IL-10 and display an immunoregulatory phenotype and function in response to Escherichia coli. Eur J Immunol 42: 1512–1522.

44. Schreibelt G, Benitez-Ribas D, Schuurhuis D, Lambeck AJ, van Hout-Kuijer M, et al. (2010) Commonly used prophylactic vaccines as an alternative for synthetically produced TLR ligands to mature monocyte-derived dendritic cells. Blood: 564–74.

45. Larange A, Antonios D, Pallardy M, Kerdine-Romer S (2012) Glucocorticoids inhibit dendritic cell maturation induced by Toll-like receptor 7 and Toll-like receptor 8. J Leukoc Biol 91: 105–117.

46. Shale M, Ghosh S (2009) How intestinal epithelial cells tolerise dendritic cells and its relevance to inflammatory bowel disease. Gut 58: 1291–1299.

47. Harry RA, Anderson AE, Isaacs JD, Hilkens CM (2010) Generation and characterisation of therapeutic tolerogenic dendritic cells for rheumatoid arthritis. Ann Rheum Dis. Nov; 69 (11): 2042–2050.

48. Raïch-Regue D, Grau-Lopez L, Naranjo-Gomez M, Ramo-Tello C, Pujol-Borrell R, et al. (2012) Stable antigen-specific T-cell hyporesponsiveness induced by tolerogenic dendritic cells from multiple sclerosis patients. Eur J Immunol 42: 771–782.

23

The Association between Race and Crohn's Disease Phenotype in the Western Cape Population of South Africa, Defined by the Montreal Classification System

Abigail Basson[1]*, **Rina Swart**[1], **Esme Jordaan**[2,3], **Mikateko Mazinu**[2], **Gillian Watermeyer**[4,5]

1 Dietetics Department, University of the Western Cape, Bellville, Western Cape, South Africa, **2** Biostatistics Unit, Medical Research Council of South Africa, Parow, Western Cape, South Africa, **3** Statistics and Population Studies Department, University of the Western Cape, Bellville, Western Cape, South Africa, **4** Department of Gastroenterology, Groote Schuur Hospital, Cape Town, Western Cape, South Africa, **5** Department of Medicine, University of Cape Town, Cape Town, Western Cape, South Africa

Abstract

Background: Inter-racial differences in disease characteristics and in the management of Crohn's disease (CD) have been described in African American and Asian subjects, however for the racial groups in South Africa, no such recent literature exists.

Methods: A cross sectional study of all consecutive CD patients seen at 2 large inflammatory bowel disease (IBD) referral centers in the Western Cape, South Africa between September 2011 and January 2013 was performed. Numerous demographic and clinical variables at diagnosis and date of study enrolment were identified using an investigator administered questionnaire as well as clinical examination and patient case notes. Using predefined definitions, disease behavior was stratified as 'complicated' or 'uncomplicated'.

Results: One hundred and ninety four CD subjects were identified; 35 (18%) were white, 152 (78%) were Cape Coloured and 7(4%) were black. On multiple logistic regression analysis Cape Coloureds were significantly more likely to develop 'complicated' CD (60% vs. 9%, p = 0.023) during the disease course when compared to white subjects. In addition, significantly more white subjects had successfully discontinued cigarette smoking at study enrolment (31% vs. 7% reduction, p = 0.02). No additional inter-racial differences were found. A low proportion of IBD family history was observed among the non-white subjects.

Conclusions: Cape Coloured patients were significantly more likely to develop 'complicated' CD over time when compared to whites.

Editor: Benoit Foligne, Institut Pasteur de Lille, France

Funding: This research was supported by the 2011 Scholarship in Gastroenterology; a grant from the AstraZeneca/South African Gastroenterology Society (SAGES). http://www.sages.co.za/D_AN_ScholTravel.asp. The funders had no role in the study design, data collection and analysis, decision to publish, or preparation of the manuscript.

Competing Interests: The authors have declared that no competing interests exist.

* Email: abbasson@uwc.ac.za

Introduction

A subtype of inflammatory bowel disease (IBD), Crohn's disease (CD) is believed to result from a complex interplay between genetic susceptibility and one or more environmental triggers. The disease is characterized as a chronic immune-mediated disorder of the gastrointestinal tract which may or may not be accompanied by a variety of extraintestinal or systemic complications. Disease presentation and severity are known to vary between individuals, having important implications for disease management [1,2]. Thus, in recent years, issues of CD sub-classification by phenotype have been reviewed, and the Montreal classification system [2] (revised Vienna) is the accepted standard.

Crohn's disease is found in all racial groups worldwide. However, historically, the highest prevalence rates have been reported in white populations, particularly those of North America and Europe, with significantly lower rates seen in black and Asian populations within these or any other foreign country [3–12]. As such, the majority of reports contributing to our understanding of disease presentation and clinical course originate primarily from Western populations, leaving a paucity of literature regarding the racial variability of CD phenotype [5,12–14].

Earlier epidemiological observations have suggested that CD presents in a more severe form in African American and Asian populations compared to their white counterparts [15–17], yet findings have been inconsistent, often limited by small sample size and variations in disease classification methods. Recently however, reports indicate that the incidence of IBD in both African American and Asian populations has been steadily rising over the decades [18–22]. This increase in incidence may be attributed to one of several factors namely, changes in utilization and accessibility of hospital care (suggesting an underreporting of previous incidence rates), selection bias of IBD centers, or a true rise in the incidence among these racial groups [23]. Therefore, aspects surrounding the racial variations in CD phenotype should continue to be explored and include all non-white populations in order to further contribute towards our understanding of the environmental and genetic factors involved in the disease etiology.

The aim of our study was thus to provide a preliminary and descriptive view on disease phenotype of the racial groups in Cape Town, South Africa.

Materials and Methods

The study protocol and questionnaire were reviewed and approved by the Senate Research Ethics Committee of the University of the Western Cape (Reg no. 11/3/16), the Human Research Ethics Committee of the University of Cape Town (HREC REF: 122/2011) and the Provincial Department of Health. All participants gave written informed consent.

Design and Setting

This was a cross sectional examination (part of a larger case-control study) of all consecutive white, Cape Coloured and black CD patients seen at Groote Schuur Hospital (GSH) and Tygerberg Hospital (TBH) during normally scheduled appointments between September 2011 and January 2013. GSH and TBH manage all public-sector IBD patients within the Western Cape, South Africa. Of the 3.5 million persons who reside in the greater Cape Town area, approximately 90% rely on the public-sector health services [24]. Cape Coloureds are subjects of mixed-ancestry. The term which is non-derogatory refers to a heterogeneous ethnic group of which genome analysis has now identified South Asian, European, Indonesian and isiXhosa sub-Saharan blacks as the four predominant genetic contributors [25]. Disease diagnosis was defined by the European Crohn's and Colitis Organization (ECCO) guidelines [26].

Following informed consent, data relating to patient demographics, smoking and disease symptoms prior to diagnosis were collected via an interviewer administered questionnaire. Race was self-reported. Information relating to disease characteristics and disease course were determined via review of patient medical records as well as clinical examination by the consulting gastroenterologist. Monthly income was determined using computerized hospital records. Only patients with complete data at diagnosis were included. Patients were excluded if disease duration was less than 5 years, or had a prior diagnosis of intestinal tuberculosis. In accordance with the paper published by Epstein et al. [27] there is no gold standard in the differential diagnosis between CD and intestinal tuberculosis however as per the algorithm suggested by these authors every attempt was made to exclude a diagnosis of tuberculosis.

The Montreal classification system [2] (Table 1) was used to define age of onset, disease location and disease behavior at two time intervals; initial diagnosis and date of study enrolment. Any disease related surgical history was categorized by timing of first surgery in relation to initial diagnosis. Information on medical management included lifetime use of immunomodulator, anti-tumor necrosis factor inhibitors or 5-aminosalicylates. Complicated disease was defined as the presence of any one of the following

at diagnosis or during subsequent follow ups: stricturing CD, penetrating CD, perianal fistulas or surgical resection. Data on extraintestinal manifestations (EIMs) was divided into four categories: (1) skin, (2) ocular, (3) joint and (4) other. Skin manifestations included erythema nodosum, pyoderma gangrenosum, and neutrophilic dermatoses. Ocular manifestations included uveitis, iritis, and episcleritis. Joint manifestations included arthralgias, arthritis and axial arthropathies. The 'other' manifestations included ankylosing spondylitis and primary biliary cirrhosis.

Data Analysis

Descriptive data is presented overall as well as separately for the three racial groups (white, Cape Coloured and black) as medians (IQRs) for numerical data, and as frequencies and percentages for categorical data. The Kruskall-Wallis test was used to compare racial groups with respect to their medians for the numeric demographic variables and the Fisher's exact test was used to compare the percentages for the categorical variables. All statistical analysis included only white and Cape Coloured subjects, due to the small number of black subjects. A separate multiple logistic regression model was conducted for each phenotype (age of onset, disease location and disease behavior) to test for an association between the phenotype and racial groups (whites and Cape Coloureds), adjusting for possible confounders age of onset, gender, smoking and duration of symptom onset as appropriate. Separate contingency tables for medication use, surgical interventions and EIMs versus racial group were conducted and the Fisher's exact test was used to test for associations. No adjustments were made in the latter analysis. A generalized linear model (GEE with an unstructured correlation matrix) was used to test for an interaction between racial groups and smoking and phenotype from diagnosis to study enrolment. The standard for significance for all analysis was P<0.05.

Results

Demographic Characteristics of Subjects

Over an approximate seventeen month period, 194 CD patients meeting our inclusion criteria were identified and consented to the study, 35 (18%) were white, 152 (78%) were Cape Coloured and 7 (4%) were black. Two patients that were approached declined to participate (response rate = 99%). Demographic and baseline characteristics for each racial group are shown in Table 2. Overall, 9 (26%) white, 41 (27%) Cape Coloured and 3 (43%) black subjects were male. The median age at enrolment was 47.0 (IQR 38–57) years, the median age of disease onset was 28 (IQR 21.5–38.0) years and median disease duration was 16 (IQR 10.0–24.0) years. The majority of subjects in all racial groups were born in South Africa (95%), but individually, 100% of the Cape Coloureds compared to 77% of the white subjects, were born in South Africa (p<0.001). There was no significant difference in the level of education between the white and Cape Coloured subjects, however there was a significant difference in the median age at study enrolment [52.0 (IQR 40.0–67.5) years vs. 46.0 (IQR 38.0–55.5) years, respectively] as whites were on average six years older at study enrolment (p = 0.04). Comparing white subjects with their Cape Coloured counterparts, median disease duration [22.0 (IQR 10.5–25.0) years vs. 16.0 (IQR 10.0–24.0) years] and median duration of initial presenting symptoms [2.0 (IQR 0.6–3.5) years vs. 1.0 (IQR 0.5–3.0) years], appeared longer in the white subjects, although results did not reach statistical significance. No significant inter-racial difference was found in the smoking habits for white and Cape Coloured subjects at diagnosis (74% vs. 63%). When

Table 1. Montreal Classification Scheme.

Age at diagnosis (years)		
A1	≤16	
A2	17–40	
A3	>40	
Disease location		
L1	Isolated to the terminal ileum	
L2	Isolated to the colon	
L3	Ileum and colonic involvement	
L4*	Upper gastrointestinal tract	
Disease behavior		
B1[†]	Inflammatory; non-stricturing, non-penetrating	
B2	Stricturing	
B3	Penetrating disease, with or without stricturing, excludes perianal penetrating disease	
p[‡]	Perianal disease modifier	

*Upper gastrointestinal (GI) modifier (L4) can be added to L1–L3 when concomitant upper GI disease present.
[†]B1 category should be considered "interim" until a pre-specified time has elapsed from time of diagnosis. Suggested time period is between 5–10 years.
[‡]"p" is added to B1–B3 when concomitant perianal disease is present.

comparing the change in smoking habits from time of diagnosis to study enrolment for the racial groups, we found a significant interaction (Chi-Square = 5.4; p = 0.02), and the results indicated that the reduction of 31% smoking for whites was significant (p = 0.001), but the reduction of 6.8% Cape Coloureds smoking was not significant (p = 0.08).

Disease Characteristics between Racial Groups

On multiple logistic regression analysis there was no significant difference between Cape Coloured and white subjects with regards to disease location or disease behavior at diagnosis (p>0.05; Table 3). However after a median disease duration of 16 years, significantly more Cape Coloured subjects had developed 'complicated' CD (60% vs. 9%, p = 0.023) during the disease course

Table 2. Demographic and Baseline Characteristics of Patients.

		White (*n*=35)	Cape Coloured (*n*=152)	Black (*n*=7)	Overall (*N*=194)	p-value*
Gender, no. (%)	Males	9 (26)	41 (27)	3 (43)	53 (27)	0.88
	Females	26 (74)	111 (73)	4 (57)	141 (73)	
Age at enrolment (median and IQR), yr.[†]		52.0 (40.0, 67.5)	46.0 (38.0, 55.5)	44.0 (38.0, 46.0)	47 (38.0, 57.0)	0.04
Age at diagnosis (median and IQR), yr.		28.0 (21.5, 45.5)	28.5 (21.5, 45.5)	29.0 (26.5, 33.5)	28 (21.5, 38.0)	0.24
Disease duration (median and IQR), yr.		22.0 (10.5, 25.0)	16.0 (10.0, 24.0)	12.0 (9.5, 14.0)	16 (10.0, 24.0)	0.30
Duration presenting symptoms (median and IQR), yr.		2.0 (0.6, 3.5)	1.0 (0.5, 3.0)	1.0 (0.2, 1.0)	1.0 (0.5, 3.5)	0.58
Married, no. (%)‡		14 (40)	78 (51)	1 (14)	93 (48)	0.64
Education, no. (%)§		13 (37)	21 (14)	2 (29)	36 (18)	0.12
Born in South Africa, no. (%)		27 (77)	152 (100)	5 (71)	184 (95)	<0.001
Income per month, no. (%)						
	<R3000	30 (86)	127 (84)	6 (86)	163 (84)	0.74
	R3000–10,000	4 (11)	23 (15)	1 (14)	28 (14)	
	>R10,000	1 (3)	2 (1)	0 (0)	3 (1)	
Smoking history, no. (%)[a]	At diagnosis	26 (74)	95 (63)	6 (86)	127 (65)	0.42
	At study enrolment	15 (43)	87 (57)	2 (29)	104 (54)	0.09
Family History IBD, no. (%)[b]		5 (14)	10 (6)	0 (0)	15 (7)	0.75

IQR, interquartile range; IBD, inflammatory bowel disease.
*Statistical analysis excluding black subjects. No subjects reported being of Indian or Asian ethnicity.
[†]Age at study enrolment missing for 1 Cape Coloured subject.
[‡]Civil marriage or living with a partner.
[§]At least some tertiary education.
[a]Smoking status at diagnosis; data missing for 5 subjects. Smoking status at study enrolment; data missing for 7 subjects.
[b]Family history IBD defined as parents, siblings or offspring.

Table 3. Patient Phenotype According to Montreal Classification Scheme.

		Diagnosis					Study enrolment				
		White (n=35)	Cape Coloured (n=152)	Black (n=7)	Overall (N=194)	p-value*	White (n=35)	Cape Coloured (n=152)	Black (n=7)	Overall (N=194)	p-value*
Age at diagnosis and at enrolment, no. (%)[a]	A1	1 (3)	15 (10)	1 (14)	17 (9)	0.43†	0 (0)	0 (0)	0 (0)	0 (0)	0.84
	A2	22 (63)	113 (74)	5 (71)	140 (72)		9 (26)	50 (33)	3 (43)	62 (31)	
	A3	12 (37)	24 (16)	1 (14)	37 (19)		26 (74)	101 (67)	4 (57)	131 (68)	
Disease location, no. (%)[b]	L1	11 (31)	27 (18)	1 (14)	39 (20)	0.65‡	13 (37)	50 (33)	2 (29)	65 (33)	0.87§
	L2	6 (17)	30 (20)	1 (14)	37 (19)		10 (28)	39 (26)	0 (0)	49 (26)	
	L3	18 (52)	93 (61)	5 (72)	116 (61)		12 (34)	62 (41)	5 (71)	79 (41)	
Disease behavior, no. (%)	B1	21 (60)	81 (53)	3 (43)	105 (54)	0.21‡	21 (60)	76 (50)	2 (29)	99 (51)	0.18§
	B2	5 (14)	36 (24)	1 (14)	42 (22)		6 (17)	39 (26)	1 (14)	46 (24)	
	B3	9 (26)	35 (21)	3 (43)	47 (24)		8 (23)	37 (24)	4 (57)	49 (25)	
	p[c]	9 (26)	36 (24)	3 (43)	48 (25)	0.73‡	3 (9)	20 (13)	2 (29)	25 (13)	0.39§

*Statistical analysis excludes black patients.
†Adjusted for gender, smoking and duration of symptom onset.
‡Adjusted for gender, smoking, age of onset and duration of symptom onset.
§Adjusted for gender, smoking, disease duration and age of onset (as appropriate).
[a]Age at study enrolment; data missing for 1 Cape Coloured subject.
[b]Disease location was not confirmed by upper endoscopy, ileocolonoscopy or small bowel imaging for 2 Cape Coloured subject at diagnosis and 1 Cape Coloured subject at study enrolment. Overall, no subjects had upper gastrointestinal disease
[c]"p" is the perianal modifier added to B1-B3 when concomitant perianal disease is present.

Table 4. Patient Medical and Surgical Management and Extraintestinal Manifestations (EIMs).

		White (n=35)	Cape Coloured (n=152)	Black (n=7)	Overall (n=194)	p-value*
Medication use over disease course, no. (%)†	Corticosteroids	6 (17)	32 (21)	1 (14)	39 (20)	0.82
	5-aminosalicylates	10 (29)	60 (40)	0 (0)	70 (36)	0.32
	Immunomodulators	19 (54)	109 (72)	4 (57)	132 (68)	0.48
	Tumor necrosis factor inhibitors	1 (3)	8 (5)	0 (0)	9 (5)	1.00
Lifetime surgical intervention, no. (%)		14 (40)	86 (57)	4 (57)	104 (54)	0.16
Timing of first surgery after diagnosis, no. (%)‡	Within 1 year	6 (17)	44 (29)	2 (29)	52 (27)	0.84
	Within 1–5 years	2 (6)	17 (11)	1 (14)	20 (10)	
	After 5 years	4 (11)	21 (14)	1 (14)	26 (13)	
Type of EIM over disease course, no. (%)	Skin	3 (9)	13 (9)	2 (29)	18 (93)	1.00
	Ocular	0 (0)	2 (1)	1 (14)	3 (2)	1.00
	Joint	10 (29)	46 (30)	3 (43)	59 (30)	0.37
	Other§	1 (3)	2 (1)	0 (0)	3 (2)	0.46

*Statistical analysis excludes black patients.
†Excludes 15 patients with insufficient records of medical management.
‡Excludes 12 patients with incomplete records of surgical dates.
§Other EIM disorders included; ankylosing spondylitis and primary biliary cirrhosis.

when compared to whites (results not shown). There was however no significant inter-racial difference in terms of EIMs, surgical or medical management over disease course (Table 4).

Although the numbers were too small for meaningful analysis all black subjects developed complicated CD within a mean of 1.71 (SD±1.25) years after initial diagnosis. In addition 43% already had a penetrating disease phenotype or perianal fistulas at diagnosis. None of the black subjects reported a first degree family history of IBD, compared to 6% of the Cape Coloured and 14% of the white patients. Overall, less than 10% of patients had a family history of IBD.

Discussion

Population based epidemiological studies remain of paramount importance in piecing together the complex pathogenesis underlying CD, particularly in terms of inter-racial variations of disease phenotype. In South Africa, while a number of earlier reports are available, no such recent data exists for the population; a population broadly classified into three ethnic groups: black south African, white and Cape Coloured.

This study included all consecutive state-sector adult CD patients within the Western Cape, South Africa seen over a seventeen month period. Comparing Cape Coloured subjects with their white counterparts, a significant difference in the development of 'complicated' CD (60% vs. 9%) over time was noted. One possible explanation is the high prevalence of ongoing active smoking in Cape Coloureds at study enrolment. Cigarette smoking is a well described risk factor for the development of complicated and aggressive CD over time [28]. The rate of complicated CD in our white subjects was lower compared to that described in other populations. It is possible that the discrepancy in disease course can be attributed to differences in treatment strategies, patient compliance to medical management, or true microbial differences between populations, but these factors were not investigated. In addition, recent reports indicate that prevalence of systemic lupus erythematosus, particularly among the black and Coloured females in Cape Town, South Africa is higher than previously thought [29,30]. However in this present study, no concomitant

diagnosis of CD and systemic lupus erythematosus was found, suggesting that different factors contribute to the etiology of the two diseases.

In keeping with reports from Asia [31–44], among our Cape Coloured subjects, ileo-colonic appeared to be the most common location at diagnosis. Interestingly in contrast to white patients, Cape Coloured subjects appeared to have a shorter duration of presenting symptoms in years until diagnosis. These findings are at odds with the widely held belief that the disease is frequently overlooked in this population due to the high rates of tuberculosis and infectious diarrhea, or poor access to health care. Notably, the public-sector health care system in South Africa predominantly caters to those who are of lower socioeconomic standing. In this study, findings are likely not attributed to inter-racial differences in access to healthcare or medical treatment as there was no significant inter-racial difference in the level of income. Moreover education is considered to be a good marker of socioeconomic status and in our cohort, there was no significant inter-racial difference in the level of education.

Family history of IBD is considered one of the strongest predisposing risk factors in CD. However in our cohort 6% of the Cape Coloured and none of the black patients reported having a first degree family member with IBD. In contrast 14% of the white subjects had a positive family history, the latter compatible with Western data (10–25%) [43,45,46]. This finding may reflect racial differences in CD susceptibility mutations. A study of South African Coloureds failed to demonstrate an association with 3 nucleotide oligomerization domain (NOD-2) mutations commonly seen in the West [47]. Moreover, significant differences of allele and genotype frequencies in the -237C→T promoter polymorphisms of the *SCL11A1* gene, a gene implicated in CD susceptibility [48], were observed in South African Coloured CD patients, but not in their white and black counterparts [49]. Similar discrepancies have been observed in Japanese [50,51], Han Chinese [52–54], Korean [55], Indian [56] and Malaysian [57] populations [58,59].

A five year retrospective study [60] based on the GSH gastrointestinal clinic patient lists, found an increasing CD incidence in the Coloured population; from 0.4/100 000 per year during 1970–1974 [61] to 1.3/100 000 per year during 1975–1980. Of the 117 CD patients reviewed; 32 were Coloured and only 1 was black. In contrast, we found 152 Cape Coloured and 7 black, consecutive CD state sector patients. Given the significant socioeconomic, dietary and lifestyle changes that have taken place over the past two decades, it is likely that our findings indicate an epidemiological transition among these racial groups, a trend noted in developed and developing countries alike [5,18]. These observed trends in our Cape Coloured and black subjects lend support to both different susceptibility genes and variable environmental interactions between racial groups, implying distinctions in disease pathogenesis or risk.

Our study was limited by the small number of black subjects. It is possible that over a longer period, including patients from both, the state and private sector, a larger sample size would be drawn. Data regarding medication use has been poorly captured in the past, as this was a retrospective study, details on the type medical treatment used, duration of treatment, dosage and adherence was difficult to determine, and may have contributed to the identified inter-racial differences. Similarly, given the retrospective nature of the study, the exact parameters used to exclude tuberculosis diagnosis (i.e., histological, radiological, endoscopic), were not available to report in this paper. Our cohort may have included a higher proportion of patients with 'complicated' disease as GSH and TBH are both referral based IBD centers. Poor socioeconomic status is associated with helminth infection and in South Africa helminth infection has been shown to be protective against IBD development [62]. Therefore it is entirely possible that within our cohort this may have influenced the severity of CD between the racial groups however this was not one of the variables evaluated in the present study. The ethnic diversity of our cohort was also not representative to that of the Western Cape, as 2011 provincial estimates approximate (N = 5,822,734) 15.7% of the population as white, 48.8% as Colored and 32.9% as black (excluding Indian and Asian ethnicities) [63]. We also did not verify the self-reported race using genetic markers. However, validity of self-reported racial status has been previously acknowledged, as very low rates of discordance between self-reported racial status and genetic markers have been described [25,64,65].

Acknowledgments

We thank the Raffners, Dr. Ernesta Kunneke, Karin Fenton, Ushma Galal and Amanda Fourie for their inspiring and administrative assistance of this research

Author Contributions

Conceived and designed the experiments: AB RS GW. Performed the experiments: AB. Analyzed the data: EJ MM AB. Contributed reagents/materials/analysis tools: EJ. Contributed to the writing of the manuscript: AB RS GW EJ MM. Critical Revision manuscript: AB RS GW EJ MM. Data Interpretation: EJ MM.

References

1. Freeman Hj (2009) Long-Term Natural History Of Crohn's Disease. World J Gastroenterol 15: 1315–1318.
2. Silverberg Ms, Satsangi J, Ahmad T, Arnott I, Bernstein Cn, et al. (2005) Toward An Integrated Clinical, Molecular And Serological Classification Of Inflammatory Bowel Disease: Report Of A Working Party Of The 2005 Montreal World Congress Of Gastroenterology. Can J Gastroenterol 19: 5–36.
3. Straus Wl, Eisen Gm, Sandler Rs, Murray Sc, Sessions Jt (2000) Crohn's Disease: Does Race Matter? Am J Gastroenterol 95: 479–483.
4. Karlinger K, Györke T, Makö E, Mester Á, Tarján Z (2000) The Epidemiology And The Pathogenesis Of Inflammatory Bowel Disease. Eur J Radiol 35: 154–167.
5. Loftus Ev, Sandborn Wj (2002) Epidemiology Of Inflammatory Bowel Disease. Gastroenterol Clin North Am 31: 1–20.
6. Rogers B, Clark Lm, Kirsner Jb (1971) The Epidemiologic And Demographic Characteristics Of Inflammatory Bowel Disease: An Analysis Of A Computerized File Of 1400 Patients. J Chronic Dis 24: 743–773.
7. Mendeloff Ai, Monk M, Siegel Ci, Lilienfeld A (1966) Some Epidemiological Features Of Ulcerative Colitis And Regional Enteritis. A Preliminary Report. Gastroenterology 51: 748–756.
8. Samuels Ad, Weese Jl, Berman Pm, Kirsner Jb (1974) An Epidemiologic And Demographic Study Of Inflammatory Bowel Disease In Black Patients. Am J Dig Dis 19: 156–160.
9. Mosley Jr E, Rogers N, Scott V, Chung E, Press Jr Hc, et al. (1977) Crohn's Disease In Black Patients. J Natl Med Assoc 69: 219–222.
10. Mekhjian H, Switz D, Melnyk C, Rankin G, Brooks R (1979) Clinical Features And Natural History Of Crohn's Disease. Gastroenterology 77: 898–906.
11. Simsek H, Schuman Bm (1989) Inflammatory Bowel Disease In 64 Black Patients: Analysis Of Course, Complications, And Surgery. J Clin Gastroenterol 11: 294–298.
12. Loftus Ev (2004) Clinical Epidemiology Of Inflammatory Bowel Disease: Incidence, Prevalence, And Environmental Influences. Gastroenterology 126: 1504–1517.
13. Loftus Ev, Silverstein Md, Sandborn Wj, Tremaine Wj, Harmsen Ws, et al. (1998) Crohn's Disease In Olmsted County, Minnesota, 1940–1993: Incidence, Prevalence, And Survival. Gastroenterology 114: 1161–1168.
14. Vind I, Riis L, Jess T, Knudsen E, Pedersen N, et al. (2006) Increasing Incidences Of Inflammatory Bowel Disease And Decreasing Surgery Rates In Copenhagen City And County, 2003–2005: A Population-Based Study From The Danish Crohn Colitis Database. Am J Gastroenterol 101: 1274–1282.
15. Thia Ktj, Luman W, Jin Oc (2006) Crohn's Disease Runs A More Aggressive Course In Young Asian Patients. Inflamm Bowel Dis 12: 57–61.
16. Goldman Cd, Kodner Ij, Fry Rd, Macdermott Rp (1986) Clinical And Operative Experience With Non-Caucasian Patients With Crohn's Disease. Dis Colon Rectum 29: 317–321.
17. Paul Jr H, Barnes R, Reese Ve, Childress Mh, Scott V, et al. (1990) Crohn's Disease In Black Patients. J Natl Med Assoc 82: 709–712.
18. Molodecky Na, Soon Is, Rabi Dm, Ghali Wa, Ferris M, et al. (2012) Increasing Incidence And Prevalence Of The Inflammatory Bowel Diseases With Time, Based On Systematic Review. Gastroenterology 142: 46–54. E42.
19. Calkins Bm (1984) Trends In Incidence Rates Of Ulcerative Colitis And Crohn's Disease. Dig Dis Sci 29: 913–920.
20. Kurata Jh, Kantor-Fish S, Frankl H, Godby P, Vadheim Cm (1992) Crohn's Disease Among Ethnic Groups In A Large Health Maintenance Organization. Gastroenterology 102: 1940–1948.
21. Hou Jk, El-Serag H, Thirumurthi S (2009) Distribution And Manifestations Of Inflammatory Bowel Disease In Asians, Hispanics, And African Americans: A Systematic Review. Am J Gastroenterol 104: 2100–2109.
22. Thia Kt, Loftus Ev, Sandborn Wj, Yang S (2008) An Update On The Epidemiology Of Inflammatory Bowel Disease In Asia. Am J Gastroenterol 103: 3167–3182.
23. Basu D, Lopez I, Kulkarni A, Sellin Jh (2005) Impact Of Race And Ethnicity On Inflammatory Bowel Disease. Am J Gastroenterol 100: 2254–2261.
24. Small K (2008) Demographic And Socio-Economic Trends For Cape Town: 1996 To 2007. Unpublished Report, City Of Cape Town.
25. Patterson N, Petersen Dc, Van Der Ross Re, Sudoyo H, Glashoff Rh, et al. (2010) Genetic Structure Of A Unique Admixed Population: Implications For Medical Research. Hum Mol Genet 19: 411–419.
26. Stange E, Travis S, Vermeire S, Beglinger C, Kupcinkas L, et al. (2006) European Evidence Based Consensus On The Diagnosis And Management Of Crohn's Disease: Definitions And Diagnosis. Gut 55: I1–I15.
27. Epstein D, Watermeyer G, Kirsch R (2007) Review Article: The Diagnosis And Management Of Crohn's Disease In Populations With High-Risk Rates For Tuberculosis. Aliment Pharmacol Ther 25: 1373–1388.
28. Aldhous Mc, Satsangi J (2010) The Impact Of Smoking In Crohn's Disease: No Smoke Without Fire. Frontline Gastroenterol 1: 156–164.
29. Ayodele Oe, Okpechi Ig, Swanepoel Cr (2010) Predictors Of Poor Renal Outcome In Patients With Biopsy-Proven Lupus Nephritis. Nephrology 15: 482–490.
30. Wadee S, Tikly M, Hopley M (2007) Causes And Predictors Of Death In South Africans With Systemic Lupus Erythematosus. Rheumatology (Oxford) 46: 1487–1491.
31. Shin Dh, Sinn Dh, Kim Y, Kim Jy, Chang Dk, et al. (2011) Increasing Incidence Of Inflammatory Bowel Disease Among Young Men In Korea Between 2003 And 2008. Dig Dis Sci 56: 1154–1159.
32. Ishige T, Tomomasa T, Takebayashi T, Asakura K, Watanabe M, et al. (2010) Inflammatory Bowel Disease In Children: Epidemiological Analysis Of The Nationwide Ibd Registry In Japan. J Gastroenterol 45: 911–917.

33. Jiang L, Xia B, Li J, Ye M, Yan W, et al. (2006) Retrospective Survey Of 452 Patients With Inflammatory Bowel Disease In Wuhan City, Central China. Inflamm Bowel Dis 12: 212–217.
34. Song X, Gao X, Li M, Chen Z, Chen S, et al. (2011) Clinical Features And Risk Factors For Primary Surgery In 205 Patients With Crohn's Disease: Analysis Of A South China Cohort. Dis Colon Rectum 54: 1147–1154.
35. Cao Q, Si J, Gao M, Zhou G, Hu W, et al. (2005) Clinical Presentation Of Inflammatory Bowel Disease: A Hospital Based Retrospective Study Of 379 Patients In Eastern China. Chin Med J 118: 747–752.
36. Chow Dk, Leong Rw, Lai Lh, Wong Gl, Leung W, et al. (2008) Changes In Crohn's Disease Phenotype Over Time In The Chinese Population: Validation Of The Montreal Classification System. Inflamm Bowel Dis 14: 536–541.
37. Oriuchi T, Hiwatashi N, Kinouchi Y, Takahashi S, Takagi S, et al. (2003) Clinical Course And Longterm Prognosis Of Japanese Patients With Crohn's Disease: Predictive Factors, Rates Of Operation, And Mortality. J Gastroenterol 38: 942–953.
38. Ye Bd, Yang S, Cho Yk, Park Sh, Yang D, et al. (2010) Clinical Features And Long-Term Prognosis Of Crohn's Disease In Korea. Scand J Gastroenterol 45: 1178–1185.
39. Lawrance Ic, Murray K, Hall A, Sung Jj, Leong R (2004) A Prospective Comparative Study Of Asca And Panca In Chinese And Caucasian Ibd Patients. Am J Gastroenterol 99: 2186–2194.
40. Hisabe T, Matsui T, Sakurai T, Murakami Y, Tanabe H, et al. (2003) Anti-Saccharomyces Cerevisiae Antibodies In Japanese Patients With Inflammatory Bowel Disease: Diagnostic Accuracy And Clinical Value. J Gastroenterol 38: 121–126.
41. Leong Rw, Lawrance Ic, Chow Dk, To K, Lau Jy, et al. (2006) Association Of Intestinal Granulomas With Smoking, Phenotype, And Serology In Chinese Patients With Crohn's Disease. Am J Gastroenterol 101: 1024–1029.
42. Chow Dk, Sung Jj, Wu Jc, Tsoi Kk, Leong Rw, et al. (2009) Upper Gastrointestinal Tract Phenotype Of Crohn's Disease Is Associated With Early Surgery And Further Hospitalization. Inflamm Bowel Dis 15: 551–557.
43. Orholm M, Munkholm P, Langholz E, Nielsen Oh, Sørensen Ti, et al. (1991) Familial Occurrence Of Inflammatory Bowel Disease. N Engl J Med 324: 84–88.
44. Yang S, Yun S, Kim J, Park Jy, Kim Hy, et al. (2008) Epidemiology Of Inflammatory Bowel Disease In The Songpa-Kangdong District, Seoul, Korea, 1986–2005: A Kasid Study. Inflamm Bowel Dis 14: 542–549.
45. Peeters M, Nevens H, Baert F, Hiele M, De Meyer Am, et al. (1996) Familial Aggregation In Crohn's Disease: Increased Age-Adjusted Risk And Concordance In Clinical Characteristics. Gastroenterology 111: 597–603.
46. Bayless T, Tokayer A, Polito J, Quaskey S, Mellits E, et al. (1996) Crohn's Disease: Concordance For Site And Clinical Type In Affected Family Members-Potential Hereditary Influences. Gastroenterology 111: 573–579.
47. Zaahl Mg, Winter Ta, Warnich L, Kotze Mj (2005) Analysis Of The Three Common Mutations In The Card15 Gene (R702w, G908r And 1007fs) In South African Colored Patients With Inflammatory Bowel Disease. Mol Cell Probes 19: 278–281.
48. Hofmeister A, Neibergs Hl, Pokorny Rm, Galandiuk S (1997) The Natural Resistance-Associated Macrophage Protein Gene Is Associated With Crohn's Disease. Surgery 122: 173–179.
49. Zaahl Mg, Winter Ta, Warnich L, Kotze Mj (2006) The -237c—>T Promoter Polymorphism Of The Slc11a1 Gene Is Associated With A Protective Effect In Relation To Inflammatory Bowel Disease In The South African Population. Int J Colorectal Dis 21: 402–408.
50. Inoue N, Tamura K, Kinouchi Y, Fukuda Y, Takahashi S, et al. (2002) Lack Of Common Nod2 Variants In Japanese Patients With Crohn's Disease. Gastroenterology 123: 86–91.
51. Yamazaki K, Takazoe M, Tanaka T, Kazumori T, Nakamura Y (2002) Absence Of Mutation In The Nod2/Card15 Gene Among 483 Japanese Patients With Crohn's Disease. J Hum Genet 47: 469–472.
52. Guo Q, Xia B, Jiang Y, Qu Y, Li J (2004) Nod2 3020insc Frameshift Mutation Is Not Associated With Inflammatory Bowel Disease In Chinese Patients Of Han Nationality. World J Gastroenterol 10: 1069–1071.
53. Leong R, Armuzzi A, Ahmad T, Wong M, Tse P, et al. (2003) Nod2/Card15 Gene Polymorphisms And Crohn's Disease In The Chinese Population. Aliment Pharmacol Ther 17: 1465–1470.
54. Li M, Gao X, Guo C, Wu K, Zhang X, et al. (2008) Octn And Card15 Gene Polymorphism In Chinese Patients With Inflammatory Bowel Disease. World J Gastroenterol 14: 4923–4927.
55. Croucher Pj, Mascheretti S, Hampe J, Huse K, Frenzel H, et al. (2003) Haplotype Structure And Association To Crohn's Disease Of Card15 Mutations In Two Ethnically Divergent Populations. Eur J Hum Genet 11: 6–16.
56. Pugazhendhi S, Amte A, Balamurugan R, Subramanian V, Ramakrishna Bs (2008) Common Nod2 Mutations Are Absent In Patients With Crohn's Disease In India. Indian J Gastroenterol 27: 201–203.
57. Chua Kh, Hilmi I, Ng Cc, Eng Tl, Palaniappan S, et al. (2009) Identification Of Nod2/Card15 Mutations In Malaysian Patients With Crohn's Disease. J Dig Dis 10: 124–130.
58. Yamazaki K, Mcgovern D, Ragoussis J, Paolucci M, Butler H, et al. (2005) Single Nucleotide Polymorphisms In Tnfsf15 Confer Susceptibility To Crohn's Disease. Hum Mol Genet 14: 3499–3506.
59. Yang S, Lim J, Chang H, Lee I, Li Y, et al. (2008) Association Of Tnfsf15 With Crohn's Disease In Koreans. Am J Gastroenterol 103: 1437–1442.
60. Wright Jp, Marks In, Jameson C, Garisch Ja, Burns Dg, et al. (1983) Inflammatory Bowel Disease In Cape Town, 1975–1980. Part Ii. Crohn's Disease. S Afr Med J 63: 226–229.
61. Novis Bh, Marks In, Bank S, Louw Jh (1975) Incidence Of Crohn's Disease At Groote Schuur Hospital During 1970–1974. S Afr Med J 49: 693–697.
62. Chu Km, Watermeyer G, Shelly L, Janssen J, May Td, et al. (2013) Childhood Helminth Exposure Is Protective Against Inflammatory Bowel Disease: A Case Control Study In South Africa. Inflamm Bowel Dis 19: 614–620.
63. Statistics South Africa (October 30, 2012) Census 2011: Statistical Release (Revised) P0301.4. 2013.
64. Risch N (2006) Dissecting Racial And Ethnic Differences. N Engl J Med 354: 408–411.
65. Tang H, Quertermous T, Rodriguez B, Kardia Sl, Zhu X, et al. (2005) Genetic Structure, Self-Identified Race/Ethnicity, And Confounding In Case-Control Association Studies. Am J Hum Genet 76: 268–275.

24

Depressive Symptoms in Crohn's Disease: Relationship with Immune Activation and Tryptophan Availability

Sinan Guloksuz[1]*, Marieke Wichers[1], Gunter Kenis[1], Maurice G.V.M. Russel[2], Annick Wauters[3], Robert Verkerk[4], Baer Arts[1], Jim van Os[1,5]

1 Department of Psychiatry and Psychology, Maastricht University Medical Centre, EURON, Maastricht, The Netherlands, **2** Department of Gastroenterology and Hepatology, Medisch Spectrum Twente, Enschede, The Netherlands, **3** Laboratory of Clinical Biology, ZNA Middelheim, Antwerp, Belgium, **4** Laboratory of Medical Biochemistry, University of Antwerp, Wilrijk, Belgium, **5** King's College London, King's Health Partners, Department of Psychosis Studies, Institute of Psychiatry, London, United Kingdom

Abstract

Crohn's disease (CD) is associated with immune activation and depressive symptoms. This study determines the impact of anti-tumor necrosis factor (TNF)-α treatment in CD patients on depressive symptoms and the degree to which tryptophan (TRP) availability and immune markers mediate this effect. Fifteen patients with CD, eligible for anti-TNF-α treatment were recruited. Disease activity (Harvey-Bradshaw Index (HBI), Crohn's Disease Activity Index (CDAI)), fatigue (Multidimensional Fatigue Inventory (MFI)), quality of life (Inflammatory Bowel Disease Questionnaire (IBDQ)), symptoms of depression and anxiety (Symptom Checklist (SCL-90), Beck Depression Inventory (BDI), Hamilton Depression Rating Scale (HDRS)), immune activation (acute phase proteins (APP)), zinc and TRP availability were assessed before treatment and after 2, 4 and 8 weeks. Anti-TNF-α increased IBDQ scores and reduced all depression scores; however only SCL-90 depression scores remained decreased after correction for HBI. Positive APPs decreased, while negative APPs increased after treatment. After correction for HBI, both level and percentage of γ fraction were associated with SCL-90 depression scores over time. After correction for HBI, patients with current/past depressive disorder displayed higher levels of positive APPs and lower levels of negative APPs and zinc. TRP availability remained invariant over time and there was no association between SCL-90 depression scores and TRP availability. Inflammatory reactions in CD are more evident in patients with comorbid depression, regardless of disease activity. Anti-TNF-α treatment in CD reduces depressive symptoms, in part independently of disease activity; there was no evidence that this effect was mediated by immune-induced changes in TRP availability.

Editor: Marianna Mazza, Catholic University of Sacred Heart of Rome, Italy

Funding: Sinan Guloksuz and Jim van Os are supported by the European Community's Seventh Framework Programme under Grant agreement no. HEALTH-F2-2009-241909 (Project EU-GEI). The funders had no role in study design, data collection and analysis, decision to publish, or preparation of the manuscript.

* E-mail: sguloksuz@yahoo.com

Introduction

Crohn's disease (CD) has been associated with an increased prevalence of psychopathology. In addition, it is proposed that CD is more likely to occur in subjects with predisposing personality traits, such as high level of neuroticism and introversion [1]. Previous studies show mixed results concerning the temporal relationship between the onset of gastrointestinal complaints and symptoms of mental disorder [2,3,4,5,6,7,8]. However, once present, bouts of disease activity and symptoms of anxiety and depression tend to co-occur. Elevated levels of inflammatory mediators have been implicated in the pathophysiology of CD. The immune response in CD patients typically has been considered majorly as Th1-type, assessed by elevated expression of interleukin (IL)-12, tumor necrosis factor (TNF)-α and interferon (IFN)-γ, which are pro-inflammatory cytokines that increase macrophage and natural killer cell activation, antigen presenting cell function, and lead to the production of other pro-inflammatory mediators [9,10,11]. In addition, the role of Th-17-mediated response in pathophysiology of CD has recently been implicated [11].

Considering that the presence of depression predicts lower remission rates and decreases the time to retreatment of CD [12], it is plausible to hypothesize that there is an interaction between depression and CD. A growing body of evidence also supports the notion that immune-modulation plays a role in pathogenesis of depression [13,14,15]. Administration of the pro-inflammatory cytokine IFN-α in humans triggers the development of depressive symptoms in up to 45% of participants [16]. Furthermore, increased production of IL-6, IL-1β, IFN-γ and TNF-α, as well as signs of an acute phase response, i.e. increased production of positive acute phase proteins (APPs) and decreased production of negative APPs, are associated with depression [13,14,17,18,19,20,21]. The observation of higher levels of positive APPs accompanied by low levels of negative APPs supports the notion that depression is inflammatory-related. Likewise, zinc, which plays a role in inflammatory mechanisms as a key antioxidant, has been reported at reduced levels in patients with depression [21,22]. In addition, increased levels of complement factors C3c and C4, as well as immunoglobulin M (IgM) and IgG are also observed in this disorder [23]. Immune activation may impact on mood, by decreasing the availability of peripheral tryptophan (TRP) that may cross the blood-brain-barrier [13,14,15]. TRP is the precursor of serotonin (5-HT), a neurotransmitter synthesized in the brain and important in the regulation of mood. Earlier studies show that indicators of the availability of TRP to brain, serum/plasma TRP, as well as the ratio of TRP to the sum of competing amino acids (CAA)—known to compete for the cerebral uptake mechanism of TRP —, are lower in depression [21,24,25,26,27,28].

The causal mechanism underlying the relationship between CD and mental disorder is unclear. Symptoms of depression and anxiety may represent the psychological response to disease activity. On the other hand, it may be hypothesized that activation of the inflammatory immune response causes both CD and symptoms of mental disorder, which could explain (i) the uncertain temporal relationship between onset of CD and symptoms of mental disorder, (ii) the close relationship between disease state and psychopathology, and (iii) personality differences between CD patients and controls. There is some evidence that depressive symptoms may be reduced in CD patients after infusion of anti-TNF-α, an efficient treatment for gastrointestinal symptoms in CD [12,29].

Therefore, the aim of the current study was to determine the impact of anti-TNF-α treatment in CD patients on depressive symptoms, and to examine the possibility that improvement of depressive symptoms occurs in parallel with changes in TRP availability imposed by a reduction in inflammation as reflected by levels of APPs.

Methods

Subjects

15 patients (4 men and 11 women) with CD, eligible for anti-TNF-α, infliximab (Remicade®) infusion were recruited. Inclusion criteria were: having a Harvey-Bradshaw Index (HBI) score>10 or active perianal fistula, being allergic or not responding to the following treatments: azathioprine, methotrexate and/or corticosteroids. Exclusion criteria were: age <18 and >65 years, pregnancy or intention to get pregnant within the period of treatment and up to 6 months after discontinuation of therapy, women not practicing or not willing to practice safe methods of contraception during the treatment period up to 6 months after discontinuation of therapy, lactation, human immunodeficiency virus positivity, chemotherapy or systemic antiviral treatment during the 6 months prior to study entry, presence of other serious disease (e.g. malignancy, uncontrolled myocardial disease or severe arrhythmias), tuberculosis positivity (current or past), creatinine levels over 150 mmol/L or 1.70 mg/dl, any condition which in the opinion of the (co-) investigator might interfere with the evaluation of the study objectives, patients meeting axis I criteria for mental disorders as defined by DSM-IV, except for patients meeting the criteria for a depressive or anxiety disorder.

The study was approved by the standing Medical Ethics Committee of Maastricht University, and carried out in accordance with the Declaration of Helsinki (Hong Kong Modification, 1989). Written informed consent was obtained from each subject prior to participation.

Study design

A within-subject design was used to determine (i) the effect of anti-TNF-α infusion on disease activity and markers of immune activation, (ii) effect of anti-TNF-α infusion on mood, fatigue and quality of life, (iii) effect of altered immune activation on TRP levels, and (iv) effect of TRP levels on depressive symptoms.

Patients received an infusion of anti-TNF-α, infliximab (Remicade®) (5 mg/kg bodyweight). Psychological assessments and measurements of immune activation were performed before infusion (baseline) and 2, 4 and 8 weeks after infusion. Fasting blood samples were collected between 8.00 and 10.00 AM. Blood samples were centrifuged at 1300x g for 10 minutes. Serum was then stored at $-80°C$ until assayed.

Disease activity and psychological assessments

Disease activity was assessed using the HBI [30] and the Crohn's Disease Activity Index (CDAI) [31]. The latter was assessed only at baseline, 4 and 8 weeks after infusion. Fatigue was assessed by the Multidimensional Fatigue Inventory (MFI), which is a self-report instrument consisting of five scales measuring general fatigue, physical fatigue, reduced activity, reduced motivation and mental fatigue [32]. In order to limit the number of tests applied, only core fatigue dimensions of physical and mental fatigue were included in the analyses in order to avoid overlap with depression dimensions of reduced activity and motivation. Quality of Life was measured using the Inflammatory Bowel Disease Questionnaire (IBDQ) [33]

The presence of depressive symptoms was assessed by the 17-item Hamilton Depression Rating Scale (HDRS) [34]. In addition, symptoms of depression and anxiety were assessed by self-report using the Beck Depression Inventory (BDI) [35,36] and the Symptom Checklist (SCL-90) [37]. To determine the presence of axis I mental disorder, the Structured Clinical Interview for DSM-IV axis I Disorders Version 5.0 was administered.

Determination of markers of immune activation and TRP/CAA

Immune activation was determined by using positive APPs (α_1–antitrypsin, α_1–acid glycoprotein and α_1–antichymotrypsin, haptoglobin, ceruloplasmin, fibrinogen, complement factor C3), negative APPs (albumin, transferrin) and zinc as markers of inflammation described in more detail below. Five major fractions of serum proteins were determined using the capillary zone electrophoresis technique; albumin (negative APP), α_1, α_2, β and γ globulin fractions. α_1–antitrypsin, α_1–acid glycoprotein and α_1–antichymotrypsin, all positive APPs, migrate in the α_1 zone, while haptoglobin and ceruloplasmin, also positive APPs, migrate in the α_2 zone. Fibrinogen, complement factor C3 and transferrin migrate in the β zone and immunoglobulins in the γ zone. Total serum protein determination and electrophoresis for measurement of albumin and the α, β and γ fractions were performed as described previously [38]. Transferrin concentration was analysed using immunoturbidimetry. Serum zinc levels were determined using atomic absorption spectroscopy [22]. Total TRP and CAA were assayed using high-performance liquid chromatography as explained previously [39].

Statistical analyses

Normality of distribution was ascertained by Kolmogorov-Smirnov test. Levene statistics were used to check the assumption of homogeneity of variances. Distributions of transferrin and percentages of the $\alpha1$ and $\alpha2$ fractions were log-transformed to improve normality. The data were analyzed with the Stata computer program, version 12 (Stata Corporation, College Station, TX, USA). Multilevel random regression models were fitted testing main effects and interactions, using the XTREG routine in Stata. The XTREG procedure takes into account the fact that level-one units (repeated observation level) were hierarchically clustered into level-two units (subject level). Effect sizes of explanatory variables were expressed as regression coefficients (B) from the multilevel models. Regression analyses were performed to examine the effects of time (linear and factored) on the CDAI, mental and physical fatigue, dimensions of the IBDQ, HDRS and on the anxiety and depression scales of the SCL-90 questionnaire. Effects of time on immune parameters were similarly estimated. In addition, regression analyses were used to determine associations, over time, between immune parameters and TRP/CAA ratio and between TRP/CAA ratio and measures of depression. Analyses were corrected *a priori* for age, smoking, sex, use of oral contraceptives, medication use during the study (mesalamine, corticosteroids, azathioprine and/or methotrexate), presence of past/current depression or anxiety disorder (0 = not present, 1 = present). In addition, the effect over time of past or current depression or anxiety disorder on immune parameters and TRP/CAA ratio was also investigated. Two-sided statistical significance was set at $p < 0.05$. Each hypothesis was corrected using the Simes' modification of the Bonferroni procedure for multiple testing [40]. Hereafter, the notation for corrected p-values is: p_{Simes}.

Results

Subject characteristics and missing data

The sample consisted of 15 patients, 4 men and 11 women. The mean age was 32.7 (SD = 11.4) years. Six were cigarette smokers. Seven of 11 women used oral contraceptives. All patients, except one, received concomitant medication. Ten patients were on mesalamine medication, nine used corticosteroids, seven received azathioprine and two received methotrexate medication. Six of 15 patients received the anti-TNF-α infusion for the first time. Two patients fulfilled criteria for lifetime depressive disorder and two for current depressive disorder with melancholic features. Table 1 shows disease activity and assessment of behavioral and psychopathological parameters at each time point. Immune parameters and TRP/CAA at each time point are presented in Table 2. All patients completed the study. With respect to the administered questionnaires, one observation was missing. Six observations were missing in the measurements of immune parameters (10%).

Table 2. Immune parameters and TRP/CAA at each time point.

	Baseline	Week 2	Week 4	Week 8
Albumin (mg/dl)	36.06 (6.66)	38.95 (5.54)	39.82 (8.07)	37.53 (7.55)
Albumin %	52.52 (6.91)	55.90 (5.02)	55.61 (5.71)	55.16 (4.93)
α_1 (mg/dl)	5.72 (0.94)	5.37 (0.99)	5.45 (1.20)	5.16 (1.21)
α_1%	8.53 (1.86)	7.86 (1.82)	7.85 (2.07)	7.71 (1.68)
α_2 (mg/dl)	8.86 (1.07)	7.71 (1.08)	8.15 (1.40)	8.04 (1.39)
α_2%	12.82 (1.55)	11.14 (1.38)	11.48 (1.55)	12.01 (1.58)
β (mg/dl)	7.23 (0.97)	7.23 (1.16)	7.33 (1.29)	6.90 (1.37)
β%	10.73 (1.80)	10.50 (1.90)	10.16 (1.87)	10.29 (1.74)
γ (mg/dl)	10.28 (3.15)	10.30 (2.96)	10.67 (2.99)	10.13 (2.93)
γ%	14.97 (3.88)	14.63 (3.45)	14.81 (3.16)	14.82 (3.40)
Total protein (mg/dl)	68.25 (6.93)	69.68 (7.30)	71.03 (11.91)	67.90 (11.17)
Transferrin (mg/dl)	256.79 (56.63)	271.28 (42.34)	281.29 (49.33)	257.75 (55.58)
TRP/CAA	0.11 (0.02)	0.11 (0.02)	0.12 (0.01)	0.11 (0.02)
Zinc (μg/dl)	95.30 (16.24)	91.96 (16.31)	96.36 (14.14)	89.06 (23.61)

The results were presented as mean (*sd*).
TRP/CAA: tryptophan/competing aminoacids.

Because data were missing randomly, we used the Expectation Maximization (EM) method to impute missing data.

CDAI and HBI scores significantly decreased compared to baseline after anti-TNF-α infusion at all time points (Table 3), and the association between these two measures over time was highly significant (B = 18.45, $p < 0.001$). Because of this high correlation, HBI scores were used in further analyses (Figure 1), as this was available at all four time points (CDAI being available only at three time points).

Table 1. Total scores of disease activity and psychopathological and behavioural assessments at each time point.

	Baseline	Week 2	Week 4	Week 8
HBI	8.78 (2.91)	3.33 (2.26)	3.73 (2.81)	6.03 (5.68)
CDAI	230.83 (94.75)	NA	102.02 (66.24)	144.84 (105.71)
MFI Physical Fatigue	13.87 (3.64)	11.53 (4.81)	12.20 (5.35)	11.86 (5.36)
MFI Mental Fatigue	9.40 (5.62)	7.20 (3.10)	8.27 (3.94)	9.04 (5.29)
IBDQ Bowel Symptoms	41.87 (6.00)	58.13 (6.28)	58.80 (6.10)	53.18 (12.05)
IBDQ Systemic Symptoms	19.13 (5.36)	26.67 (5.11)	26.73 (3.97)	25.44 (6.63)
IBDQ Emotional Status	61.53 (13.26)	71.27 (6.84)	73.27 (6.94)	70.09 (14.97)
IBDQ Social Functioning	24.33 (6.50)	29.93 (3.65)	30.80 (3.51)	28.78 (7.06)
HDRS	9.47 (5.58)	5.87 (5.85)	5.27 (4.15)	6.94 (7.55)
BDI	8.07 (6.86)	5.00 (5.79)	5.53 (6.31)	3.99 (3.18)
SCL-90 Depression	1.91 (0.71)	1.68 (0.64)	1.55 (0.32)	1.41 (0.32)
SCL-90 Anxiety	0.95 (0.30)	0.89 (0.20)	0.80 (0.09)	0.83 (0.10)

The results were presented as mean (*sd*).
HBI: Harvey-Bradshaw Index, CDAI: Crohn's Disease Activity Index, MFI: Multidimensional Fatigue Inventory, IBDQ: Inflammatory Bowel Disease Questionnaire, HDRS: Hamilton Depression Rating Scale, BDI: Beck Depression Inventory, SCL-90: Symptom Checklist.

Table 3. Effects of anti-TNF-α infusion on disease activity, fatigue, quality of life and mood compared to baseline reference value.

	Week 2		Week 4		Week 8		Time (linear trend)	
	B	p_{Simes}	B	p_{Simes}	B	p_{Simes}	B	P
HBI	−5.57	<0.001	−5.17	<0.001	−2.87	0.006	−0.77	NS
CDAI	NA	NA	−128.8	<0.001	−85.99	<0.001	−33.77	<0.001
MFI physical	−2.33	0.027	−1.67	NS	−2.01	NS	−0.53	NS
MFI mental	−2.20	0.012	−1.13	NS	−0.36	NS	−0.00	NS
IBDQ bowel	16.26	<0.001	16.93	<0.001	11.31	<0.001	3.46	<0.001
IBDQ systemic	7.53	<0.001	7.60	<0.001	6.31	<0.001	1.90	<0.001
IBDQ emotional	9.73	0.001	11.73	<0.001	8.55	0.003	2.77	0.008
IBDQ social	5.60	<0.001	6.47	<0.001	4.45	0.002	1.42	0.008
HDRS	−3.60	0.005	−4.20	0.001	−2.53	NS	−0.82	NS
BDI	−3.07	0.002	−2.53	0.009	−2.81	0.005	−0.81	0.016
SCL-90 Depression	−3.00	0.019	−4.67	<0.001	−5.08	<0.001	−1.71	<0.001
SCL-90 Anxiety	−0.80	NS	−1.40	0.004	−0.93	NS	−0.34	0.032

HBI: Harvey-Bradshaw Index, CDAI: Crohn's Disease Activity Index, MFI: Multidimensional Fatigue Inventory, IBDQ: Inflammatory Bowel Disease Questionnaire, HDRS: Hamilton Depression Rating Scale, BDI: Beck Depression Inventory, SCL-90: Symptom Checklist.

Effects of anti-TNF-α on fatigue, quality of life and mood

Administration of anti-TNF-α significantly increased scores on all dimensions of quality of life and reduced depression scores measured by the HDRS, BDI and SCL-90 (Table 3). Anxiety, measured by the SCL-90, was significantly decreased only at one time point, namely 4 weeks after infusion. Physical and mental fatigue was decreased only at 2 weeks after infusion. Because of the impact that disease activity may have on mood, analyses were performed again corrected for HBI score (Table 4). IBDQ scores with respect to bowel symptoms, systemic symptoms and social functioning remained significantly increased with respect to baseline. In addition, depressive symptom score measured by SCL-90 remained significantly decreased at 4 and 8 weeks after infusion, and also showed a significant reduction linear trend over time. Reductions in fatigue scores, BDI scores, HDRS scores and

SCL-90 anxiety scores no longer were significant after correction for disease activity.

Effects of anti-TNF-α on immune parameters and TRP/CAA

Table 5 shows the changes in immune parameter and TRP/CAA ratio compared to baseline after anti-TNF-α infusion. Serum transferrin, albumin and the percentage of the albumin fraction were significantly increased after infusion, whereas α₁ and α₂ fractions and the percentages of α₁, α₂ and β fractions were significantly decreased. There was no variation in TRP/CAA ratio compared to baseline after anti-TNF-α infusion. A higher HBI score was associated significantly with a lower TRP/CAA ratio (B = − 0.0009, p = 0.031) over time. There were no significant associations between changes in immune parameters over time and the TRP/CAA ratio (results not shown).

Effects of changes in TRP/CAA ratio and immune parameters over time on depressive symptoms

As the SCL-90 depression score was most sensitive to mood changes after infusion of anti-TNF-α (Figure 2), the association between mood changes and immune parameters was examined in more detail. Table 6 shows the association over time between SCL-90 depression scores on the one hand and immune parameters as well as TRP/CAA on the other, before and after correction for HBI scores. Overall percentage of γ was associated with SCL-90 depression scores over time (B = 1.15, p_{Simes} = 0.001). After correction for disease activity, both level of γ fraction and percentage of γ were associated with SCL-90 depression scores over time (B = 0.90, p_{Simes} = 0.005 and B = 1.18, p_{Simes} = 0.001).

Effects of current/past depressive disorder on TRP/CAA ratio and immune parameters over time

After correction for disease activity, overall levels of zinc (B = −24.28, p_{Simes}<0.001) albumin fraction (B = −7.02, p_{Simes}<0.001) and the percentage of the albumin fraction (B = −7.56, p_{Simes}<0.001) were significantly lower and levels of α₂ (B = 1.15, p_{Simes}<0.001), β (B = 0.64, p_{Simes} = 0.005) and γ

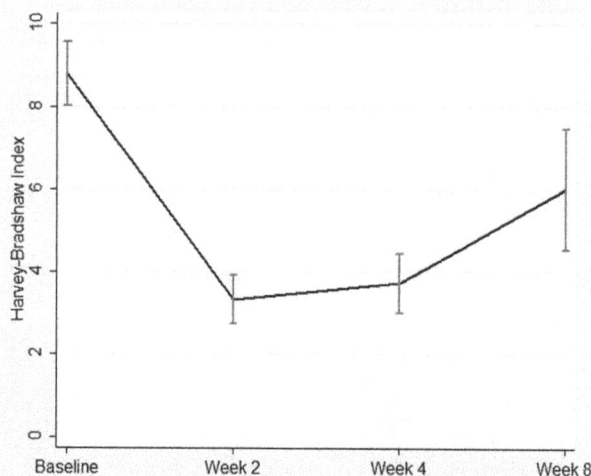

Figure 1. Overtime course of Harvey Bradshaw Index. The line represents the mean score and the error bars represent the standard error at each time point.

Table 4. Effects of anti-TNF-α on fatigue, quality of life and mood compared to baseline scores, corrected for disease activity.

	Week 2		Week 4		Week 8		Time (linear trend)	
	B	P$_{Simes}$	B	P$_{Simes}$	B	P$_{Simes}$	B	P
MFI physical	0.72	NS	1.17	NS	−0.41	NS	−0.17	NS
MFI mental	0.81	NS	1.68	NS	1.35	NS	0.45	NS
IBDQ bowel	9.12	<0.001	10.28	<0.001	7.44	<0.001	1.85	0.006
IBDQ systemic	3.49	0.012	3.84	0.004	4.17	<0.001	1.14	0.003
IBDQ emotional	3.25	NS	5.71	NS	5.19	NS	1.66	NS
IBDQ social	3.07	NS	4.16	0.007	3.40	0.014	0.98	0.024
HDRS	0.25	NS	−0.61	NS	−0.42	NS	−0.22	NS
BDI	−1.58	NS	−1.16	NS	−2.07	NS	−0.53	NS
SCL-90 Depression	−1.97	NS	−3.72	0.016	−4.58	0.001	−1.51	<0.001
SCL-90 Anxiety	−0.10	NS	−0.73	NS	−0.51	NS	−0.21	NS

MFI: Multidimensional Fatigue Inventory, IBDQ: Inflammatory Bowel Disease Questionnaire, HDRS: Hamilton Depression Rating Scale, BDI: Beck Depression Inventory, SCL-90: Symptom Checklist.

(B = 2.02, p$_{Simes}$ = 0.028) fractions and those of the percentages of α$_2$ (B = 0.18, p$_{Simes}$<0.001), β (B = 1.23, p$_{Simes}$ = 0.002) and γ (B = 3.39, p$_{Simes}$<0.001) fractions were significantly higher in subjects with a current/past depressive disorder. Current/past depressive disorder had no influence on overall TRP/CAA ratio.

Discussion

To the best of our knowledge, this is the first prospective study investigating the impact of anti-TNF-α (infliximab) infusion on disease activity, quality of life, fatigue and depressive symptoms along with its possible relation to immune parameters and the TRP/CAA ratio in CD patients. The principal findings of this study were as follows: (i) scores of depression scales were decreased after anti-TNF-α infusion and this effect was to a degree, but not entirely, reducible to disease activity; (ii) there was no change in

the TRP/CAA ratio after anti-TNF-α infusion and neither scores of depression scales, nor immune parameters were associated with TRP/CAA ratio; (iii) immune activation was higher in patients with current/past depressive disorder.

The association between the immune system and depression comes from several lines of evidence, including the induction of sickness behavior (which resembles core features of major depression in patients such as sleep disturbances, anergia and anhedonia) in animals treated with inflammatory agents, and the high comorbidity of inflammation related medical disorders - e.g. CD, rheumatoid arthritis, psoriasis and treatments with immune modulators-with psychopathology [13,14,41] Moreover, it was shown that treatment of CD with anti-TNF-α reduces not only disease activity but also depressive symptoms [8,29,42]. The present findings, showing decrement in depressive symptom scores

Table 5. Effects of anti-TNF-α infusion on immune parameters and TRP/CAA compared to baseline reference value.

	Week 2		Week 4		Week 8		Time (linear trend)	
	B	P$_{Simes}$	B	P$_{Simes}$	B	P$_{Simes}$	B	P
Albumin	2.88	NS	3.76	**0.005**	1.47	NS	0.53	NS
Albumin %	3.38	**<0.001**	3.10	**<0.001**	2.65	**<0.001**	0.77	**0.001**
α$_1$	−0.35	NS	−0.27	NS	−0.56	**0.009**	−0.16	**0.019**
Log α$_1$%	−0.09	**0.005**	−0.09	**0.003**	−0.10	**0.001**	−0.03	**0.002**
α$_2$	−1.15	**<0.001**	−0.71	**0.004**	−0.82	**0.001**	−0.20	**0.034**
Log α$_2$%	−0.17	**<0.001**	−0.15	**<0.001**	−0.10	**<0.001**	−0.03	**0.016**
β	−0.00	NS	0.09	NS	−0.33	NS	−0.09	NS
β%	−0.23	NS	−0.57	**0.003**	−0.44	**0.020**	−0.17	**0.007**
γ	0.01	NS	0.39	NS	−0.15	NS	−0.01	NS
γ%	−0.34	NS	−0.17	NS	−0.15	NS	−0.03	NS
Total protein	1.42	NS	2.78	NS	−0.35	NS	0.03	NS
Log transferrin	0.07	NS	0.10	**0.010**	0.01	NS	0.01	NS
Zinc	−3.34	NS	2.97	NS	−6.24	NS	−1.28	NS
TRP/CAA	0.00	NS	0.01	NS	0.00	NS	0.00	NS

TRP/CAA: tryptophan/competing aminoacids.

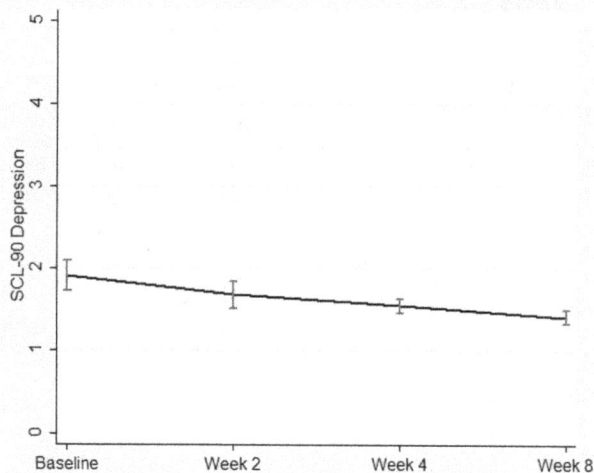

Figure 2. Overtime course of SCl-90 Depression. The line represents the mean score and the error bars represent the standard error at each time point.

Table 6. Association between SCL-90 depression scores and immune parameters and TRP/CAA over time.

	SCL-90 Depression[a]		SCL-90 Depression[b]	
	B	P_{Simes}	B	P_{Simes}
Albumin	−0.07	NS	0.09	NS
Albumin %	−0.46	NS	−0.19	NS
α_1	0.11	NS	0.09	NS
Log α_1%	−4.25	NS	−5.82	NS
α_2	1.26	NS	0.63	NS
Log α_2%	6.98	NS	−2.75	NS
β	0.56	NS	0.98	NS
β%	−0.34	NS	−0.45	NS
γ	0.69	NS	0.90	**0.005**
γ%	1.15	**0.001**	1.18	**0.001**
Total protein	0.07	NS	0.11	NS
Log transferrin	−9.67	NS	−4.35	NS
Zinc	0.03	NS	0.04	NS
TRP/CAA	17.70	NS	48.21	NS

[a]without correction for disease activity [b]corrected for disease activity
SCL-90: Symptom Checklist, TRP/CAA: tryptophan/competing aminoacids.

measured by SCL-90, BDI, and HDRS in patients with CD after anti-TNF-α treatment, are in agreement with these previous reports. Considering that depressive symptom scores measured by SCL-90 remained significantly decreased after correction for HBI scores compared to baseline, it is plausible that the decrease in depressive symptoms maybe mediated in part through changes in the immune system rather than only through reductions in psychological distress due to reduced disease activity. The differences between these three scales are likely related to differences in the constructs underlying the scales. [43] The HDRS in fact taps into various symptom groups that may be associated with the nuclear depression syndrome, particularly somatic symptoms. Although the HDRS is widely used, the SCL-90 is a more unidimensional measure of the nuclear depression syndrome, whereas the BDI assesses attitudes and cognitions which are mostly stable overtime. Given these differences, the SCL-90 was chosen for further analysis.

In addition, it was found that decrements in depressive symptom scores after anti-TNF-α infusion followed the reduction of inflammation as defined by an increase in negative APPs (albumin) and a decrease in positive APPs (α₁ and α₂ fractions). Research suggests that an imbalance of the immune system plays a role in depression through several interacting mechanisms [13]. There is some evidence that serotonin neurotransmission may play a role in the pathogenesis of depression and given the fact that TRP depletion decreases mood in vulnerable people, much attention has been focused on the degradation of TRP by the indoleamine 2,3 dioxygenase (IDO) enzyme, which is predominantly induced by IFN-γ and TNF-α [13,44]. In contrast to earlier studies showing decreased TRP/CAA ratios in patients with depression [21,24,25,26,27] and correlations between depressive symptoms and TRP levels in IFN-γ induced depression [45,46], we did not find any increase in TRP/CAA ratio over time and there was no association over time between SCL-90 depressive symptom scores and TRP/CAA ratio after infusion of anti-TNF-α. Considering the earlier findings showing decreased TRP/CAA ratio in IFN-γ induced depression,the fall in TRP may explain the role of immune mediators in depression,albeit partially. It has been argued that IFN-γ induced depression is associated with induction of IDO that increases levels of kynurenine (KYN), which in turn

leads to formation of neurotoxic metabolites, 3-hydroxykynurenine and quinolinic acid, rather than just TRP degradation by itself [13,39,44,47,48,49]. Furthermore, it has been demonstrated there was no relationship between response to antidepressant treatment and TRP/CAA ratio in a large group of patients with major depression [50]. In the light of these findings, it can be speculated that the reduction in depressive symptom scores in our sample is maybe associated with restoration of balance in KYN pathway rather than changes in TRP/CAA ratio.

Similar to the findings of the current study demonstrating invariant TRP/CAA ratio after treatment with anti-TNF-α, it was shown adalimumab, which is also a TNF-α antagonist, exerts its immune-suppressant effect without influencing IDO activity and TRP levels in patients with rheumatoid arthritis [51]. Furthermore, the present study also failed to find an association between immune parameters and TRP/CAA ratio over time. Consequently, it may be reasoned that TNF-α antagonists exert effects on disease activity and depressive symptoms through several different pathways, for example nuclear factor kappa B modulation of cell survival and apoptosis, corticotrophin releasing factor, vasopressin, brain-derived neurotrophic factor [13,14,52,53].

In the current study it was demonstrated that, even after correction for disease activity, levels and percentages of positive APPs (α₂, β, γ) were higher, while levels and percentages of albumin and levels of zinc were lower in patients with a current or past depressive episode. In other words, an inflammatory reaction was more evident in patients with depression, and not solely dependent on disease activity. The association between SCL-90 depression scores and γ fraction after correction for disease activity also fortifies this notion. There are numerous studies showing that depression exacerbates CD and predicts lower remission rates in CD [5,6,7,12]. In order to clarify the additive effect of depression on immune activation and disease activity in CD, studies comparing immune parameters between CD patients with and without depression are required.

In agreement with previous studies evaluating CD patients, improvement in quality of life after anti-TNF-α infusion was demonstrated by increases across all domains of IBDQ [8,54,55]. Likewise, in line with previous studies, anti-TNF-α infusion decreased physical and mental fatigue at week 2. Nevertheless, decreases in fatigue scores were no longer significant after correction for disease activity. Contrary to this latter finding, it has been suggested that fatigue in CD is secondary to depression rather than a primary manifestation of disease activity [56].

The strength of this prospective study is that it has not only analysed the effect of anti-TNF-α treatment on depressive symptoms in CD patients, but also concentrated on the underlying immune mechanism by measuring TRP/CAA ratio and immune parameters with corrections for disease activity. Although the study design allowed us to use patients as their own controls over a time period of 8 weeks, the sample size was rather small which may have caused type-II errors. We carefully evaluated the presence of axis I mental disorder using the Structured Clinical Interview for DSM-IV axis I Disorders Version 5.0 in this sample. Two patients fulfilled criteria for lifetime depressive disorder and two for current depressive disorder with melancholic features. Since the presence of depressive disorder is a likely confounder, all analyses were corrected for this variable. We did not specifically collect information about patients' psychotropic treatment plan, however this likely overlaps with presence of mental disorder. Other limitations also apply. In the present study, TRP availability to the brain was estimated by the peripheral TRP/CAA ratio. Various previous studies measured brain tryptophan availability using the same TRP/CAA ratio. [21,24,25,26,28,39,50,57]. Given that plasma TRP concentrations correlate poorly with those in cerebrospinal fluid (CSF), the TRP/CAA ratio gives us a more reliable measure of brain TRP availability taking into account the fact that CAA is competing for the cerebral uptake of TRP [57]. For a more direct approach, TRP and its metabolites would have

to be measured in CSF, which might provide a better estimate [58]. However, lumbar puncture in these patients ethically would be considered invasive, given lifetime chronic illness requiring major medical diagnostic testing and interventions over the course of the illness. As explained previously, measurement of IDO activity, along with its products and the ratio between neurotoxic and neuroprotective metabolites may allow for a more direct test of the question whether a decrease in depressive symptom scores after anti-TNF-α is due to changes in TRP and its metabolites, or whether several other mechanisms are involved. Another approach to understand the effect of TNF-α antagonists on depression may be to evaluate the effect of anti-TNF-α treatment on treatment response and immune markers in patients with depression. This approach may help to eliminate other potential confounders originating from the nature of autoimmune disorders like CD requiring use of concomitant medication influencing immune parameters. Ongoing studies evaluating the efficacy of drugs with antagonist properties at TNF-α, namely infliximab and minocycline, for treatment of treatment resistant depression and bipolar depression along with the relationship between efficacy and inflammatory markers will hopefully shed more light on the association between TNF-α system and depression [59,60].

Notwithstanding its limitations, this study does suggest that anti-TNF-α infusion in patients with CD reduces depressive symptoms, in part independently of disease activity, and that the effect on depressive symptoms is not associated with immune-induced changes in TRP availability to the brain, as estimated indirectly by serum TRP/CAA ratio.

Author Contributions

Conceived and designed the experiments: MW JvO MR. Performed the experiments: GK AW RV. Analyzed the data: SG MW JvO. Wrote the paper: SG JvO. Recruited the participants: MR.

References

1. Robertson DA, Ray J, Diamond I, Edwards JG (1989) Personality profile and affective state of patients with inflammatory bowel disease. Gut 30: 623–626.
2. Helzer JE, Chammas S, Norland CC, Stillings WA, Alpers DH (1984) A study of the association between Crohn's disease and psychiatric illness. Gastroenterology 86: 324–330.
3. North CS, Alpers DH, Helzer JE, Spitznagel EL, Clouse RE (1991) Do life events or depression exacerbate inflammatory bowel disease? A prospective study. Ann Intern Med 114: 381–386.
4. Kurina LM, Goldacre MJ, Yeates D, Gill LE (2001) Depression and anxiety in people with inflammatory bowel disease. J Epidemiol Community Health 55: 716–720.
5. Camara RJ, Schoepfer AM, Pittet V, Begre S, von Kanel R (2011) Mood and nonmood components of perceived stress and exacerbation of Crohn's disease. Inflammatory bowel diseases 17: 2358–2365.
6. Mardini HE, Kip KE, Wilson JW (2004) Crohn's disease: a two-year prospective study of the association between psychological distress and disease activity. Digestive diseases and sciences 49: 492–497.
7. Mittermaier C, Dejaco C, Waldhoer T, Oefferlbauer-Ernst A, Miehsler W, et al. (2004) Impact of depressive mood on relapse in patients with inflammatory bowel disease: a prospective 18-month follow-up study. Psychosomatic medicine 66: 79–84.
8. Banovic I, Gilibert D, Cosnes J (2009) Perception of improved state of health and subjective quality of life in Crohn's disease patients treated with Infliximab. Journal of Crohn's & colitis 3: 25–31.
9. Papadakis KA, Targan SR (2000) Role of cytokines in the pathogenesis of inflammatory bowel disease. Annu Rev Med 51: 289–298.
10. Plevy SE, Landers CJ, Prehn J, Carramanzana NM, Deem RL, et al. (1997) A role for TNF-alpha and mucosal T helper-1 cytokines in the pathogenesis of Crohn's disease. J Immunol 159: 6276–6282.
11. Strober W, Zhang F, Kitani A, Fuss I, Fichtner-Feigl S (2010) Proinflammatory cytokines underlying the inflammation of Crohn's disease. Current opinion in gastroenterology 26: 310–317.
12. Persoons P, Vermeire S, Demyttenaere K, Fischler B, Vandenberghe J, et al. (2005) The impact of major depressive disorder on the short- and long-term outcome of Crohn's disease treatment with infliximab. Alimentary pharmacology & therapeutics 22: 101–110.

13. Dantzer R, O'Connor JC, Freund GG, Johnson RW, Kelley KW (2008) From inflammation to sickness and depression: when the immune system subjugates the brain. Nature reviews Neuroscience 9: 46–56.
14. Miller AH, Maletic V, Raison CL (2009) Inflammation and its discontents: the role of cytokines in the pathophysiology of major depression. Biological psychiatry 65: 732–741.
15. Leonard B, Maes M (2012) Mechanistic explanations how cell-mediated immune activation, inflammation and oxidative and nitrosative stress pathways and their sequels and concomitants play a role in the pathophysiology of unipolar depression. Neuroscience and biobehavioral reviews 36: 764–785.
16. Van Gool AR, Kruit WH, Engels FK, Stoter G, Bannink M, et al. (2003) Neuropsychiatric side effects of interferon-alfa therapy. Pharm World Sci 25: 11–20.
17. Maes M, Wauters A, Neels H, Scharpe S, Van Gastel A, et al. (1995) Total serum protein and serum protein fractions in depression: relationships to depressive symptoms and glucocorticoid activity. J Affect Disord 34: 61–69.
18. Sluzewska A, Rybakowski J, Bosmans E, Sobieska M, Berghmans R, et al. (1996) Indicators of immune activation in major depression. Psychiatry Res 64: 161–167.
19. Leonard BE (2001) The immune system, depression and the action of antidepressants. Prog Neuropsychopharmacol Biol Psychiatry 25: 767–780.
20. Licinio J, Wong ML (1999) The role of inflammatory mediators in the biology of major depression: central nervous system cytokines modulate the biological substrate of depressive symptoms, regulate stress-responsive systems, and contribute to neurotoxicity and neuroprotection. Mol Psychiatry 4: 317–327.
21. Maes M, Verkerk R, Vandoolaeghe E, Van Hunsel F, Neels H, et al. (1997) Serotonin-immune interactions in major depression: lower serum tryptophan as a marker of an immune-inflammatory response. European archives of psychiatry and clinical neuroscience 247: 154–161.
22. Maes M, De Vos N, Demedts P, Wauters A, Neels H (1999) Lower serum zinc in major depression in relation to changes in serum acute phase proteins. Journal of affective disorders 56: 189–194.
23. Song C, Dinan T, Leonard BE (1994) Changes in immunoglobulin, complement and acute phase protein levels in the depressed patients and normal controls. J Affect Disord 30: 283–288.

24. Maes M, Meltzer HY, Scharpe S, Bosmans E, Suy E, et al. (1993) Relationships between lower plasma L-tryptophan levels and immune-inflammatory variables in depression. Psychiatry research 49: 151–165.

25. Maes M, Scharpe S, Meltzer HY, Okayli G, Bosmans E, et al. (1994) Increased neopterin and interferon-gamma secretion and lower availability of L-tryptophan in major depression: further evidence for an immune response. Psychiatry research 54: 143–160.

26. Maes M, Wauters A, Verkerk R, Demedts P, Neels H, et al. (1996) Lower serum L-tryptophan availability in depression as a marker of a more generalized disorder in protein metabolism. Neuropsychopharmacology: official publication of the American College of Neuropsychopharmacology 15: 243–251.

27. Cowen PJ, Parry-Billings M, Newsholme EA (1989) Decreased plasma tryptophan levels in major depression. Journal of affective disorders 16: 27–31.

28. Maes M, De Ruyter M, Hobin P, Suy E (1986) The diagnostic performance of the L-tryptophan/competing amino acids ratio in major depression. Acta psychiatrica Belgica 86: 257–265.

29. Minderhoud IM, Samsom M, Oldenburg B (2007) Crohn's disease, fatigue, and infliximab: is there a role for cytokines in the pathogenesis of fatigue? World journal of gastroenterology: WJG 13: 2089–2093.

30. Harvey RF, Bradshaw JM (1980) A simple index of Crohn's-disease activity. Lancet 1: 514.

31. Yoshida EM (1999) The Crohn's Disease Activity Index, its derivatives and the Inflammatory Bowel Disease Questionnaire: a review of instruments to assess Crohn's disease. Can J Gastroenterol 13: 65–73.

32. Smets EM, Garssen B, Bonke B, De Haes JC (1995) The Multidimensional Fatigue Inventory (MFI) psychometric qualities of an instrument to assess fatigue. J Psychosom Res 39: 315–325.

33. Russel MG, Pastoor CJ, Brandon S, Rijken J, Engels LG, et al. (1997) Validation of the Dutch translation of the Inflammatory Bowel Disease Questionnaire (IBDQ): a health-related quality of life questionnaire in inflammatory bowel disease. Digestion 58: 282–288.

34. Hamilton M (1967) Development of a rating scale for primary depressive illness. Br J Soc Clin Psychol 6: 278–296.

35. Beck AT, Steer RA (1984) Internal consistencies of the original and revised Beck Depression Inventory. J Clin Psychol 40: 1365–1367.

36. Bosscher RJ, Koning H, Van Meurs R (1986) Reliability and validity of the Beck Depression Inventory in a Dutch college population. Psychol Rep 58: 696–698.

37. Derogatis LR, Rickels K, Rock AF (1976) The SCL-90 and the MMPI: a step in the validation of a new self-report scale. Br J Psychiatry 128: 280–289.

38. Van Hunsel F, Wauters A, Vandoolaeghe E, Neels H, Demedts P, et al. (1996) Lower total serum protein, albumin, and beta- and gamma-globulin in major and treatment-resistant depression: effects of antidepressant treatments. Psychiatry research 65: 159–169.

39. Wichers MC, Koek GH, Robaeys G, Verkerk R, Scharpe S, et al. (2005) IDO and interferon-alpha-induced depressive symptoms: a shift in hypothesis from tryptophan depletion to neurotoxicity. Molecular psychiatry 10: 538–544.

40. Simes RJ (1986) An improved Bonferroni procedure for multiple tests of significance. Biometrika 73: 751–754.

41. Irwin MR, Miller AH (2007) Depressive disorders and immunity: 20 years of progress and discovery. Brain Behav Immun 21: 374–383.

42. Loftus EV, Feagan BG, Colombel JF, Rubin DT, Wu EQ, et al. (2008) Effects of adalimumab maintenance therapy on health-related quality of life of patients with Crohn's disease: patient-reported outcomes of the CHARM trial. The American journal of gastroenterology 103: 3132–3141.

43. Cusin C, Yang H, Yeung A, Fava M (2010) Rating scales for depression. In: Baer L, Blais MA, editors. Handbook of clinical rating scales and assessment in psychiatry and mental health (Current clinical psychiatry).New York: Humana Press. pp. 7–35.

44. Wichers MC, Maes M (2004) The role of indoleamine 2,3-dioxygenase (IDO) in the pathophysiology of interferon-alpha-induced depression. Journal of psychiatry & neuroscience: JPN 29: 11–17.

45. Capuron L, Ravaud A, Neveu PJ, Miller AH, Maes M, et al. (2002) Association between decreased serum tryptophan concentrations and depressive symptoms in cancer patients undergoing cytokine therapy. Molecular psychiatry 7: 468–473.

46. Capuron L, Neurauter G, Musselman DL, Lawson DH, Nemeroff CB, et al. (2003) Interferon-alpha-induced changes in tryptophan metabolism. relationship to depression and paroxetine treatment. Biological psychiatry 54: 906–914.

47. Myint AM, Kim YK (2003) Cytokine-serotonin interaction through IDO: a neurodegeneration hypothesis of depression. Medical hypotheses 61: 519–525.

48. Raison CL, Dantzer R, Kelley KW, Lawson MA, Woolwine BJ, et al. (2010) CSF concentrations of brain tryptophan and kynurenines during immune stimulation with IFN-alpha: relationship to CNS immune responses and depression. Molecular psychiatry 15: 393–403.

49. Maes M, Leonard BE, Myint AM, Kubera M, Verkerk R (2011) The new '5-HT' hypothesis of depression: cell-mediated immune activation induces indoleamine 2,3-dioxygenase, which leads to lower plasma tryptophan and an increased synthesis of detrimental tryptophan catabolites (TRYCATs), both of which contribute to the onset of depression. Progress in neuro-psychopharmacology & biological psychiatry 35: 702–721.

50. Porter RJ, Mulder RT, Joyce PR, Luty SE (2005) Tryptophan and tyrosine availability and response to antidepressant treatment in major depression. Journal of affective disorders 86: 129–134.

51. Kurz K, Herold M, Winkler C, Klotz W, Russe E, et al. (2011) Effects of adalimumab therapy on disease activity and interferon-gamma-mediated biochemical pathways in patients with rheumatoid arthritis. Autoimmunity 44: 235–242.

52. Soczynska JK, Kennedy SH, Goldstein BI, Lachowski A, Woldeyohannes HO, et al. (2009) The effect of tumor necrosis factor antagonists on mood and mental health-associated quality of life: novel hypothesis-driven treatments for bipolar depression? Neurotoxicology 30: 497–521.

53. Kenis G, Prickaerts J, van Os J, Koek GH, Robaeys G, et al. (2011) Depressive symptoms following interferon-alpha therapy: mediated by immune-induced reductions in brain-derived neurotrophic factor? The international journal of neuropsychopharmacology/official scientific journal of the Collegium Internationale Neuropsychopharmacologicum 14: 247–253.

54. van Balkom BP, Schoon EJ, Stockbrugger RW, Wolters FL, van Hogezand RA, et al. (2002) Effects of anti-tumour necrosis factor-alpha therapy on the quality of life in Crohn's disease. Alimentary pharmacology & therapeutics 16: 1101–1107.

55. Lichtenstein GR, Bala M, Han C, DeWoody K, Schaible T (2002) Infliximab improves quality of life in patients with Crohn's disease. Inflammatory bowel diseases 8: 237–243.

56. Banovic I, Gilibert D, Cosnes J (2010) Crohn's disease and fatigue: constancy and co-variations of activity of the disease, depression, anxiety and subjective quality of life. Psychology, health & medicine 15: 394–405.

57. Christmas DM, Potokar J, Davies SJ (2011) A biological pathway linking inflammation and depression: activation of indoleamine 2,3-dioxygenase. Neuropsychiatric disease and treatment 7: 431–439.

58. van Donkelaar EL, Blokland A, Ferrington L, Kelly PA, Steinbusch HW, et al. (2011) Mechanism of acute tryptophan depletion: is it only serotonin? Molecular psychiatry 16: 695–713.

59. Raison CL, Rutherford RE, Woolwine BJ, Shuo C, Schettler P, et al. (2012) A Randomized Controlled Trial of the Tumor Necrosis Factor Antagonist Infliximab for Treatment-Resistant Depression: The Role of Baseline Inflammatory Biomarkers. Archives of general psychiatry: 1–11.

60. Savitz J, Preskorn S, Teague TK, Drevets D, Yates W, et al. (2012) Minocycline and aspirin in the treatment of bipolar depression: a protocol for a proof-of-concept, randomised, double-blind, placebo-controlled, 2×2 clinical trial. BMJ open 2: e000643.

25

Prioritisation and Network Analysis of Crohn's Disease Susceptibility Genes

Daniele Muraro[1]*, Douglas A. Lauffenburger[2], Alison Simmons[1]

1 Weatherall Institute of Molecular Medicine, University of Oxford, Oxford, United Kingdom, **2** Department of Biological Engineering, Massachusetts Institute of Technology, Cambridge, Massachusetts, United States of America

Abstract

Recent Genome-Wide Association Studies (GWAS) have revealed numerous Crohn's disease susceptibility genes and a key challenge now is in understanding how risk polymorphisms in associated genes might contribute to development of this disease. For a gene to contribute to disease phenotype, its risk variant will likely adversely communicate with a variety of other gene products to result in dysregulation of common signaling pathways. A vital challenge is to elucidate pathways of potentially greatest influence on pathological behaviour, in a manner recognizing how multiple relevant genes may yield integrative effect. In this work we apply mathematical analysis of networks involving the list of recently described Crohn's susceptibility genes, to prioritise pathways in relation to their potential development of this disease. Prioritisation was performed by applying a text mining and a diffusion based method (GRAIL, GPEC). Prospective biological significance of the resulting prioritised list of proteins is highlighted by changes in their gene expression levels in Crohn's patients intestinal tissue in comparison with healthy donors.

Editor: David L Boone, University of Chicago, United States of America

Funding: DM and AS gratefully acknowledge the Sir Jules Thorn Charitable Trust for financial support through grant HBRWGDO. DL gratefully acknowledges the Institute for Collaborative Biotechnologies through grant W911NF-09-0001 from the United States Army Research Office; the content of the information does not necessarily reflect the position or the policy of the Government, and no official endorsement should be inferred. The funders had no role in study design, data collection and analysis, decision to publish, or preparation of the manuscript.

Competing Interests: The authors have declared that no competing interests exist.

* Email: Daniele.Muraro@ndm.ox.ac.uk

Introduction

Biological functions are rarely a consequence of the activity of a single molecule and arise from the interactions between multiple components of biological systems. Since the completion of the human genome project in 2003, high-throughput techniques have generated a large amount of molecular-interaction data in the human cells. The need to analyse the role of associated interaction networks at a system-wide level, rather than focusing on single interactions, led to a change in perspective in the investigation of biological systems and to the development of Systems Biology approaches [1]. During the past decade, significant contributions have been made to curate databases of validated network maps at different levels (protein-interaction, regulatory, metabolic and RNA networks), these often comprising thousands of nodes and links [2], [3]. Investigation of networks of such dimension cannot be easily performed by intuitive reasoning and quantitative approaches are needed to explore their emerging properties more objectively. Recent progresses in network theory have encouraged the application of network based approaches in the study of molecular interaction networks. Although incompleteness in knowledge should suggest caution as these networks are a proxy of the actual interactome, integration with independent functional data may support the biological viability of their topology [4].

When a network-based viewpoint is applied to disease, the disease phenotype is associated with global perturbed networks instead of single failing components [5], [6]. Starting from the underlying assumption that a disease is rarely a consequence of abnormality in single genes, but depends on the indirect perturbation of an interaction network, it should be clarified whether genes and proteins associated with disease are placed randomly in the interactome, or there are correlations between their function and their network topology [7]. Understanding how defects in such networks influence the progression of disease may provide useful information when selecting targets for drug development.

Genetic studies have revealed numerous susceptibility gene variants in common diseases such as Crohn's, but the function of individual gene variants in disease induction remains unclear. Here we use a list of Crohn's susceptibility genes to prioritise genes to serve as a seed to define a putative Crohn's disease network. We then use graph theory to probe hypotheses about its topological structure and to analyse how proteins implicated as being linked to Crohn's disease by this network may relate with their neighbours in the rest of the proteome. Biological relevance of the prioritised list and of its associated interactions is supported by microarray and functional classification data.

This article is organised as follows. First, we prioritise a list of candidate disease genes obtained from literature GWAS reports by applying both a diffusion-based and a text-mining approach. The relevance of our prioritised list is next examined by comparison with differentially expressed genes in biopsies from patients with

Crohn's disease. We then build a proteome interaction network of the associated prioritised proteins and we investigate its topological, functional features and relationships with other proteins in the proteome. Correlation between topological localisation and functional role supports the biological relevance of the datasets interactions. The network associated with disease shows enrichment in hubs nearest neighbours and topological segregation of the prioritised list. In the light of our observations, we conclude by highlighting proteins in the network associated with disease with noteworthy topological and functional properties that may warrant further experimental investigation.

Results and Discussion

In what follows we prioritise a list of candidate genes associated with Crohn's disease and test its enrichment among the set of differentially expressed genes in patients affected by Crohn's disease. We then build a molecular interaction network from this list and test correlations between the network topology and its functional organisation. In each section we first provide a brief review of the relevant methods, we then describe in more detail our particular application. The technical details of the methods applied are described either in the section Methods or in (Information S1).

Prioritisation of genes associated with Crohn's disease

Genome-Wide Association Studies have identified a large number of candidate disease genes for Crohn's but the role of each in disease pathogenesis is unclear [8]. In order to reduce the number of candidate genes and to identify the disease module, several tools from bioinformatics and biomathematics have been proposed. Such methods rely upon different assumptions and can be classified in three main categories as pairwise, neighbourhood and diffusion based methods [9]. Pairwise methods assume that proteins associated with disease tend to directly interact with each other. In this category, linkage methods select genes located in the linkage interval of genes whose protein product is a first neighbour of proteins associated with disease. Other pairwise methods analyse relatedness between two genes by applying text mining and assessing a score to the association depending on the degree of similarity in the text describing them within article abstracts [10]. Neighbourhood based methods rely upon the hypothesis that cellular components associated with the same disease tend to cluster together [8].

In diffusion based methods, random walkers are released from a set of known disease genes and diffuse along the links of the proteome; in such a way, nodes that are more connected to disease proteins are more frequently visited and prioritised [11]. All of these methods depend on the topological structure of the interactome; but, while linkage and neighbourhood based methods rely upon a particular topological metric, such as pairwise or nearest interactions, diffusion based methods adopt the full information of the network topology. Diffusion-based methods have been recently applied and shown to achieve the state-of-the-art predictive performance [12], [13], [14], [15]; in addition, combining predictions made by different methods in a 'consensus method' yielded to Pareto optimal performance in the precision-recall objectives [15].

Accounting for the results of this comparative analysis, we selected 171 SNPs and 354 genes associated with Crohn's disease from the Catalog of Published Genome-Wide Association Studies [16] and in a recent published GWAS by Jostins et al. [17] and we performed prioritisation of these genes using both a diffusion based method and a pairwise text mining algorithm (see Methods

section). We finally selected a consensus list from the results of the prioritisation algorithms, together with the training set of known genes, to obtain a sub-list of 99 genes. From this list we built a sub-network associated with Crohn's disease by selecting all interactions containing at least one protein identified by prioritisation; in such a way, we also considered indirect interactions among proteins associated with disease, as suggested by Rossin et al. [8]. This sub-network is shown in Figure 1. The list of the prioritised proteins and the interactions in the network associated with disease are reported in an Excel workbook in the (Workbook S1). Support for involvement of this protein network as being implicated in Crohn's disease related inflammation was then obtained by comparing our list with genes whose expression has been identified as being differentially regulated in intestinal tissue from patients with Crohn's. We used publicly available microarray data from a study whose aim was to investigate differential intestinal gene expression in patients with Crohn's disease (CD) and controls (see Methods section). As a result of this selection we found that 4926 genes of the 41616 measured in the microarray were differentially expressed of which 28 were part of the 99 prioritised genes. A Fisher's exact test shows enrichment in differentially expressed genes among the prioritised ones with p-value equal to $7.55 \cdot 10^{-6}$, thus supporting the association of the prioritised list to Crohn's disease. Interestingly not all the genes of the training set, although associated with Crohn's disease, are differentially expressed; this suggesting that differential expression should be combined with other criteria, such as functional and topological, to support selection of candidate proteins as associated with disease. The list of Entrez IDs of the prioritised list together with their p-values is reported in Workbook S1.

Topological characterisation of the network associated with Crohn's disease

We analysed the global and local topological organisation of the sub-network that we have built in the previous section. Characteristic graph-theoretical distributions and metrics show signatures of hierarchical modularity and preferential attachment; these properties resemble the ones of other biological networks, this supporting the biological viability of the network that we associated with Crohn's disease (see Information S1, Figure S1 and Table S1). The density of this network is approximately three times higher than in the NCBI proteome network suggesting a higher tendency of the disease proteins to interact among themselves than among proteins that are not associated with disease.

Since disease is often caused by perturbation in the communication between bio-molecules [18], [19], investigating how such changes at the local level can affect the network structure may provide insight into its robustness and highlight which components are critical to maintain a correct functioning. Analysis of network robustness by node removal (failure-attack tolerance) shows robustness to removal of nodes with low degree and susceptibility to deletion of highly connected nodes; this reflects the key role played by hub proteins in maintaining the connectivity of this biological network. A detailed description of this analysis is reported in the Information S1 (see also Figures S2 and S3).

We then investigated if proteome hubs are over-represented in the network associated with Crohn's and we analysed if the number of hubs in the list of prioritised proteins is over-represented when compared to the total number of hubs in the NCBI proteome. The p-value obtained by a hypergeometric distribution does not show a significant over-representation (see Table 1). We then considered the list of proteins in the network associated with Crohn's, including the first neighbours of the

(a)

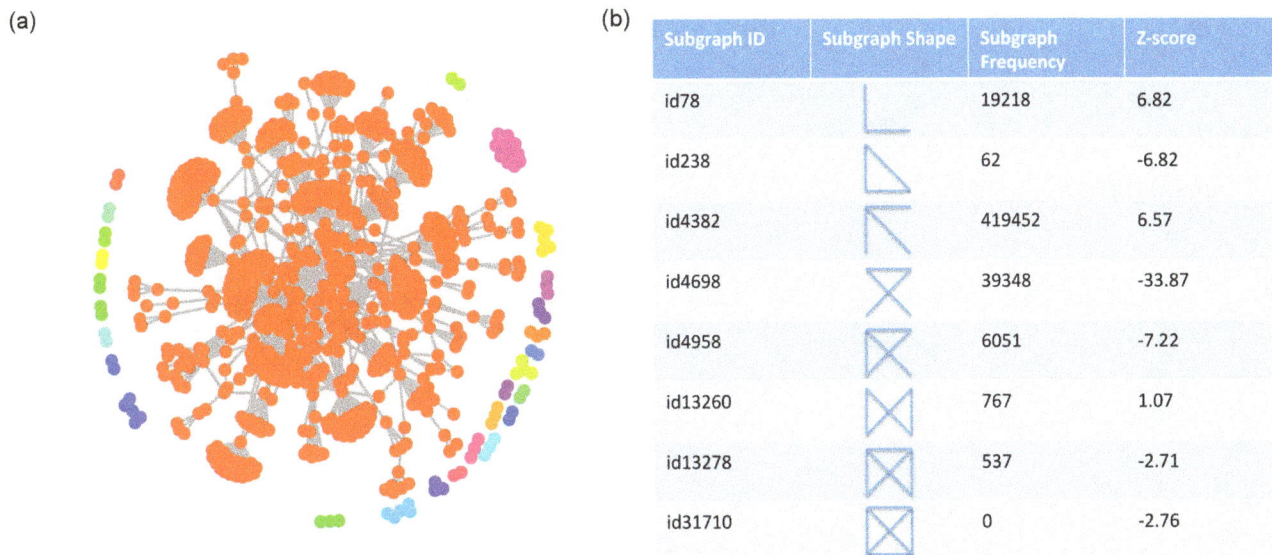

(b)

Subgraph ID	Subgraph Shape	Subgraph Frequency	Z-score
id78		19218	6.82
id238		62	-6.82
id4382		419452	6.57
id4698		39348	-33.87
id4958		6051	-7.22
id13260		767	1.07
id13278		537	-2.71
id31710		0	-2.76

Figure 1. Network associated with Crohn's disease and motifs. (a) Representation of the protein interaction network obtained by prioritisation. The network presents 28 connected components, each one being highlighted using a different colour. The giant component, namely the connected subgraph that contains the majority of the entire graph's nodes, is shown in red. (b) Sub-graphs frequency and z-scores in the network associated with Crohn's. Considering the threshold |Z-score| > 2, subgraphs id78 and id4382 are over-represented (motifs), whereas subgraphs id238, id4698, id4958, id13278, id31710 are under-represented (anti-motifs).

prioritised list, and analysed their over-representation in a similar manner; in this case, hub over-representation is significant, suggesting Crohn's disease susceptibility genes tend to directly interact with proteome hubs.

The global features of preferential attachment and hierarchical modularity suggest the presence of sub-graphs characterising the network at a local level. We now address the problem of identifying such topological modules and analysing their potential correlation with proteins associated with disease. More specifically, we searched for over-represented subgraphs (motifs) when compared to randomised versions of the same network. Algorithms for the search of network motifs explore the full combinatorial set of graphs of a given dimension. Since the computational time grows exponentially with graph dimension, small motifs comprising three or four nodes are usually analysed [20]. Several tools have been developed to identify network motifs, such as Mfinder [21], MAVisto [22], FANMOD [23]. A well established tool developed for network motif search is Mfinder [21]. Beginning with a selected edge, Mfinder searches for all the subgraphs of a given dimension comprising it. All the sets of visited nodes are then stored in a hash table, this reducing the searching time as the searching tree is stopped when a set of nodes has been already visited. Motif over-representation is then evaluated by comparing the frequency of motifs in the real network with a set of

randomly generated networks. In the default mode random networks preserve the degree distribution of the nodes and are generated using a switching method, namely edges are switched while keeping the number of incoming edges, outgoing edges and mutual edges of each node of the input network. We investigated the presence of motifs and anti-motifs in the network associated with disease by applying Mfinder with the default conditions. Because of the computational time required, we analysed motifs of three or four nodes only and evaluated their over-representation over 1000 random networks. According to the default Z-score threshold (Z-score = 2), the network associated with Crohn's contains 2 motifs (with motif ids id78 and id4382) and 5 anti-motifs (with motif ids id238, id4698, id4958, id13278, id31710), (Figure 1b). Interestingly, cliques composed of four nodes are under-represented, suggesting that such a high level of connectivity is not likely in realistic biological networks. We then analysed which prioritised proteins were more frequently associated with motifs and we found, in order of frequency, PRDM1, ATF4 and FASLG. Notwithstanding the degree distribution of the network associated with Crohn's was preserved when generating random networks, two of these proteins are highly connected, FASLG being the fourth most connected protein in the prioritised list and ATF4 the thirteenth. ATF4 is also one of the known proteins associated with Crohn's disease, see Table S2.

Table 1. Hubs distribution.

Proteins list	N. proteins	N. Hubs	p-value
NCBI Human PPI network proteins	10486	2685	–
Prioritised proteins	99	31	$1.18{\cdot}10^{-1}$
Disease network proteins	807	563	$<2.20{\cdot}10^{-16}$

Table summarising the number of hub proteins in the NCBI proteome, in the list of prioritised proteins and in the same list together with their first neighbours (Disease network proteins). Over-representation of hubs is statistically significant when considering first neighbours of the prioritised list (Hypergeometric distribution p-values).

(a)

Biological Process

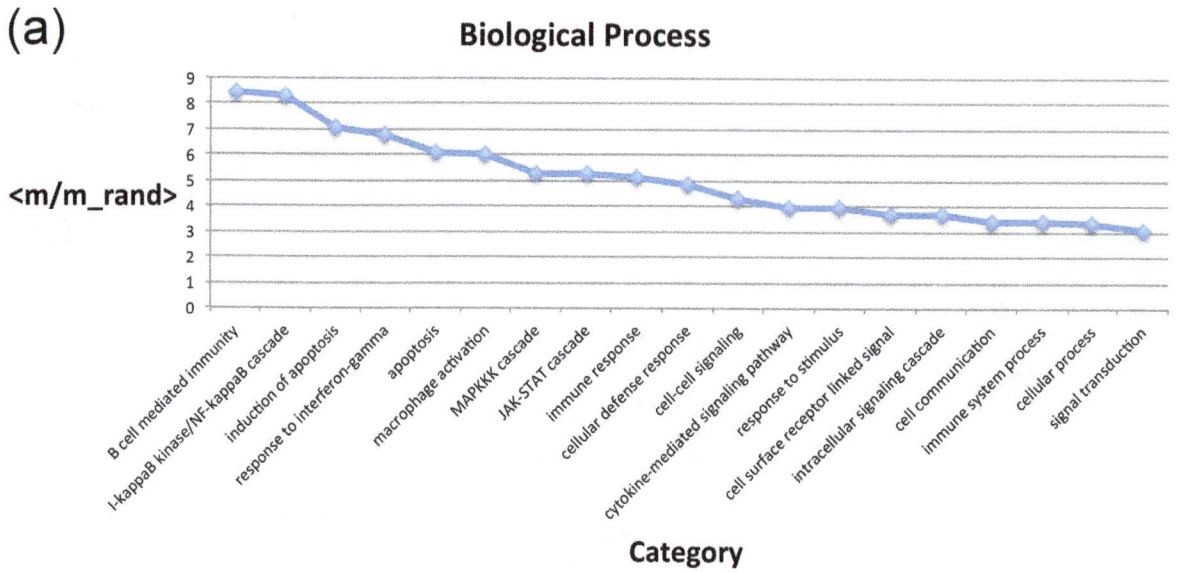

(b)

Protein Class

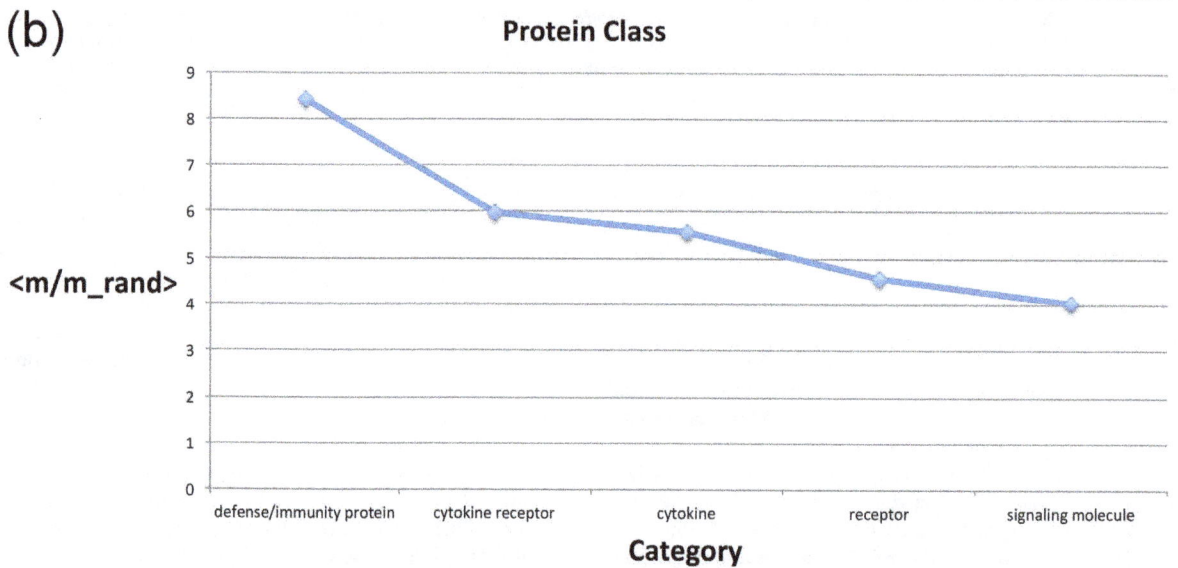

(c)

Pathway/Molecular Function

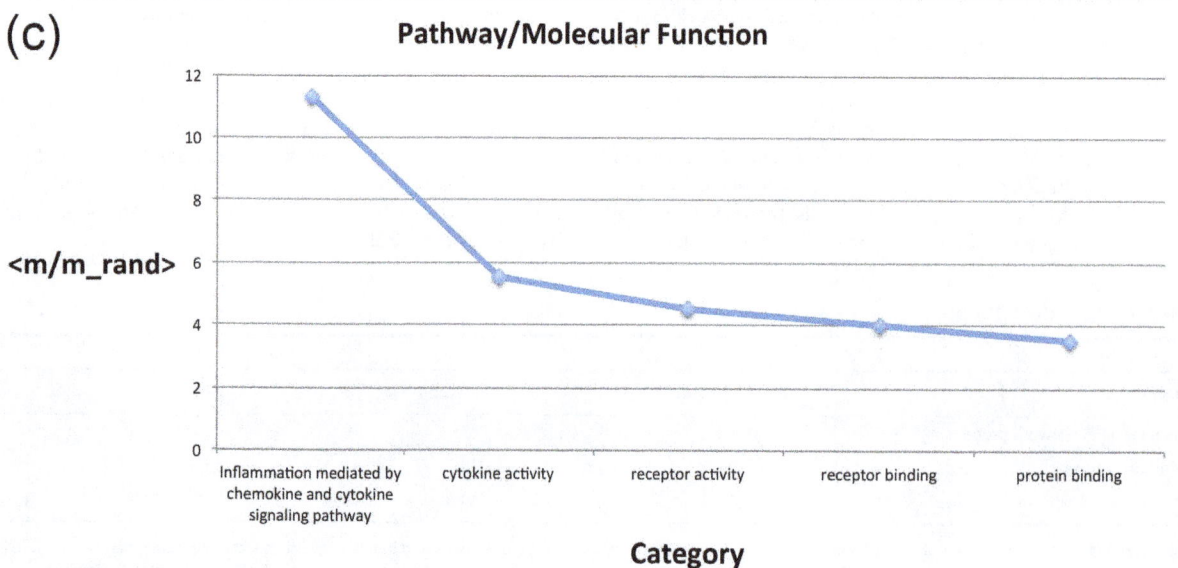

Figure 2. Topological segregation. Series of plots representing the segregation functions of over-represented categories in the network associated with Crohn's sorted from the most to the least segregated category. (a) categories within biological processes; (b) categories within protein classes; (c) categories within molecular functions and pathways.

Functional classification and topological segregation of enriched categories

Based on the assumption that proteins with similar functional properties interact with one another, protein interaction maps have been frequently used to generate hypotheses on the functional role of proteins of unknown functional classification [24], [25]. A systematic graph-theoretical study built from this premise was proposed in [4] on four datasets that approximate the protein interaction network of yeast *Saccharomyces cerevisiae*. In order to determine how well such datasets characterise the protein interaction network of *Saccharomyces cerevisiae*, the authors investigated the relationship between the topology of the protein interaction maps and the known functional properties of the protein. In all four datasets strong correlations were found between the network's structure and the functional role and sub-cellular localisation of its protein constituents. By measuring the tendency of proteins to interact with other proteins of the same functional or localisation class they concluded that most functional classes appear as relatively segregated sub-networks of the full protein interaction network.

In the spirit of this analysis, we examined whether the protein network that we associated with Crohn's disease leads to a similar correlation with the functional properties of the prioritised proteins. We performed a functional classification by applying the PANTHER (Protein ANalysis THrough Evolutionary Relationships) Classification System [26]. Here proteins have been functionally classified according to molecular function (the function of the protein by itself or with directly interacting proteins at a biochemical level, e.g. a protein kinase); biological process (the function of the protein in the context of a larger network of proteins that interact to accomplish a process at the level of the cell or organism, e.g. mitosis) or pathway (similar to biological process, but a pathway also explicitly specifies the relationships between the interacting molecules). We asked whether enriched categories presented a correlation with network topology being topologically segregated. Categories comprising less than 10 proteins were not considered in this analysis as they are too few to perform a statistical characterisation. Topological segregation was evaluated by calculating the segregation function $\bar{m}^\lambda$ per functional class λ in the enriched categories (see Methods section). This function represents how many times it is more likely that proteins in a particular functional category interact with neighbours belonging to the same category than with proteins randomly placed in the network. The evaluation of the topological segregation is reported in Figure 2. Particularly interconnected classes are the ones related to inflammation ('Inflammation mediated by chemokine and cytokine signalling pathway') and to the immune system ('defense/immunity protein'). Correlation between topology and functional organisation further supports the biological relevance of the network topology. Evaluation of the topological segregation of the prioritised list by Eq. (1) in the Methods section returned a value of 3.21 showing tendency of these proteins to aggregate.

Conclusions

In this work we have prioritised a list of genes associated with Crohn's disease and developed a graph-theoretical analysis of the molecular interaction network resulting from this list. Prioritisation was performed by applying both a diffusion based method (GPEC) [11] and a pairwise text mining algorithm (GRAIL: Gene Relationships Across Implicated Loci) [10] with available software. The relevance of the prioritised list was supported by enrichment in differentially expressed genes in microarray data between biopsies taken from patients with Crohn's disease and healthy controls. By analysing the network associated with Crohn's from a graph-theoretical perspective, we have shown that it presents hierarchical modularity and density higher than in the NCBI proteome network, this suggesting a higher tendency of the disease proteins to interact among themselves than among proteins that are not associated with disease. Finally we have analysed the relationships among the topology of this network and the functional properties of its proteins. To test if prioritised proteins associated with the same functional class are more likely to interact among each other than with other proteins we have calculated their segregation function and we have highlighted a correlation between functional role and their topological location, this being also in agreement with the global modular organisation of the disease network. A small number of the prioritised proteins demonstrated both noteworthy functional and topological properties which are discussed below. STAT3 and JAK2 are present in 11 and 15 over-represented and topologically segregated functional categories respectively; they interact in the same signaling path 'JAK-STAT cascade', they were both differentially expressed in Crohn's tissue and they are highly interconnected with hubs as first neighbours, besides being highly interconnected proteins themselves in the network associated with disease, see Table 2. Vitamin D receptor (VDR) represents a strong positional candidate susceptibility gene for inflammatory bowel disease (IBD) [27] and is part of the training set (see Table S2); it is highly interconnected in the network associated with disease and also highly interconnected with hubs as a first neighbour (see Table 2); in addition, it is present in 6 over-represented and topologically segregated functional categories. PRDM1 is the protein which is most frequently present in network motifs and the adjusted p-value associated to its differential expression, although not being under the arbitrary statistical threshold of 0.05, is still significant being 0.08; it is also highly interconnected with hubs as a first neighbour (see Table 2). FASLG is present in 22 over-represented and topologically segregated functional categories, it is one of the proteins that occur most frequently in network motifs, it is also highly interconnected in the network associated with Crohn's and highly interconnected with hubs as a first neighbour (see Table 2). ATF4 is a protein of the training set and is part of the unfolded protein response (UPR) pathway which has been recently emerged in IBD pathophysiology [28], [29], [30]; it is one of the proteins most frequently associated with network motifs and it is highly interconnected with hubs as a first neighbour (see Table 2). A table listing the over-represented functional categories of the proteins just mentioned is reported in Table S3. Selected proteins combining functional and topological information may constitute candidates to investigate novel interactions between proteins directly associated to a causal mutation and proteins whose perturbation may be indirectly relevant in affecting the disease phenotype.

Methods

Prioritisation algorithms

171 SNPs and 354 genes associated with Crohn's disease were downloaded from the Catalog of Published Genome-Wide Association Studies [16] and from a recent published GWAS by Jostins et al. [17]. Genes and SNPs association is given by the locus list defined by the NHGRI GWAS catalogue [16], whose annotation was applied by Jostins et al., and that reports the strongest SNP and genes reported by the author(s) of the publication per locus window. Prioritisation was derived by the consensus of two algorithms, namely a diffusion based method (GPEC) [11] and a pairwise text mining algorithm (GRAIL: Gene Relationships Across Implicated Loci) [10] using as input SNPs rs numbers and Entrez IDs respectively with available software. GRAIL has two input sets of disease regions in the form of genomic regions around associated SNPs: a collection of seed regions and a collection of query regions. Genes in query regions are evaluated for relationships to genes in seed regions, and query regions are then assigned a significance score. When examining a set of regions for relationships between implicated genes, as in this case, the query regions and the seed regions are identical. GRAIL ranks genes by text similarity calculating gene relatedness as the degree of similarity in the text describing them within PubMed article abstracts; the algorithm then assigns a p-value to each gene by evaluating the number of other disease regions with related genes. By querying all human genes within the database, GRAIL associated 156 of the 171 SNPs to 174 genes with a p-value less than 0.1. We then applied GPEC on the list of genes reported from the collection of GWAS as follows. Prioritisation with GPEC was performed through a random walk with restart algorithm along a gene or protein relationship network. Nodes in the network were represented by Entrez Gene IDs, UniProt ACs, or official symbols for genes and proteins. A set of training genes, whose role in disease is verified in the literature, was specified together with a set of candidate genes which was defined as the list of genes associated with Crohn's disease from GWAS. The list of the candidate genes is reported in Workbook S1, whereas the list of training genes, together with a list of literature references, is listed in Table S2. A human protein-protein interaction network was downloaded from the NCBI Entrez Gene FTP site (ftp://ftp.ncbi.nlm.nih.gov/gene/GeneRIF/interactions.gz) which integrates three databases: Biomolecular Interaction Network Database [31], Biological General Repository for Interaction Datasets [32], Human Protein Reference database [33]. As a result a network of 10,486 genes and 50,791 interactions was built and employed to define the graph on which the random walk was defined. Random walkers were then initialised in the set of training genes and allowed to diffuse along the protein interaction network until they reached a steady state, which is numerically approximated by repeating the iterations until the difference between the vector of probabilities at time t and at time $t+1$, where the i-th element represents the probability of the walker being at node i at a fixed time, is smaller than a threshold value (whose default value is set to 10^{-6}). As a result of the GPEC algorithm run a set of 212 genes were identified at steady state. We finally selected a consensus list from the results of the prioritisation algorithms, together with the training set of known genes, to obtain a sub-list of 99 genes.

Microarray dataset

The microarray dataset analysed is available at Gene Expression Omnibus (http://www.ncbi.nlm.nih.gov/geo/ accession number GSE20881). 172 biopsies from CD and control subjects were studied. Endoscopic biopsies were taken at ileocolonoscopy from four specific anatomical locations, these being terminal ileum, sigmoid colon, ascending colon, descending colon [34]. The groups of CD and healthy samples were compared in order to identify genes that are differentially expressed across experimental conditions using the interactive web tool GEO2R (http://www.ncbi.nlm.nih.gov/geo/geo2r). GEO2R performs comparisons on original submitter-supplied processed data tables using the GEOquery and limma R packages from the Bioconductor project (http://www.bioconductor.org). The Benjamini and Hochberg false discovery rate method was selected by default to adjust p-values for multiple testing. We used these values as the primary statistics by which to interpret results, selecting as differentially expressed genes those whose p-value was less than 0.05.

Categories enrichment

Enrichment was performed by applying a statistical over-representation test to the prioritised proteins using as a reference list the set of all genes in the genome classified in the PANTHER database. Each list is compared to the reference list using the binomial test [35] for each molecular function, biological process, or pathway term in PANTHER; Bonferroni correction is applied for multiple testing. PANTHER mapped 97 of the 99 disease proteins into different categories and assigned a p-value to each category. Categories with a p-value minor than 0.01 were considered over-represented; their chart representations are reported in Figures S4–S7 and their lists in Workbook S1.

Table 2. Selected proteins.

Protein name	N. neighbours	N. hub neighbours	p-value
STAT3	112	99	$<2.2 \cdot 10^{-16}$
JAK2	91	74	$<2.2 \cdot 10^{-16}$
VDR	53	50	$<2.2 \cdot 10^{-16}$
PRDM1	13	10	$1.5 \cdot 10^{-4}$
FASLG	41	38	$<2.2 \cdot 10^{-16}$
ATF4	25	18	$1.5 \cdot 10^{-6}$

Table summarising the number of hub first neighbours in the selected proteins listed in section 'Results and discussion'. P-values represent the probability that the number of neighbour hubs is due to random choice and are calculated using a Fisher's exact test which compares the total number of hubs in the NCBI proteome with the number of hubs in the neighbours of the selected proteins. Of the 10486 proteins listed in the NCBI protein interaction network 2685 have a number of first neighbours which is strictly higher than the average; connectivity with these hubs is over-represented for the 6 proteins presented.

Classification by cellular component returned a number of classified proteins that was too low for a statistical analysis, for completeness these are reported in Workbook S1.

Evaluation of the topological segregation

The presence of topological segregation was evaluated by calculating its segregation function for each enriched category; this is defined as follows. Given a protein i belonging to the functional class λ the segregation function is given by

$$m_i^\lambda(d) : = \frac{M_i^\lambda(d)}{M_i(d)}$$

where $M_i^\lambda(d)$ denotes the number of proteins at distance d from protein i and belonging to the functional class λ and $M_i(d)$ denotes the total number of proteins at distance d from protein i. We then denote by $m^\lambda(d)$ the average of all $m_i^\lambda(d)$ belonging to the same class λ:

$$m^\lambda(d) : = \langle m_i^\lambda(d) \rangle$$

If proteins of a functional class λ were randomly distributed, then (see [4])

$$m^\lambda(d) = m_{rand}^\lambda : = N^\lambda/N,$$

for any d, where N^λ denotes the total number of proteins belonging to the functional class λ and N is the total number of proteins in the protein network. Defining

$$\bar{m}^\lambda : = \langle m^\lambda(d)/m_{rand}^\lambda \rangle, \tag{1}$$

where the average is taken over the distance, a random distribution would return $\bar{m}^\lambda = 1$.

Supporting Information

Figure S1 Topological distributions. Characteristic graph-theoretical distributions of the NCBI human protein-protein interaction network and of the protein interaction network obtained by prioritisation. (a), (b) average clustering coefficient distributions; (c), (d) topological coefficient distributions. A formal definition of these distributions is reported in the Appendix.

Figure S2 Failure-attack tolerance to node removal. Series of plots representing how the number of interactions and the number of secondary extinctions vary when removing nodes randomly (black circles), from the highest to the lowest degree (red circles) and from the lowest to the highest degree (green circles). (a) Number of interactions in the network associated with Crohn's against percentage of removed nodes; (b) Number of secondary extinctions in the network associated with Crohn's against percentage of removed nodes; (c) Number of interactions in a random network against percentage of removed nodes; (d) Number of secondary extinctions in a random network against percentage of removed nodes.

Figure S3 Failure-attack tolerance to SNP removal. Plots representing how the number of interactions varies when removing nodes associated with the SNPs locus windows (blue) and when removing the same number of nodes from the highest to the lowest degree (red circles) and from the lowest to the highest degree (green circles).

Figure S4 Enriched biological processes. Chart summarising the biological precesses that are enriched in the prioritised list of proteins. P-value threshold was set to 0.01.

Figure S5 Enriched protein classes. Chart summarising the protein classes that are enriched in the prioritised list of proteins. P-value threshold was set to 0.01.

Figure S6 Enriched molecular functions. Chart summarising the molecular functions that are enriched in the prioritised list of proteins. P-value threshold was set to 0.01.

Figure S7 Enriched pathways. Chart summarising the pathways that are enriched in the prioritised list of proteins. P-value threshold was set to 0.01.

Table S1 Topological metrics. Table summarising the topological properties of the disease network and of 30 Erdős-Rényi networks with the same number of nodes and edges. All the listed properties in the disease network are significantly different from random with p-values, calculated from z-scores, smaller than $2 \cdot 10^{-4}$. μ and σ are respectively mean values and standard deviations of the graph metrics.

Table S2 Training set. Table listing the Entrez IDs included in the training set with their literature references.

Table S3 Segregated enriched categories. Table summarising the segregated enriched categories containing STAT3, JAK2, VDR, FASLG (see section 'Results and discussion' in the main text). ATF4 and PRDM1 are not reported not being present in such categories.

Workbook S1 Network associated with Crohn's disease and enrichment tables. Workbook containing the candidate SNPs and Entrez IDs (Sheet 1), the prioritised Entrez IDs (Sheet 2), the network associated with Crohn's disease (Sheet 3), the NCBI proteome network (Sheet 4), the interactions among the proteins associated with the 28 prioritised and differentially expressed genes (Sheet 5) and the enrichment tables in biological processes (Sheet 6), protein classes (Sheet 7), molecular functions (Sheet 8), pathways (Sheet 9), cellular components (Sheet 10).

Information S1 Supplementary Text and Supplementary Tables.

Acknowledgments

We thank Professor Charlotte Deane for helpful comments.

Author Contributions

Conceived and designed the experiments: DM DL AS. Performed the experiments: DM. Analyzed the data: DM. Contributed reagents/materials/analysis tools: DM. Wrote the paper: DM DL AS.

References

1. Ideker T, Galitski T, Hood L (2001) A new approach to decoding life: systems biology. Annu Rev Genomics Hum Genet 2: 343–72.
2. Ideker T, Krogan NJ (2012) Differential network biology. Mol Syst Biol 8: 565.
3. Zhu X, Gerstein M, Snyder M (2007) Getting connected: analysis and principles of biological networks. Genes Dev 21(9):1010–24.
4. Yook SH, Oltvai ZN, Barabasi AL (2004) Functional and topological characterization of protein interaction networks. Proteomics 4(4):928–42.
5. Pawson T, Linding R (2008) Network medicine. FEBS Lett 582(8):1266–70.
6. Kreeger PK, Lauffenburger DA (2010) Cancer systems biology: a network modeling perspective. Carcinogenesis 31(1):2–8.
7. Vidal M, Cusick ME, Barabasi AL (2011) Interactome networks and human disease. Cell 144(6):986–98.
8. Rossin EJ, Lage K, Raychaudhuri S, Xavier RJ, Tatar D, et al. (2011) Proteins Encoded in Genomic Regions Associated with Immune-Mediated Disease Physically Interact and Suggest Underlying Biology. PLoS Genet 7(1): e1001273.
9. Barabasi AL, Gulbahce N, Loscalzo J (2011) Network medicine: a network-based approach to human disease. Nat Rev Genet 12: 56–68.
10. Raychaudhuri S, Plenge RM, Rossin EJ, Ng AC, International Schizophrenia Consortium, et al. (2009) Identifying Relationships among Genomic Disease Regions: Predicting Genes at Pathogenic SNP Associations and Rare Deletions. PLoS Genet 5(6): e1000534.
11. Le DH, Kwon YK (2012) GPEC: a Cytoscape plug-in for random walk-based gene prioritization and biomedical evidence collection. Comput Biol Chem 37: 17–23.
12. Zhang SW, Shao DD, Zhang SY, Wang YB (2014) Prioritization of candidate disease genes by enlarging the seed set and fusing information of the network topology and gene expression. Mol Biosyst 10(6):1400–8.
13. Valentini G, Paccanaro A, Caniza H, Romero AE, Re M (2014) An extensive analysis of disease-gene associations using network integration and fast kernel-based gene prioritization methods. Artif Intell Med 61(2): 63–78.
14. Zhu J, Qin Y, Liu T, Wang J, Zheng X (2013) Prioritization of candidate disease genes by topological similarity between disease and protein diffusion profiles. BMC Bioinformatics 14 Suppl 5:S5.
15. Navlakha S, Kingsford C (2010) The power of protein interaction networks for associating genes with diseases. Bioinformatics 26, 1057–1063.
16. Hindorff LA, MacArthur J, Morales J, Junkins HA, Hall PN, et al. (2012) A Catalog of Published Genome-Wide Association Studies. Available: www.genome.gov/gwastudies. Accessed 2012 October.
17. Jostins L, Ripke S, Weersma RK, Duerr RH, McGovern DP, et al. (2012) Host-microbe interactions have shaped the genetic architecture of inflammatory bowel disease. Nature 491, 119–124.
18. Nussinov R, Panchenko AR, Przytycka T (2011) Physics approaches to protein interactions and gene regulation. Phys Biol 8(3):030301.
19. Yadav G, Babu S (2012) NEXCADE: Perturbation Analysis for Complex Networks. PLoS ONE 7(8): e41827.
20. Mirzasoleiman B, Jalili M (2011) Failure Tolerance of Motif Structure in Biological Networks. PLoS ONE 6(5): e20512.
21. Kashtan N, Itzkovitz S, Milo R, Alon U (2004) Efficient sampling algorithm for estimating subgraph concentrations and detecting network motifs. Bioinformatics 20: 1758–1746.
22. Schreiber F, Schwöbbermeyer H (2005) MAVisto: a tool for the exploration of network motifs. Bioinformatics 21: 3572–3574.
23. Wernicke S, Rasche F (2006) FANMOD: a tool for fast network motif detection. Bioinformatics 22: 1152–1153.
24. Tong AH, Drees B, Nardelli G, Bader GD, Brannetti B, et al. (2002) A combined experimental and computational strategy to define protein interaction networks for peptide recognition modules. Science 295(5553):321–4.
25. Schwikowski B, Uetz P, Fields S, et al (2000) A network of protein-protein interactions in yeast. Nat Biotechnol 18(12):1257–61.
26. Mi H, Muruganujan A, Thomas PD (2013) PANTHER in 2013: modeling the evolution of gene function, and other gene attributes, in the context of phylogenetic trees. Nucleic Acids Res. 41(Database issue):D377-86. http://www.pantherdb.org
27. Simmons JD, Mullighan C, Welsh KI, Jewell DP (2000) Vitamin D receptor gene polymorphism: association with Crohn's disease susceptibility. Gut 47(2):211–4.
28. Fritz T1, Niederreiter L, Adolph T, Blumberg RS, Kaser A (2011) Crohn's disease: NOD2, autophagy and ER stress converge. Gut 60(11):1580–8.
29. Kaser A, Blumberg RS (2010) Endoplasmic reticulum stress and intestinal inflammation. Mucosal Immunol 3: 11–16.
30. Kaser A, Blumberg RS (2009) Endoplasmic reticulum stress in the intestinal epithelium and inflammatory bowel disease. Semin Immunol 21: 156–63.
31. Bader GD, Betel D, Hogue CWV (2003) BIND: the Biomolecular Interaction Network Database. Nucleic Acids Res, 31, pp. 248–250.
32. Breitkreutz BJ, Stark C, Reguly T, Boucher L, Breitkreutz A, et al. (2008) The BioGRID interaction database: 2008 update. Nucleic Acids Res 36, pp. D637–D640.
33. Keshava Prasad TS, Goel R, Kandasamy K, Keerthikumar S, Kumar S, et al. (2009) Human protein reference database - 2009 update. Nucleic Acids Res 37, pp. D767–D772.
34. Noble CL, Abbas AR, Lees CW, Cornelius J, Toy K, et al. (2010) Characterization of intestinal gene expression profiles in Crohn's disease by genome-wide microarray analysis. Inflamm Bowel Dis 16(10):1717–28.
35. Cho RJ, Campbell MJ (2000) Transcription, genomes, function. Trends Genetics 16: 409–415.

Permissions

List of Contributors

Maria de Lourdes Setsuko Ayrizono and Cláudio Saddy Rodrigues Coy
Coloproctology Unit, Surgery Department, University of Campinas (UNICAMP), Medical School, Sao Paulo, Brazil

Raquel Franco Leal
Coloproctology Unit, Surgery Department, University of Campinas (UNICAMP), Medical School, Sao Paulo, Brazil
Laboratory of Cell Signaling, Internal Medicine Department, University of Campinas (UNICAMP), Medical School, Sao Paulo, Brazil

Marciane Milanski, Mariana Portovedo and Lício Augusto Velloso
Laboratory of Cell Signaling, Internal Medicine Department, University of Campinas (UNICAMP), Medical School, Sao Paulo, Brazil

Cilene Bicca Dias
Coloproctology Unit, Surgery Department, University of Campinas (UNICAMP), Medical School, Sao Paulo, Brazil
Laboratory of Cell Signaling, Internal Medicine Department, University of Campinas (UNICAMP), Medical School, Sao Paulo, Brazil
Doctoral CAPES fellowship, Post graduate Program in Surgery Sciences, Faculty of Medical School, University of Campinas, Sao Paulo, Brazil

Vivian Horita and Luciana Rodrigues Meirelles
Department of Pathology, University of Campinas (UNICAMP), Medical School, Sao Paulo, Brazil

Núria Planell
Department of Gastroenterology and Bioinformatics Platform, CIBERehd, Barcelona, Spain

Julia Seiderer, Cornelia Tillack, Florian Beigel, Christian Steib and Stephan Brand
Department of Medicine II - Grosshadern, Ludwig-Maximilians-University, Munich, Germany

Christoph Fries, Matthias Friedrich and Julia Diegelmann
Department of Medicine II - Grosshadern, Ludwig-Maximilians-University, Munich, Germany
Department of Preventive Dentistry and Periodontology, Ludwig- Maximilians-University, Munich, Germany

Corinna Bayrle
Department of Preventive Dentistry and Periodontology, Ludwig- Maximilians-University Munich, Germany

Jürgen Glas
Department of Medicine II - Grosshadern, Ludwig-Maximilians-University, Munich, Germany
Department of Preventive Dentistry and Periodontology, Ludwig- Maximilians-University, Munich, Germany
Department of Human Genetics, Rheinisch-Westfälische Technische Hochschule (RWTH), Aachen, Germany

Martin Wetzke
Department of Pediatrics, Hannover Medical School, Hannover, Germany

Torsten Olszak
Department of Medicine II - Grosshadern, Ludwig-Maximilians-University, Munich, Germany
Division of Gastroenterology, Brigham and Women's Hospital, Harvard Medical School, Boston, Massachusetts, United States of America

Darina Czamara
Max-Planck-Institute of Psychiatry, Munich, Germany

Debby Laukens, Harald Peeters and Martine De Vos
Department of Gastroenterology, Ghent University, Ghent, Belgium

Michel Georges, Cécile Libioulle, Cynthia Sandor and Myriam Mni
Unit of Animal Genomics, GIGA-R and Faculty of Veterinary Medicine, University of Liège, Liège, Belgium

Bert Vander Cruyssen and Dirk Elewaut
Department of Rheumatology, Ghent University, Ghent, Belgium

Irina Costea
Public Health Agency of Canada, Montreal, Canada
Research Centre, Sainte-Justine Hospital, Montreal, Canada

Philippe Lambrette
Research Centre, Sainte-Justine Hospital, Montreal, Canada

David R. Mack
Division of Gastroenterology, Hepatology and Nutrition, Children's Hospital of Eastern Ontario, Ottawa, Canada

David Israel
Department of Gastroenterology, Hepatology and Nutrition, British Columbia's Children's Hospital, Vancouver, Canada

Kenneth Morgan
Department of Human Genetics, McGill University and the Research Institute of the McGill University Health Center, Montreal, Canada

Alfreda Krupoves
Research Centre, Sainte-Justine Hospital, Montreal, Canada
Department of Preventive and Social Medicine, University of Montreal, Montreal, Canada

Ernest Seidman
Department of Medicine, McGill University and the Research Institute of the McGill University Health Center, Montreal, Canada

Colette Deslandres and Devendra K. Amre
Research Centre, Sainte-Justine Hospital, Montreal, Canada
Department of Pediatrics, University of Montreal, Montreal, Canada

Guy Grimard
Research Centre, Sainte-Justine Hospital, Montreal, Canada
Division of Orthopedics, Department of Pediatrics, University of Montreal, Montreal, Canada

Emile Levy
Research Centre, Sainte-Justine Hospital, Montreal, Canada
Department of Nutrition, University of Montreal, Montreal, Canada

Alexandra Wolf, Stephan Schleder, Andrea Dirmeier and Frank Klebl
Department of Internal Medicine I, University of Regensburg, Regensburg, Germany

Anja Schirbel
Department of Pathobiology, Lerner Research Institute, Cleveland Clinic Foundation, Cleveland, Ohio, United Sates of America

Florian Rieder
Department of Internal Medicine I, University of Regensburg, Regensburg, Germany
Department of Pathobiology, Lerner Research Institute, Cleveland Clinic Foundation, Cleveland, Ohio, United Sates of America
Department of Gastroenterology, Cleveland Clinic Foundation, Cleveland, Ohio, United Sates of America

Rocio Lopez
Department of Quantitative Health Sciences, Cleveland Clinic Foundation, Cleveland, Ohio, United Sates of America

Andre Franke, Philip Rosenstiel and Stefan Schreiber
Institute of Clinical Molecular Biology and Department of General Internal Medicine, Christian-Albrechts-University, Kiel, Germany

Nir Dotan
Glycominds Ltd., Lod, Israel

Gerhard Rogler
Departement of Internal Medicine, Clinic for Gastroenterology and Hepatology, University Hospital Zuerich, Zuerich, Switzerland

Fiona Blanco-Kelly
Department of Clinical Immunology, Hospital Clínico San Carlos, Madrid, Spain

María Teruel, Lina M. Díaz-Gallo and Javier Martín
Instituto Parasitología y Biomedicina "López Neyra", C. S. I. C., Granada, Spain

María Gómez-García
Servicio de Digestivo, Hospital Universitario Virgen de las Nieves, Granada, Spain

Miguel A. López-Nevot
Servicio de Inmunología , Hospital Universitario Virgen de las Nieves, Granada, Spain

Luis Rodrigo
Servicio de Digestivo, Hospital Universitario Central de Asturias, Oviedo, Spain

Antonio Nieto
Servicio de Inmunología, Hospital Puerta del Mar, Ca´diz, Spain

Carlos Cardeña
Servicio de Digestivo, Hospital Clínico San Cecilio, Granada, Spain

Guillermo Alcain
Servicio de Digestivo, Hospital Virgen de la Victoria, Málaga, Spain

Manuel Díaz-Rubio
Digestive Department, Hospital Clínico San Carlos, Madrid, Spain

Oscar Fernandez
Servicio de Neurología, Instituto de Neurociencias Clínicas, Hospital Carlos Haya, Málaga, Spain
Members of the Red Española de Esclerosis Múltiple (REEM)

Rafael Arroyo
Multiple Sclerosis Unit, Neurology Department, Hospital Clínico San Carlos, Madrid, Spain
Members of the Red Española de Esclerosis Múltiple (REEM)

Emilio G. de la Concha and Elena Urcelay
Department of Clinical Immunology, Hospital Clínico San Carlos, Madrid, Spain
Members of the Red Española de Esclerosis Múltiple (REEM)

Fuencisla Matesanz and Antonio Alcina
Instituto Parasitología y Biomedicina "López Neyra", C. S. I. C., Granada, Spain
Members of the Red Española de Esclerosis Múltiple (REEM)

Tianyi Zhang, Bowen Song and Wei Zhu
Department of Applied Mathematics and Statistics, Stony Brook University, Stony Brook, New York, United States of America

Xiao Xu
Department of Medicine, Stony Brook University, Stony Brook, New York, United States of America

Ellen Li
Department of Medicine, Stony Brook University, Stony Brook, New York, United States of America
Department of Medicine, Washington University-St. Louis School of Medicine, Saint Louis, Missouri, United States of America

Qing Qing Gong, Christopher Morando, Themistocles Dassopoulos and Rodney D. Newberry
Department of Medicine, Washington University-St. Louis School of Medicine, Saint Louis, Missouri, United States of America

Steven R. Hunt
Department of Surgery, Washington University-St. Louis School of Medicine, Saint Louis, Missouri, United States of America

Jens Kelsen, Anders Dige, Jørgen Agnholt, Lisbet A. Christensen, Jens F. Dahlerup and Christian L. Hvas
Gastro-Immuno Research Laboratory (GIRL), Department of Medicine V, Aarhus University Hospital, Aarhus, Denmark

Heinrich Schwindt and Finn S. Pedersen
Institute of Molecular Biology, Aarhus University, Aarhus, Denmark

Francesco D'Amore
Department of Hematology, Aarhus University Hospital, Aarhus, Denmark

Irina Dinu, Qi Liu, Noha Sharaf Eldin, Erin Kreiter, Xuan Wu, Shahab Jabbari and Yutaka Yasui
School of Public Health, University of Alberta, Edmonton, Alberta, Canada

Surakameth Mahasirimongkol and Katsushi Tokunaga
Department of Human Genetics, School of International Health, Graduate School of Medicine, University of Tokyo, Tokyo, Japan

Hideki Yanai
Department of Human Genetics, School of International Health, Graduate School of Medicine, University of Tokyo, Tokyo, Japan
Fukujuji Hospital, Japan Anti-Tuberculosis Association, Kiyose, Japan

Julia Seiderer, Cornelia Tillack, Simone Pfennig, Florian Beigel, Maria Weidinger, Burkhard Göke, Thomas Ochsenkühn and Stephan Brand
Department of Medicine II - Grosshadern, Ludwig-Maximilians-University, Munich, Germany

Julia Diegelmann
Department of Medicine II - Grosshadern, Ludwig-Maximilians-University, Munich, Germany
Department of Preventive Dentistry and Periodontology, Ludwig- Maximilians-University, Munich, Germany

Jürgen Glas
Department of Medicine II - Grosshadern, Ludwig-Maximilians-University, Munich, Germany
Department of Preventive Dentistry and Periodontology, Ludwig- Maximilians-University, Munich, Germany
Department of Human Genetics, RWTH (Rheinisch-Westfälische Technische Hochschule), Aachen, Germany

Matthias Jürgens
Department of Medicine II - Grosshadern, Ludwig-Maximilians-University, Munich, Germany
Division of Gastroenterology, University of Leuven, Leuven, Belgium

Torsten Olszak
Department of Medicine II - Grosshadern, Ludwig-Maximilians-University, Munich, Germany
Division of Gastroenterology, Hepatology and Endoscopy, Brigham and Women's Hospital, Harvard Medical School, Boston, Massachusetts, United States of America

Rüdiger P. Laubender
Institute of Medical Informatics, Biometry and Epidemiology (IBE), Ludwig-Maximilians-University, Munich, Germany

Bertram Müller-Myhsok and Darina Czamara
Max-Planck-Institute of Psychiatry, Munich, Germany

Peter Lohse
Institute of Clinical Chemistry - Grosshadern, Ludwig-Maximilians-University, Munich, Germany

Shufang Xu, Lu Song, Xiaobing Wang and Fengming Yi
Department of Gastroenterology, Zhongnan Hospital of Wuhan University School of Medicine, Wuhan, People's Republic of China

Feng Zhou, Liping Chen and Bing Xia
Department of Gastroenterology, Zhongnan Hospital of Wuhan University School of Medicine, Wuhan, People's Republic of China
Hubei Clinical Center and Key Laboratory for Intestinal and Colorectal Diseases, and Hubei Key Laboratory of Immune Related Diseases, Wuhan, People's Republic of China

Rui Zhou
Hubei Clinical Center and Key Laboratory for Intestinal and Colorectal Diseases, and Hubei Key Laboratory of Immune Related Diseases, Wuhan, People's Republic of China

Jinsheng Tao
BGI-Shenzhen, Bei Shan Industrial Zone, Yantian District, Shenzhen, People's Republic of China

Siew Chien NG
Institute of Digestive Disease, Department of Medicine and Therapeutics, Li Ka Shing Institute of Health Sciences, The Chinese University of Hong Kong, Hong Kong, People's Republic of China

Zhihua Ran
Department of Gastroenterology, Renji Hospital, Shanghai Institute of Digestive Disease, Shanghai Jiao Tong University School of Medicine, Shanghai, People's Republic of China

Susan E. Alters, Bryant McLaughlin, Benjamin Spink, Tigran Lachinyan, Chia-wei Wang, Vladimir Podust, Volker Schellenberger and Willem P. C. Stemmer
Amunix Inc., Mountain View, California, United States of America

Hilbert S. de Vries, Rene H. M. te Morsche, Wilbert H. M. Peters and Dirk J. de Jong
Department of Gastroenterology and Hepatology, Radboud University NijmegenMedical Center, Nijmegen, The Netherlands

Iris D. Nagtegaal
Department of Pathology, Radboud University Nijmegen Medical Center, Nijmegen, The Netherlands

Martijn G. H. van Oijen
Department of Gastroenterology and Hepatology, Radboud University NijmegenMedical Center, Nijmegen, The Netherlands
Department of Gastroenterology and Hepatology, University Medical Center Utrecht, Utrecht, The Netherlands

Erik Corona, Joel T. Dudley and Atul J. Butte
Lucile Packard Children's Hospital, Stanford, California, United States of America
Department of Pediatrics, Stanford University School of Medicine, Stanford, California, United States of America

Nirmala Akula and Francis J. McMahon
Mood and Anxiety Section, Human Genetics Branch, National Institute of Mental Health, National Institutes of Health, Department of Health and Human Services, Bethesda, Maryland, United States of America

Donald Seto and Jeffrey Solka
School of Systems Biology, College of Science, George Mason University, Fairfax, Virginia, United States of America

Ancha Baranova
School of Systems Biology, College of Science, George Mason University, Fairfax, Virginia, United States of America
Research Center for Medical Genetics, RAMS, Moscow, Russian Federation

Michael A. Nalls and Andrew Singleton
Molecular Genetics Section, Laboratory of Neurogenetics, Intramural Research Program, National Institute on Aging, Bethesda, Maryland, United States of America

Luigi Ferrucci and Toshiko Tanaka
Longitudinal Studies Section, Clinical Research Branch, Intramural Research Program, National
Institute on Aging, National Institutes of Health, Baltimore, Maryland, United States of America

Stefania Bandinelli
Geriatric Unit, Azienda Sanitaria di Firenze, Florence, Italy

Yoon Shin Cho, Young Jin Kim, Jong-Young Lee and Bok-Ghee Han
Center for Genome Science, National Institute of Health, Seoul, Korea

Isabelle Cleynen, Wouter Van Moerkercke, PaulRutgeerts and Severine Vermeire
Department of Gastroenterology, KU Leuven, Leuven, Belgium

Jestinah M. Mahachie John and Kristel Van Steen
Systems and Modeling Unit, Department of Electrical Engineering and Computer Science, University of Liège, Liège, Belgium
Bioinformatics and Modeling, GIGA-R, University of Liège Liège, Belgium

Liesbet Henckaerts
Department of Medicine, UZ Leuven, Leuven, Belgium

Franc͜oise Merlin
Université Paris Diderot, UMR843, Paris, France
UMR843, INSERM, Paris, France

Camille Jung and Jean-Pierre Hugot
Université Paris Diderot, UMR843, Paris, France
UMR843, INSERM, Paris, France
Service de Gastroentérologie Pédiatrique, Hôpital Robert Debrè, APHP, Paris, France

Jean-Pierre Cezard
Service de Gastroentérologie Pédiatrique, Hôpital Robert Debrè, APHP, Paris, France

Jean-Frédéric Colombel and Gwenola Vernier-Massouille
Service de Gastroentérologie, Hôpital Claude Huriez, Université de Lille, Lille, France

Marc Lemann, Matthieu Allez and Jean-Marc Gornet
Service de Gastroentérologie, Hôpital Saint-Louis, AP-HP, Université Paris- Diderot, Paris, France

Laurent Beaugerie, Jacques Cosnes and Jean-Pierre Gendre
Department of Gastroenterology, Hôpital Saint-Antoine, AP-HP, and UPMC Univ Paris 06, Paris, France

Frank M. Ruemmele
Université Paris Descartes and Service de Gastroentérologie Pédiatrique, Hôpital Necker Enfants-Malades, APHP, Paris, France

Dominique Turck
Service de Gastroentérologie Pédiatrique, Hôpital Jeanne de Flandre, Universitéde Lille 2, Lille, France

Habib Zouali and Gilles Thomas
CEPH/Fondation Jean Dausset, Paris, France

Christian Libersa
Centre D'Investigation Clinique 9301, Hôpital Cardiologique, INSERM, Lille, France

Philippe Dieude
Université Paris Diderot and Service de Rhumatologie, Hôpital Bichat, Paris, France

Nadem Soufir
Université Paris Diderot and Service de Biochimie Génétique, Hôpital Bichat, Paris, France

Sara Szymanska, Nilminie Rathnayake, Anders Gustafsson and Annsofi Johannsen
Department of Dental Medicine, Division of Periodontology, Karolinska Institutet, Huddinge, Sweden

Mikael Lördal
Department of Medicine, Division of Gastroenterology and Hepathology at Karolinska Institutet, Huddinge, Sweden
Stockholm Gastro Center, Sophiahemmet, Stockholm, Sweden

Julia Seiderer, Giulia Pasciuto and Stephan Brand
Department of Medicine II - Grosshadern, University of Munich, Munich, Germany

Julia Diegelmann
Department of Medicine II - Grosshadern, University of Munich, Munich, Germany
Department of Preventive Dentistry and Periodontology, University of Munich, Munich, Germany

Jürgen Glas
Department of Medicine II - Grosshadern, University of Munich, Munich, Germany
Department of Preventive Dentistry and Periodontology, University of Munich, Munich, Germany
Department of Human Genetics, Rheinisch-Westfälische Technische Hochschule (RWTH) Aachen, Aachen, Germany

Darina Czamara, Christiane Wolf and Bertram Müller-Myhsok
Max-Planck-Institute of Psychiatry, Munich, Germany

Martin Wetzke
Center for Pediatrics, Hannover Medical School, Hannover, Germany

Torsten Olszak
Department of Medicine II - Grosshadern, University of Munich, Munich, Germany
Division of Gastroenterology, Brigham & Women's Hospital, Harvard Medical School, Boston, United States of America

Tobias Balschun and Andre Franke
Institute of Clinical Molecular Biology, Christian-Albrechts-University, Kiel, Germany

Jean-Paul Achkar
Department of Pathobiology, Lerner Research Institute, Cleveland Clinic, Cleveland, Ohio, United States of America
Department of Gastroenterology and Hepatology, Digestive Disease Institute, Cleveland Clinic, Cleveland, Ohio, United States of America

M. Ilyas Kamboh
Department of Human Genetics, Graduate School of Public Health, University of Pittsburgh, Pittsburgh, Pennsylvania, United States of America

Richard H. Duerr
Department of Human Genetics, Graduate School of Public Health, University of Pittsburgh, Pittsburgh, Pennsylvania, United States of America
Division of Gastroenterology, Hepatology and Nutrition, School of Medicine, University of Pittsburgh, Pittsburgh, Pennsylvania, United States of America

Satish Keshav
John Radcliffe Hospital, University of Oxford, Oxford, United Kingdom

Tomáš Vaňásek
Hepato-Gastroenterologie HK, Hradec Králové , Czech Republic

Yaron Niv
Rabin Medical Center, Petach Tikva, Israel

Robert Petryka
NZOZ Vivamed, Zespół Lekarzy Specjalistów, Warszawa, Poland

Stephanie Howaldt
Praxis für Innere Medizin, Hamburg, Germany

Mauro Bafutto
Instituto Goiano de Gastroenterologia e Endoscopia Digestiva Ltda., Goia^nia, Brazil,

István Rácz
Petz Alada´r County and Teaching Hospital, Györ, Hungary

David Hetzel
Royal Adelaide Hospital, Adelaide, Australia

Ole Haagen Nielsen
Department of Gastroenterology, Herlev Hospital, Herlev, Denmark

Séverine Vermeire
UZ Gasthuisberg, Leuven, Belgium

Walter Reinisch
Allgemeines Krankenhaus Wien, Universitätsklinik für Innere Medizin III, Klinische Abteilung für Gastroenterologie und Hepatologie, Vienna, Austria

Per Karlén
Department of Clinical Science and Education, Karolinska Institutet, Södersjukhuset, Stockholm, Sweden

Stefan Schreiber
Department of Medicine I, Christian Albrechts University, University Hospital Schleswig Holstein, Kiel, Germany

Thomas J. Schall and Pirow Bekker
ChemoCentryx, Inc., Mountain View, California, United States of America

David Schwarzmaier, Toni Weinhaga and Georg Varga
Department of Pediatric Rheumatology and Immunology, University Children's Hospital Münster, Münster, NRW, Germany

Dirk Foell
Department of Pediatric Rheumatology and Immunology, University Children's Hospital Münster, Münster, NRW, Germany
Interdisciplinary Center of Clinical Research, University of Münster, Münster, NRW, Germany

Jan Däbritz
Department of Pediatric Rheumatology and Immunology, University Children's Hospital Münster, Münster, NRW, Germany
Interdisciplinary Center of Clinical Research, University of Münster, Münster, NRW, Germany
The Royal Children's Hospital Melbourne, Murdoch Children's Research Institute, Parkville, VIC, Australia

Raquel Cabezón and Carolina España
Department of Gastroenterology, Hospital Clínic de Barcelona, IDIBAPS, Barcelona, Spain

Elena Ricart and Julián Panés
Department of Gastroenterology, Hospital Clínic de Barcelona, IDIBAPS, Barcelona, Spain
Centro de Investigación Biomédica en Red de Enfermedades Hepáticas y Digestivas (CIBERehd) and Centre Esther Koplowitz, Barcelona, Spain

Daniel Benitez-Ribas
Centro de Investigación Biomédica en Red de

Enfermedades Hepáticas y Digestivas (CIBERehd) and Centre Esther Koplowitz, Barcelona, Spain

Abigail Basson and Rina Swart
Dietetics Department, University of the Western Cape, Bellville, Western Cape, South Africa

Mikateko Mazinu
Biostatistics Unit, Medical Research Council of South Africa, Parow, Western Cape, South Africa

Esme Jordaan
Statistics and Population Studies Department, University of the Western Cape, Bellville, Western Cape, South Africa

Gillian Watermeyer
Department of Gastroenterology, Groote Schuur Hospital, Cape Town, Western Cape, South Africa
Department of Medicine, University of Cape Town, Cape Town, Western Cape, South
Africa

Sinan Guloksuz, Marieke Wichers, Gunter Kenis and Baer Arts
Department of Psychiatry and Psychology, Maastricht University Medical Centre, EURON, Maastricht, The Netherlands

Maurice G.V.M. Russel
Department of Gastroenterology and Hepatology, Medisch Spectrum Twente, Enschede, The Netherlands

Annick Wauters
Laboratory of Clinical Biology, ZNA Middelheim, Antwerp, Belgium

Robert Verkerk
Laboratory of Medical Biochemistry, University of Antwerp, Wilrijk, Belgium

Jim van Os
Department of Psychiatry and Psychology, Maastricht University Medical Centre, EURON, Maastricht, The Netherlands
King's College London, King's Health Partners, Department of Psychosis Studies, Institute of Psychiatry, London, United Kingdom

Daniele Muraro and Alison Simmons
Weatherall Institute of Molecular Medicine, University of Oxford, Oxford, United Kingdom

Douglas A. Lauffenburger
Department of Biological Engineering, Massachusetts Institute of Technology, Cambridge, Massachusetts, United States of America

Index

www.ingramcontent.com/pod-product-compliance
Lightning Source LLC
Chambersburg PA
CBHW080537200326
41458CB00012B/4462